Neuromuscular Block
in Perioperative and Intensive Care

Edited by

David G. Silverman, MD
Professor of Anesthesiology
Director of Departmental Clinical Research
Yale University School of Medicine
Attending Anesthesiologist
Yale-New Haven Hospital
New Haven, Connecticut

◆ *With six additional contributors*

J.B. Lippincott Company
Philadelphia

Acquisitions Editor: Mary K. Smith
Assistant Editor: Anne Geyer
Production Editor: Virginia Barishek
Indexer: Maria Coughlin
Interior Designer: Arlene Putterman
Cover Designer: William T. Donnelley
Production: P.M. Gordon Associates, Inc.
Compositor: Pine Tree Composition, Inc.
Printer/Binder: R.R. Donnelley & Sons Company/Crawfordsville

Copyright © 1994, by J.B. Lippincott Company.
All rights reserved. No part of this book may be used or reproduced in any manner whatsoever without written permission except for brief quotations embodied in critical articles and reviews. Printed in the United States of America. For information write J.B. Lippincott Company, 227 East Washington Square, Philadelphia, Pennsylvania 19106.

6 5 4 3 2 1

Library of Congress Cataloging-in-Publication Data

Neuromuscular block : in perioperative and intensive care / edited by
  David G. Silverman ; with six additional contributors.
    p. cm.
  Includes biographical references and index.
  ISBN 0-397-51377-1
  1. Neuromuscular blocking agents. 2. Therapeutics, Surgical.
  3. Critical care medicine. I. Silverman, David G.
  [DNLM: 1. Neuromuscular Blocking Agents—pharmacology.
  2. Neuromuscular Blocking Agents—therapeutic use. 3. Neuromuscular Junction—drug effects. 4. Synaptic Transmission—drug effects.
  QV 140 N4939 1994]
  RD83.5.N48 1994
  615'.781—dc20
  DNLM/DLC
  for Library of Congress   94-15674
                                                                  CIP

Every effort has been made to ensure drug selections and dosages are in accordance with current recommendations and practice. Because of ongoing research, changes in government regulations and the constant flow of information on drug therapy, reactions and interactions, the reader is cautioned to check the package insert for each drug for indications, dosages, warnings, and precautions, particularly if the drug is new or infrequently used.

To the animals sacrificed for the advancement of medical care. May they be used wisely, sparingly, and mercifully.

◆ Contributors

◆ **RICHARD R. BARTKOWSKI,** MD, PhD
Professor of Anesthesiology, Director of Departmental Research,
Jefferson Medical College;
Attending Anesthesiologist, Jefferson University Medical Center,
Philadelphia, Pennsylvania

◆ **SORIN J. BRULL,** MD
Associate Professor of Anesthesiology, Director of Resident Education,
Department of Anesthesiology, Yale University School of Medicine;
Attending Anesthesiologist and member Pharmacy Comm. on ICU Relaxant Use,
Yale-New Haven Hospital,
New Haven, Connecticut

◆ **FRANÇOIS DONATI,** MD, PhD, FRCPC
Professor and Chairman, Department of Anaesthesia,
University of Montreal,
Montreal, Quebec, Canada

◆ **RAJINDER K. MIRAKHUR,** MD, PhD, FFARCS
Senior Lecturer and Consultant in Anaesthetics,
Department of Anaesthesia, The Queen's University of Belfast,
Belfast, Northern Ireland, United Kingdom

◆ **HENRY ROSENBERG,** MD
Professor and Chairman, Department of Anesthesiology,
Hahnemann University;
Chairman, Department of Anesthesiology,
Hahnemann University Hospital,
Philadelphia, Pennsylvania

◆ **DAVID G. SILVERMAN,** MD
Professor of Anesthesiology, Director of Departmental Clinical Research,
Yale University School of Medicine; Attending Anesthesiologist and member
Pharmacy Comm. on ICU Relaxant Use,
Yale-New Haven Hospital,
New Haven, Connecticut

◆ **FRANK G. STANDAERT,** MD
Special Expert, National Institute of Mental Health,
National Institutes of Health,
Rockville, Maryland

◆ Foreword

In the 138 years since Claude Bernard's report on the essential physiologic action of curare on the neuromuscular junction in 1856, major advances have been made with respect to our understanding of the neuromuscular junction and the pharmacology of neuromuscular blocking agents. Much of the progress in this field has occurred in the past decade. Today, perioperative medicine and intensive care medicine necessitate considerable knowledge of the physiology and pharmacology of neuromuscular transmission and neuromuscular relaxants. Not only should the anesthesiologist be an expert in the action and side effects of a family of drugs that is such an essential component of intraoperative care, but surgeons, internists, and intensivists should be well informed about the use and potential misuse of these agents in intensive care settings.

This book brings together in one volume the major issues that one should consider when using neuromuscular blocking agents. Each chapter begins with a concise description of relevant information; this is followed by questions (and answers) that are often asked in the operating theater and/or intensive care unit. The authors of the various chapters are world-renowned experts in their respective fields. For the purpose of cohesiveness, they have adhered to a uniform format. This optimizes readability and minimizes repetition. The essays at the end of each chapter provide a unique means for these authorities to help the reader put facts and issues into perspective.

Early chapters focus nicely upon the anatomy and physiology of neuromuscular transmission, mechanisms of neuromuscular block, and means of neuromuscular assessment. The chapters that follow expand on this basis to detail the overall and individual effects of depolarizing and nondepolarizing relaxants. The text concludes with a clear presentation of relevant neuromuscular disorders and disease states. New problems concerning the usage of succinylcholine have been clearly addressed. Potential pharmacologic interactions are effectively summarized. Critical issues concerning the potential use and misuse of relaxants—including those newly appreciated in intensive care settings—are carefully detailed and thoughtfully discussed.

There has been a need for a text that provides an up-to-date, integrated assessment of the scientific basis and clinical aspects of neuromuscular block. There is no doubt that this is such a book. The authors have succeeded in putting together a detailed, stimulating, and practical text that provides the basis for developing a rational approach to the clinical use of neuromuscular blocking agents in the myriad settings encountered in anesthesia and intensive care medicine.

Luke M. Kitahata, M.D., Ph.D.
Professor of Anesthesiology
Yale University
New Haven, Connecticut

◆ Preface

Within the past decade, there have been marked changes in the nature of neuromuscular blocking agents. In the early 1980s, relaxants of intermediate duration (atracurium and vecuronium) became available. They were followed by long-acting agents with reduced side effects (doxacurium and pipecuronium). In 1992, the first short-acting nondepolarizing drug (mivacurium) became available in the United States. Soon after, the first nondepolarizing agent with a rapid onset (rocuronium) was introduced.

The diversity of neuromuscular blocking agents (and of more sophisticated means to monitor their effects) has enabled us to optimize neuromuscular block in the perioperative and intensive care settings. Unfortunately, the news is not all positive: the long-term use of relaxants in intensive care settings has been implicated in a mounting number of cases of residual weakness and myopathy; in 1993, the F.D.A. declared that the routine use of succinylcholine, a mainstay of relaxant administration, was contraindicated in children and adolescents.

Although the requirements for neuromuscular block in the OR and ICU differ, these settings share the need for a working knowledge of neuromuscular anatomy, monitoring, and pharmacology in health and disease and in the presence of myriad other medications. This text has been designed to address these issues and to relate them to perioperative and intensive care patients. Our primary aim is to provide a thorough understanding of neuromuscular block and of means to optimize its efficacy and safety. In addition, we have sought to provide a basis for integrating and applying the wealth of new information that is being generated. Each chapter consists of a detailed review (with key points italicized) and a more expansive analysis of relevant discussion topics. These topics address issues germane to clinical care, simulate the "selective topics" encountered on oral examinations, and delve into more remote areas that we think are critical to a full understanding of relevant issues. Each chapter is designed to stand on its own; however, to maintain cohesiveness and avoid repetition, we commonly refer to material in other sections.

I am delighted and honored by the willingness of leading authorities to lend their expertise and names to this text. Although Drs. Bartkowski, Brull,

Donati, Mirakhur, Rosenberg, and Standaert are highly accomplished and well-respected authors in their own "write," they willingly have adhered to the style that I had selected for this book. I owe much of my understanding of neuromuscular block to each of them.

I also would like to take this opportunity to thank Drs. Paul Barash, Nicholas Greene, and Luke Kitahata. The Department of Anesthesiology at Yale has been fortunate not only to have an outstanding leader and teacher in our chairman, Paul Barash, but also to have two distinguished former chairmen on our faculty. The opportunities that I have had to discuss manuscripts with Dr. Greene have provided me with an insight into the writing process that is available to only a limited few. An outstanding scientist, Dr. Kitahata willingly has shared his keen perception and research skills with members of our Department. I also feel that I have been fortunate to have Ms. Jacki Fitzpatrick as a secretary; she stood by me despite innumerable revisions and was invaluable in bringing this book to completion. Likewise, Mary K. Smith, Peg Forster, Anne Geyer, and Stephanie Reilly of Lippincott and Mary McDonald of P.M. Gordon Associates have demonstrated great patience with this somewhat petulant and forever-revising author.

Most of all, I would like to thank my family. My wife, Sally, my children, Tyler and Charlotte, and my mother know how important they are to me and how I appreciate their willingness to have shared me with this text. My greatest thanks and admiration belong to my father—an outstanding role model before his debilitating stroke in 1984, and a continuing source of pride and inspiration despite his severe disabilities.

David G. Silverman, M.D.

◆ Contents

1 Anatomy and Physiology of Neuromuscular Transmission 1
DAVID G. SILVERMAN | FRANK G. STANDAERT

2 Mechanisms of Neuromuscular Block 11
DAVID G. SILVERMAN | FRANK G. STANDAERT

3 Features of Neurostimulation 23
DAVID G. SILVERMAN | SORIN J. BRULL

4 Patterns of Stimulation 37
DAVID G. SILVERMAN | SORIN J. BRULL

5 Monitoring of Evoked Responses 51
DAVID G. SILVERMAN | SORIN J. BRULL

6 Requirements for Relaxation and Recovery in the Perioperative and ICU Settings: Responses to Neurostimulation and Clinical Signs 64
DAVID G. SILVERMAN

7 Pharmacokinetics and Pharmacodynamics of Nondepolarizing Relaxants: Onset 78
DAVID G. SILVERMAN | RICHARD R. BARTKOWSKI

8 Pharmacokinetics and Pharmacodynamics of Nondepolarizing Relaxants: Maintenance and Recovery 95
DAVID G. SILVERMAN | RICHARD R. BARTKOWSKI

9 Effects of Other Agents on Nondepolarizing Relaxants 104
DAVID G. SILVERMAN | RAJINDER K. MIRAKHUR

10 Effects of Patient Status and Conditions on Nondepolarizing Relaxants 123
DAVID G. SILVERMAN | RAJINDER K. MIRAKHUR

11 Systemic and Long-Term Effects of Nondepolarizing Relaxants 143
DAVID G. SILVERMAN | RICHARD R. BARTKOWSKI

12 Nondepolarizing Relaxants of Long Duration 171
DAVID G. SILVERMAN | RAJINDER K. MIRAKHUR

13 Intermediate-Acting Relaxants of the 1980s 184
DAVID G. SILVERMAN | RAJINDER K. MIRAKHUR

14 Nondepolarizing Relaxants of the 1990s 200
DAVID G. SILVERMAN | RAJINDER K. MIRAKHUR

15 Reversal of Nondepolarizing Block 217
DAVID G. SILVERMAN | RAJINDER K. MIRAKHUR

16 Neuromuscular Effects of Depolarizing Relaxants 239
DAVID G. SILVERMAN | FRANÇOIS DONATI

17 Factors Affecting Pseudocholinesterase and the Pharmacokinetics and Pharmacodynamics of Succinylcholine 255
DAVID G. SILVERMAN | FRANÇOIS DONATI

18 Undesirable Effects of Succinylcholine 276
DAVID G. SILVERMAN | FRANÇOIS DONATI

19 Malignant Hyperthermia: Etiology, Risks, and Assessment of Susceptibility 297
DAVID G. SILVERMAN | HENRY ROSENBERG

20 Malignant Hyperthermia: Signs, Symptoms, and Treatment 314
DAVID G. SILVERMAN | HENRY ROSENBERG

21 Myasthenia Gravis and the Myasthenic Syndrome 324
DAVID G. SILVERMAN

22 Nerve Injury, Burns, and Trauma 332
DAVID G. SILVERMAN

23 Other Muscle Disorders 349
DAVID G. SILVERMAN | HENRY ROSENBERG

Index 358

1

DAVID G. SILVERMAN | FRANK G. STANDAERT

Anatomy and Physiology of Neuromuscular Transmission

The difficulties encountered in learning neuromuscular physiology as it relates to neurostimulation and monitoring may be attributable, in part, to failure to discriminate among terms and definitions. A nerve *bundle* (e.g., the ulnar nerve) consists of 10–1,000 *fibers,* each of which is the axon of an individual neuron. Each fiber arborizes into multiple *branches,* each of which is associated with a neuromuscular junction (NMJ) and a muscle fiber cell.[1–4] These function as a *motor unit:* stimulation of the nerve fiber results in "all-or-none" firing of all of its branches, causing contraction of all the muscle cells in the unit. The contraction seen clinically is a graded response made up of the quantal responses of hundreds of individual cells.

In addition to endogenous excitation, nerve fibers may be depolarized by an exogenous source (i.e., a nerve stimulator). *Depolarization* overcomes the resting membrane potential (−90 mV) and generates a *nerve action potential.* The individual fibers have *different thresholds* for firing in response to an exogenous current. The differences may be attributable to factors such as the fiber's distance from the stimulating electrode. Not all fibers of a given bundle will fire at a given stimulating current unless a "maximal" or "supramaximal" current is provided.

When it reaches the *nerve terminal,* the nerve action potential causes a conformational change in the protein of the *presynaptic membrane* channels (Fig. 1-1) such that the membrane binds Ca^{2+},[5] which enters by "fast" ("P") and then "slow" ("L") calcium channels. *Fast calcium channels* play the more prominent role during depolarization, undergoing a conformational change in response to the voltage changes generated by Na^+ entry. *Slow calcium channels* then allow for the entry of additional Ca^{2+}. The entering Ca^{2+} is critical to the release of acetylcholine (ACh).[5–7] It binds to *synaptophysin;* the resulting change in this glycoprotein allows ACh-containing vesicles to fuse with "docking" proteins in the presynaptic membrane and discharge their contents into the junctional cleft.[7–11] *Each vesicle holds a quantum* (2,000–10,000 molecules of ACh). A nerve impulse causes 200–400 quanta to be released, such that 400,000–4,000,000 ACh molecules enter the

1

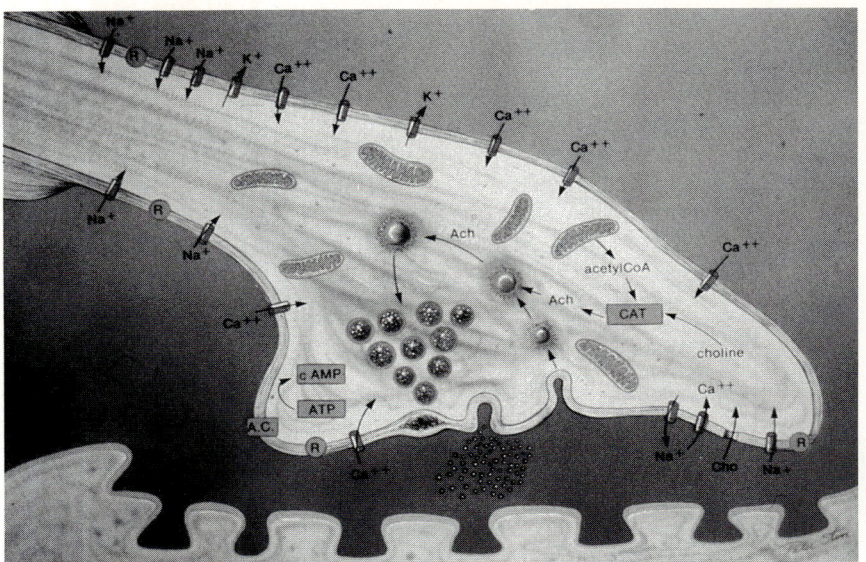

FIGURE 1-1 Illustration of the presynaptic nerve terminal, which is specialized for the synthesis, mobilization, and release of acetylcholine. Its surface is lined with cation channels and cholinoceptors (R). It contains choline acetyltransferase (CAT) for synthesis of ACh, much of which is stored in vesicles.

cleft.[12-20] These molecules depolarize the end-plate to a degree that is sufficient to generate an *end-plate potential*. This, in turn, triggers a muscle action potential (MAP). Lesser degrees of ACh release (e.g., random release of a quantum) generate a *miniature* end-plate potential that is not capable of triggering an MAP.

The end-plate of each NMJ contains millions of *postsynaptic receptor channels*[21-24] and normally is the only region that is sensitive to ACh. It typically is situated around the midportion of the muscle fiber and is aligned opposite the presynaptic nerve terminal. Each receptor consists of *five subunits* (two alpha, one beta, one delta, one epsilon) arranged in a rosette (Fig. 1-2). Both *alpha subunits* must be occupied concurrently by ACh (or an exogenous depolarizing agent such as succinylcholine) for "all-or-none" opening of a given receptor channel to occur.[25-27] The neighboring subunits (e.g., beta, delta, epsilon) influence the conformational changes induced by binding to the alpha receptors[25]; the two alpha receptor sites have different binding coefficients.[26] Each open channel contributes to an ion flux by allowing passage of Na^+ and Ca^{2+}, and exit of K^+ at the end-plate for approximately 1 msec.[22] When at least 5–20% of the channels of a given NMJ are open, the *summated end-plate potential typically reaches threshold* (approximately –45 mV) and elicits an MAP.[28,29] *Repolarization* occurs when ACh diffuses

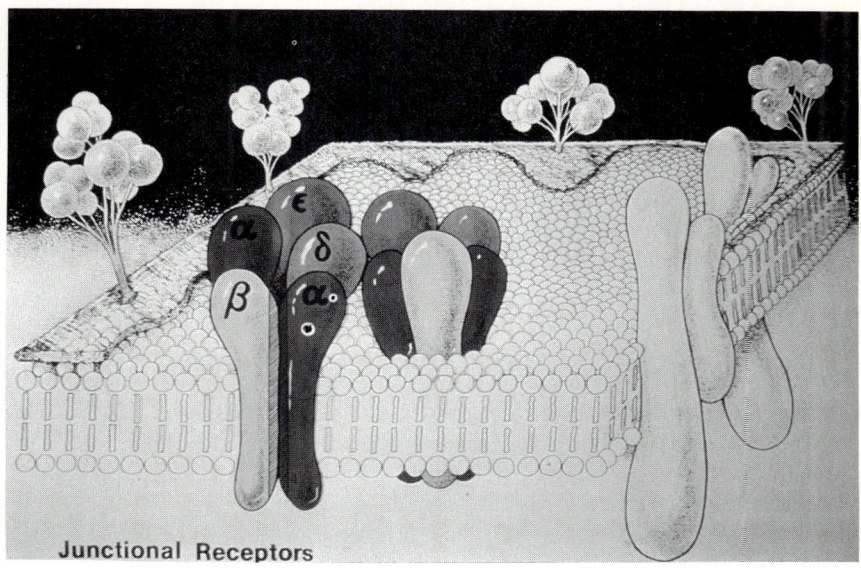

FIGURE 1-2 Postjunctional membrane (end-plate). The two structures in the center represent receptors. Each member of the pair is made of five subunits (two alphas, one beta, one delta, one epsilon) arranged in a circle around a channel. The structure at the right represents Na-K-ATPase, another molecule that crosses from one side of the membrane to the other. The balloonlike structures at the periphery represent acetylcholinesterase, which metabolizes acetylcholine in the neuromuscular junction. (Reproduced with permission from Standaert FG: Neuromuscular physiology. In Miller RD (ed): Anesthesia, 3rd ed. New York, Churchill Livingstone, 1990, pp 659–684.)

away from the receptor to be metabolized within milliseconds to acetate and choline by acetylcholinesterase.[24,30,31]

The muscle surrounding the end-plate is rich in voltage-sensitive Na^+ channels.[32] It has been proposed that, at the border of the end-plate, a *perijunctional rim of dual-gated Na^+ channels* initiates and modulates the MAP. In the resting state, the lower gate of an Na^+ channel is open and the voltage-dependent upper gate is closed.[28,32,33] Depolarization of the end-plate opens the voltage-dependent upper gate and permits *"all-or-none" generation of the MAP*. The upper gate remains open for the duration of end-plate depolarization. However, the time-dependent *lower ("inactivation") gate closes soon after the upper gate opens;* this terminates the MAP, even if there is persistent end-plate depolarization. The lower gate remains closed until the end-plate returns toward normal polarization, i.e., until the resting voltage gradient is restored. This *prevents continuous MAP generation;* i.e., a new MAP cannot be generated while the Na^+ channels are inactivated. Thus, the muscle cannot be re-excited, even though the end-plate remains depolarized. The "refractory period" lasts between 1.5 and 3.0 msec.

The MAP allows *entry of* Ca^{2+} into the muscle cell and its release from the *sarcoplasmic reticulum*. The accumulated Ca^{2+} opposes *troponin* inhibition of muscle contraction; *myosin* becomes free to interact with *actin,* and the muscle fiber contracts. Rapid extrusion and reuptake of Ca^{2+} return the muscle to the resting state. The MAP lasts from 5 to 10 msec; fiber contraction may last for as long as 150 msec.

The aforementioned events are affected by the *rate of neurostimulation* (Chaps. 3 and 4). When individual stimuli are delivered at a rate that allows the muscle to return to its resting state, the evoked response constitutes a "*single twitch*." Alternatively, rapid stimulation may lead to a summated, *tetanic response*. Tetanic stimulation induces two distinct phenomena:

1. By 20 Hz (20 stimuli/sec, with a 50-msec interval between each stimulus), the *individual muscle contractions fuse,* since the next MAP is generated before the contraction in response to the prior MAP is completed. This provides a smoother, stronger contraction that is more effective at overcoming muscle elastic forces than is a single twitch. Thus, the amplitude of the tetanic response is greater than that for a single twitch.[34]
2. Rapid stimulation depletes the supply of the readily releasable ACh, such that the nerve terminal must "mobilize" its stores. In normal settings (i.e., in the absence of relaxants or toxins), the response to tetanic stimulation typically can be maintained for rates as fast as 70–100 Hz: *the use-dependent rundown of ACh release*[35-39] *is offset by increased formation and packaging of ACh* as a result of positive feedback at presynaptic cholinoceptors.[40,41] Higher rates and/or marked prolongation of tetanic stimulation result in *fade* of the evoked response; i.e., the nerve terminal is incapable of releasing sufficient quanta to maintain repetitive end-plate depolarization.[35-38] Such fade is the hallmark of nondepolarizing block (Chaps. 2 and 4).

Discussion Questions ◆

a. What is meant by the "*innervation ratio*"? What is its significance?
b. What is the role of the Na^+/K^+ pump in the *motor nerve?*
c. Briefly summarize the roles of *sodium* in the *presynaptic nerve terminal.*
d. Compare the sensitivities of fast and slow Ca^{2+} *channels at the presynaptic nerve terminal* to: nerve firing, divalent ions, catecholamines, and calcium channel blockers.
e. How does Ca^{2+} promote *ACh release* from the presynaptic terminal?
f. Distinguish between "miniature" and "summated" *end-plate potentials.*
g. How would the summated *end-plate potential* be affected by prolongation of the nerve action potential by an agent that delays the *efflux of* K^+ (e.g., *4-aminopyridine*)?
h. What are the *durations* of the following: (1) The typical *impulse* deliv-

ered by a nerve stimulator? (2) The *"refractory periods"* of the motor nerve and NMJ? (3) The muscle action potential? (4) Muscle contraction? Discuss the significance of the relative times with respect to rates of neurostimulation.
i. How do *tonic and twitch-type muscle fibers* differ from one another with respect to *rate of contraction*, ability to *sustain contraction*, and *susceptibility to muscle relaxants*?
j. Why might muscles of the *diaphragm of a premature neonate* be more prone to fatigue than those of older children?
k. Explain why, even in the absence of neuromuscular block, the evoked contractile ("twitch") response to a single stimulus is of a lesser magnitude than the *summated (tetanic) response* to rapid stimulation.

Answers ◆

a. The number of muscle fibers innervated by a single nerve fiber and its branches constitutes the *innervation ratio*. This ratio may be determined by dividing the number of muscle fibers in a muscle by the number of motor axons in the nerve supplying that muscle.[1] *The lower the innervation ratio, the more precise the regulation,* and hence the finer the control of muscle movements.[3,4]
b. In the resting state, a *resting potential* of approximately –90 mV exists across the cell membrane. This potential is maintained by the K^+ *difference* between inside and outside, a difference that is threatened by leakage and permeability changes in ion channels. The Na^+/K^+ *pump* maintains the ionic gradients by pumping Na^+ out and bringing K^+ in.
c. Na^+ causes depolarization, which in turn causes the voltage-dependent Ca^{2+} channels to open and allow the influx of Ca^{2+}. Na^+ also appears to be critical to a rate-limiting step in the terminal's synthesis of ACh, being involved in the uptake of choline and in the activity of choline acetyltransferase.[42–44]
d. *Fast Ca^{2+} channels*, which "open" with Na^+ influx during depolarization, are *voltage dependent;* they tend to be sensitive to divalent ions (e.g., Mg^{2+}) but not to organic drugs. *Slow Ca^{2+} channels* are sensitive to cyclic AMP, which is generated by activation of adrenergic receptors.[45] Their activity increases in the presence of alpha-adrenergic agents; and they tend to be *inhibited by Ca^{2+} channel blockers* (but not divalent ions). This inhibition of slow Ca^{2+} channels by Ca^{2+} channel blockers contributes to the slight augmentation of neuromuscular block that may be noted with these agents (Chap. 9).
e. *Calcium entry into the presynaptic terminal* permits ACh release and mobilization by a number of mechanisms,[5–13,46,47] including the following: (1) Ca^{2+} binds to synaptophysin; the resulting change in this glycoprotein allows the vesicle to fuse with a "docking protein" and thereby

discharge its contents into the junctional cleft. (2) Ca^{2+} binds with calmodulin to activate calcium/calmodulin-dependent protein kinase II; this reduces the affinity of synapsin for actin, thereby facilitating movement of stored ACh toward the junction for release.[46,47] The role of Ca^{2+} is such that changes in quantal release of ACh are proportional to the fourth power of a change in Ca^{2+} concentration.[6]

f. A *miniature end-plate potential* is a small, brief voltage (approximately 0.5 mV) that may be noted at the muscle end-plate in response to release of a single quantum of ACh even when the nerve is not stimulated. It is not adequate to generate a muscle action potential.[13,16,48,49] A *summated end-plate potential* is the cumulative effect of multiple miniature end-plate potentials.[13,15,16,18–20,49] The synchronized release of multiple quanta (as a result of nerve firing) typically generates a summated end-plate potential that is well beyond the end-plate's threshold. This in turn causes generation of the (all-or-none) muscle action potential.

g. *4-Aminopyridine* and related agents that *oppose K^+ efflux* result in prolongation of the nerve action potential, with *increased entry of Ca^{2+}*.[50,51] This allows increased release of ACh and thus prolongation of the end-plate potential.[15] Although 4-aminopyridine may reverse nondepolarizing block, it does not restore normal function, and it elicits central and autonomic excitation.

h. (1) The typical *pulse duration* of an impulse delivered by a nerve stimulator is 0.1–0.3 msec. (2) The *refractory period of the motor nerve* is ≤1 msec and the period of relative NMJ unresponsiveness is 1.5–3 msec[52,53]; hence, the nerve theoretically can respond to stimulation as frequent as 1,000 impulses/sec (1,000 Hz) and the NMJ can transmit 333–667 impulses/sec. (3) The *muscle action potential* lasts 5–10 msec; hence, individual MAPs may be generated as frequently as 200 times/sec. (4) The *resultant muscle contraction* lasts for up to 150 msec; hence, there is an interval during which the muscle is capable of a subsequent MAP while it is still contracting as a result of a prior MAP. At rates above 5–10 Hz (5–10 stimuli/sec), each subsequent MAP may elicit a contractile response that is superimposed on the prior one, producing a *summated (tetanic) contraction*.

i. The muscles of the human body differ with respect to *fiber type*.[54] They may be broadly classified as "tonic" and "twitch" types. *Tonic fibers* undergo slow sustained contraction. Of relevance to the anesthesiologist, this type is found in the extraocular muscles and may cause increased intraocular pressure in response to succinylcholine (Chap. 18). Tonic fibers have several NMJs per cell; i.e., they are multiply innervated with a low innervation ratio. This allows for precisely regulated movement.

Twitch fibers typically are innervated by a single nerve terminal and respond to nerve firing with more rapid contraction. Three subtypes of "twitch fibers" can be identified according to histochemical staining, electromyographic activity, and/or end-plate activity.[55,56]

Type I (slow-twitch or "red") fibers are rich in myoglobin. They undergo relatively slow contraction and relaxation, have a relatively high oxidative capacity, and are relatively resistant to fatigue. Slow-twitch fibers constitute a major portion of the adductor pollicis muscle and soleus muscles, approximately 50% of the gastrocnemius and abductor digiti quinti muscles, and less than 20% of the orbicularis oculi muscle[54,57,58]. Slow-twitch fibers tend to be particularly susceptible to nondepolarizing relaxants,[57-62] preferentially losing their ability to sustain contractions in the presence of partial block with *d*-tubocurarine (but not with the depolarizing relaxant decamethonium).[62] The sensitivity of slow-twitch fibers to nondepolarizing relaxant may be due to relatively greater perfusion,[63] a smaller ACh quantum content (which would make them more susceptible to competitive block),[37,64] and/or fewer receptors.[65]

Type II fibers, which are faster than Type I fibers, are divided into two subgroups. *Type IIA (intermediate) fibers* combine fast contraction and resistance to fatigue. *Type IIB fibers* have high contraction speeds but are not suited for sustained work as they have fewer mitochondria.

Type II fibers tend to "drop out" during an otherwise sustained contraction even without a nondepolarizing relaxant.[56] The faster fibers are particularly susceptible to a depolarizing relaxant such as decamethonium, which slows their contractions.[58,60,66-69] The contraction time of the thyroarytenoid (an adductor of the vocal cords) is particularly short,[70-72] while that of the posterior cricoarytenoid (an abductor) is longer[70-72] but nevertheless relatively fast compared to other muscles of the body. The potential impact of these differences on the response to relaxants is discussed in Chapters 3 and 16.

j. The *resistance of a muscle to fatigue* correlates with its proportion of *high-oxidative (e.g., Type I) muscle fibers*. The *diaphragm of premature infants* (<37 weeks' gestation) has only 10% Type I fibers, whereas the diaphragms of full-term newborns and children more than 8 months old have 25% and 55% Type I fibers, respectively.[73] Likewise, the intercostal muscles of premature, full-term, and older infants have 19%, 46%, and 65% Type I fibers, respectively.[73]

k. Despite "complete depolarization" of its motor nerve upon *single twitch* stimulation at supramaximal current, the muscle does not achieve maximal contraction because the evoked response to a single twitch is too brief to overcome the inertia of the series elastic components of the muscle's contractile apparatus. *A maximal response is attained during tetanic stimulation,* since there is time for the inertia to be overcome. It takes approximately 350 msec to develop maximal tension at the start of a tetanic response and 150 msec for tension to disappear after tetanic stimulation.[74]

References ◆

1. Buchthal F, Schmalbruch H: Motor unit of mammalian muscle. Physiol Rev 60:90–142, 1980
2. Birks R, Huxley HE, Katz B: The fine structure of the neuromuscular junction of the frog. J Physiol (Lond) 150:134–144, 1960
3. Carlsöö S: Motor units and action potentials in masticatory muscles. Acta Morphol Neerl Scand 2:13–19, 1958
4. Feinstein B, Lindegard B, Nyman E, Wohlfart G: Morphologic studies of motor units in normal human muscles. Acta Anat (Basel) 23:127–142, 1955
5. Parnas J, Parnas H: The "Ca-voltage" hypothesis for neurotransmitter release. Biophys Chem 29:85–93, 1988
6. Dodge FA Jr, Rahamimoff R: Cooperative action of Ca ions in transmitter release at the neuromuscular junction. J Physiol (Lond) 193:419, 1967
7. Bowman WC: Pharmacology of Neuromuscular Function, 2nd ed. Wright, London, 1990
8. Burgoyne RD: Secretory vesicle-associated proteins and their role in exocytosis. Annu Rev Physiol 52:647–569, 1990
9. Marshall IG: Prejunctional aspects of neuromuscular transmission: physiology, biochemistry and pharmacology. Curr Opin Anaesth 4:577–582, 1991
10. Slater C, Vincent A: Structure and development of the neuromuscular junction. In Vincent A, Wray D (eds): Neuromuscular Transmission. Manchester, England, Manchester University Press, 1990, pp 1–26
11. Marshall IG, Parsons SM: The vesicular acetylcholine transport system. Trends Neurosci 10:174–177, 1987
12. Ceccarelli B, Hurlbut WP: Vesicle hypothesis of the release of quanta of acetylcholine. Physiol Rev 60:396–441, 1980
13. DelCastillo J, Katz B: Quantal components of the end-plate potential. J Physiol 124:560–573, 1954
14. Dunant Y: On the mechanism of acetylcholine release. Prog Neurobiol 26:55–92, 1986
15. Katz B, Miledi R: Estimates of quantal content during "chemical potentiation" of transmitter release. Proc R Soc Lond 205:369–378, 1979
16. Katz B: Quantal mechanism of neural transmitter release. Science 173:123–126, 1971
17. Martin AR: Quantal nature of synaptic transmission. Physiol Rev 46:51–66, 1966
18. Unsworth CD, Johnson RG: Acetylcholine and ATP are co-released from the electromotor nerve terminals of *Narcine brasiliensis* by an exocytotic mechanism. Proc Natl Acad Sci USA 87:553–557, 1990
19. Van der Kloot W: Acetylcholine quanta are released from vesicles by exocytosis (and why some think not). Neuroscience 24:1–7, 1988
20. Zucker S, Lando L, Fogelson A: Can presynaptic depolarization release transmitter without calcium influx? J Physiol (Paris) 81:237–245, 1986
21. Barrantes FJ: Muscle endplate cholinoreceptors. Pharmacol Ther 38:331, 1988
22. Dreyer F: Acetylcholine receptor. Br J Anaesth 54:115–130, 1982
23. Land BR, Salpeter EE, Salpeter MM: Acetylcholine receptor site density affects the rising phase of miniature endplate currents. Proc Natl Acad Sci USA 77:3736, 1980
24. Peper K, Bradley RJ, Dreyer F: The acetylcholine receptor at the neuromuscular junction. Physiol Rev 62:1271–1340, 1982
25. Pedersen SE, Cohen JB: *d*-Tubocurarine binding sites are located at α-γ and α-δ subunit interfaces of the nicotinic acetylcholine receptor. Proc Natl Acad Sci USA 87:2785–2789, 1990
26. Blount P, Merlie JP: Molecular basis of the two nonequivalent ligand binding sites of the muscle nicotinic acetylcholine receptor. Neuron 3:349–357, 1989

27. Sheridan RE, Lester HA: Rates and equilibria at the acetylcholine receptor of *Electrophorus* electroplaques. J Gen Physiol 70:187–219, 1977
28. Standaert FG: Neuromuscular physiology. In Miller RD (ed): Anesthesia, 3rd ed. New York, Churchill Livingstone, 1990, pp 659–684
29. Waud BE, Waud DR: The margin of safety of neuromuscular transmission in the muscle of the diaphragm. Anesthesiology 37:417–422, 1972
30. Anderson CR, Stevens CF: Voltage clamp analysis of acetylcholine produced end-plate current fluctuations at frog neuromuscular junction. J Physiol 235:655–691, 1973
31. Katz B, Miledi R: The binding of acetylcholine to receptors and its removal from the synaptic cleft. J Physiol 231:549–574, 1973
32. Betz WJ, Caldwell JH, Kinnamon SC: Increased sodium conductance in the synaptic region of rat skeletal muscle fibres. J Physiol (Lond) 352:189–202, 1984
33. Katz AM, Messineo FC, Herbette L: Ion channels in membranes. Circulation 65:I2–I10, 1982
34. Edwards RHT, Young A, Hosking GP, Jones DA: Human skeletal muscle function: description of tests and normal values. Clin Sci 52:283–290, 1977
35. Blackman JG: Stimulus frequency and neuromuscular block. Br J Pharmacol 20:5–16, 1963
36. Brooks VB, Theis RE: Reduction of quantum content during neuromuscular transmission. J Physiol (Lond) 162:298–310, 1962
37. Elmqvist D, Quastel DMJ: A quantitative study of end-plate potentials in isolated human muscle. J Physiol (Lond) 178:505–529, 1965
38. Kurihara T, Brooks JE: The mechanism of neuromuscular fatigue: a study of mammalian muscle using excitation-contraction uncoupling. Arch Neurol 32:168–174, 1975
39. Storella RJ, Ackerman TS, Katul ZJ: Tetanic fade and acetylcholine release. Anesthesiology 79:A923, 1993
40. Bowman WC, Prior C, Marshall IG: Presynaptic receptors in the neuromuscular junction. Ann NY Acad Sci 604:69–81, 1990
41. Van der Kloot W: The regulation of quantal size. Prog Neurobiol 36:93–130, 1991
42. Beach RL, Vaca K, Pilar G: Ionic and metabolic requirements for high affinity choline uptake and acetylcholine synthesis in nerve terminals at a neuromuscular junction. J Neurochem 34:1387, 1980
43. Standaert FG: Release of transmitter at the neuromuscular junction. Br J Anaesth 54:131–145, 1982
44. Tucek S: Acetylcholine Synthesis in Neurons. New York, John Wiley & Sons, Inc, 1978
45. Salvatore A, Del Pozo E, Carlos R, Baeyens JM: Differential effects of calcium channel blocking agents on pancuronium- and suxamethonium-induced neuromuscular blockade. Br J Anaesth 60:495–499, 1988
46. De Lorenzo RJ: Role of calmodulin in neurotransmitter release and synaptic function. Ann NY Acad Sci 356:92, 1980
47. McGuinness TL, Greengard P: Protein phosphorylation and synaptic transmission. In Sellin LC, Libelius R, Thesleff S (eds): Neuromuscular Junction. Amsterdam, Elsevier, 1988, pp 111–124
48. Katz B, Miledi R: Transmitter leakage from motor nerve endings. Proc R Soc Lond [Biol] 196:59–72, 1977
49. Boyd IA, Martin AR: Spontaneous subthreshold activity at mammalian neuromuscular junction. J Physiol (Lond) 132:61, 1956
50. Beaufort TM, Wierda JMKH, Kruyswijk JE, Agoston S: 2,4-Diaminopyridine: clinical evaluation of a recently synthesized 4-aminopyridine derivative for reversal of competitive neuromuscular blockade. Eur J Anaesthesiol 7:453–457, 1990
51. Thesleff S: Aminopyridines and synaptic transmission. Neuroscience 5:1413, 1980
52. Epstein RA, Jackson SH: Repetitive muscle depolarization from single indirect stimulation in anesthetized man. J Appl Physiol 28:407–410, 1970
53. Epstein RA, Jackson SH, Wyte SR: The effects of nondepolarizing relaxants and anticholinesterases on the neuromuscular refractory period of anesthetized man. Anesthesiology 31:69–77, 1969
54. Johnson MA, Polgar W, Weightman D, Appleton D: Data on the distribution of fibre types in thirty-six human muscles: an autopsy study. J Neurol Sci 18:111–129, 1973

55. Ellisman MH, Rash JE, Staehelin LA, Porter KR: Studies of excitable membranes. J Cell Biol 68:752, 1976
56. Warmolds JR, Engel WK: Open-biopsy electromyography. Arch Neurol 27:512, 1972
57. Secher NH, Robe N, Secher O: Effect of tubocurarine on human soleus and gastrocnemius muscles. Acta Anaesthesiol Scand 26:231–234, 1982
58. Paton WDM, Zaimis EJ: The action of d-tubocurarine and of decamethonium on respiratory and other muscles in the cat. J Physiol 112:311–331, 1951
59. Jewell Pa, Zaimis E: A differentiation between red and white muscles in the cat based on responses to neuromuscular blocking agents. J Physiol (Lond) 124:417, 1954
60. Alderson AM, MacLagan J: The action of decamethonium and tubocurarine on the respiratory and limb muscles of the cat. J Physiol (Lond) 173:38–56, 1964
61. Zaimis E: Motor end plate differences as a determining factor in the mode of action of neuromuscular blocking substances. J Physiol 122:238–251, 1953
62. Molbech S, Johansen SH: Endurance time in static work during partial curarization. J Appl Physiol 27:44, 1969
63. Andersen P: Capillary density in skeletal muscle of man. Acta Physiol Scand 95:203, 1975
64. Jenkinson DH: The antagonism between tubocurarine and substances which depolarize the motor end-plate. J Physiol (Lond) 152:309, 1960
65. Sterz R, Pagala M, Peper K: Postjunctional characteristics of the endplates in mammalian fast and slow muscles. Pflugers Arch 398:48–54, 1983
66. Secher NH, Rube N, Molbech S: The voluntary muscle contraction pattern in man. In De Potter J-C (ed): Adapted Physical Activities. Editions de l'Universite de Bruxelles, 1981, p 225
67. Choi WW, Gergis SD, Sokoll MD: Effects of succinylcholine chloride on the response of fast and slow muscle in the cat. Acta Anaesthesiol Scand 28:516–520, 1984
68. Muir AW, Houston J, Green KL, Marshall RJ, Bowman WC, Marshall IG: Effects of a new neuromuscular blocking agent (Org 9426) in anaesthetized cats and pigs and in isolated nerve-muscle preparations. Br J Anaesth 63:400–410, 1989
69. Muir AW, Marshall RJ: Comparative neuromuscular blocking effects of vecuronium, pancuronium, ORG 6368 and suxamethonium in the anaesthetized domestic pig. Br J Anaesth 59:622–629, 1987
70. Hast MH: The primate larynx: a comparative physiological study of intrinsic muscles. Acta Otolaryngol (Stockh) 67:84–92, 1969
71. Martensson A, Skoglund CR: Contraction properties of intrinsic laryngeal muscles. Acta Physiol Scand 60:318–336, 1964
72. Sanders I, Aviv J, Kraus WM, Racenstein MM, Biller HF: Transcutaneous electrical stimulation of the recurrent laryngeal nerve in monkeys. Ann Otol Rhinol Laryngol 96:38–42, 1987
73. Keens TG, Bryan AC, Levison H, Ianuzzo CD: Developmental pattern of muscle fiber types in human ventilatory muscles. J Appl Physiol 44:909–913, 1978
74. Epstein RA, Epstein RM: The electromyogram and the mechanical response of indirectly stimulated muscle in anesthetized man following curarization. Anesthesiology 38:212–223, 1973

2
DAVID G. SILVERMAN | FRANK G. STANDAERT
Mechanisms of Neuromuscular Block

Nondepolarizing and depolarizing relaxants share structural similarities with acetylcholine (ACh) (Fig. 2-1).[1] This allows them to occupy ACh receptor sites. Nondepolarizing relaxants (NDRs) primarily prevent receptor activation by ACh, whereas depolarizing relaxants primarily activate ACh receptors, opening the receptor channel for passage of Na^+ and Ca^{2+} into the cell and K^+ out of it.

◆ NONDEPOLARIZING BLOCK

Nondepolarizing relaxants are charged *quaternary nitrogen* compounds that cause *flaccid paralysis* by competing with ACh at the alpha subunits of junctional cholinoceptors. They are large, bulky, relatively inflexible molecules that contain at least one quaternary ammonium group. The NDRs are of two basic *structural types:* vecuronium, pancuronium, pipecuronium, and rocuronium are aminosteroidal compounds; *d*-tubocurarine, metocurine, atracurium, doxacurium, and mivacurium are benzylisoquinolonium ("curariform") compounds (Chaps. 12–14).

NDRs occupy the cholinoceptors with high affinity without appreciable agonist activity. They thereby compete with ACh by decreasing the probability of ACh binding to receptor sites and causing channel opening. They "jump" on and off receptors, exerting an appreciable effect within milliseconds.[2-5] It takes two agonist molecules to open a given channel but only one antagonist to prevent it from opening.

Traditionally thought to act exclusively by binding to one or both alpha subunits of *postsynaptic receptors,* NDRs also act by occupying *presynaptic cholinoceptors* and/or by *occluding the postsynaptic receptor channel.*

Key features of *nondepolarizing block* are outlined below and detailed in Chapter 4:

1. It is a *competitive block* that may be offset by increased amounts of ACh.
2. There is a *wide margin of safety* such that ≥75% of receptors must be

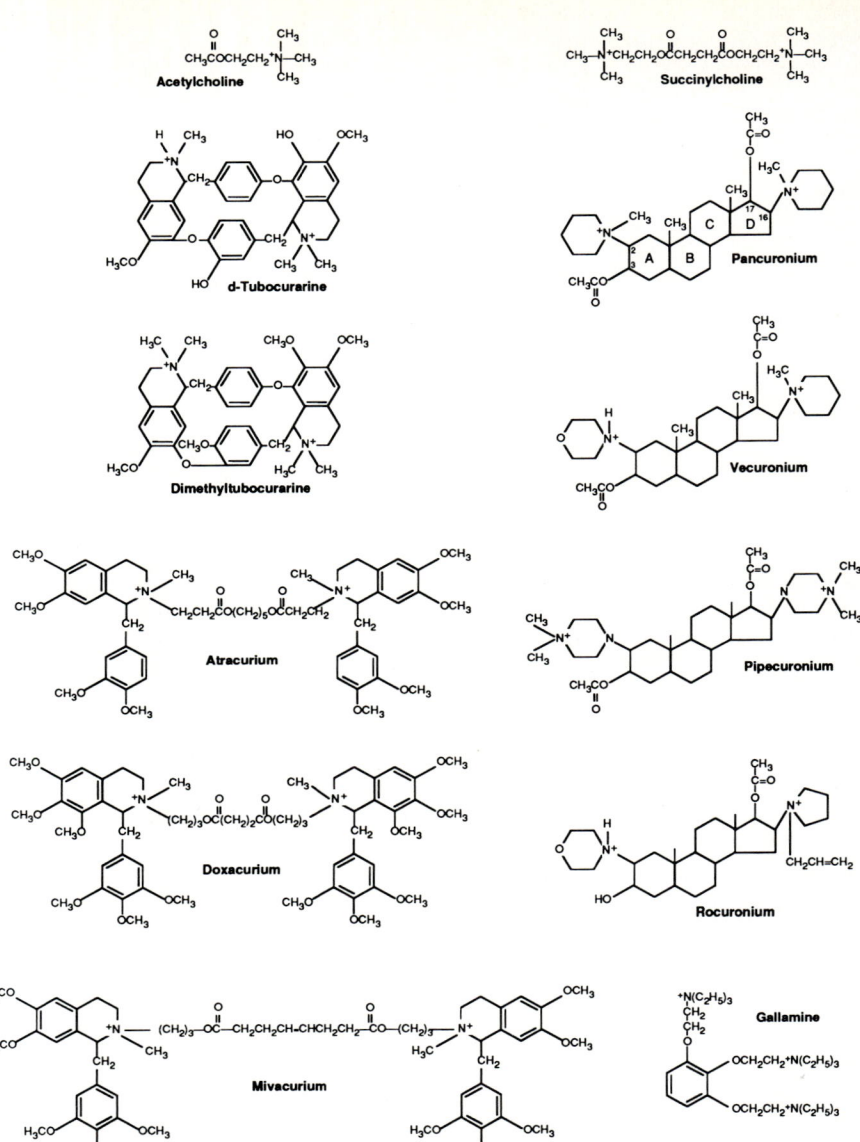

FIGURE 2-1 Acetylcholine and neuromuscular blocking agents. Each molecule contains at least one charged N^+ for electrostatic binding to a cholinoceptor. Although d-tubocurarine is shown as a bisquaternary structure, it may also have a monoquaternary configuration.[1] Like tubocurarine, vecuronium and rocuronium tend to acquire a second positive charge at physiologic pH. They thus are illustrated as bisquaternary structures, even though they may exist as monoquaternary molecules. Notice the 4-ring (androstane) core that is a component of each member of the steroidal series; the four rings are labeled A–D in the drawing for pancuronium. Four sites on these rings are primarily responsible for differences among steroidal agents; these are labeled *2, 3, 16,* and *17* on the drawing for pancuronium.

occupied by an NDR before there is significant twitch height depression.[6–9]
3. There is a *narrow range of receptor occupancy* over which detectable changes in twitch height occur (approximately 76–92%).[5–8]
4. It is characterized by *fade* in response to rapid (e.g., train-of-four and tetanic) stimulation; i.e., the amplitude of the evoked responses steadily declines in response to rapid stimulation. Fade is noted at lesser degrees of receptor occupancy[7,9–13] and lower plasma concentrations of relaxant[14] than is depression of the single twitch.
5. It is characterized by a period of *posttetanic facilitation,* with posttetanic twitch responses of greater magnitude than the pretetanic responses.

Most investigators have attributed *fade* to a presynaptic effect of NDRs. *Presynaptic binding* of NDRs to cholinoceptors prevents the rapid ACh mobilization that is required to maintain adequate ACh release during rapid stimulation[15–45]; it may oppose the cation movement required for ACh mobilization and release. It appears that low doses of an NDR can prevent channel opening of the presynaptic "positive feedback" receptors[15,23,41] (which are similar to, but not identical with, the postsynaptic end-plate receptors).[44] The propensity for presynaptic block differs among NDRs: hexamethonium > gallamine > tubocurarine > vecuronium > atracurium > pancuronium.[15,16,23,46–48] However, the relative differences among agents may be minimal once deep block is established.[49]

The *mechanisms of fade* are not clear-cut. The generally accepted belief that the degree of *fade* is related to propensity for presynaptic binding. In addition, a *"multiple compartment" hypothesis* attributes the propensity for fade to the distribution of relaxant to different pharmacokinetic compartments, each of which has a different propensity for fade.[50,51] There also is evidence that fade may be noted in the context of selective *postsynaptic occupancy*[52]; snake venoms with virtually pure postsynaptic affinity may cause fade.[52] Such postsynaptic effects may be the result of binding to other than classic postsynaptic receptors.[53,54]

◆ DEPOLARIZING BLOCK

Like ACh, depolarizing relaxants activate the cholinoceptors in the neuromuscular junction (NMJ).[55] However, in contrast to ACh, *succinylcholine (SCh) and decamethonium* are *not* hydrolyzed by acetylcholinesterase in the NMJ. Succinylcholine is simply two ACh molecules hooked tail to tail. Each of the ACh components contains an ester link which is susceptible to hydrolysis by pseudocholinesterase in the plasma but not by acetylcholinesterase in the NMJ. Decamethonium has a similar internitrogen distance; however, it is not susceptible to ester hydrolysis in the plasma, and its clearance is dependent on renal elimination.

The persistence of these agents in the NMJ allows them to bind repeatedly to the receptors, thereby causing *prolonged end-plate depolarization*. The persistent depolarized state then prompts the *dual-gated Na$^+$ channels* which rim the end-plate (Chap. 1) to "accommodate" by closing their lower (inactivation) gates. *Flaccid paralysis* ensues until the end-plate returns toward normal polarization and the "gates" return to their resting states so that a subsequent MAP may be initiated (Chap. 16).

As is the case for NDRs, depolarizing relaxants also exert a *presynaptic effect*[56]; they depolarize the unmyelinated nerve endings and may activate presynaptic cholinoceptors.[19] Such effects may be blocked by small doses of nondepolarizing drugs and by diphenylhydantoin (a known suppressor of motor nerve terminal repetitive discharging),[57] presumably by a presynaptic mechanism.[58]

The *onset of SCh* may be characterized by (1) a transient increase of *muscle tension*[59-66] as the initial depolarization of individual end-plates gives rise to individual muscle fiber contractions, and (2) synchronous (possibly repetitive) firing of all muscle cells in a motor unit (*"fasciculations"*), the result of SCh-induced depolarization of the presynaptic nerve terminals.[15,41,58,67,68]

Depolarizing block abates as drug leaves the NMJ. In addition, persistent SCh-induced influx of Na$^+$ through the open receptor channels may be offset by increased activity of the Na$^+$/K$^+$ pump, and the end-plate current may return toward baseline, even if the depolarizing relaxant is still present.[69]

◆ CHANNEL BLOCK AND DESENSITIZATION

Receptors may be "taken out of the pool" by channel block and/or desensitization. *Channel block* entails direct occlusion of the receptor channel.[70,71] Open-channel (use-dependent) block involves physical occlusion of an opened receptor channel, typically by a positively charged or neutral molecule. Closed-channel block involves occlusion of the channel mouth independent of channel opening. *Desensitization* classically develops when the receptor channel no longer opens in respone to agonists on its alpha subunits. Desensitization may entail conformational changes as a result of such varied factors as binding of an agonist, antagonist, or other drug to a site in the receptor other than the ACh binding site, distortion of the channel, or disruption of sub end-plate mechanisms (as by a slim molecule such as SCh that can slip through the channel).[71-78] Such changes, which may occur pre- as well as postsynaptically, may account for *phase 2 block* with a depolarizing relaxant (Chap. 16).[79-81]

Channel block and desensitization also may contribute to the neuromuscular blocking effects of NDRs[51,82,83] as well as to the neuromuscular block that may accompany cholinesterase inhibitors,[69] volatile anesthetics,[84] and a myriad of other drugs that may be used in perioperative and intensive care settings.[73,83,85]

◆ LABORATORY MODELS

Insight into the nature of a block may be gained by measuring end-plate currents in a number of laboratory models, including the rat *hemidiaphragm preparation*.[41,86,87] This model is useful for comparing the effects of different agents, and recently was used to confirm the similar effects of rocuronium and vecuronium.[88,89] *Postjunctional effects* are evidenced by a reduction in the amplitude of a single end-plate current or of the first end-plate current in a train. *Prejunctional effects* are indicated by a rundown (decline) of end-plate current amplitudes in the "plateau" portion of the train.[15,28,88–90]

◆ SITES OF INJECTION

Although relaxants typically are administered intravenously (IV), they may be given by other routes. Intramuscular (IM) injection of SCh has been used effectively when IV access is unavailable. After 2–3 times the typical IV dose, adequate systemic levels are reached 3–4 minutes after IM administration of SCh (vs. 1–1.5 minutes after IV administration) (Chap. 16).

Of note, *relaxants may be effective at the site of IM infiltration*. Local injection of 1 mL (0.05 mg) of pancuronium into the middle of the *masseter muscle* provided relaxation for reduction after a mandibular dislocation.[91]

Discussion Questions ◆

a. What is meant by the *"margin of safety"* with respect to nondepolarizing block?
b. Do all of the *end-plates within a given muscle* respond identically to a nondepolarizing relaxant?
c. Briefly describe how *fade* may be induced by competitive binding of a nondepolarizing relaxant to *presynaptic cholinoceptors*.
d. Compare the nondepolarizing agents *hexamethonium, d-tubocurarine,* and *pancuronium* with respect to propensity for *presynaptic block* and channel block.
e. *d*-Tubocurarine induces tetanic fade; *magnesium* tends to simply decrease the magnitude of the end-plate potential. How might this difference be accounted for by their different *presynaptic actions?*
f. Does *persistent depolarization* of the end-plate (as by *succinylcholine*) ensure repeated or continuous triggering of muscle action potentials? Why or why not?
g. Do the same *number of receptors* need to be occupied to achieve neuromuscular block with *succinylcholine* and *d-tubocurarine?*

h. How do *receptors in denervated muscle* differ from traditional receptors? How does this affect the patient's sensitivity to depolarizing and nondepolarizing relaxants?

i. What is meant by the statement that the developing muscles of the fetus have more than one *type of cholinoceptor*?

Answers ◆

a. A *margin of safety* exists because activation of only a small percentage of receptors is required for effective neuromuscular transmission; i.e., a summated end-plate potential that is capable of triggering an MAP is generated by the opening of a small percentage of receptor channels. In their classic studies, Paton and Waud noted that to "produce a threshold block to indirect stimulation once every 10 sec (i.e., single twitch at 0.1 Hz), a *fractional occupancy* by the antagonist of 0.76 ± 0.05 was required; for nearly complete block, including block of the more resistant NMJs, an occupancy of 0.917 ± 0.16 was required."[6] The margin of safety is particularly evident at the diaphragm, where transmission occurs upon opening of as few as 5–10% of the millions of receptors that line the typical end-plate,[73,92] i.e., with as much as 0.90–0.95 fractional occupancy by antagonist.

b. The *sensitivities of end-plates to nondepolarizing block are not identical*; there is a normal distribution of sensitivities even among the individual fibers of the same muscle group. For example, some NMJs that transfer impulses from the ulnar nerve to the adductor pollicis muscle fail to transmit at a level of relaxant that produces *75% receptor occupancy*; hence, we begin to see depression of adductor pollicis twitch height at this degree of occupancy. Other end-plates are more "resistant" and are not blocked until approximately *92% occupancy* is attained; hence, total loss of the adductor pollicis twitch response is not attained until this degree of occupancy is achieved. Remember, the decline in twitch height between 75% and 92% receptor occupancy does not represent a progressive decline in the ability of each end-plate to transmit a stimulus. Instead, it is due to an increasing number of end-plates becoming unable to generate an MAP in response to a given stimulus (an *"all-or-none" effect* at each muscle cell). Hence, there is transmission to fewer of the fibers that compose the adductor pollicis muscle and consequently a weaker contractile response to neurostimulation. To summarize, a strong contraction results from MAP generation in the majority of motor units composing a muscle group; a weaker contraction suggests that the end-plates of fewer motor units are depolarized sufficiently to generate an MAP.

c. *Nondepolarizing relaxants* appear to enhance use-dependent rundown of ACh release by blocking the *presynaptic cholinoceptors* that are responsible for increased "mobilization" of ACh in response to rapid stimulation. The presynaptic terminal thus may not be able to maintain a level of ACh release that is sufficient to depolarize the end-plate sufficiently to trigger an MAP. This rundown of ACh release results in *fade* of the tetanic response.

d. *Hexamethonium* causes the greatest degree of *presynaptic block,* and it is associated with a relatively large degree of postsynaptic *channel block* as compared to "traditional" *postsynaptic receptor block.* In contrast, *pancuronium* causes relatively little presynaptic block and relatively little channel block, but has a high degree of postsynaptic receptor affinity. *Tubocurarine* is intermediate with respect to these features. These differences among agents alter responses during neuromuscular monitoring. Consistent with their relative amounts of presynaptic block, hexamethonium causes the most and pancuronium causes the least amount of *fade.*

e. Mg^{2+} blocks the entry of Ca^{2+} and so reduces the number of quanta released, regardless of the rate of stimulation; i.e., it does not selectively compromise rate-related "mobilization" and hence does not cause fade.[25] Alternatively, an NDR with presynaptic binding (e.g., *d*-tubocurarine) or other agents that decrease vesicle filling (e.g., vesamicol) produce a significant decrease in the number of "refilled" quanta available for release in response to rapid stimulation, and hence cause fade.[19,93,94]

f. *Persistent end-plate depolarization* does not ensure continuous generation of *MAPs*. With persistent end-plate depolarization, the lower (time-dependent) Na^+ gate of the *perijunctional rim of Na^+ channels* closes and remains closed. Thus, after initial contraction, the muscle remains flaccid following administration of a depolarizing relaxant. A subsequent MAP cannot be generated until the lower gate opens (i.e., until after the end-plate depolarization dissipates).

g. It has been documented that >70% *occupancy* is required before even the more susceptible NMJs are blocked by a *nondepolarizing relaxant.*[6] Alternatively, only *5–20% of receptors* need to be opened in the presence of a *depolarizing agent* such as SCh to trigger an MAP and cause closing of the inactivation gates of the Na^+ channels which rim the end-plate.

h. *Denervation* causes loss of neural trophic factor and loss of muscle activity, leading to proliferation of cholinoceptors that vary in type and location from standard junctional receptors[83,95–102] (Chap. 22). These *extrajunctional receptors* (EJRs) proliferate along the entire muscle surface, well beyond the insulating zone of sodium channels that rims the end-plate (Chap. 1). The EJRs and sodium channels are not segregated; that is, there is no zone where there are only sodium channels and no receptors. The absence of the insulating rim of sodium channels with their inactivation gates allows EJR activation to trigger repetitive contractions and *contractures*. It also should be noted that EJRs contain a *gamma subunit* rather than an *epsilon subunit*.[103–105] This alters their responses to depolarizing and nondepolarizing agents.[106–110] Most notably, EJRs have a smaller single-channel conductance and a longer burst duration time than typical receptors. They respond to lower concentrations of agonists than do normal receptors, and a high concentration of NDR is required to block an agonist's effect. Thus, it is easy to set off EJR-induced contractures and produce hyperkalemia upon administration of a depolarizing agent, but it is difficult to prevent these phenomena by pretreatment with an NDR (Chap. 22).

i. As the fetus develops, *extrajunctional receptors* (with a *gamma subunit*) are gradually replaced with junctional receptors (with an epsilon subunit). During early infancy, the EJRs progressively disappear and only junctional receptors are present in normal children and adults. This development is stimulated by increased neural activity.[103,111] Of note, infants are not particularly prone to exaggerated SCh-induced increases in serum K$^+$, presumably because their EJRs are relatively few in number.

References ◆

1. Everett AJ, Lowe LA, Wilkinson S: Revision of structure of (+)- tubocurarine chloride and chondracurine. J Chem Soc (Chem Commun) 1:1020–1021, 1970
2. Armstrong DL, Lester HA: The kinetics of tubocurarine action and restricted diffusion within the synaptic cleft. J Physiol (Lond) 294:365–386, 1979
3. Colquhoun D, Sheridan RE: The effect of tubocurarine competition on the kinetics of agonist action on the nicotinic receptor. Br J Pharmacol 75:77–86, 1982
4. McCarthy MP, Stroud RM: Conformational states of the nicotinic acetylcholine receptor from *Torpedo californica* induced by the binding of agonists, antagonists, and local anesthetics: equilibrium measurements using tritium-hydrogen exchange. Biochemistry 28:40–48, 1989
5. Sheridan RE, Lester HA: Rates and equilibria at the acetylcholine receptor of *Electrophorus* electroplaques. J Gen Physiol 70:187–219, 1977
6. Paton WDM, Waud DR: The margin of safety of neuromuscular transmission. J Physiol (Lond) 191:59–90, 1967
7. Waud BE, Waud DR: The relation between the response to "train-of-four" stimulation and receptor occlusion during competitive neuromuscular block. Anesthesiology 37:413–416, 1972
8. Waud BE, Waud DR: The margin of safety of neuromuscular transmission in the muscle of the diaphragm. Anesthesiology 37:417–422, 1972
9. Lee C: Train-of-4 quantitation of competitive neuromuscular block. Anesth Analg 54:649–653, 1975
10. Gissen AJ, Katz RL: Twitch, tetanus and posttetanic potentiation as indices of nerve-muscle block in man. Anesthesiology 30:481–487, 1969
11. Paton WDM, Zaimis EJ: The action of *d*-tubocurarine and decamethonium on respiratory and other muscles in the cat. J Physiol (Lond) 112:311–331, 1951
12. Rosenblueth A, Morison RS: Curarization, fatigue and Wedensky inhibition. Am J Physiol 119:236–256, 1937
13. Waud BE, Waud DR: The relation between tetanic fade and receptor occlusion in the presence of competitive neuromuscular block. Anesthesiology 35:456–464, 1971
14. Torda TA, Graham GG, Tsui D: Neuromuscular sensitivity to atracurium in humans. Anaesth Intensive Care 18:62–68, 1990
15. Bowman WC: Prejunctional and postjunctional cholinoceptors at the neuromuscular junction. Anesth Analg 59:935–943, 1980

16. Bowman WC, Webb SN: Tetanic fade during partial transmission failure produced by nondepolarizing neuromuscular blocking drugs in the cat. Clin Exp Pharmacol Physiol 3:545–555, 1976
17. Blackman JG: Stimulus frequency and neuromuscular block. Br J Pharmacol 20:5–16, 1963
18. Brooks VB, Theis RE: Reduction of quantum content during neuromuscular transmission. J Physiol (Lond) 162:298–310, 1962
19. Bowman WC, Prior C, Marshall IG: Presynaptic receptors in the neuromuscular junction. Ann NY Acad Sci 604:69–81, 1990
20. Bowman WC, Marshall IG, Gibb AJ, Harborne AJ: Feedback control of transmitter release at the neuromuscular junction. Trends Pharmacol Sci 9:16–20, 1988
21. Bowman WC, Marshall IG, Gigg AJ: Is there feedback control of transmitter release at the neuromuscular junction? Semin Anesthesiol 3:275–283, 1984
22. Bowman WC: The neuromuscular junction: recent developments. Eur J Anaesthesiol 2:59–93, 1985
23. Baker T, Aguero A, Stanec A, Lowndes HE: Prejunctional effects of vecurcnium in the cat. Anesthesiology 65:480–484, 1986
24. Elmqvist D, Quastel DMJ: A quantitative study of endplate potentials in isolated human muscle. J Physiol (Lond) 178:505–529, 1965
25. Foldes FF, Chaudhry IA, Kinjo M, Nagashima H: Inhibition of mobilization of acetylcholine: the weak link in neuromuscular transmission during partial neuromuscular block with d-tubocurarine. Anesthesiology 71:218–223, 1989
26. Galindo A: Prejunctional effect of curare: its relative importance. J Neurophysiol 34:289–301, 1971
27. Graham GG, Morris R, Pybus DA, Torda TA, Woodey R: Relationship of train-of-four ratio to twitch depression during pancuronium-induced neuromuscular blockade. Anesthesiology 65:579–583, 1986
28. Gibb AJ, Marshall IG: Pre- and post-junctional effects of d-tubocurarine and other nicotinic antagonists during repetitive stimulation in the rat. J Physiol (Lond) 351:275–297, 1984
29. Glavinovic MI: Presynaptic action of curare. J Physiol (Lond) 290:499–506, 1979
30. Hubbard JI, Wilson DF, Miyamoto M: Reduction of transmitter release by d-tubocurarine. Nature 223:531–533, 1969
31. Hutter OF: Post-tetanic restoration of neuromuscular transmission blocked by d-tubocurarine. J Physiol 118:216–227, 1952
32. Kurihara T, Brooks JE: The mechanism of neuromuscular fatigue. Arch Neurol 32:168–174, 1975
33. Lilleheil G, Naess K: A presynaptic effect of d-tubocurarine in the neuromuscular junction. Acta Physiol Scand 52:120–136, 1961
34. Miyamoto MD: The actions of cholinergic drugs on motor nerve terminals. Pharmacol Rev 29:221–247, 1978
35. Magleby KL, Pallotta BS, Terrar DA: The effect of (+)- tubocurarine on neuromuscular transmission during repetitive stimulation in the rat, mouse, and frog. J Physiol (Lond) 312:97–113, 1981
36. Power SJ, Jones RM: Relationship between single twitch depression and train-of-four fade: influence of relaxant dose during onset and spontaneous offset of neuromuscular blockade. Anesth Analg 66:633–636, 1987
37. Riker WF: Prejunctional effects of neuromuscular blocking and facilitatory drugs. In Katz RL (ed): Muscle Relaxants. New York, American Elsevier, 1975, pp 59–102
38. Riker WF, Standaert FG: The action of facilitatory drugs and acetylcholine on neuromuscular transmission. Ann NY Acad Sci 135:163–176, 1966
39. Riker WF, Roberts J, Standaert FG, Fujimori H: The motor nerve terminal as the primary focus for drug-induced facilitation of neuromuscular transmission. J Pharmacol Exp Ther 121:286–312, 1957
40. Standaert FG: The action of d-tubocurarine on the motor nerve terminal. J Pharmacol Exp Ther 143:181–186, 1964
41. Standaert FG: Release of transmitter at the neuromuscular junction. Br J Anaesth 54:131–145, 1982

42. Baker T, Guzzi MS, Ross RM, Lowndes HE: A structure-activity relationship (SAR) difference between pre-junctional and post-junctional nicotinic receptors. Anesthesiology 73:A915, 1990
43. Storella RJ, Ackerman TS, Katul ZJ: Tetanic fade and acetylcholine release. Anesthesiology 79:A923, 1993
44. Deneris ES, Connolly J, Rogers SW, et al: Pharmacological and functional diversity of neuronal nicotinic acetylcholine receptors. Trends Pharmacol Sci 12:34, 1991
45. Wessler I: Control of transmitter release from the motor nerve by presynaptic nicotinic and muscarinic autoreceptors. Trends Pharmacol Sci 10:110–114, 1989
46. Robbins R, Donati F, Bevan DR, et al: Differential effects of myoneural blocking drugs on neuromuscular transmission in infants. Br J Anaesth 56:1095–1099, 1984
47. Pearce AC, Casson WR, Jones RM: Factors affecting train-of-four fade. Br J Anaesth 57:602–606, 1985
48. Williams NE, Webb SN, Calvey TN: Differential effects of myoneural blocking drugs on neuromuscular transmission. Br J Anaesth 52:1111–1115, 1980
49. Gibson FM, Mirakhur RK: Tetanic fade following administration of non-depolarizing neuromuscular blocking drugs. Anesth Analg 68:759–762, 1989
50. Bartkowski RR, Epstein RH: Relationship between train-of-four ratio and first-twitch depression during neuromuscular blockade: a pharmacokinetic/dynamic explanation. J Pharmacokinet Biopharm 18:335–346, 1990
51. Storella RJ, Slomowitz SA, Rosenberg H: Relationships between block-of-twitch and train-of-four fade in the mouse phrenic nerve-diaphragm preparation. Can J Anaesth 38:401–407, 1991
52. Bradley RJ, Edge MT, Chau WC: The α-neurotoxin erabutoxin b causes fade at the rat end-plate. Eur J Pharmacol 176:11–21, 1990
53. Colquhoun D, Dreyer F, Sheridan RE: The actions of tubocurarine at the frog neuromuscular junction. J Physiol (Lond) 293:247–284, 1979
54. Katz B, Miledi R: A reexamination of curare action at the motor end plate. Proc R Soc Lond [Biol] 203:119–133, 1978
55. Burns BD, Paton WDM: Depolarization of the motor end plate by decamethonium and acetylcholine. J Physiol (Lond) 115:41–73, 1951
56. Standaert FG, Adams JE: The actions of succinylcholine on the mammalian motor nerve terminal. J Pharmacol Exp Ther 149:113–123, 1965
57. Raines A, Standaert FG: Pre- and postjunctional effects of diphenylhydantoin at the cat soleus neuromuscular junction. J Pharmacol Exp Ther 153:361–366, 1966
58. Hartman GS, Fiamengo SA, Riker WF: Succinylcholine: mechanism of fasciculations and their prevention by d-tubocurarine or diphenylhydantoin. Anesthesiology 65:405–413, 1986
59. Leary NP, Ellis FR: Masseteric muscle spasm as a normal response to suxamethonium. Br J Anaesth 64:488–492, 1990
60. Plumley MH, Bevan JC, Saddler JM, Donati F, Bevan DR: Dose-related effects of succinylcholine on the adductor pollicis and masseter muscles in children. Can J Anaesth 37:15–20, 1990
61. Saddler JM, Bevan JC, Plumley MH, Polomeno RC, Donati F, Bevan DR: Jaw muscle tension after succinylcholine in children undergoing strabismus surgery. Can J Anaesth 37:21–25, 1990
62. Smith CE, Donati F, Bevan DR: Effects of succinylcholine at the masseter and adductor pollicis muscles in adults. Anesth Analg 69:158–162, 1989
63. Van Der Spek AFL, Fang WB, Ashton-Miller JA, Stohler CS, Carlson DS, Schork MA: Increased masticatory muscle stiffness during limb flaccidity associated with succinylcholine administration. Anesthesiology 69:11–16, 1988
64. Van Der Spek AFL, Fang WB, Ashton-Miller JA, Stohler CS, Carlson DS, Schork MA: The effects of succinylcholine on mouth opening. Anesthesiology 67:459–465, 1987
65. Van Der Spek AFL, Reynolds PI, Fang WB, Ashton-Miller JA, Stohler CS, Schork MA: Changes in resistance to mouth opening induced by depolarizing and nondepolarizing neuromuscular relaxants. Br J Anaesth 64:21–27, 1990
66. Kimura I, Kondoh T, Kimura M: Changes in intracellular Ca^{2+} produced in the mouse diaphragm by neuromuscular blocking drugs. J Pharm Pharmacol 42:626–631, 1990

67. Blaber LC: The effect of facilitatory concentrations of decamethonium on the storage and release of transmitter at the neuromuscular junction of the cat. J Pharmacol Exp Ther 175:664–672, 1970
68. Alderson AM, MacLagan J: The action of decamethonium and tubocurarine on the respiratory and limb muscles of the cat. J Physiol (Lond) 173:38–56, 1964
69. Creese R, Head SD, Jenkinson DF: The role of the sodium pump during prolonged endplate currents in guinea-pig diaphragm. J Physiol (Lond) 384:377–403, 1987
70. Albuquerque EX, Akaike A, Shaw KP, Rickett DL: The interaction of anticholinesterase agents with the acetylcholine receptor-ionic channel complex. Fundam Appl Toxicol 4:S27–S33, 1984
71. Gage PW, Hammill OP: Effects of anesthetics on ion channels in synapses. Int Rev Physiol (Neurophysiol) 25:1–46, 1981
72. Neubig RR, Boyd ND, Cohen JB: Conformations of *Torpedo* acetylcholine receptor associated with ion transport and desensitization. Biochemistry 21:3460–3467, 1982
73. Peper K, Bradley RJ, Dreyer F: The acetylcholine receptor at the neuromuscular junction. Physiol Rev 62:1271–1340, 1982
74. Standaert FG, Dretchen KL: Cyclic nucleotides in neuromuscular transmission. Anesth Analg 60:91, 1981
75. Standaert FG: Donuts and holes: molecules and muscle relaxants. Semin Anesthesiol 3:251–261, 1984
76. Sakmann B, Patlak J, Neher E: Single acetylcholine-activated channels show burst-kinetics in presence of desensitizing concentrations of agonist. Nature 286:71–73, 1980
77. Churchill-Davidson HC, Christie TH, Wise RP: Dual neuromuscular block in man. Anesthesiology 21:144–149, 1960
78. Unwin N, Toyoshima C, Kubalek E: Arrangement of the acetylcholine receptor subunits in the resting and desensitized states, determined by cryoelectron microscopy of crystallized *Torpedo* postsynaptic membranes. J Cell Biol 107:1123, 1988
79. Katz B, Thesleff S: A study of the "desensitization" produced by acetylcholine at the motor end-plate. J Physiol (Lond) 138:63–80, 1957
80. Lee C: Dose relationships of phase II, tachyphylaxis and train-of-four fade in suxamethonium-induced dual neuromuscular block in man. Br J Anaesth 47:841–845, 1975
81. Waud DR: The nature of "depolarization block." Anesthesiology 29:1014–1024, 1968
82. Colquhoun D, Sheridan RE: Modes of action of gallamine at the neuromuscular junction. Br J Pharmacol 66:78–79P, 1979
83. Dreyer F: Acetylcholine receptor. Br J Anaesth 54:115–130, 1982
84. Brett RS, Dilger JP, Yland KF: Isoflurane causes "flickering" of the acetylcholine receptor channel: observations using the patch clamp. Anesthesiology 69:161–170, 1988
85. Lingle CJ, Steinbach JH: Neuromuscular blocking agents. Int Anaesthesiol Clin 26:288–301, 1986
86. Barstad JAB, Lilliheil G: Transversely cut diaphragm preparations from the rat. Arch Int Pharmacodyn Ther 175:373–390, 1968
87. Glavinovic MI: Voltage clamping of unparalyzed cut rat diaphragm for study of transmitter release. J Physiol (Lond) 310:145–158, 1975
88. Muir AW, Houston J, Green KL, Marshall RJ, Bowman WC, Marshall IG: Effects of a new neuromuscular blocking agent (Org 9426) in anaesthetized cats and pigs and in isolated nerve-muscle preparations. Br J Anaesth 63:400–410, 1989
89. Tian L, Mehta MP, Prior C, Marshall IG: Relative pre- and postjunctional effects of a new vecuronium analogue, Org 9426, at the rat neuromuscular junction. Br J Anaesth 69:284–287, 1992
90. Gibb AJ, Marshall IG: Examination of the mechanisms involved in tetanic fade produced by vecuronium and related analogues in the rat diaphragm. Br J Pharmacol 90:511–521, 1987
91. Videira RLR: Injection of pancuronium into the masseter muscle for difficult reduction of mandibular dislocation (letter). Anesthesiology 79:191, 1993
92. Barrantes FJ: Muscle endplate cholinoreceptors. Pharmacol Ther 38:331, 1988
93. Marshall IG: Prejunctional aspects of neuromuscular transmission: physiology, biochemistry and pharmacology. Curr Opin Anaesth 4:577–582, 1991

94. Marshall IG, Parsons SM: The vesicular acetylcholine transport system. Trends Neurosci 10:174–177, 1987
95. Martyn JAJ, White DA, Gronert GA, Jaffe RS, Ward JM: Up-and-down regulation of skeletal muscle acetylcholine receptors: effects on neuromuscular blockers. Anesthesiology 76:822–843, 1992
96. Thesleff S: Effects of motor innervation on the chemical sensitivity of skeletal muscle. Physiol Rev 40:734–752, 1960
97. Brenner HR, Rudin W: On the effect of muscle activity on the end-plate membrane in denervated mouse muscle. J Physiol (Lond) 410:501–512, 1989
98. Levitt-Gilmour TA, Salpeter MM: Gradient of extrajunctional acetylcholine receptors early after denervation of mammalian muscle. J Neurosci 6:1606, 1986
99. Goldman D, Brenner HR, Heinemann S: Acetylcholine receptor alpha-, beta-, gamma-, and delta-subunit mRNA levels are regulated by muscle activity. Neuron 1:329, 1988
100. Schuetze SM: Embryonic and adult acetylcholine receptors: molecular basis of developmental changes in ion channel properties. Trends Neurosci 9:386–388, 1986
101. Laufer R, Changeux JP: Activity-dependent regulation of gene expression in muscle and neuronal cells. Mol Neurobiol 3:1, 1989
102. Fambrough DM: Control of acetylcholine receptors in skeletal muscle. Physiol Rev 59:165–227, 1979
103. Goudsouzian NG, Standaert FG: The infant and myoneural junction. Anesth Analg 65:1208–1217, 1986
104. Gu Y, Hall ZW: Characterization of acetylcholine receptor subunits in developing and denervated mammalian muscle. J Biol Chem 263:12878–12885, 1988
105. Gu Y, Franco A Jr, Gardner PD, Lansman JB, Forsayeth JR, Hall ZW: Properties of embryonic and adult muscle acetylcholine receptors transiently expressed in COS cells. Neuron 5:147–157, 1990
106. Lorkovic H: Sensitivity of rodent skeletal muscles to dicholines: dependence on innervation and age. Neuropharmacology 28:373–377, 1989
107. Reiser G, Miledi R: Changes in the properties of synaptic channels opened by acetylcholine in denervated frog muscle. Brain Res 479:83, 1989
108. Morris CE, Wong BS, Jackson MB, et al: Single-channel currents activated by curare in cultured embryonic rat muscle. J Neurosci 3:2525, 1983
109. Trautmann A: Curare can open and block ionic channels associated with cholinergic receptors. Nature 298:272, 1982
110. Jenkinson DH, Nichols JG: Contractures and permeability changes produced by acetetylcholine in depolarized denervated muscle. J Physiol (Lond) 159:111–127, 1961
111. Standaert FG: Basic chemistry of acetylcholine receptors. Anesthesiol Clin North Am 11:205–218, 1993

3

DAVID G. SILVERMAN | SORIN J. BRULL

Features of Neurostimulation

In the clinical setting, neurostimulation typically is delivered by a 9-volt, adjustable-current *nerve stimulator* via subcutaneous needles (typically at currents <10 mA) or via surface *electrodes*[1,2] coated with a conductive gel such as silver–silver chloride (at 30–70 mA). The *strength of the stimulus* depends on its duration (pulse width) and the current that reaches the nerve fiber (Fig. 3-1).[3-5]

As summarized in Table 3-1, a nerve stimulator should generate an *impulse* that is: (1) <0.5 msec (*typically 0.1–0.2 msec*) *in duration* in order to avoid direct muscle or repetitive nerve stimulation (by extending beyond the refractory period of the nerve)[6,7]; (2) *monophasic and rectangular* (i.e., square-wave pattern), because a biphasic pulse might cause a burst of action potentials; and (3) *constant current,* in order to provide consistent stimulation—i.e., once the rheostat is set for delivery of a given current, the stimulator should be able to maintain this current by changing its voltage in response to varying resistances (impedance) up to at least 5,000 ohms.

Impedance is influenced by a multitude of factors,[8-11] most notably electrode contact with skin. When stainless steel needle electrodes are used, tissue impedance generally is between 500 and 2,000 ohms.[6] Acceptable levels also can be obtained with surface electrodes[4,12] as long as the skin is adequately prepared. The effect of tissue resistance can be markedly reduced by rubbing an electrolyte into the skin, lightly abrading (decorrifying) the skin, lightly rubbing with alcohol, and/or applying a paste (and waiting a few minutes for osmosis or "curing") (Fig. 3-2).[10-15] When such preparation is performed, the threshold for an evoked twitch response generally is <15 mA.[12]

Nevertheless, *a constant current is not always maintained* in the clinical setting. Some stimulators are incapable of maintaining current output in the face of even a small increase in resistance; that is, the impedance often is beyond an "acceptable" range.[16-21] In such cases, the output will fall off progressively.[13,17,19]

The stimulating current required for effective depolarization of all fibers of a nerve bundle is called the *maximal current*. Below this current, the relationship between the number of nerve fibers recruited and the intensity of stimulating current is sigmoidal (Fig. 3-3).[4,5,20] When monitoring absolute

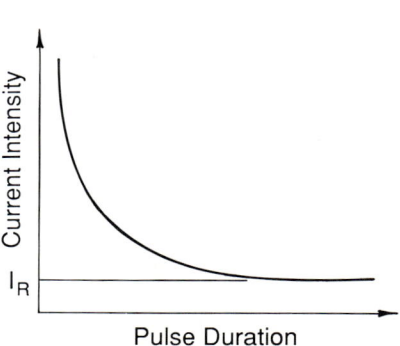

FIGURE 3-1 Relationship between pulse duration and stimulating current. The magnitude of the stimulus (i.e., the electrical charge, in coulomb, illustrated by the curve) is a function of the pulse duration and stimulating current. The current intensity required to achieve a given electrical charge increases exponentially as the pulse duration is decreased. The rheobase current, I_R, is that stimulating current required to reach threshold at the longest pulse duration. (Reproduced with permission from Brull SJ, Silverman DG: Neuromuscular block monitoring. In Ehrenwerth J, Eisenkraft JE (eds): Anesthesia Equipment: Principles and Applications. St. Louis, Mosby–Year Book, 1993, pp 297–318.)

twitch height, the stimulus intensity should be *supramaximal* (i.e., 10–20% higher than maximal current) to *ensure consistent recruitment of all fibers* despite minor variations of skin impedance over time. As discussed later, a supramaximal stimulus is not necessarily required when relative responses are compared during train-of-four or double-burst stimulation.

A *supramaximal current* generally is achieved at *2.5–3 times the threshold current*.[4] However, especially if skin impedance is >5,000 ohms, *surface electrodes may fail to deliver a supramaximal current reliably*[4,12,16,18] and thereby may fail to recruit all the fibers in a given nerve bundle. Older nerve stimulators may be unable to deliver more than 30 mA,[4,12,16,18] especially in

TABLE 3-1
Desirable Features of a Nerve Stimulator

ESSENTIAL

- Square-wave impulse, <0.5 msec duration
- Ability to maintain selected current for duration of impulse (i.e., constant current, variable voltage)
- Durability
- Battery-powered
- Multiple patterns of stimulation: single twitch, train-of-four, double-burst, tetanus, posttetanic count
- Adjustable current output

OPTIONAL

- Polarity output indicator
- High-output (up to 80-100 mA) socket for transcutaneous stimulation and low-output (<5 mA) socket for subcutaneous nerve localization
- Audible or visual signal with each stimulus delivered
- Indicators for excessive impedance, lead disconnect, low battery

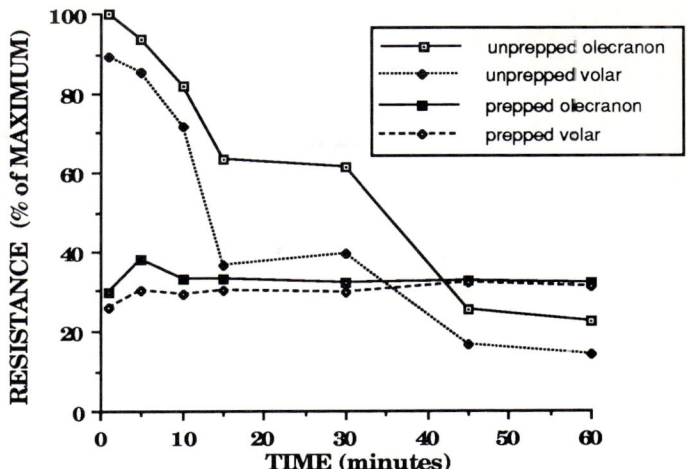

FIGURE 3-2 Effect of cleansing and abrading the skin (with Omni Prep, D. O. Weaver & Co., Aurora, CO) on skin resistance. Without prior prepping, resistance at surface electrodes remains elevated for 10–30 minutes after electrode application over the olecranon groove and volar forearm. (Reproduced with permission from Brull SJ, Silverman DG: Neuromuscular block monitoring. In Ehrenwerth J, Eisenkraft JE (eds): Anesthesia Equipment: Principles and Applications. St. Louis, Mosby–Year Book, 1993, pp 297–318.)

the setting of increased skin impedance (Fig. 3-4).[16] Other devices may deliver a pulse of only 0.1 msec duration and thereby achieve less than maximal recruitment.[5,22]

Although not essential, it is preferable to place the *negative electrode* closer to the nerve.[23–25] One should ensure that the other (positive) electrode is not placed at a site where it is likely to induce firing of another nerve (thus distorting assessment). The effect of *skin temperature* must be appreciated. Peripheral cooling decreases the amplitude of the evoked responses (Chap. 10). Local heating results in decreased electrode impedance, electrode-to-skin impedance, and tissue impedance.[26] However, direct heating actually may decrease electromyogram amplitudes by compromising the signal source and increasing cutaneous blood flow.[26]

For *ulnar nerve stimulation,* one electrode typically is placed proximal to the wrist on the radial side of the flexi carpi ulnaris and the other may be placed more than 2 cm proximally on the volar forearm or over the olecranon groove at the elbow. The ulnar nerve predominantly innervates the *adductor pollicis, abductor digiti quinti* (minimi), and *interosseous muscles* and contributes to innervation of the abductor pollicis brevis (with the median nerve). As detailed in Chapter 5, these muscles have different sensitivi-

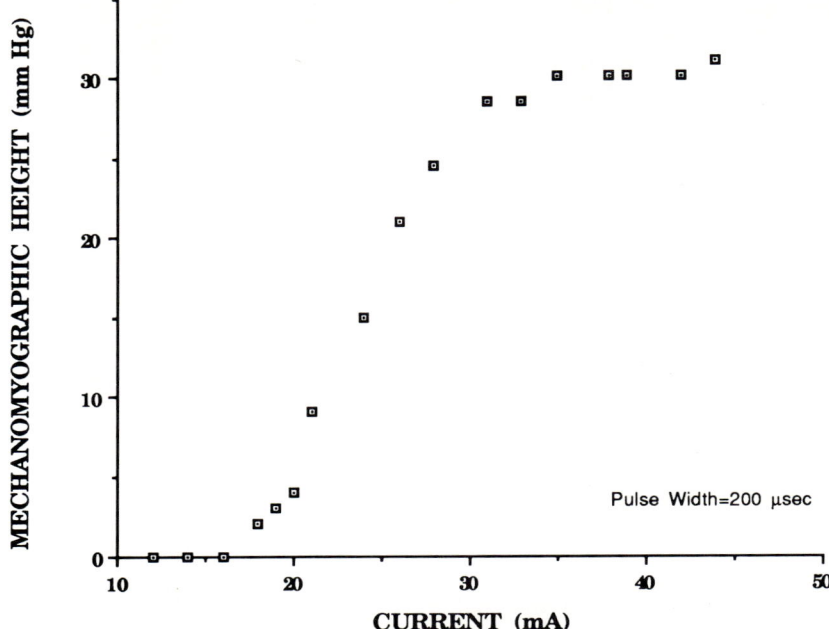

FIGURE 3-3 Effect of stimulating current on amplitude of the evoked muscular response, as measured by mechanomyographic single "twitch" heights, at a fixed pulse duration in a healthy volunteer. Little change is noted with currents above 35 mA.

ties to neuromuscular relaxants. The adductor pollicis is largely composed of Type I fibers, which are particularly sensitive to nondepolarizing relaxants (Chap. 1, question i).

Other potential sites of stimulation include (1) the *posterior tibial nerve* behind the medial malleolus (where plantar flexion of the big toe[27] and foot may be monitored); (2) the *peroneal* and *lateral popliteal nerves* (dorsiflexion of the foot); and (3) the *facial nerve* as it leaves the stylomastoid foramen near the tragus, 2–3 cm posterior to the lateral border of the orbit (contraction of the orbicularis oculi muscle), and the facial nerve below the lip (contraction of the orbicularis oris muscle). Recently, a means has been introduced for monitoring vocal cord adduction in response to recurrent laryngeal nerve stimulation,[28] but this has been limited to investigative settings.

The *adductor pollicis,* the most commonly monitored peripheral muscle, is more sensitive than the *airway/respiratory muscles* to *nondepolarizing relaxants* (NDRs).[29–44] Approximately 1.5–2 times more relaxant is required to completely relax the diaphragm and laryngeal muscles than the adductor pollicis. In awake volunteers receiving tubocurarine, *vital capacity* remained

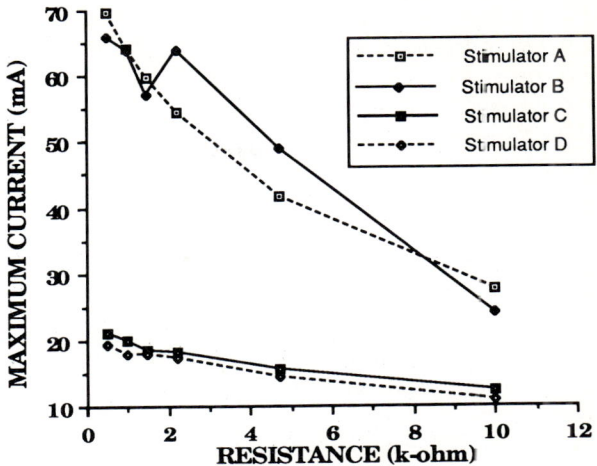

FIGURE 3-4 Ability of four nerve stimulators (obtained from different manufacturers) to generate a constant current despite variations in resistance (in vitro). Note that two of the four stimulators tested were unable to reliably deliver a supramaximal stimulus even at the lowest resistance. The two stimulators capable of reliably delivering a high enough current typically lost this ability at an external resistance beyond 3,000 ohms. (Reproduced with permission from Brull SJ, Silverman DG: Neuromuscular block monitoring. In Ehrenwerth J, Eisenkraft JE (eds): Anesthesia Equipment: Principles and Applications. St. Louis, Mosby–Year Book, 1993, pp 297–318.)

at 90% of control when grip strength decreased to 20% of control.[45] In anesthetized patients, the dose required for adductor pollicis twitch depression was approximately 60% of that necessary for a comparable reduction in maximal inspiratory force.[46] These findings have been supported by laboratory data demonstrating that the diaphragm can function with only 10% of the receptor pool available, whereas in most peripheral muscles at least 20% of the receptors are necessary to obtain a normal twitch response.[40] Similar "sparing" of infra-epiglottic airway muscles was noted during comparison of twitch depression at the adductor pollicis and larynx after vecuronium,[32] atracurium,[39] and rocuronium.[37] In contrast, the *muscles of the oropharynx have sensitivities similar to that of the peripheral muscles*. In fact, the ED_{95} at the masseter muscle is slightly less than that for the adductor pollicis muscle.[47] Likewise, the medial rectus abdominis appears to be relatively sensitive (i.e., it has a lower ED_{95} than muscles of the hand[48]). Thus, the *relative sensitivities* appear to be: diaphragm and larynx < adductor pollicis and several pharyngeal muscles < masseter and rectus abdominis.

The *decreased sensitivity* of the diaphragm and laryngeal muscles to

NDRs is offset in part by a *more rapid onset*. *Onset of* and *recovery from* depolarizing and nondepolarizing relaxants are more rapid in airway, respiratory, and facial muscles.[31–33,38,41,46,49–54] Thus, maximum block may be attained at the diaphragm before it is reached at the adductor pollicis. Likewise, during recovery, when T_1 of the adductor pollicis returned to 25% of its baseline height after vecuronium, the twitch height of the diaphragm had returned to 75% of its baseline value.[41] The airway muscles have better perfusion, different fiber types, and may have significant ultrastructural differences at the end-plate (i.e., quantity and quality of receptors).[55,56] The *relative times for recovery* appear to be: diaphragm, larynx, rectus abdominis < adductor pollicis and many pharyngeal muscles. As discussed in Chapter 5, the abductor digiti quinti muscle of the hand and the orbicularis oculi muscle of the face have sensitivities and time courses which resemble those of the diaphragm and larynx.

The relative importance of sensitivity and rate of onset differs at the larynx and diaphragm. For *laryngeal muscles, decreased sensitivity predominates;* e.g., a 0.04 mg · kg^{-1} IV bolus of vecuronium caused 55% depression of twitch height at the larynx (in 3.3 minutes) and 89% depression at the adductor pollicis (5.7 minutes).[31] Similarly, 0.25 mg · kg^{-1} of rocuronium caused 37% depression at the larynx (in 1.6 minutes) and 69% depression at the adductor pollicis (in 3.0 minutes).[43] At the *diaphragm,* the *differing sensitivities and time courses offset themselves* after a *rapid IV bolus* of an NDR: a 0.07 mg · kg^{-1} bolus dose of vecuronium provided 95% block at the diaphragm and 95% block at the adductor pollicis (i.e., the ED$_{95}$ requirements for single bolus injection were equivalent) (Fig. 3-5).[32] This offset is in contrast to the clearly higher ED$_{95}$ of the diaphragm when it is determined during recovery or after slow, cumulative (as opposed to single bolus) dosing.[29,32,35,36,41,51]

The relative effects of sensitivity and rate of onset are slightly different for *depolarizing relaxants.* The *diaphragm* appears to be less sensitive to both depolarizing and nondepolarizing relaxants.[57] The effect of the diaphragm's decreased sensitivity to depolarizing agents is at least partially offset by faster onset.[50] Thus, the maximal degrees of block at the diaphragm and periphery are similar.[54] In contrast, *laryngeal muscles* demonstrate increased, as opposed to decreased, sensitivity to depolarizing relaxants.[50,53] Thus, the faster onset of depolarizing relaxants at the larynx is "unopposed"; this leads to rapid onset of relatively deep block of the laryngeal muscles. It has been shown that fast-twitch fibers (e.g., thyroarytenoid) are highly sensitive to depolarizing, but not nondepolarizing, relaxants (Chap. 1, question i; Chap. 16).

Discussion Questions ◆

a. Why might one prefer surface to needle *electrodes?*
b. What limits the utility of very large *surface electrodes?*

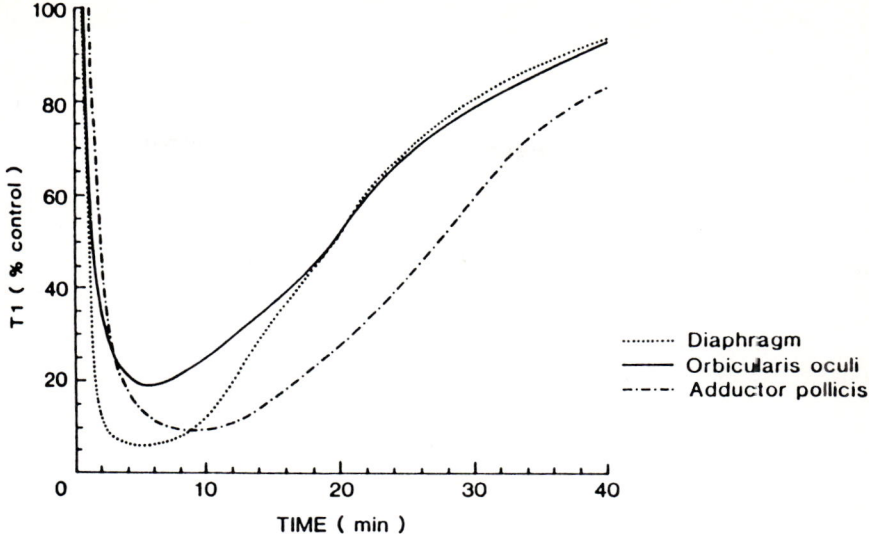

FIGURE 3-5 T_1 of the train-of-four obtained at three muscles after a bolus dose of vecuronium, 0.07 mg · kg^{-1}. Although the diaphragm is less sensitive than the adductor pollicis muscle to relaxant, it attains the same depth of block because the onset of block at the diaphragm is more rapid (see text). The time course at the diaphragm is more closely reflected by that at the orbicularis oculi muscle. (Reproduced with permission from Donati F, Meistelman C, Plaud B: Vecuronium neuromuscular blockade at the diaphragm, the orbicularis oculi, and adductor pollicis muscles. Anesthesiology 73:870–875, 1990.)

c. What is the effect of stimulating *current intensity* on single *twitch height*?
d. What is the effect of stimulating *current intensity* on the ratio of the fourth to first twitch (T_4/T_1) during *train-of-four monitoring*?
e. During *ulnar nerve stimulation,* why should we monitor the movement of the *thumb* rather than the movement of the *fourth and fifth digits*?
f. Briefly compare the *adductor pollicis and diaphragm muscles* with respect to ED$_{95}$, rate of onset, and rate of recovery. How do these differences affect onset of *intubating conditions* after a large bolus dose (e.g., 4 × ED$_{95}$) of a nondepolarizing relaxant?
g. Does complete loss of *adductor pollicis* twitch height as a result of a nondepolarizing relaxant imply complete *vocal cord* relaxation? Explain.
h. Why might it be argued that, although there is *sparing of respiratory muscles* during low-dose *nondepolarizing block,* there is not necessarily sparing of ventilatory function?
i. If, during a neurosurgical procedure, the surgeon wishes to identify the

facial nerve and its roots by direct stimulation, can you still administer a *relaxant*?
j. If a surgeon wishes to monitor *cortical or spinal motor evoked potentials*, can you still administer a *relaxant*?
k. Are the *extrinsic muscles of the eye* sensitive to nondepolarizing relaxants?
l. Why might it be preferable to monitor the *orbicularis oculi* muscle (as opposed to the adductor pollicis) during *onset* of block?
m. Why might it be preferable to monitor the *adductor pollicis* muscle during *recovery* from block?

Answers ◆

a. *Needle electrodes* may be (1) a source of local irritation, pain (in awake subjects), infection, and nerve damage (especially if they are placed intraneurally); (2) a site for diathermy burns (because they provide good contact for exit of high-frequency current); and (3) a conduit for high currents that reach the threshold for repetitive nerve stimulation and/or direct muscle stimulation (which are considerably higher than that for nerve firing).[7,58,59] If the nerve stimulator is inadvertently electrically grounded while the indifferent electrode of the electrocautery unit has a defective ground, the needle electrodes can become the ground, and a third-degree burn can result.[60]

b. Although *large conducting areas* decrease resistance, discomfort, and the potential for local burns, they may not be practical because they may markedly decrease current density (such that a supramaximal stimulus cannot be delivered), and they also may cause stimulation of multiple nerves.

c. *As the stimulating current intensity is increased toward maximal*, more fibers reach threshold and the magnitude of the evoked twitch response increases in a sigmoidal fashion.

d. As a general rule, a change in *stimulating current* intensity has a similar effect on the T_1 and T_4 responses to *train-of-four stimulation* (as well as on the D_1 and D_2 responses to *double-burst stimulation*, described in Chap. 4).[18,20,61,62] Hence, the relationship among the twitches evoked during train-of-four remains relatively consistent at different currents. This may best be appreciated if we distinguish between the effects of stimulating current on the motor nerve as opposed to the neuromuscular junction (NMJ). If a *motor nerve fiber* fires in response to the first of the four twitches (T_1), then it will fire in response to the fourth twitch (T_4); T_1 and T_4 constitute identical "all-or-none" stimuli. However, depolarization of the motor nerve does not guarantee effective transmission across the NMJ, for NMJ transmission is more sensitive to neuromuscular block for T_4 than for T_1. If the T_4/T_1 ratio is 0.1, then for every ten motor nerve firings that elicit a muscle action potential in response to T_1, only one will elicit an MAP in response to T_4. This is the case regardless of the current that elicited nerve fiber firing.

If *low-current testing* is desired, it should be performed at ≥10 mA above the T_4 threshold so as to recruit enough motor fibers to enable accurate detection and measurement of T_4.[20,61,63,64] At ≥10 mA above the T_4 threshold, the mean T_4/T_1 ratio remains relatively consistent at different currents (although there is greater variability).[20,61,62] The accuracy of testing at low current intensity facilitates testing of awake patients, since discomfort is related to the intensity of the stimulating current.[5,65,66]

e. *The site of ulnar nerve stimulation* is remote from the *adductor pollicis* muscle; thus the nerve stimulator does not depolarize this muscle directly. Alternatively, an electrode for ulnar nerve stimulation can directly stimulate the *muscles to the fourth and fifth digits*. The resultant movement of these fingers might be misinterpreted as due to transmission across the NMJ and thus falsely suggest inadequate block of the NMJ.

f. A *higher dose* of relaxant apparently is required to block the NMJs of the *diaphragm* (i.e., the diaphragm has a higher ED_{95}). Thus, the diaphragm has a wider margin of safety. Alternatively, the *onset* of, and *recovery* from, block are more rapid at the diaphragm, probably as a result of better perfusion. Because a large bolus dose of relaxant will provide complete paralysis of airway as well as peripheral muscles, the diaphragm's faster time course may predominate after a dose that is 4 times the ED_{95}. A dose of this magnitude will more than compensate for the diaphragm's lesser sensitivity. Thus, paralysis of the diaphragm may be achieved before total paralysis of the adductor pollicis is obtained.[32]

g. The *dose of NDR* that is required for ablation of the evoked muscle contraction is 50–100% higher for *laryngeal muscles* than for the *adductor pollicis*. While the response to single twitch stimulation at the adductor pollicis is lost after a dose of relaxant that causes 90–92% receptor occupancy, a greater dose is required for paralysis of laryngeal muscles. Thus, it is possible to have *vocal cord movement* despite loss of the adductor pollicis response. This may be important during *laser surgery* on the vocal cords, when vocal cord movement is particularly undesirable. To decrease the likelihood of coughing or vocal cord movement, one may increase the dose of relaxant to ablate evoked responses of the adductor pollicis not only in response to *twitch* and *tetanus*, but also in response to *posttetanic count* (Chap. 5).[67,68]

h. Even though *respiratory muscles* are less sensitive to NDRs than the adductor pollicis, the *ability to breathe deeply and to cough* may be partially impaired after low doses of relaxant. *Ventilatory efforts* often entail sustained contraction (which is more sensitive to nondepolarizing block). In addition, *pharyngeal muscles* do not share the decreased sensitivity of the diaphragm and vocal cords. Thus, even though diaphragmatic function may be adequate, weakening of the pharyngeal muscles may pose a threat to upper airway integrity and handling of secretions (Chap. 6).[69–71] Administration of 12 mg of *d*-tubocurarine to volunteers caused a minor decrease in vital capacity (4.8 to 4.4 L) but a doubling of *airway resistance* (0.5 to 1.0 cm $H_2O \cdot L^{-1} \cdot sec^{-1}$).[69] It also should be noted that sensitivities to relaxants vary markedly among patients[72–74]: a safe dose in one patient may result in a significant degree of block in another.

i. Yes, it is possible to administer a neuromuscular blocking agent to a patient who is undergoing *intracranial stimulation of the facial nerve* (e.g., with a 60-Hz, constant voltage monopolar stimulator). Such direct stimulation elicited a response that was noted 12 minutes before a response to train-of-four stimulation of the ulnar nerve (via forearm electrodes) during recovery from atracurium, 0.2–0.5 mg $\cdot$ kg^{-1}. Upon return of a detectable T_1 at the adductor pollicis, the facial response had recovered to 76% of baseline amplitude. Upon return of a detectable T_4, the facial response was 87% of baseline amplitude.[75]

j. NDR-induced block may reduce, in a dose-dependent manner, the response to transcranial magnetic stimulation during monitoring of *cortical motor evoked potentials*. However, a significant decline in amplitude was not noted until the T_4/T_1 ratio was ≤0.1 (unless the potentials themselves decreased to 0.2 of baseline).[76,77] The effect on the amplitude of the evoked response is greater than the effect on latency. The former has been attributed to a reduction in the number of motor units responding to evoked motor nerve activity.[76,77] If amplitude is to be measured and neuromuscular relaxation is required for optimal anesthetic management, then one should maintain a constant degree of relaxation so as not to change its impact during the study period. Fortunately, the effect of neuromuscular block on the evoked potentials is of lesser magnitude than the decline of the direct electromyogram[76,77] and the latter may be used as a guide. Several investigators have cited the feasibility of motor evoked potential recording during titrated, "controlled" neuromuscular block.[78–81]

k. *The extrinsic muscles of the eye* are more sensitive to *NDRs* than are those of the extremities.[82] On testing in the postanesthesia care unit, *visual disturbances* have been noted in up to 71% of patients who received long-acting relaxants[83,84] (they are far less common after short-acting relaxants).[85] Likewise, visual disturbances often are noted after the small amounts of an NDR that may be used as a *defasciculating* (or *priming*) *dose*.[86,87] Of note, the sensitivity of eye muscles to *depolarizing relaxant* is unique, in that the muscle undergoes prolonged contractions with a resulting increase of *intraocular pressure* (Chap. 18).

l. It may be argued that it is preferable to monitor the *orbicularis oculi response to facial nerve stimulation* (as opposed to the adductor pollicis response to ulnar nerve stimulation) during onset of a nondepolarizing block. The sensitivity of this muscle, and the time course of the relaxant effect, more closely reflect the response at the diaphragm and larynx.[21,31,32,39,75,88] However, the electrodes for facial nerve stimulation may stimulate the orbicularis oculi or neighboring muscles directly and thus give a false indication of adequate neuromuscular transmission. This can be minimized by (1) placing the recording electrodes near the midportion and insertion of the muscle[32]; (2) placing the stimulating electrodes laterally over the temporal branch of the facial nerve, anterior to the earlobe[32]; and/or (3) utilizing needle electrodes.

Similarly, one may elect to monitor EMG responses at the *hypothenar eminence,* since the sensitivity and time course of the abductor digiti quinti (minimi) more closely resemble those of the diaphragm and larynx than do the responses of the adductor pollicis (Chap. 5).[89–91]

m. The increased sensitivity and slower time course at the *adductor pollicis* make monitoring at this site preferable during recovery.[32] *Airway patency* and adequate ventilation require more than the diaphragm[70,92]; the muscles responsible for upper airway patency tend to recover more slowly than the diaphragm and laryngeal muscles. Thus, it is important to assess the degree of block at a peripheral muscle that is less likely to underestimate the amount of remaining block at muscles responsible for maintenance of an unobstructed airway (e.g., pharyngeal muscles).

References ◆

1. Kopman AF: A safe surface electrode for peripheral-nerve stimulation. Anesthesiology 44:343–345, 1976
2. Pue AF: Disposable EKG pads for peripheral nerve stimulation (corresp). Anesthesiology 45:107–108, 1976
3. Mortimer JT: Electrical excitation of nerve. In Agnew WF, McCreery DB (eds): Neural Prosthesis. Englewood Cliffs, NJ, Prentice-Hall, 1990
4. Kopman AF, Lawson D: Milliamperage requirements for supramaximal stimulation of the ulnar nerve with surface electrodes. Anesthesiology 61:83–85, 1984
5. Silverman DG, Garcia RM, O'Connor TZ, Brull SJ: Effect of pulse width and current intensity on EMG twitch height and subjective discomfort. Anesthesiology 77:A957, 1992
6. Epstein RA, Wyte SR, Jackson SH, Sitter S: The electromechanical response to stimulation by the Block-Aid Monitor. Anesthesiology 30:43–47, 1969
7. Epstein RA, Jackson SH: Repetitive muscle depolarization from single indirect stimulation in anesthetized man. J Appl Physiol 28:407–410, 1970
8. Yamamoto Y, Yamamoto T: Dynamic system for the measurement of electrical skin impedance. Med Biol Eng Comput 17:135–137, 1979
9. Hary D, Bekey GA, Antonelli DJ: Circuit models and simulation analysis of electromyographic signal sources: I. The impedance of EMG electrodes. IEEE Trans Biomed Eng BME-34:91–97, 1987
10. Fuhrer MJ, Yegge B: Effects of skin impedance changes accompanying functional electrical stimulation of the peroneal nerve. Arch Phys Med Rehabil 53:276–281, 1972
11. Yamamoto T, Yamamoto Y: Analysis for the change of skin impedance. Med Biol Eng Comput 15:219–227, 1977
12. Beemer GH, Reeves JH, Bjorksten AR: Accurate monitoring of neuromuscular blockade using a peripheral nerve stimulator—a review. Anaesth Intensive Care 18:490–496, 1990
13. Brull SJ, Silverman DG: Monitoring of neuromuscular block. In Ehrenwerth J, Eisenkraft

JB (eds): Anesthesia Equipment: Principles and Applications. St. Louis, Mosby–Year Book, 1992
14. Zipp P, Hennemann K, Grunwald R, Rohmert W: Bioelectrode jellies for long-term monitoring. Eur J Appl Physiol 45:131–145, 1980
15. Olson WH, Schmincke DR, Henley BL: Time and frequency dependence of disposable ECG electrode-skin impedance. Med Instrum 13:269–272, 1979
16. Mylrea KC, Hameroff SR, Calkins JM, Blitt CD, Humphrey LL: Evaluation of peripheral nerve stimulators and relationship to possible errors in assessing neuromuscular blockade. Anesthesiology 60:464–466, 1984
17. Zeh DW, Katz RL: A new nerve stimulator for monitoring neuromuscular blockade and performing nerve blocks. Anesth Analg 57:13–17, 1978
18. Brull SJ, Ehrenwerth J, Silverman DG: Stimulation with submaximal current for train-of-four monitoring. Anesthesiology 72:629–632, 1990
19. Beemer GH, Reeves JH: An evaluation of eight peripheral nerve stimulators for monitoring neuromuscular blockade. Anaesth Intensive Care 16:464–477, 1988
20. Silverman DG, Connelly NR, O'Connor TZ, Garcia RM, Brull SJ: Accelographic train-of-four fade at near-threshold currents. Anesthesiology 76:34–38, 1992
21. Stiffel P, Hameroff SR, Blitt CD, Cork RC: Variability in assessment of neuromuscular blockade. Anesthesiology 52:436–437, 1980
22. Werner MU: Is the Relaxograph (NMT-100) a reliable pediatric monitor of neuromuscular transmission? Anesthesiology 73:A913, 1990
23. Hudes E, Lee KC: Clinical use of nerve stimulators in anaesthesia. Can J Anaesth 34:525–534, 1987
24. Berger JJ, Gravenstein JS, Munson ES: Electrode polarity and peripheral nerve stimulation. Anesthesiology 56:402–404, 1982
25. Rosenberg H, Greenhow DE: Peripheral nerve stimulator performance: the influence of output polarity and electrode placement. Can Anaesth Soc J 25:424–426, 1978
26. Zipp P: Temperature dependent alterations of the surface-EMG and ECG: an investigation of the electrical transfer characteristics of the human skin. Eur J Appl Physiol 37:275–288, 1977
27. Sopher MJ, Sears DH, Walts LF: Neuromuscular function monitoring comparing the flexor hallucis brevis and adductor pollicis muscles. Anesthesiology 69:129–131, 1988
28. Donati F, Plaud B, Meistelman C: A method to measure elicited contraction of laryngeal adductor muscles during anesthesia. Anesthesiology 74:827–832, 1991
29. Donati F, Antzaka C, Bevan DR: Potency of pancuronium at the diaphragm and the adductor pollicis muscle in humans. Anesthesiology 65:1–5, 1986
30. Debaene B, Guesde R, Clergue F, Lienhart A: Plasma concentration-response relationship of pancuronium for the diaphragm and the adductor pollicis in anesthetized man. Anesthesiology 73:A887, 1990
31. Donati F, Meistelman C, Plaud B: Vecuronium neuromuscular blockade at the adductor muscles of the larynx and adductor pollicis. Anesthesiology 74:833–837, 1991
32. Donati F, Meistelman C, Plaud B: Vecuronium neuromuscular blockade at the diaphragm, the orbicularis oculi, and adductor pollicis muscles. Anesthesiology 73:870–875, 1990
33. Derrington MC, Hindocha N: Comparison of neuromuscular block in the diaphragm and hand after administration of tubocurarine, pancuronium and alcuronium. Br J Anaesth 64:294–299, 1990
34. Geris SD, Sokoll MD, Methar M, Keminotsu O, Rudd GD: Intubation conditions after atracurium and suxamethonium. Br J Anaesth 55:835–836S, 1983
35. Laycock JRD, Donati F, Bevan DR: Potency of atracurium and vecuronium at the diaphragm and adductor pollicis muscle in humans. Br J Anaesth 59:1321P, 1987
36. Lebrault C, Chauvin M, Guirimand F, Duvaldestin P: Relative potency of vecuronium on the diaphragm and the adductor pollicis. Br J Anaesth 63:389–392, 1989
37. Plaud B, Meistelman C, Donati F: Organon 9426 neuromuscular blockade at the adductor muscles of the larynx and adductor pollicis in man. Anesthesiology 75:A784, 1991
38. Tran DQ, Amaki Y, Ohta Y, Nagashima H, Duncalf D, Foldes FF: Simultaneous *in vivo* measurement of NM block on three muscles. Anesthesiology 57:A276, 1982
39. Ungureanu D, Meistelman C, Frossard J: Monitoring orbicularis oculi is an accurate indi-

cator of vocal cords relaxation in atracurium induced neuromuscular blockade. Anesthesiology 75:A797, 1991
40. Waud BE, Waud DR: The margin of safety of neuromuscular transmission in the muscle of the diaphragm. Anesthesiology 37:417–422, 1972
41. Chauvin M, Lebrault C, Duvaldestin P: The neuromuscular blocking effect of vecuronium on the human diaphragm. Anesth Analg 66:117–122, 1987
42. Paton WDM, Zaimis EJ: The action of d-tubocurarine and of decamethonium on respiratory and other muscles in the cat. J Physiol 112:311–331, 1951
43. Meistelman C, Plaud B, Donati F: Rocuronium (ORG 9426) neuromuscular blockade at the adductor muscles of the larynx and adductor pollicis in humans. Can J Anaesth 39:665–669, 1992
44. Taylor DB, Prior RD, Bevan JA: The relative sensitivities of diaphragm and other muscles of the guinea pig to neuromuscular blocking agents. J Pharmacol Exp Ther 143:137–191, 1963
45. Foldes FF, Monte AP, Brunn HM Jr, Wolfson B: Studies with muscle relaxants in unanesthetized subjects. Anesthesiology 22:230–236, 1961
46. Wymore ML, Eisele JH: Differential effects of d-tubocurarine on inspiratory muscles and two peripheral muscle groups in anesthetized man. Anesthesiology 48:360–362, 1978
47. Smith CE, Donati F, Bevan DR: Differential effects of pancuronium on masseter and adductor pollicis muscle in humans. Anesthesiology 71:57–61, 1989
48. Gerber HR, Johansen SH, Mortimer JT, Yodlowski E: Frequency sweep electromyogram and voluntary effort in volunteers after d-tubocurarine. Anesthesiology 46:35–39, 1977
49. Curran MJ, Ali HH, Savarese JJ, Shash AM, Basta SJ: Comparative evoked thumb and jaw force measurement using accelerometry. Anesthesiology 69:A472, 1988
50. Meistelman C, Plaud B, Donati F: Neuromuscular effects of succinylcholine on the vocal cords and adductor pollicis muscles. Anesth Analg 73:278–282, 1991
51. Pansard JL, Chauvin M, Lebrault C, Gauneau P, Duvaldestin P: Effect of an intubating dose of succinylcholine and atracurium on the diaphragm and the adductor pollicis in humans. Anesthesiology 67:326–330, 1987
52. Saddler JM, Bevan JC, Plumley MH, Polomeno RC, Donati F, Bevan DR: Jaw muscle tension after succinylcholine in children undergoing strabismus surgery. Can J Anaesth 37:21–25, 1990
53. Smith CE, Donati F, Bevan DR: Effects of succinylcholine at the masseter and adductor pollicis muscles in adults. Anesth Analg 69:158–162, 1989
54. Lee CH: Some characteristics of neuromuscular block in the respiratory musculature in anaesthetized man. Can Anaesth Soc J 23:125–134, 1976
55. Johnson MA, Polgar W, Weightman D, Appleton D: Data on the distribution of fibre types in thirty-six human muscles: an autopsy study. J Neurol Sci 18:111–129, 1973
56. Keens TG, Bryan AC, Levison H, Ianuzzo CD: Developmental pattern of muscle fiber types in human ventilatory muscles. J Appl Physiol Respirat Environ Exercise Physiol 44:909–913, 1978
57. Smith CE, Donati F, Bevan DR: Potency of succinylcholine at the diaphragm and adductor pollicis muscle in man. Anesth Analg 67:625–630, 1988
58. Gray JA: Nerve stimulators and burns. Anesthesiology 42:231–232, 1975
59. Lippmann M, Fields WA: Burns of the skin caused by a peripheral nerve stimulator. Anesthesiology 40:82–84, 1974
60. Paulus DA: Electrical signals. Probl Anesth 1:21–27, 1987
61. Silverman DG, Brull SJ: Prospective assessment of double burst monitoring at 10 mA above their respective thresholds. Can J Anaesth 40:502–506, 1993
62. Helbo-Hansen H, Bang U, Nielsen HK, Skovgaard LT: The accuracy of train-of-four monitoring at varying stimulating currents. Anesthesiology 76:199–203, 1992
63. Lawson D: Doctor . . . Are you sure the patient is paralyzed? Anesthesiology 73:574, 1990
64. Sosis MB: Train-of-four ratio is not always independent of stimulating current (letter). Anesthesiology 73:573–574, 1990
65. Connelly NR, Silverman DG, O'Connor TZ, Brull SJ: Subjective responses to train-of-four and double burst stimulation in awake patients. Anesth Analg 70:650–653, 1990
66. Edwards RHT, Young A, Hosking GP, Jones DA: Human skeletal muscle function: description of tests and normal values. Clin Sci 52:283–290, 1977
67. Fernando PUE, Viby-Mogensen J, Bonsu AK, Tamilarasan A, Muchhal KK, Lambourne A:

Relationship between posttetanic count and response to carinal stimulation during vecuronium-induced neuromuscular blockade. Acta Anaesthesiol Scand 31:593–596, 1987
68. Ridley SA, Hatch DJ: Post-tetanic count and profound neuromuscular blockade with atracurium infusion in paediatric patients. Br J Anaesth 60:31–35, 1988
69. Dodgson BG, Knill RL, Clement JL: Curare increases upper airway resistance while reducing ventilatory muscle strength (abstract). Can Anaesth Soc J 28:505–506, 1981
70. Gal TJ, Smith TC: Partial paralysis with d-tubocurarine and the ventilatory response to CO_2: an example of respiratory sparing? Anesthesiology 45:22–28, 1976
71. Pavlin EG, Holle RH, Schoene RB: Recovery of airway protection compared with ventilation in humans after paralysis with curare. Anesthesiology 70:381–385, 1989
72. Katz RL: Neuromuscular effects of d-tubocurarine, edrophonium and neostigmine in man. Anesthesiology 28:327–336, 1967
73. Matteo RS, Spector S, Horowitz PE: Relation of serum d-tubocurarine concentration to neuromuscular blockade in man. Anesthesiology 41:440, 1974
74. Silverman DG, Swift CA, Dubow HD, O'Connor TZ, Brull SJ: Variability of onset within and among relaxant regimens. J Clin Anesth 4:28–33, 1992
75. Ho LC, Crosby G, Sundaram P, Ronner SF, Ojemann RG: Ulnar train-of-four stimulation in predicting face movement during intracranial facial nerve stimulation. Anesth Analg 69:242–244, 1989
76. Sloan TB, Erian R: Effect of vecuronium-induced neuromuscular blockade on cortical motor evoked potentials. Anesthesiology 78:966–973, 1993
77. Sloan TB, Erian R: Effect of atracurium-induced neuromuscular block on cortical motor-evoked potentials. Anesth Analg 76:979–984, 1993
78. Adams DC, Emerson RG, Heyer EJ, McCormick PC, Carmel PW, Stein BM, Farcy JP, Gallo EJ: Monitoring of intraoperative motor-evoked potentials under conditions of controlled neuromuscular blockade. Anesth Analg 77:913–918, 1993
79. Edmonds HL, Markku PJ, Paloheimo PJ, et al: Transcranial magnetic motor evoked potentials (tcMMEP) for functional monitoring of motor pathways during scoliosis surgery. Spine 14:683–686, 1989
80. Kalkman CJ, Drummond JC, Kennely NA, et al: Intraoperative monitoring of tibialis anterior muscle motor evoked responses to transcranial electrical stimulation during partial neuromuscular blockade. Anesth Analg 73:584–589, 1992
81. Jellinek D, Jewkes D, Symon L: Noninvasive intraoperative monitoring of motor evoked potentials under propofol anesthesia: effects of spinal surgery on the amplitude and latency of motor evoked potentials. Neurosurgery 29:551–557, 1991
82. Paton WDM: The principles of neuromuscular block. Anaesthesia 8:151–174, 1953
83. Henegan C, McAuliffe R, Thomas D, Radford P: Morbidity after outpatient anaesthesia. Anaesthesia 36:4–9, 1981
84. Hannington-Kiff JG: Residual post-operative paralysis. Proc R Soc Med 63:73–76, 1970
85. Sosis M, Goldberg ME, Marr AT, Cubler AJ, Larijani GE: Atracurium and vecuronium do not affect extraocular muscle function after outpatient surgery. Anesth Analg 66:S164, 1987
86. Howardy-Hansen P, Moller J, Hansen B: Pretreatment with atracurium: the influence on neuromuscular transmission and pulmonary function. Acta Anaesthesiol Scand 31:642–644, 1987
87. Taboada JA, Rupp SM, Miller RD: Refining the priming principle for vecuronium rapid-sequence induction of anesthesia. Anesthesiology 64:243–247, 1986
88. Caffrey RR, Warren ML, Becker KE Jr: Neuromuscular blockade monitoring comparing the orbicularis oculi and adductor pollicis muscles. Anesthesiology 65:95–97, 1986
89. Kalli I: Effect of surface electrode position on the compound action potential evoked by ulnar nerve stimulation during isoflurane anaesthesia. Br J Anaesth 65:494–499, 1990
90. Katz RL: Electromyographic and mechanical effects of suxamethonium and tubocurarine on twitch, tetanic and post-tetanic responses. Br J Anaesth 45:849–859, 1973
91. Dupuis JY, Martin R, Tétrault JP: Clinical, electrical and mechanical correlations during recovery from neuromuscular blockade with vecuronium. Can J Anaesth 37:192–196, 1990
92. de Troyer A, Bastenier J, Delhez L: Function of respiratory muscles during partial curarization in humans. J Appl Physiol Respirat Environ Exercise Physiol 49:1049–1056, 1980

4

DAVID G. SILVERMAN | SORIN J. BRULL

Patterns of Stimulation

Neurostimulation in perioperative and intensive care settings may include single twitch, train-of-four, double-burst, and tetanic patterns of impulse repetition. Both depolarizing and nondepolarizing block cause depression of the evoked muscle response. In addition, nondepolarizing block is characterized by fade in response to the rapid repetitive stimulation of train-of-four, double-burst, and tetanic stimulating patterns. The differences between the responses to nondepolarizing block and traditional "phase 1" depolarizing block are illustrated in Figure 4-1. The remainder of this chapter focuses on the responses that typify nondepolarizing block and also occur during the "phase 2" block that may evolve in certain settings during administration of a depolarizing agent (Chap. 16).

◆ SINGLE TWITCH STIMULATION

Single twitch stimulation is the simplest form of neurostimulation. Unfortunately, the magnitude of a muscle response to one-time nerve firing is difficult to evaluate over time. It is important to compare a value to a *prerelaxant baseline* twitch height at the same (typically supramaximal) stimulating current. In addition, the clinically useful range of single twitch responses is limited: twitch tension is not reduced until at least 75–80% of the receptors are occupied by *nondepolarizing relaxant* (NDR), and the twitch response disappears completely once 90–95% of the receptors are blocked.[1-3] Simplifying the relationship, we can say that at between 75% and 95% receptor occupancy, twitch height decreases by roughly 25% for each 5% occupancy. (Remember, however, that the response is sigmoidal and hence is most rapid between 80% and 90% occupancy and less so at the extremes.)

◆ TETANIC STIMULATION

Tetanus involves serial stimulation at high frequency (i.e., ≥30 Hz) to provide *repetitive nerve firing* with *repetitive generation of muscle action potentials* (MAPs) and *sustained muscle contraction*. The sustained muscle contraction allows summation of individual twitch responses, such that *elastic forces* are more readily overcome,[4,5] with peak tension typically being attained in approximately 350 msec.[4] Tetanus most commonly is delivered for 5 seconds at 50 Hz. At this rate, the muscular contraction is completely fused and approaches that which may be achieved with maximal voluntary effort.[6] Stimulation at 50 Hz is more sensitive to receptor occlusion than stimulation at 20–30 Hz.[2,7] Higher frequencies may elicit responses that are even more sensitive to receptor occlusion.[7,8] However, at supraphysiologic rates of stimulation (e.g., above 70–200 Hz),[6,9] even normal neuromuscular transmission may fatigue.

A major feature of nondepolarizing block is *fade* in response to rapid (e.g., tetanic) stimulation. With rapid stimulation, there is an attempt to mobilize increased amounts of acetylcholine (ACh) presynaptically, but there

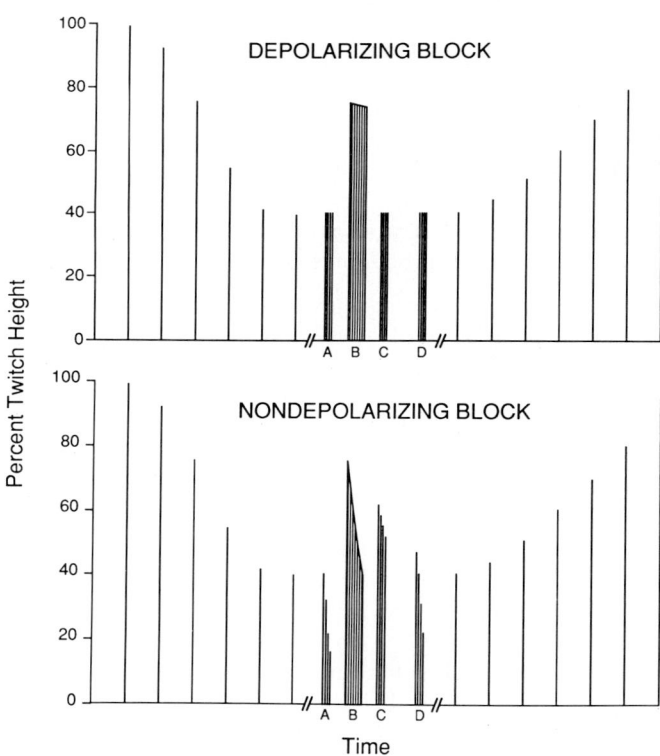

FIGURE 4-1. Patterns of neuromuscular block. Depolarizing block causes decreased single-twitch height, but it does not cause fade in response to rapid (train-of-four or tetanic) stimulation or post-tetanic facilitation. Nondepolarizing block not only causes decreased single-twitch height, but also fade in response to train-of-four (A) and tetanic stimulation (B) and facilitation of subsequent neuromuscular transmission (posttetanic facilitation; C and D). (Reproduced with permission from Brull SJ, Silverman DG: Neuromuscular block monitoring. In Ehrenwerth J, Eisenkraft JE (eds): Anesthesia Equipment: Principles and Applications. St. Louis, Mosby–Year Book, 1993, pp 297–318.)

nevertheless may be a *decline in the amount of ACh* that is available to be released with each impulse (Chap. 1). In the absence of an NDR, this decline generally is of relatively little clinical consequence unless supraphysiologic rates are delivered, since there is a wide margin of safety within the neuromuscular junction (NMJ). In the presence of an NDR, the release of ACh presynaptically is compromised to a much greater degree, and the response to ACh postsynaptically is compromised by competition for postsynaptic receptors.

◆ POSTTETANIC FACILITATION

Although in the presence of an NDR *ACh mobilization* may not be adequate to sustain tetanus without fade, it nevertheless provides for increased evoked responses on subsequent stimulation, presumably owing to increased ACh release by the nerve terminal.[4,10-23] Thus, when the response to a single stimulus is depressed by nondepolarizing block, it will be increased following tetanic stimulation[4,15,19]; this is most commonly referred to as *posttetanic facilitation* (PTF) or posttetanic *potentiation* (see Fig. 4-1).

Posttetanic facilitation may be characterized by (1) an increase in twitch tension, (2) a decrease in fade in response to train-of-four and double-burst stimulation,[22] and (3) a decreased latency period between the beginning of an MAP and the rise in muscle tension.[24] *Theories for the mechanism of PTF* include the following:

1. The intense tetanic stimulus induces *increased mobilization and release of ACh*, which results in an increase in subsequent end-plate potentials.[14,15]
2. During high-frequency stimulation, Ca^{2+} enters the nerve terminal faster than it can be pumped out and promotes subsequent ACh mobilization and release.
3. The motor nerve terminal itself becomes superexcitable,[25] such that its minimal gradient requirement for excitation (i.e., its time constant for accommodation) is decreased.[26]
4. Tetanus-induced displacement of relaxant from the postsynaptic receptor.[20] This *displacement* (or *knock-off* or *decurarization*) theory is disputed by evidence that relaxant binds too briefly to be "knocked off" and that no significant change in the response to exogenous ACh occurs when PTF is at its peak.[14]
5. Washout of NDR from the NMJ as a result of a tetanus-induced increase in blood flow.
6. Increased responsiveness of the muscle fibers themselves.

Posttetanic facilitation serves as the basis for *posttetanic count* (Chap. 5), but also may distort subsequent monitoring by giving a *false underestimation of block:* during a continuous infusion, PTF generally abates by 2 minutes,[22,27] whereas during recovery from a bolus dose of relaxant, it may exert its effect considerably longer and give a false impression of "adequate" recovery.[20,23] The greater effect during recovery (vs. continuous infusion) may be attributed to a larger NMJ to plasma gradient in this setting.

◆ TRAIN-OF-FOUR STIMULATION

Train-of-four neurostimulation consists of four stimuli delivered at 2 Hz.[11-13,16] When a nondepolarizing block is present, *fatigue (fade)* is noted at relatively slow (1–2 Hz) as well as fast (e.g., 50 Hz) rates of neurostimulation.[12,16] The nadir of the electromyographic (EMG) response typically is reached at the fourth impulse during stimulation at 2 Hz and at the eighth impulse during tetanic stimulation at 50 Hz.[16,28] With both patterns of stimulation, maximal fade typically occurs at approximately the same plasma concentration of relaxant.[29] Thus, train-of-four monitoring may obviate the need for tetanic stimulation, since stimulation at 2 Hz is sufficient to elicit fade comparable to that noted during tetanus (see Fig. 4-1).[10,12,16,29,30] However, the close agreement may not hold for all settings.[31-33]

Train-of-four monitoring also obviates the need for a prerelaxant baseline twitch height determination, by permitting comparison of the fourth twitch to the first twitch (T_4/T_1). Train-of-four thus serves as its *own control*. In the absence of nondepolarizing block, the T_4/T_1 ratio is approximately 1.0. At 70% receptor occupancy,[2] T_4 typically will start to decrease selectively; i.e., *fade* is seen. The amplitude of T_4 may decrease by as much as 25% before T_1 has an appreciable decrease from baseline (at approxi-

TABLE 4-1
Relationships Between Receptor Occupancy and Neuromuscular Monitoring

% of Receptors Blocked	Twitch (% Normal)	T_4 (% Normal)	T_4/T_1 Ratio	Tetanus
100	0%	0%	—	
95	0%	0%	—	
	0%	0%	T_1 lost	
90	10%	0%	T_2 lost	
	20%	0%	T_3 lost	
80	25%	0%	T_4 lost	Onset of fade at 30 Hz
	80–90%	55–65%	0.60–0.70	
	95%	65–70%	0.70–0.75	
75	100%	75–100%	0.75–1.0	
	100%	90–100%	0.90–1.0	Sustained at 50 Hz
50	100%	100%	1.0	Onset of fade at 100 Hz
30	100%	100%	1.0	Onset of fade at 200 Hz

The values in this table, which are approximations, illustrate some important relationships: fade occurs at a lesser degree of receptor occupancy than does twitch height depression, and the transition from light block (5% depression of twitch height) to deep block (e.g., 95% depression) constitutes a change from approximately 80% receptor occupancy to approximately 90% receptor occupancy (or a decrease in free receptors from 20% to 10%).

mately 75–80% receptor occupancy). The relative declines in T_4 and T_1 then tend to parallel one another such that when T_4 disappears, T_1 has declined by 75%, to approximately 25% of its baseline height. T_3 is lost when T_1 is 15–20% of its baseline height. T_2 is lost when T_1 is 10–15% of baseline.[16] As for single twitch stimulation, T_1 is lost when there is 90–95% receptor occupancy (Table 4-1).[1-3,16]

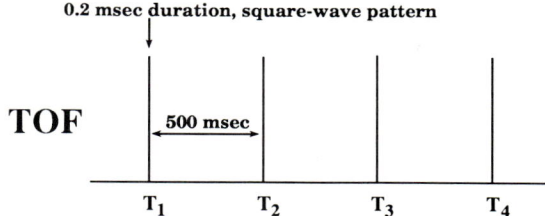

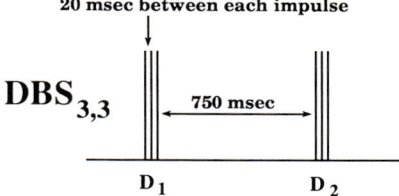

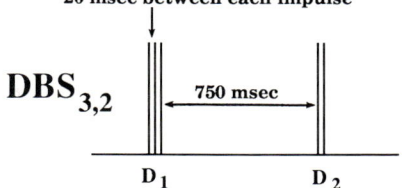

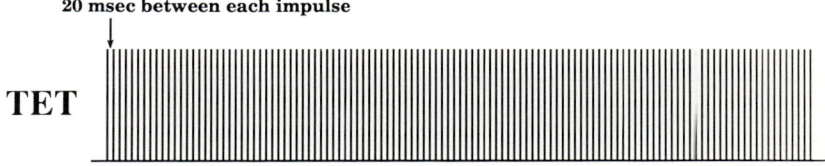

FIGURE 4-2 Comparison of stimulating patterns for train-of-four, $DBS_{3,3}$, $DBS_{3,2}$, and tetanus at 50 Hz. The impulses comprising single twitch, the four twitches of train-of-four, the two mini-tetanic bursts of DBS, and the 5 seconds of tetanus are identical with respect to duration (e.g., 200 μsec) and pattern (e.g., square-wave). (Reproduced with permission from Brull SJ, Silverman DG: Neuromuscular block monitoring. In Ehrenwerth J, Eisenkraft JE (eds): Anesthesia Equipment: Principles and Applications. St. Louis, Mosby–Year Book, 1993, pp 297–318.)

The increased sensitivity of T_4/T_1 compared to single twitch may be especially prominent, and especially important, during recovery.[34–39] The relatively slow changes during recovery (vs. onset) allow the delineation of fade. Following spontaneous recovery to ≥90% of baseline single twitch tension, the T_4/T_1 ratio was still only 0.44 and 0.56 after vecuronium and atracurium, respectively[34]; however, the ratio was higher (i.e., the degree of fade was less) during accelerated recovery after a reversal agent.[10]

◆ DOUBLE-BURST STIMULATION

Double-burst stimulation (DBS) entails delivery of *two mini-tetanic bursts* of stimuli; each burst consists of two to four impulses (each of which has a standard pulse duration of 0.2 msec) at a rate of 50 Hz. The two bursts are separated by 0.75 second. For $DBS_{3,3}$, the first burst consists of three pulses at 50 Hz; after the 0.75-second pause, there is a second burst, which likewise consists of three impulses (Figs. 4-2 and 4-3). Several investigators have shown that the D_2/D_1 of $DBS_{3,3}$ and the T_4/T_1 of the train-of-four response correlate highly when assessed mechanographically[40–42] and have indicated that DBS is preferable to train-of-four monitoring because DBS fade may be more readily detected than train-of-four fade by visual or tactile means (i.e., without the aid of a mechanical recording device).[41–48] Drenck et al. reported that absence of fade on qualitative assessment of the train-of-four response was associated with a 48% chance of missing actual fade (as confirmed by mechanographic testing), whereas qualitative assessment of the DBS was associated with only a 9% chance of missing such fade.[45]

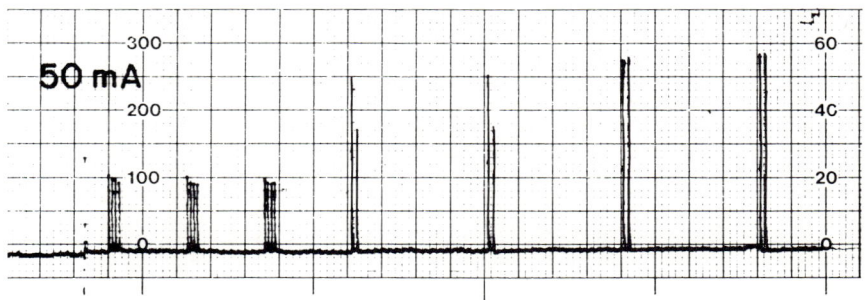

FIGURE 4-3 Evoked responses of train-of-four (every 12 seconds), $DBS_{3,2}$ and $DBS_{3,3}$ (every 20 seconds) in an unmedicated volunteer. Although the magnitude of the individual responses is greater for DBS, the T_4/T_1 ratio of train-of-four and the D_2/D_1 ratio of $DBS_{3,3}$ are virtually equivalent; the D_2/D_1 of $DBS_{3,2}$ is lower as a result of its second burst being of shorter duration than its first burst. (Reproduced with permission from Brull SJ, Silverman DG: Neuromuscular block monitoring. In Ehrenwerth J, Eisenkraft JE (eds): Anesthesia Equipment: Principles and Applications. St. Louis, Mosby–Year Book, 1993, pp 297–318.)

Two possible reasons for the *increased sensitivity of DBS* are (1) the overcoming of muscle elastic forces by mini-tetanic (DBS) as opposed to twitch (train-of-four) stimulation, and (2) the lack of intervening stimuli between D_1 and D_2 as opposed to the intervening stimuli between T_1 and T_4 during train-of-four (i.e., T_2 and T_3 may compromise visual or tactile comparison of T_1 to T_4). Another potential advantage of DBS is during assessment of deep block, since D_1 is still detected at slightly deeper levels of block than is T_1 (i.e., when single twitch is absent but a response to tetanus is detectable, and the posttetanic count is 7).[49]

Discussion Questions ◆

a. How does increasing the *rate of stimulation* from 0.1 Hz to 1.0 Hz affect the **apparent** *depth of block*?
b. How does increasing the *rate of stimulation* from 0.1 to 1.0 Hz affect the **apparent** *rate of block onset*?
c. Why might it be preferable to wait for 100% depression of *single twitch* at 0.1 Hz prior to *tracheal intubation* in a setting where any patient movement or coughing would be unacceptable?
d. Why might *tetanic stimulation* provide a better indication of *inspiratory capacity* than single twitch stimulation?
e. Is *fade* in response to tetanic stimulation pathognomonic of block with a nondepolarizing relaxant?
f. What is occurring to the *end-plate current* when one sees *fade* of a contractile response during tetanus at 50 Hz in the presence of a nondepolarizing block?
g. Compare the T_4/T_1 ratio before and immediately *after tetanic stimulation* in the context of nondepolarizing block.
h. Is the height of the *first twitch of train-of-four* at 20-second intervals the same as that of *individual twitches* at 0.1 Hz (in the context of nondepolarizing block)?
i. Why might *train-of-four stimulation* be preferable to *tetanic stimulation* for assessing the degree of block?
j. For a given degree of T_1 depression as a result of nondepolarizing block, is the T_4/T_1 ratio the same during *onset* and *recovery*? Why?
k. What is the total duration of the first "burst" of impulses during $DBS_{3,3}$?
l. Do the mechanographic responses to $DBS_{3,3}$ and $DBS_{3,2}$ correlate with the mechanographic response to *train-of-four*? What is the effect of the shortened second impulse of $DBS_{3,2}$ on the relationship between $DBS_{3,2}$ and $DBS_{3,3}$?

Answers ◆

a. Single (perhaps more accurately "serial") twitch stimulation at *0.1 Hz* means a single impulse is delivered by a nerve stimulator every 10 seconds. This slow rate of stimulation is relatively nondisturbing to the NMJ. As the *rate of single twitch stimulation* is increased above 0.1 Hz, we typically see fade (fatigue) of the evoked response during nondepolarizing block.[16,31,50–52] Although stimulation at 1.0 Hz may provide a quicker assessment of rapidly changing levels of block,[53–55] such a relatively *fast rate of stimulation may be associated with significant fade*[13,30,56] *and increased blood flow* to the stimulated NMJ (and hence increased delivery of relaxant).[57–59] The apparent dose requirements for tubocurarine decreased by a factor of 3 as the stimulus frequency increased from 0.1 to 1.0 Hz.[60]

b. Increasing the *stimulus frequency* (e.g., from 0.1 Hz to 1.0 Hz or to train-of-four at brief intervals) results in *faster onset* of neuromuscular depression at the site of stimulation for depolarizing[51,61,62] and nondepolarizing[16,30,50,51,60,61,63–65] block. This may be attributed to a combination of increased delivery of relaxant (increased blood flow) and fatigue (especially for nondepolarizing agents). Alternatively, it has been shown that serial tetanic stimulation (at 1- to 2-minute intervals) actually may delay the apparent onset of block, presumably due to posttetanic facilitation.[66]

c. Compared to more rapid rates of neurostimulation, monitoring the *adductor pollicis* response to single twitch stimulation at 0.1 Hz provides a desirable *"safety factor" for intubation* in settings in which patient movement is unacceptable. Even so, it was noted that ideal intubating conditions were not reliably observed until 30 seconds after 100% adductor pollicis depression was achieved (at 0.1 Hz).[67] If it is not necessary to ensure "ideal" conditions—without any movement—then a lesser degree of block may be acceptable at 0.1 Hz,[67–70] or one may use a faster rate of neurostimulation or monitor at a muscle whose time course and sensitivity more closely resemble those of the diaphragm and larynx. Regardless of the rate of stimulation used to monitor onset in a given patient, it is preferable to use the dose estimated during the slow twitch mode as it is more likely to be sufficient to paralyze the (less sensitive) vocal cords and diaphragm.

d. The degree of block that causes *tetanic fade* is similar to that which decreases *inspiratory capacity*. Both are more sensitive to block than is depression of single twitch height. Breathing to inspiratory capacity involves a prolonged and maintained (tetanic-like) effort.

e. In addition to being characteristic of block with an NDR, *fade* may also be a manifestation of a *phase 2 block* with a depolarizing relaxant (Chap. 16).[71–74] It may also occur during the use of potent *inhalational anesthetics* in the absence of nondepolarizing agents.[9,75,76] Moreover, at supraphysiologic rates of stimulation (e.g., >100 Hz), fade may be elicited in the absence of drugs.[6,9]

f. *Fade* of the contractile response to *tetanus* is due to a *decline of the* *end-plate current* to below the threshold required for generation of a muscle action potential. NDRs decrease presynaptic mobilization of ACh and reduce the postsynaptic margin of safety (Chap. 2). These factors impinge on the end-plate current. When the presynaptic rundown of ACh release becomes sufficient to prevent the end-plate current from reaching the MAP threshold, then an MAP will no longer be generated, the muscle fiber will not contract, and the response to tetanic stimulation will fade.

g. In the context of *nondepolarizing block,* the effect of *posttetanic facilitation* on T_4 is far more noticeable than its effect on T_1.[22] The T_4/T_1 ratio increases toward 1.0 as the increased release of ACh overcomes relaxant-induced fade. However, the duration of this effect appears to be the same for T_1 and T_4.[22] These effects persist slightly longer when higher-frequency stimuli (i.e., 100-Hz tetanus) are used.[22]

h. The *heights of T_1 (of train-of-four)* and *single twitch* are the same so long as neither train-of-four nor single (serial) twitch stimulation is repeated so frequently as to elicit fatigue (fade) of evoked responses. As noted above, rapid stimulation may alter the apparent onset of block; i.e., train-of-four stimulation at 10-second intervals and single twitch stimulation at 0.5–1.0 Hz may result in acceleration of apparent onset (as compared to stimulation at 0.1 Hz). For example, train-of-four stimulation at 10-second intervals resulted in a 25% decrease in the calculated ED_{95} for mivacurium,[77] and train-of-four stimulation at 12-second intervals accelerated the onset of atracurium from 3.35 minutes to 1.98 minutes.[61]

i. *Train-of-four stimulation is far less painful than tetanus and is not associated with prolonged posttetanic effects* (e.g., *posttetanic facilitation*). In some cases, *train-of-four monitoring may actually be more sensitive* than tetanus.[10,16,17,31,78,79] In the context of nondepolarizing block, both train-of-four and tetanic neurostimulation are rapid enough to result in muscle fatigue (manifested by *fade*).[10,13,16,30,80] However, in contrast to train-of-four, tetanus increases responses (perhaps by causing *ACh mobilization*) during and after its application.[4,10–13,16–18] This might tend to offset fade during tetanus, and causes facilitation after tetanus (PTF). Train-of-four may offer another advantage from a technical standpoint: *a strong tetanic contraction may overload a transducer* that is not designed for tension exceeding 8–10 kg. Overload may damage the transducer and mask fade that may be occurring in the overload range.[4,81]

Alternatively, *there are settings in which tetanus may be more sensitive than train-of-four:* (1) Following neostigmine reversal of pancuronium block, in the context of 1 MAC of enflurane or isoflurane, there was marked tetanic fade despite a T_4/T_1 >0.70.[82] (2) If, after adequate reversal, a second dose of neostigmine was given, the resultant degree of tetanic fade was greater than for train-of-four.[83] (3) Serial tetanic stimulation at 100 Hz (at 15- to 60-second intervals) was more sensitive than train-of-four stimulation after nondepolarizing block in the presence of isoflurane.[32,33] It should be noted that high-frequency tetanic stimulation increases the neuromuscular refractory period, thereby decreasing the ability of the muscle to respond to stimuli.[4] Perhaps this effect is additive to the effects of inhalational agents.

j. The relationship between T_4 and T_1 does not remain consistent throughout the course of a neuromuscular block. For a given degree of T_1 depression, the T_4/T_1 *ratio is lower during spontaneous recovery than after reversal*[10] *or during onset.*[34–39] Typically T_4 is not noted until T_1 has recovered to 20–35% of its baseline size.[16,84–87] It has been suggested that the *rate of binding* is faster (and unbinding slower) at (1) presynaptic sites responsible for fade (than at postsynaptic sites responsible for depression of twitch height and peak tetanic tension)[35,37,88] (Chap. 2), and/or at (2) fibers with a greater propensity for fade (than at fibers that do not tend to demonstrate fade).[39,89] Both theories are consistent with the observation that gradual changes in NDR concentration noted during spontaneous recovery and during slow intravenous infusion are associated with fade.[90]

k. The first *burst of impulses during* $DBS_{3,3}$ requires approximately 40 msec: 20 msec between pulses 1 and 2 and 20 msec between pulses 2 and 3 (50 Hz = 50 pulses/sec = 1 pulse/20 msec); the effect of the individual pulse durations (0.2 msec) is negligible. This mini-tetanic stimulus is sufficient to allow summation of the muscle fiber's contractile responses and to induce fade comparable to that seen after the serial twitches of train-of-four.

l. $DBS_{3,3}$ produces a pattern of *mechanical fade* that is virtually equivalent to that of *train-of-four.*[40–42] Alternatively, $DBS_{3,2}$ has "increased mechanical fade." Even in the unblocked state, the second burst produces a muscle contraction of lesser magnitude; its briefer duration (two rather than three stimuli in the second burst) overcomes less elastic forces. In the absence of block, the D_2/D_1 ratio of $DBS_{3,2}$ is 0.8 while that of $DBS_{3,3}$ is 1.0, and the T_4/T_1 is 1.0. Changes in $DBS_{3,2}$ correlate with, but thus are not identical to, changes in train-of-four.

References ◆

1. Paton WDM, Waud DR: The margin of safety of neuromuscular transmission. J Physiol 191:59–90, 1967
2. Waud BE, Waud DR: The relation between the response to "train-of-four" stimulation and receptor occlusion during competitive neuromuscular block. Anesthesiology 37:413–416, 1972
3. Waud BE, Waud DR: The margin of safety of neuromuscular transmission in the muscle of the diaphragm. Anesthesiology 37:417–422, 1972
4. Epstein RA, Epstein RM: The electromyogram and the mechanical response of indirectly

stimulated muscle in anesthetized man following curarization. Anesthesiology 38:212–223, 1973
5. Edwards RHT, Young A, Hosking GP, Jones DA: Human skeletal muscle function: description of tests and normal values. Clin Sci 52:283–290, 1977
6. Merton PA: Voluntary strength and fatigue. J Physiol 123:553–564, 1954
7. Waud BE, Waud DR: The relation between tetanic fade and receptor occlusion in the presence of competitive neuromuscular block. Anesthesiology 35:456–464, 1971
8. Gissen AJ, Katz RL: Twitch, tetanus and posttetanic potentiation as indices of nerve-muscle block in man. Anesthesiology 30:481–487, 1969
9. Stanec A, Heyduk J, Stanec G, Orkin LR: Tetanic fade and post-tetanic tension in the absence of neuromuscular blocking agents in anesthetized man. Anesth Analg 57:102–107, 1978
10. Ali HH, Savarese JJ, Lebowitz PW, Ramsey FM: Twitch, tetanus and train-of-four as indices of recovery from nondepolarizing neuromuscular blockade. Anesthesiology 54:294–297, 1981
11. Ali HH, Utting JE, Gray TC: Quantitative assessment of residual antidepolarizing block (Part I). Br J Anaesth 43:473–477, 1971
12. Ali HH, Utting JE, Gray TC: Quantitative assessment of residual antidepolarizing block (Part II). Br J Anaesth 43:478–485, 1971
13. Ali HH, Utting JE, Gray C: Stimulus frequency in the detection of neuromuscular block in humans. Br J Anaesth 42:967–978, 1970
14. Hutter OF: Post-tetanic restoration of neuromuscular transmission blocked by d-tubocurarine. J Physiol 118:216–227, 1952
15. Liley AW, North KAK: An electrical investigation of effects of repetitive stimulation on mammalian neuromuscular junction. J Neurophysiol 16:509–527, 1953
16. Lee C: Train-of-4 quantitation of competitive neuromuscular block. Anesth Analg 54:649–653, 1975
17. Lee C, Barnes A, Katz RL: Neuromuscular sensitivity to tubocurarine: a comparison of 10 parameters. Br J Anaesth 48:1045–1051, 1976
18. Magelby KL: The effect of repetitive stimulation on facilitation of transmitter release at the frog neuromuscular junction. J Physiol 234:327–352, 1973
19. Katz RL: Electromyographic and mechanical effects of suxamethonium and tubocurarine on twitch, tetanic and post-tetanic responses. Br J Anaesth 45:849–859, 1973
20. Feldman SA, Tyrrell MF: A new theory on the termination of action of the muscle relaxants. Proc R Soc Med 63:692–695, 1970
21. Hughes JR, Morrell RM: Posttetanic changes in the human neuromuscular system. J Appl Physiol 11:51–57, 1957
22. Brull SJ, Connelly NR, O'Connor TZ, Silverman DG: Effect of tetanus on subsequent neuromuscular monitoring in patients receiving vecuronium. Anesthesiology 74:64–70, 1991
23. Brull SJ, Silverman DG: Tetanus-induced changes in apparent recovery following bolus doses of atracurium or vecuronium. Anesthesiology 77:642–645, 1992
24. Botelho SY, Cander L: Post-tetanic potentiation before and during ischemia in intact human skeletal muscle. J Appl Physiol 6:221–228, 1953
25. Zucker S, Lando L, Fogelson A: Can presynaptic depolarization release transmitter without calcium influx? J Physiol (Paris) 81:237–245, 1986
26. Ushiyama J, Brooks CM: Minimal-gradient requirements of motoneurons during posttetanic potentiation. Am J Physiol 220:1949–1955, 1971
27. Silverman DG, Garcia RM, Grosso LM, Brull SJ: Consistency of response to tetanic stimulations at two and five-minute intervals. Anesthesiology 77:A958, 1992
28. Lee C, Katz RL: Fade of neurally evoked compound electromyogram during neuromuscular block by d-tubocurarine. Anesth Analg 56:271–275, 1977
29. Torda TA, Graham GG, Tsui D: Neuromuscular sensitivity to atracurium in humans. Anaesth Intensive Care 18:62–68, 1990
30. Blackman JG: Stimulus frequency and neuromuscular block. Br J Pharmacol 20:5–16, 1963
31. Ali HH, Savarese JJ: Monitoring of neuromuscular function. Anesthesiology 45:216–249, 1976
32. Baurain MJ, d'Hollander AA, Melot C, Dernovoi BS, Barvais L: Effects of residual concentrations of isoflurane on the reversal of vecuronium-induced neuromuscular blockade. Anesthesiology 74:474–478, 1991
33. Caldwell JE, Laster MJ, Magorian T, Heier T, Yasuda N, Lynam DP, Eger EI II, Weiskopf

RB: The neuromuscular effects of desflurane, alone and combined with pancuronium or succinylcholine in humans. Anesthesiology 74:412–418, 1991
34. Foldes FF, Nagashima H, Boros M, Tassonyi E, Fitzal S, Agoston S: Muscular relaxation with atracurium, vecuronium and duador under balanced anaesthesia. Br J Anaesth 55:97S–103S, 1983
35. Graham GG, Morris R, Pybus DA, Torda TA, Woodey R: Relationship of train-of-four ratio to twitch depression during pancuronium-induced neuromuscular blockade. Anesthesiology 65:579–583, 1986
36. Pearce AC, Casson WR, Jones RM: Factors affecting train-of-four fade. Br J Anaesth 57:602–606, 1985
37. Power SJ, Jones RM: Relationship between single twitch depression and train-of-four fade: influence of relaxant dose during onset and spontaneous offset of neuromuscular blockade. Anesth Analg 66:633–636, 1987
38. Robbins R, Donati F, Bevan DR, et al: Differential effects of myoneural blocking drugs on neuromuscular transmission in infants. Br J Anaesth 56:1095–1099, 1984
39. Storella RJ, Slomowitz SA, Rosenberg H: Relationships between block-of-twitch and train-of-four fade in the mouse phrenic nerve-diaphragm preparation. Can J Anaesth 38:401–407, 1991
40. Brull SJ, Connelly NR, Silverman DG: Correlation of train-of-four and double-burst stimulation ratios at varying amperages. Anesth Analg 71:489–492, 1990
41. Engbaek J, Ostergaard D, Viby-Mogensen J: Double burst stimulation (DBS): a new pattern of nerve stimulation to identify residual neuromuscular block. Br J Anaesth 62:274–278, 1989
42. Ueda N, Viby-Mogensen J, Olsen NV, Drenck NE, Tsuda H, Muteki T: The best choice of double burst stimulation pattern for manual evaluation of neuromuscular transmission. J Anesth 3:94–99, 1989
43. Brull SJ, Silverman DG: Visual assessment of train-of-four and double burst-induced fade at submaximal stimulating currents. Anesth Analg 73:627–632, 1991
44. Brull SJ, Garcia RM, Silverman DG: Visual and tactile assessment of neuromuscular fade. Anesthesiology 77:A926, 1992
45. Drenck NE, Ueda N, Olsen NV, Engbaek J, Jensen E, Skovgaard LT, Viby-Mogensen J: Manual evaluation of residual curarization using double burst stimulation: a comparison with train-of-four. Anesthesiology 70:578–581, 1989
46. Gill SS, Donati F, Bevan DR: Clinical evaluation of double-burst stimulation: its relationship to train-of-four stimulation. Anaesthesia 45:543–548, 1990
47. Saddler JM, Bevan JC, Donati F, Bevan DR, Pinto SR: Comparison of double-burst and train-of-four stimulation to assess neuromuscular blockade in children. Anesthesiology 73:401–403, 1990
48. Ueda N, Muteki T, Tsuda H, Inoue S, Nishina H: Is the diagnosis of significant residual neuromuscular blockade improved by using double-burst nerve stimulation? Eur J Anaesthesiol 8:213–218, 1991
49. Braude N, Vyvyan HAL, Jordan MJ: Intraoperative assessment of atracurium-induced neuromuscular block using double burst stimulation. Br J Anaesth 67:574–578, 1991
50. Ali HH, Savarese JJ: Stimulus frequency is essential information (letter). Anesthesiology 50:76, 1979
51. Preston JB, van Maanen EF: Effects of frequency of stimulation on the paralyzing dose of neuromuscular blocking agents. J Pharmacol Exp Ther 107:165–171, 1953
52. Silverman DG, Swift CA, Dubow HD, O'Connor TZ, Brull SJ: Variability of onset within and among relaxant regimens. J Clin Anesth 4:28–33, 1992
53. Hughes R, Payne JP: Clinical assessment of atracurium using the single twitch and tetanic responses of the adductor pollicis muscles. Br J Anaesth 55:47S-52S, 1983
54. Naguib M, Gyasi HK, Abdulatif M, Absood GH: Rapid tracheal intubation with atracurium—a comparison of priming intervals. Can Anaesth Soc J 33:150–155, 1986
55. Viby-Mogensen J: Neuromuscular monitoring. In Miller RD (ed): Anesthesia. New York, Churchill Livingstone, 1990
56. Wislicki L: Effects of rate of stimulation and of fatigue on the response to neuromuscular blocking agents. Br J Pharmacol 13:138–143, 1958
57. Goudsouzian NG, Martyn J, Rudd GD, Liu LMP, Lineberry CG: Continuous infusion of atracurium in children. Anesthesiology 64:171–174, 1986

58. Goat VA, Yeung ML, Blakeney C, Feldman SA: The effect of blood flow upon the activity of gallamine triethiodide. Br J Anaesth 48:69–73, 1976
59. Saxena PR, Dhasmana KM, Prakash O: A comparison of systemic and regional hemodynamic effects of d-tubocurarine, pancuronium, and vecuronium. Anesthesiology 59:102–108, 1983
60. Ali HH, Savarese JJ: Stimulus frequency and dose-response curve to d-tubocurarine in man. Anesthesiology 52:36–39, 1980
61. Curran MJ, Donati F, Bevan DR: Onset and recovery of atracurium and suxamethonium-induced neuromuscular blockade with simultaneous train-of-four and single twitch stimulation. Br J Anaesth 59:989–994, 1987
62. Connelly NR, Silverman DG, Brull SJ: Temporal correlation of succinylcholine-induced fasciculations to loss of twitch response at different stimulating frequencies. J Clin Anesth 4:190–193, 1992
63. Ali HH, Basta SJ, Savarese JJ, Gargarian M, Scott RFP, Sunder N, Gionfriddo M: Single twitch and train-of-four responses for atracurium and vecuronium. Anesth Analg 64:A187, 1985
64. Lee C, Katz RL: Neuromuscular pharmacology: a clinical update and commentary. Br J Anaesth 52:173–188, 1980
65. Savarese JJ, Ali HH, Antonio RP: The clinical pharmacology of metocurine: dimethyl-tubocurarine revisited. Anesthesiology 47:277–284, 1977
66. Wali FA, Bradshaw EG, Suer AH: Clinical assessment of neuromuscular blockade produced by vecuronium using twitch, train of four, tetanus and post-tetanic twitch responses of the adductor pollicis muscle. Acta Anaesthesiol Belg 39:35–42, 1988
67. Bencini A, Newton DEF: Rate of onset of good intubating conditions, respiratory depression and hand muscle paralysis after vecuronium. Br J Anaesth 56:959–965, 1984
68. Agoston S, Salt P, Newton D, Bencini A, Boomsma P, Erdmann W: The neuromuscular blocking action of ORG NC45, a new pancuronium derivative, in anaesthetized patients. Br J Anaesth 52:53S–59S, 1980
69. Mirakhur RK, Ferres CJ, Clarke RSJ, Bali IM, Dundee JW: Clinical evaluation of ORG NC45. Br J Anaesth 55:119–124, 1983
70. Debaene B, Meistelman C, Lienhart A, Donati F: Le monitorage de l'oeil permet de prévoir précocément de bonnes conditions d'intubation trachéale. Ann Fr Anesth Reanim 10:A24, 1991
71. Katz RL, Ryan JF: The neuromuscular effects of suxamethonium in man. Br J Anaesth 41:381–390, 1969
72. Lee C: Dose relationships of phase II, tachyphylaxis and train-of-four fade in suxamethonium-induced dual neuromuscular block in man. Br J Anaesth 47:841–845, 1975
73. Ramsey FM, Lebowitz PW, Savarese JJ, Ali HH: Clinical characteristics of long-term succinylcholine neuromuscular blockade during balanced anesthesia. Anesth Analg 59:110–116, 1980
74. Savarese JJ, Ali HH, Murphy JD, Padget C, Lee C-M, Ponitz J: Train-of-four nerve stimulation in the management of prolonged neuromuscular blockade following succinylcholine. Anesthesiology 42:106–111, 1975
75. Cohen PJ, Heisterkamp CV, Skovsted P: The effect of general anaesthesia on the response to stimulus in man. Br J Anaesth 42:543–547, 1970
76. Miller RD, Eger EI II, Way WL, et al: Comparative neuromuscular effects of forane and halothane alone and in combination with d-tubocurarine in man. Anesthesiology 35:38–42, 1971
77. Maddineni VR, Mirakhur RK, Cooper R, McCoy E: Potency estimation of mivacurium: comparison of two different modes of nerve stimulation. Br J Anaesth 70:694–695, 1993
78. Ali HH, Kitz RJ: Evaluation of recovery from nondepolarizing neuromuscular block, using a digital neuromuscular transmission analyzer: preliminary report. Anesth Analg 52:740–745, 1973
79. Dupuis JY, Martin R, Tétrault JP: Clinical, electrical and mechanical correlations during recovery from neuromuscular blockade with vecuronium. Can J Anaesth 37:192–196, 1990
80. Rosenblueth A, Morison RS: Curarization, fatigue and Wedensky inhibition. Am J Physiol 119:236–256, 1937

81. Freund FG, Merati JK: A source of errors in assessing neuromuscular blockade. Anesthesiology 39:540–542, 1973
82. Dernovoi B, Agoston S, Barvais L, Baurain M, Lefebvre R, d'Hollander A: Neostigmine antagonism of vecuronium paralysis during fentanyl, halothane, isoflurane, and enflurane anesthesia. Anesthesiology 66:698–701, 1987
83. Goldhill DR, Wainwright AP, Stuart CS, Flynn PJ: Neostigmine after spontaneous recovery from neuromuscular blockade: effect on depth of blockade monitored with train-of-four and tetanic stimuli. Anaesthesia 44:293–299, 1989
84. Kopman AF: Tactile evaluation of train-of-four count as an indicator of reliability of antagonism of vecuronium- or atracurium-induced neuromuscular blockade. Anesthesiology 75:588–593, 1991
85. O'Hara DA, Fragen RJ, Shanks CA: Reappearance of the train-of-four after neuromuscular blockade induced with tubocurarine, vecuronium or atracurium. Br J Anaesth 58:1296–1299, 1986
86. O'Hara DA, Fragen RJ, Shanks CA: Comparison of visual and measured train-of-four recovery after vecuronium induced neuromuscular blockade using two anaesthetic techniques. Br J Anaesth 58:1300–1302, 1986
87. Gibson FM, Mirakhur RK, Clarke RSJ, Brady MM: Quantification of train-of-four responses during recovery of block from non-depolarising muscle relaxants. Acta Anaesthesiol Scand 31:655–657, 1987
88. Bowman WC: Prejunctional and postjunctional cholinoceptors at the neuromuscular junction. Anesth Analg 59:935–943, 1980
89. Bartkowski RR, Epstein RH: Relationship between train-of-four ratio and first-twitch depression during neuromuscular blockade: a pharmacokinetic/dynamic explanation. J Pharmacokinet Biopharm 18:335–346, 1990
90. Bowman WC, Webb SN: Tetanic fade during partial transmission failure produced by non-depolarizing neuromuscular blocking drugs in the cat. Clin Exp Pharmacol Physiol 3:545–555, 1976

5

DAVID G. SILVERMAN | SORIN J. BRULL

Monitoring of Evoked Responses

We can qualitatively assess the evoked muscle responses to neurostimulation by visual and tactile means (i.e., subjectively), or we can quantify them objectively with an electromyogram or mechanomyogram.

◆ VISUAL AND TACTILE MEANS

Unfortunately, *visual and tactile assessments often fail to identify fade* in response to train-of-four stimulation at moderate degrees of block (i.e., they often fail to identify block which causes a T_4/T_1 <0.70 and even as low as 0.30).[1-11] Likewise, tetanic fade was not detected reliably unless the tetanic fade ratio was ≤0.30.[12] Nevertheless, subjective means are employed most commonly because of the cost and the elaborate setup associated with mechanographic devices.

When no twitch response is noted by visual or tactile assessment, we can safely assume that mechanographic height is less than 10% of baseline.[13] At such a deep level of block, we can evaluate the *posttetanic count* (PTC).[14-24] It has long been appreciated that posttetanic facilitation can be observed even in the context of 100% twitch depression.[25,26] The PTC delineates the degree of block by recording the number of twitches in response to serial stimulation at 1 Hz beginning *3 seconds after tetanus* (5 seconds at 50 Hz). The greater the number of posttetanic counts, the less deep the block; i.e., the *number of PTC twitches is inversely related to the depth of block* (Table 5-1).

The PTC is most helpful in assessing depths of block that abolish the response to single twitch, train-of-four, and even tetanic stimulation—i.e., to assess depths of block that cause >92% receptor occupancy (Chap. 4). The PTC may also be used to assess posttetanic facilitation and fade when a response to twitch or train-of-four stimulation is still apparent. Since in the presence of nondepolarizing block the response to stimulation at 1 Hz will fade progressively until it is no longer apparent, one may gain an appreciation of depth of block simply by counting the PTC "rather than endeavoring

TABLE 5-1
Posttetanic Count (PTC) and Approximate Time Until Recovery of Detectable Twitch Response

	Recovery Time (min)	
No. of Posttetanic Counts	Atracurium or Vecuronium[14,21]	Pancuronium[20,24]
0	>9	>37
1	9	37
2	7	30
4	4	20
6	2	10
8	0–2	5

PTC was assessed during recovery from nondepolarizing block when no response to single twitch or train-of-four stimulation was apparent.

to estimate the TOF ratio which is difficult without complex monitoring equipment."[22]

The utility of the PTC is a consequence of its being more sensitive to the presence of unoccupied (i.e., unblocked) receptors than single twitch, train-of-four, or tetanus monitoring. During recovery from atracurium, PTC was first noted (PTC = 1) at a plasma concentration of 1.15 mg $\cdot$ L^{-1}, while 50% recovery of twitch height was not noted until the level had decreased to 0.217 mg $\cdot$ L^{-1}.[23]

The PTC has been assessed at 6- to 8-minute intervals[15,22] and as frequently as every 2 minutes.[18,19] There is evidence to suggest that, in the presence of a stable neuromuscular junction (NMJ) to plasma concentration gradient, the NMJ returns to its pretetanic baseline state within this time.[27,28] As for other stimulating patterns, assessment of the PTC is unreliable in the context of hypothermia.[29]

When a twitch response is apparent, an appreciation of the depth of block may be attained by *counting the responses to train-of-four*[13] or double-burst (DBS)[30] stimulation. Because it elicits a greater degree of contraction, the first impulse (D_1) of DBS remains detectable at a greater depth of block than the first twitch (T_1) of train-of-four. Such counting may be particularly helpful in assessing whether to deepen a block. It may also serve as a guide for determining when, and with what agent, to reverse (Chap. 15) the effects of a nondepolarizing relaxant (NDR) at the end of surgery (even though precise assessment is not possible unless a mechanographic device is employed[31-34]). T_4 typically reappears when T_1 has returned to 20–30% of its baseline height.[13,31-33] However, it has been reported to reappear when T_1 has returned to as little as $13\% \pm 4\%$[31] or as much as $33\% \pm 6\%$ of baseline.[32] T_4 typically is not detected tactilely until T_1 has returned to approximately 30–35% of baseline.[13]

◆ ELECTROMYOGRAPHY

An electromyogram (EMG) records the electrical signal that is generated by the muscle action potential(s) (MAPs) under its recording electrodes. The *amplitude of the compound MAP* (of the integrated EMG) is proportional to the number of motor units that generate an MAP. It may be measured as the first major deflection or the rectified EMG integrated response; these measurements appear to be highly correlated.[35,36] The *duration and morphology* of the compound MAP reflect the synchrony of contraction (Fig. 5-1, Table 5-2).

EMG recording electrodes typically are placed near the midportion or *"motor point,"* over the tendinous insertion of the muscle, and at a slightly remote "indifferent" site. EMG monitoring of the hand muscles may evaluate any or all of the following: adductor pollicis, abductor pollicis brevis, first dorsal interosseous, and abductor digiti quinti (minimi) muscles (Fig. 5-2, Table 5-2). Although typically innervated by the ulnar nerve, these muscles vary with respect to contributions by the median nerve.[37] It is appealing to monitor the EMG of the same muscle that is assessed mechanomyographically; hence the *adductor pollicis* often is selected. However, the EMG of the adductor pollicis is very sensitive to electrode positioning and at times has poorly defined morphology,[36,38–40] and it is subject to dual (ulnar and median) innervation.[36]

Many believe that monitoring of the *first dorsal interosseous muscle* is preferable for EMG: the responses of the first dorsal interosseous *exhibit good morphology*,[36,38] with a large peak-to-peak amplitude[36] and relatively little baseline drift.[41] Since the first dorsal interosseous muscle lies on the dorsal side of the hand, the electrodes are easy to affix and maintain and are seldom disturbed by hand movement.[36] The sensitivity of this muscle to NDRs more closely parallels that of the adductor pollicis than does the sensitivity of the *abductor digiti quinti muscle*.[36,42]

The *abductor digiti quinti is less sensitive to relaxant* than the adductor pollicis or first dorsal interosseous. The time course of neuromuscular block at the abductor digiti quinti more closely *parallels changes at the diaphragm and larynx*.[36,42–44] During recovery, a T_4/T_1 of 0.7 (and possibly lower) at the adductor pollicis corresponded to a T_4/T_1 of 0.9 at the abductor digiti quinti.[45] The mechanographic T_4/T_1 at the adductor pollicis consistently was approximately 0.2 below the abductor digiti quinti EMG T_4/T_1.[45] Unfortunately, although the abductor digiti quinti clearly demonstrates a detectable response to ulnar nerve stimulation,[38,39] this response is prone to stimulus artifact[41] and its morphology is very sensitive to electrode positioning.

◆ MECHANOMYOGRAPHY

A mechanomyogram (MMG) measures the *evoked contractile response* of the stimulated muscle by force translation or accelerography. The classic MMG device, the *adductor pollicis force translation monitor*, employs a

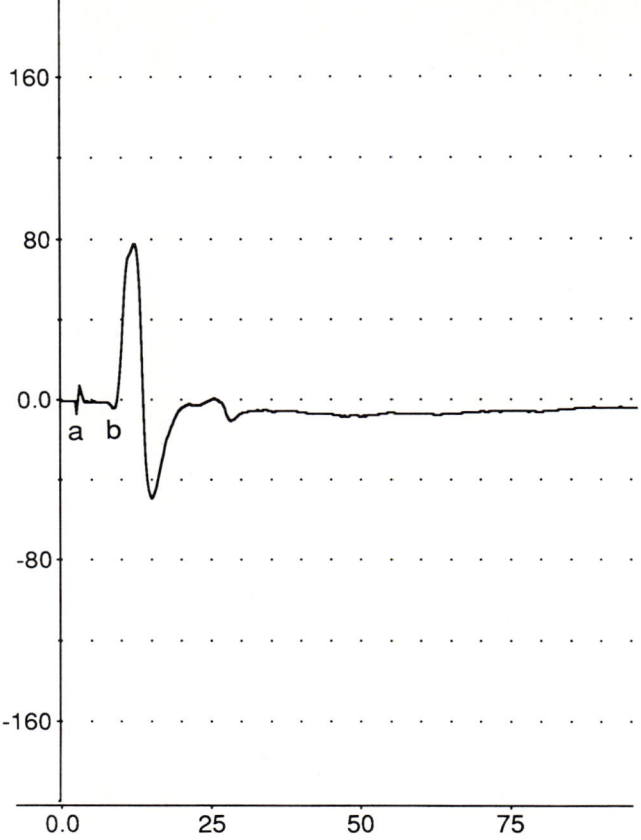

FIGURE 5-1 EMG tracing obtained in a healthy volunteer with a Quantum 84 monitor (Cadwell Laboratories, Kennewick, Wash.). Time (in milliseconds) is illustrated on the *x*-axis, compound muscle action potential (in millivolts) on the *y*-axis. *a* = stimulus artifact, *b* = onset of EMG response. Motor latency is provided by *b* minus *a*. Duration and morphology of the compound MAP are assessed during a gated window that encompasses the interval between the first deflection and the time when the MAP returns to the isoelectric line (time epoch). (Courtesy of Cadwell Laboratories, Kennewick, Wash.)

force transducer. The thumb is placed in a ring with a resting *preload of 200–300 gm,* in order to attain optimal muscle fiber stretch.[46,47] *Isometric contraction* of the adductor pollicis muscle in response to ulnar nerve stimulation is translated into an electrical signal that can be displayed on an interfaced pressure monitor and recorded. *Key features of adductor pollicis force translation* include: aligning the direction of thumb movement with the

TABLE 5-2
Relative Locations of Electrodes During Electromyographic Monitoring

Muscle	Site of Active Recording Electrode	Site of Reference Recording Electrode
Abductor digiti quinti	Medial aspect of hypothenar eminence	Fifth finger
Adductor pollicis	Thenar eminence	Anywhere on thumb
First dorsal interosseous	Dorsal groove between first finger and thumb	Base or proximal phalanx of index finger or thumb
Orbicularis oculi	Lateral brow	Middle of brow or inferior to eye
Diaphragm	8th or 9th intercostal space, anterior axillary line	8th or 9th intercostal space, midaxillary line
Flexor hallucis brevis	Medial plantar foot	Between active electrode and big toe

transducer and securing its position, applying a consistent amount of baseline tension, employing a transducer and monitor with adequate monitoring range, and zeroing the monitor before stimulation.

Instead of a force transducer, *accelerography* uses a miniature acceleration (piezoelectric) transducer to determine the *rate of angular acceleration* of the thumb (adductor pollicis muscle) in response to ulnar stimulation. This is based on the constant relationship (Newton's second law) between force and acceleration so long as mass is constant ($F = m \times a$). Clinical trials have indicated that accelerography provides T_4/T_1 ratios similar to those of force translation.[48-53] However, the accelerographic T_4/T_1 typically is greater than 1.0 in the absence of neuromuscular block; this may be attributable to thumb movement or to failure of the *unsecured thumb (without preload)* to return to its baseline position after the first of the four contractions of train-of-four.[54]

The *EMG and MMG* tend to detect similar degrees of block, but are not identical.[9,42-46,55-60] The differences between the T_4/T_1 ratio provided by EMG and by MMG primarily are due to the nature of what is monitored and, when different muscles are assessed, the responses of the given muscles to relaxant. The *MMG is influenced by the nature of muscle contraction.* The EMG focuses on electrical events; however, it, too, may be influenced by the preload tension provided by an adductor pollicis monitor.[46] The intertechnique differences are exaggerated when the EMG monitors a muscle with a different response to NDRs. For example, the abductor digiti quinti and orbicularis oculi are less sensitive to relaxant than is the adductor pollicis, and they demonstrate a faster time course.

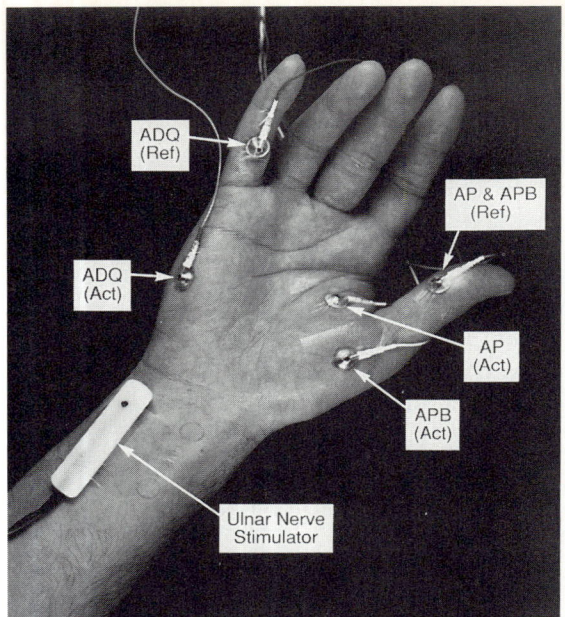
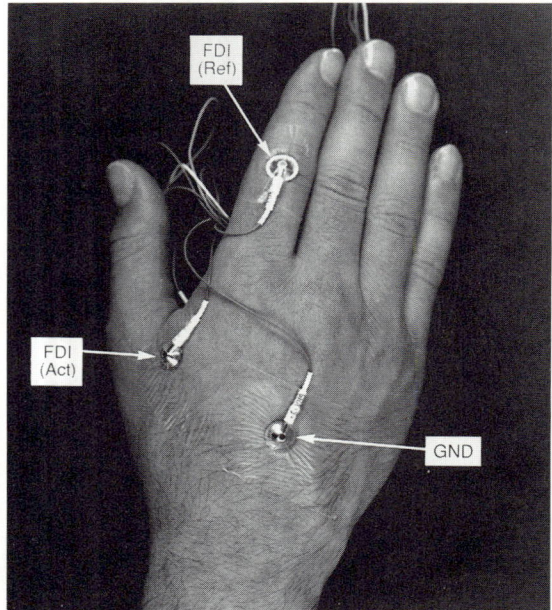

FIGURE 5-2 Example of electrode placement for electromyographic monitoring of responses to stimulation of the ulnar nerve on the (**A**) palmar and (**B**) dorsal surfaces of the hand. *Act* = active electrode, *Ref* = reference electrode, *ADQ* = abductor digiti quinti, *AP* = adductor pollicis, *APB* = abductor pollicis brevis, *FDI* = first dorsal interosseous.

The following illustrate the *varying relationships:*

1. During recovery from atracurium or vecuronium, an MMG T_4/T_1 of 0.70 at the adductor pollicis corresponded to an EMG T_4/T_1 of 0.90 at the abductor digiti quinti.[42,45,57]
2. When the EMG at the first dorsal interosseous was compared to the MMG at the adductor pollicis, virtually equal cutoffs were noted.[55]
3. Likewise, EMG and MMG T_4/T_1 ratios were nearly identical during general anesthesia with *d*-tubocurarine.[46]
4. The MMG and EMG of the adductor pollicis were similar during atracurium-induced block during nitrous-narcotic anesthesia,[43] but the MMG was found to be more sensitive than the EMG of the same muscle to an infusion of vecuronium.[58]
5. The MMG of the adductor pollicis was more sensitive than the thenar EMG to alcuronium.[59]
6. During metocurine-induced block, the MMG of the adductor pollicis was similar to the EMG of the first dorsal interosseous when resting tension was applied, but the *EMG suggested a greater degree of block* when performed without resting tension.[60]

Discussion Questions ◆

a. When T_4/T_1 is 0.5, is *fade* reliably detected *by visual or tactile* evaluation (without the aid of a mechanogram)?
b. Why might assessment of the *posttetanic count* be helpful during eye surgery or laser surgery on the vocal cords?
c. What is meant by the *"compound muscle action potential"*?
d. How might one be able to distinguish the *EMG* response to direct muscle stimulation from that of nerve-to-muscle transmission?
e. How do the *muscles of the hypothenar eminence* (e.g., abductor digiti quinti) *differ from the adductor pollicis* with respect to sensitivity to nondepolarizing relaxants?
f. Why do the *EMG* and *MMG* exhibit different responses to *dantrolene?*
g. Why might it be preferable to monitor the initial *fade* noted during response to *tetanic stimulation* as opposed to the amount of fade at the end of 5 seconds?
h. Will a *force transducer* with a maximum linear response of 2 kg provide accurate assessment of the response to *tetanus?* Why or why not?
i. Why might an *EMG* be more sensitive than an *MMG* to *tetanic fade?*
j. Compare the changes in heights of *MMG and EMG responses* during the course of 5-second, 50-Hz *tetanic stimulation* in the absence of neuromuscular block.
k. In the *unblocked NMJ*, why do we see *posttetanic "facilitation"* of the contractile response but not of the EMG response?

l. What is a *"gel bridge"* during *EMG monitoring?*
m. Describe the relative *locations* of the active recording electrode, reference electrode, and grounding electrode during *EMG monitoring.*
n. To what degree, if any, is the magnitude of the evoked twitch response affected by resting *thumb tension?*

Answers ◆

a. It has been reported that, when simply relying on visual or tactile evaluation, experienced observers do not reliably identify fade associated with an MMG T_4/T_1 ratio as low as 0.3.[1-11] This limitation has been partially overcome by newer means of assessment such as DBS,[4-6,61,62] since the fade of the sequential bursts of DBS is easier to detect than the fade between the first and fourth responses of train-of-four. It also has been shown that qualitative evaluation of fade was no better during tetanus.[12] Tetanic fade was detected reliably only when the tetanic fade ratio was ≤0.3.[12]

b. The *posttetanic count* may be particularly helpful during surgery in which any muscle movement is unacceptable. Because the diaphragm and laryngeal adductor muscles are less sensitive to relaxants than the adductor pollicis muscle, ablation of the single twitch at the adductor pollicis does not necessarily guarantee absence of *coughing or cord movement.* To more reliably ensure absence of all movement, the PTC should be zero.[17] During narcotic-relaxant anesthesia, one of 25 and five of 25 patients coughed mildly in response to carinal stimulation when the PTC was reduced to 0 and 1, respectively, whereas 23 of 25 coughed when response to single twitch stimulation (without preceding tetanic stimulation) was still evident.[17]

c. The *compound muscle action potential* is the cumulative signal that is generated by the individual MAPs that are produced by the individual muscle fibers of the muscle under study.

d. If the muscle were stimulated directly, the *EMG* would show an abnormally short *latency* between the stimulus artifact and the MAP. The normal latency for hypothenar muscles is approximately 9 msec on ulnar stimulation at the elbow and 4–5 msec from the wrist, with a typical conduction velocity of 53 m · sec^{-1}.[36,63] For intraoperative monitoring, the EMG typically is gated to integrate the signal from 3 msec after the stimulus artifact to approximately 16 msec after the stimulus artifact.

e. The muscles of the *hypothenar eminence* (e.g., abductor digiti quinti) are *more resistant* to NDRs than the *adductor pollicis,* and they tend to recover faster (Chap. 3). In a study of seven volunteers receiving vecuronium, when respiratory function returned to normal, the MMG T_4/T_1 of the adductor pollicis was >0.5, but the EMG T_4/T_1 of the hypothenar muscle was >0.90.[45] Thus, the *muscles of the hypothenar eminence more closely resemble those of the larynx and diaphragm.*

f. *Dantrolene* affects muscle contraction (by modulation of Ca^{2+} levels responsible for myofibril contraction) but does not affect the nerve or NMJ. Hence, the *EMG* remains normal while the *MMG* becomes depressed.[64]

g. There are two major reasons why it may be preferable to monitor the *initial fade of a tetanic response:* (1) The tetanic stimulus promotes mobilization of ACh and may cause *"recovery during tetanus"*; the resulting fade pattern that is noted after the initial decline from peak tetanic tension (termed "pseudofade") may lead to underestimation of the degree of fade.[65] (2) Force transducers are sensitive to the thumb repositioning that might occur during peak contraction, and thus subsequent assessments may be distorted.

h. A transducer with a maximum linear response of 2 kg will underestimate the force of a tetanic response in a large number of cases. In the absence of neuromuscular blocking agents, *peak tetanic tension* commonly is in excess of 5–10 kg,[66,67] averaging 7.1 ± 2.2 kg in one such study.[67] Thus, peak tetanic tension will be underestimated, and fade (e.g., from 10 kg to 2 kg) might not be appreciated.[66] Furthermore, such forces may damage a transducer that is not designed to withstand them. *Transducer overload* should be suspected when the maximal recorded tetanic force is less than 2 to 3 times twitch tension.[65]

i. During *tetanic stimulation,* the *EMG fade response* may be more sensitive than the *MMG fade response.* The contractile response summates to overcome elastic forces, reaching a maximum at 350 msec. Hence, the MMG response might transiently continue to increase despite a decrease in end-plate potentials and a possible decrease in the generation of MAPs (which results in fade of the EMG response).[65] Alternatively, muscle fatigue would impact on the MMG.

j. Over the time course of 5-second, 50-Hz *tetanic stimulation* in the unblocked setting, the *EMG maintains a response of constant magnitude.* Because the MAP and subsequent refractory period of hand muscles last 5–10 msec, the individual EMG responses may be identified even for frequencies exceeding 100 Hz (so long as the EMG is gated accordingly). In contrast, because the *contractile response may last for 150 msec,* stimulation at 7–10 Hz may result in *summated contractile tension.* The *MMG response increases to a plateau* (asymptote) as elastic forces are overcome.

k. The "stretching" that results from the *overcoming of elastic forces* in response to tetanic stimulation actually persists for several seconds after cessation of tetanus, such that a single twitch may evoke an *exaggerated posttetanic contractile response.* This amplification of the posttetanic MMG response (but not EMG response) despite absence of nondepolarizing block may also be due to summation of contraction in response to repetitive posttetanic firing. These responses are different from the posttetanic facilitation that is noted in the presence of nondepolarizing block. In the latter cases, the tetanic stimulus causes mobilization of ACh, which can then compete more effectively with the NDR (Chap. 4).

l. A *gel bridge* occurs when electrode gel spreads to cover the skin between two electrodes. This will lead to decreased neurostimulation and smaller evoked responses.

m. The *active recording electrode* should be placed above the end-plate region, which typically is near the middle of the muscle. The *reference recording electrode* should be placed at a site devoid of significant muscle activity (e.g., a tendon). The grounding electrode is most often placed midway between the stimulating and recording electrodes (Table 5-2).

n. The *height of the evoked twitch response* is influenced by the resting *preload*, especially between 50 and 200 gm. At 50, 100, 200, and 300 gm, the developed tensions were 313, 371, 400, and 410 gm, respectively.[47]

The presence of preload may also influence the EMG. In the presence of 250–300 gm of thumb preload, the determined ED_{95} for metocurine and tubocurarine were higher than ED_{95} values obtained without preload; i.e., *as for the MMG, in the absence of preload the EMG tended to overestimate sensitivity to neuromuscular block.* This may be attributable simply to technical changes as a result of altered distances between recording electrodes and the underlying muscles.[46,60]

References ◆

1. Bevan DR, Smith CE, Donati F: Postoperative neuromuscular blockade: a comparison between atracurium, vecuronium, and pancuronium. Anesthesiology 69:272–276, 1988
2. Beemer GH, Rozenthal P: Postoperative neuromuscular function. Anaesth Intensive Care 14:41–45, 1986
3. Brull SJ, Silverman DG: Visual assessment of train-of-four and double burst-induced fade at submaximal stimulating currents. Anesth Analg 73:627–632, 1991
4. Brull SJ, Silverman DG: Visual and tactile assessment of neuromuscular fade. Anesth Analg 77:352–355, 1993
5. Drenck NE, Ueda N, Olsen NV, Engbaek J, Jensen E, Skovgaard LT, Viby-Mogensen J: Manual evaluation of residual curarization using double burst stimulation: a comparison with train-of-four. Anesthesiology 70:578–581, 1989
6. Gill SS, Donati F, Bevan DR: Clinical evaluation of double-burst stimulation: its relationship to train-of-four stimulation. Anaesthesia 45:543–548, 1990
7. Lennmarken C, Lofstrom JB: Partial curarization in the postoperative period. Acta Anaesthesiol Scand 28:260–262, 1984
8. Pedersen T, Viby-Mogensen J, Bang U, Olsen NV, Jensen E, Engbaek J: Does perioperative tactile evaluation of the train-of-four response influence the frequency of postoperative residual neuromuscular blockade? Anesthesiology 73:835–839, 1990
9. Tammisto T, Wirtavuori K, Linko K: Assessment of neuromuscular block: comparison of three clinical methods and evoked electromyography. Eur J Anaesthesiol 5:1–8, 1988
10. Viby-Mogensen J, Jensen NH, Engbaek J, Ording H, Skovgaard LT, Chraemmer-Jorgen-

sen B: Tactile and visual evaluation of the response to train-of-four nerve stimulation. Anesthesiology 63:440–443, 1985
11. Viby-Mogensen J, Jorgensen BC, Ording H: Residual curarization in the recovery room. Anesthesiology 50:539–541, 1979
12. Dupuis JY, Martin R, Tessonnier JM, Tetrault JP: Clinical assessment of the muscular response to tetanic nerve stimulation. Can J Anaesth 37:397–400, 1990
13. Kopman AF: Tactile evaluation of train-of-four count as an indicator of reliability of antagonism of vecuronium- or atracurium-induced neuromuscular blockade. Anesthesiology 75:588–593, 1991
14. Bonsu AK, Viby-Mogensen J, Fernando PUE, Muchhal A, Tamilarasan A, Lambourne A: Relationship of post-tetanic count and train-of-four response during intense neuromuscular blockade caused by atracurium. Br J Anaesth 59:1089–1092, 1987
15. Engbaek J, Ostergaard D, Skovgaard LT, Viby-Mogensen J: Reversal of intense neuromuscular blockade following infusion of atracurium. Anesthesiology 72:803–806, 1990
16. Eriksson LI, Lennmarken C, Staun P, Viby-Mogensen J: Use of post-tetanic count in assessment of a repetitive vecuronium-induced neuromuscular block. Br J Anaesth 65:487–493, 1990
17. Fernando PUE, Viby-Mogensen J, Bonsu AK, Tamilarasan A, Muchhal KK, Lambourne A: Relationship between posttetanic count and response to carinal stimulation during vecuronium-induced neuromuscular blockade. Acta Anaesthesiol Scand 31:593–596, 1987
18. Gwinnutt CL, Meakin G: Use of the post-tetanic count to monitor recovery from intense neuromuscular blockade in children. Br J Anaesth 61:547–550, 1988
19. Gwinnutt CL, Walker RWM, Meakin G: Antagonism of intense atracurium-induced neuromuscular block in children. Br J Anaesth 67:13–16, 1991
20. Howardy-Hansen P, Viby-Mogensen J, Gottschau A, Skovgaard LT, Chraemmer-Jorgensen B, Engbaek J: Tactile evaluation of the posttetanic count (PTC). Anesthesiology 60:372–374, 1984
21. Muchhal KK, Viby-Mogensen J, Fernando PUE, Tamilarasan A, Bonsu AK, Lambourne A: Evaluation of intense neuromuscular blockade caused by vecuronium using posttetanic count (PTC). Anesthesiology 66:846–849, 1987
22. Ridley SA, Braude N: Post-tetanic count and intense neuromuscular blockade with vecuronium in children. Br J Anaesth 61:551–556, 1988
23. Torda TA, Graham GG, Tsui D: Neuromuscular sensitivity to atracurium in humans. Anaesth Intensive Care 18:62–68, 1990
24. Viby-Mogensen J, Howardy-Hansen P, Chraemmer-Jorgensen B, Ording H, Engbaek J, Nielsen A: Posttetanic count (PTC): a new method of evaluating an intense nondepolarizing neuromuscular blockade. Anesthesiology 55:458–461, 1981
25. Brown GL, von Euler US: The after effects of a tetanus on mammalian muscle. J Physiol 93:39–60, 1938
26. Wali FA, Bradshaw EG, Suer AH: Clinical assessment of neuromuscular blockade produced by vecuronium using twitch, train of four, tetanus and post-tetanic twitch responses of the adductor pollicis muscle. Acta Anaesthesiol Belg 39:35–42, 1988
27. Brull SJ, Connelly NR, O'Connor TZ, Silverman DG: Effect of tetanus on subsequent neuromuscular monitoring in patients receiving vecuronium. Anesthesiology 74:64–70, 1991
28. Silverman DG, Brull SJ: The effect of a tetanic stimulus on the response to subsequent tetanic stimulation. Anesth Analg 76:1284–1287, 1993
29. Eriksson LI, Viby-Mogensen J, Lennmarken C: The effect of peripheral hypothermia on a vecuronium-induced neuromuscular block. Acta Anaesthesiol Scand 35:387–392, 1991
30. Braude N, Vyvyan HAL, Jordan MJ: Intraoperative assessment of atracurium-induced neuromuscular block using double burst stimulation. Br J Anaesth 67:574–578, 1991
31. O'Hara DA, Fragen RJ, Shanks CA: Reappearance of the train-of-four after neuromuscular blockade induced with tubocurarine, vecuronium or atracurium. Br J Anaesth 58:1296–1299, 1986
32. Gibson FM, Mirakhur RK, Clarke RSJ, Brady MM: Quantification of train-of-four responses during recovery of block from non-depolarising muscle relaxants. Acta Anaesthesiol Scand 31:655–657, 1987

33. Mirakur RK, Gibson FM, Clarke RSJ, Brady MM: Monitoring of neuromuscular block with atracurium, vecuronium, pancuronium and *d*-tubocurarine using train-of-four stimulation. Anesthesiology 65:A110, 1986
34. O'Hara DA, Fragen RJ, Shanks CA: Comparison of visual and measured train-of-four recovery after vecuronium induced neuromuscular blockade using two anaesthetic techniques. Br J Anaesth 58:1300–1302, 1986
35. Pugh ND, Kay B, Healy TEJ: Electromyography in anaesthesia: a comparison between two methods. Anaesthesia 39:574–577, 1984
36. Kalli I: Effect of surface electrode position on the compound action potential evoked by ulnar nerve stimulation during isoflurane anaesthesia. Br J Anaesth 65:494–499, 1990
37. Williams PL, Warwick R, Dyson M, Bannister LH: Gray's Anatomy, 37th ed. Edinburgh, Churchill Livingstone, 1993, pp 1133–1137
38. Halevy J, Brull SJ, Booke J, Garcia R, Silverman DG: Dual innervation of hand muscles: potential influence on monitoring of neuromuscular blockade. Anesthesiology 75:A814, 1991
39. Brull SJ, Garcia RM, Halevy J, Booke J, Silverman DG: Comparative EMG responses during ulnar nerve stimulation. Anesthesiology 77:A566, 1992
40. Kalli I: Optimal electrode site on the hand for evoked EMG monitoring. Anesthesiology 73:A911, 1990
41. Kalli I: Effect of surface electrode positioning on the compound action potential evoked by ulnar nerve stimulation in anaesthetized infants and children. Br J Anaesth 62:188–193, 1989
42. Kopman AF: The relationship of evoked electromyographic and mechanical responses following atracurium in humans. Anesthesiology 63:208–211, 1985
43. Ali HH, DeCesare R: Evoked EMG, integrated EMG (IEMG) and mechanical response. Anesthesiology 71:A396, 1989
44. Katz RL: Electromyographic and mechanical effects of suxamethonium and tubocurarine on twitch, tetanic and post-tetanic responses. Br J Anaesth 45:849–859, 1973
45. Dupuis JY, Martin R, Tétrault JP: Clinical, electrical and mechanical correlations during recovery from neuromuscular blockade with vecuronium. Can J Anaesth 37:192–196, 1990
46. Kopman AF: The effect of resting muscle tension on the dose-effect relationship of *d*-tubocurarine: does preload influence the evoked EMG? Anesthesiology 69:1003–1005, 1988
47. Donlon JV, Savarese JJ, Ali HH: Cumulative dose-response curves for gallamine: effect of altered resting thumb tension and mode of stimulation. Anesth Analg 58:377–381, 1979
48. May O, Kirkegaard-Nielson H, Werner MU: The acceleration transducer—an assessment of its precision in comparison with a force displacement transducer. Acta Anaesthesiol Scand 32:239–243, 1988
49. Ueda N, Muteki T, Poulsen A, Espensen JL: Clinical assessment of a new neuromuscular transmission monitoring system (Accelograph[R]). J Anesth 3:90–93, 1989
50. Viby-Mogensen J, Jensen E, Werner M, Nielsen HK: Measurement of acceleration: a new method of monitoring neuromuscular function. Acta Anaesthesiol Scand 32:45–48, 1988
51. Werner MU: A methods-comparison study of acceleration, EMG and force responses during recovery from a non-depolarizing block in children. Anesthesiology 73:A911, 1990
52. Werner MU: Monitoring of neuromuscular transmission in infants and children: a comparison between an acceleration responsive transducer and a force displacement transducer. Anesthesiology 69:A474, 1988
53. Werner MU, Kierkegaard-Nielsen H, May O, Djernes M: Assessment of neuromuscular transmission by the evoked acceleration response: an evaluation of the accuracy of the acceleration transducer in comparison with a force displacement transducer. Acta Anaesthesiol Scand 32:395–400, 1988
54. Silverman DG, Connelly NR, O'Connor TZ, Garcia RM, Brull SJ: Accelographic train-of-four fade at near-threshold currents. Anesthesiology 76:34–38, 1992
55. Engbaek J, Ostergaard D, Viby-Mogensen J, Skovgaard LT: Clinical recovery and train-of-four ratio measured mechanically and electromyographically following atracurium. Anesthesiology 71:391–395, 1989
56. Eon B, Blache JL, Aknin P, Francois G: Quantitative comparisons of evoked electromyo-

graphic and mechanical responses of the adductor pollicis muscle during a regional neuromuscular blockade technique with vecuronium. Anesthesiology 69:A469, 1988
57. Weber S, Muravchick S: Electrical and mechanical train-of-four responses during depolarizing and nondepolarizing neuromuscular blockade. Anesth Analg 65:771–776, 1986
58. Hyman SA, Berman ML, Rogers WD, Smith DW: Electrical versus mechanical assessment of neuromuscular blockade during vecuronium infusion. Anesth Analg 68:S130, 1989
59. Meretoja OA, Werner MU, Wirtavuori K, Luosto T: Comparison of thumb acceleration and thenar EMG in a pharmacodynamic study of alcuronium. Acta Anaesthesiol Scand 33:545–548, 1989
60. Kopman AF: The dose-effect relationship of metocurine: the integrated electromyogram of the first dorsal interosseous muscle and the mechanomyogram of the adductor pollicis compared. Anesthesiology 68:604–607, 1988
61. Engbaek J, Ostergaard D, Viby-Mogensen J: Double burst stimulation (DBS): a new pattern of nerve stimulation to identify residual neuromuscular block. Br J Anaesth 62:274–278, 1989
62. Ueda N, Viby-Mogensen J, Olsen NV, Drenck NE, Tsuda H, Muteki T: The best choice of double burst stimulation pattern for manual evaluation of neuromuscular transmission. J Anesth 3:94–99, 1989
63. Eaton LM, Lambert EH: Electromyography and electric stimulation of nerves in diseases of motor unit: observations on myasthenic syndrome associated with malignant tumors. JAMA 163:1117–1124, 1957
64. Flewellen EH, Nelson TE, Jones WP, Arens JF, Wagner DL: Dantrolene dose-response in awake man: implications for management of malignant hyperthermia. Anesthesiology 59:275–280, 1983
65. Epstein RA, Epstein RM: The electromyogram and the mechanical response of indirectly stimulated muscle in anesthetized man following curarization. Anesthesiology 38:212–223, 1973
66. Freund FG, Merati JK: A source of errors in assessing neuromuscular blockade. Anesthesiology 39:540–542, 1973
67. Stanec A, Heyduk J, Stanec G, Orkin LR: Tetanic fade and post-tetanic tension in the absence of neuromuscular blocking agents in anesthetized man. Anesth Analg 57:102–107, 1978

6

DAVID G. SILVERMAN

Requirements for Relaxation and Recovery in the Perioperative ICU Settings: Responses to Neurostimulation and Clinical Signs

No single form of assessment is ideal for monitoring the response to and recovery from neuromuscular blocking agents in intraoperative, postoperative, and ICU settings. Within each of these settings, requirements differ, and the relevance of evoked responses and clinical signs also varies.

◆ MONITORING RELAXATION INTRAOPERATIVELY

Anesthesiologists most commonly rely on assessments of thumb adduction in response to ulnar nerve stimulation in order to supplement their clinical impression as to the adequacy of relaxation for tracheal intubation, surgical intervention, and subsequent recovery. Stimulating patterns and means of assessment are detailed in Chapters 3 through 5. The following addresses perioperative requirements.

Adequate conditions for *tracheal intubation* generally are obtained when there is 90–95% depression of the adductor pollicis response to single twitch stimulation of the ulnar nerve at 0.1 Hz. So long as a dose sufficient to block the vocal cords and diaphragm is administered (e.g., $\geq 2 \times$ the ED_{95} at the adductor pollicis [Chap. 3]), relaxation of the airway musculature typically is adequate by the time this degree of adductor pollicis twitch depression is attained. If any movement (e.g., coughing) would be intolerable, then one may seek to confirm a deeper level of block with ablation of the response to single twitch, tetanic stimulation, and posttetanic count at the adductor pollicis. One also may seek to confirm ablation of responses of the abductor digiti quinti muscle (in response to ulnar nerve stimulation) or at the orbicularis oculi muscle (in response to facial nerve stimulation), since, like the diaphragm, these muscles have relatively decreased sensitivity to relaxants (Chap. 3).

Intraoperatively, 75–95% *depression of adductor pollicis twitch height* typically is associated with adequate *abdominal relaxation*,[1-9] especially if an inhalational anesthetic has been used. If total paralysis is required (e.g., for laser surgery on the vocal cords), then a deeper level of block should be confirmed as described above.

Readiness for reversal will depend primarily on which relaxant has been given and whether or not recovery from it is compromised. When *normal recovery is under way* for a given relaxant, then we can count the responses to train-of-four stimulation and assess the T_4/T_1 ratio (or the D_2/D_1 ratio of double-burst stimulation) (Chaps. 4 and 5). As a general rule of thumb, I withhold reversal agent until there is at least one response to train-of-four stimulation during recovery from a short-acting nondepolarizing relaxant (NDR) such as mivacurium, at least one or two responses during recovery from an NDR of intermediate duration, and at least two to three responses during recovery from an NDR of long duration (Chap. 15).

Adequacy of *recovery and/or reversal* (i.e., "readiness for extubation") typically is assessed by monitoring the T_4/T_1 ratio (or the D_2/D_1 ratio) and evaluating clinical signs. It is generally believed that a T_4/T_1 ratio greater than 0.70 at the adductor pollicis muscle is required for *adequate recovery* (see below).[10-12] However, it should be remembered that "the thumb twitch is an artificial contraction elicited by electric shocks. Respiratory movement, by contrast, results from tetanic volleys of nerve impulses of variable frequency. . . ."[8] The relationship of T_4/T_1 to clinical signs is described in the following discussion of clinical parameters.

Tidal volume (VT) is a relatively insensitive indicator of neuromuscular block. It typically remains near normal until there is detectable twitch height depression (i.e., ≥75% receptor occlusion), a decrease in T_4/T_1 to less than 0.6,[13] and markedly decreased grip strength.[14] Provided that upper airway integrity is maintained, *end-tidal* CO_2[15] and the ventilatory response to CO_2[16] are relatively unaffected by residual block; a relatively small fraction of maximal diaphragmatic function is needed for a near-normal VT. It appears that weakened respiratory muscles are able to sustain the normal respiratory cycle with "relative ease" (in agreement with normal pressure-volume relationships), but that "the same weakened muscles may be unable to generate sufficient force to handle mechanical challenges such as coughing and vomiting"[17] or to maintain airway patency.

Vital capacity (VC) is more sensitive to partial neuromuscular block than either VT or twitch height and is a better indicator of coughing ability.[13] More than 30 years ago it was established that the VC should be ≥20% of normal (≥15 mL · kg^{-1}) for sustained adequate ventilation by the patient with respiratory insufficiency who was maintained on mechanical ventilation.[18] Following general anesthesia with relaxant, a T_4/T_1 ratio of 0.7 corresponded to a VC of 17 mL · kg^{-1} [19] (vs. 59 mL · kg^{-1} in unmedicated volunteers[13]). However, although it is more sensitive than VT, VC is less sensitive to residual block than other parameters. A near-normal VC was attained when diaphragmatic "strength" was less than 45% of normal, hand grip was only 18% of baseline, and a few subjects were unable to swallow.[15,20] In another study, VC was 66% ± 3% of control, while inspiratory and expiratory pressures decreased to an average of 39% ± 2% of control, and hand grip strength and ability to sustain head lift for 5 seconds were abolished in volunteers receiving *d*-tubocurarine.[17]

Maximum inspiratory pressure (MIP)[13,15] is a measure of the pressure (typically expressed as –cm H_2O) generated by deep inspiration in a closed system. In the absence of neuromuscular weakness, this value may reach –100 cm H_2O. MIP is more sensitive to neuromuscular block than VT or VC, being compromised at less than 50% receptor occupancy. The MIP can be depressed to as low as 25% of normal despite a normal VT.[15] In healthy volunteers receiving *d*-tubocurarine to achieve a T_4/T_1 ratio of 0.6, MIP was ≤70% of the control value, while VC and expiratory flow rate were ≥90% of control.[13] Similarly, respiratory function was maintained and forced expiratory volume and forced vital capacity remained within 80% of baseline when MIP was decreased by 50%.[21] *Maximum expiratory pressure (MEP)* likewise is a sensitive indicator of respiratory function and coughing ability.[22]

More than 20 years ago it was reported that an MIP >–30 cm H_2O (30% of control) was required for effective weaning of patients who received mechanical ventilation because of respiratory insufficiency.[18,23] Following general anesthesia with relaxants in American Society of Anesthesiologists (ASA) class III–IV patients, a T_4/T_1 above 0.7 was associated with an MIP ≥ –22 cm H_2O.[19] Originally felt to be adequate,[19,24] an MIP of this magnitude may not be sufficient to prevent aspiration of gastric contents or airway obstruction (Table 6-1).[15,17] Pavlin[20] recommends an MIP of ≥ –50 cm H_2O as one predictor of airway adequacy. Admittedly, in clinical practice, we often settle for lesser values while remaining cognizant of the potential need for airway support.

Head lift has long been recommended as an important indicator of readiness for tracheal extubation.[25,26] Ability to maintain head lift for 5 seconds typically is associated with an ability to sustain tetanus at 50 Hz for 5 seconds and a T_4/T_1 ratio ≥0.8.[12,27–29] These values usually are indicative of an ability to generate a VC, inspiratory flow rate, expiratory flow rate, and maximum voluntary ventilation that are ≥90% of control.[28–31] An ability to sustain head lift also has been associated with an MIP >50% of control and an ability to perform airway protective maneuvers.[15] Head lift generally cannot be maintained when the T_4/T_1 ratio is less than 0.5 and/or MIP is markedly decreased[15,27,31] (see Table 6-1).

Hand grip also may be very sensitive,[14–16,31–34] but quantification re-

TABLE 6-1
Relationships Among Clinical Signs in Healthy Awake Volunteers Receiving Low Doses of Tubocurarine

Parameter	Maximum Inspiratory Pressure (cm H_2O)
Control (no relaxant)	−90
Head lift, 5 sec	−53
Leg lift, 5 sec	−50
Effective swallowing	−42
Patent airway without jaw lift	−39
Glottic closure against Valsalva to an esophageal pressure of +30 cm H_2O	−30
Vital capacity > 33% of control	−20

Data in the table are derived from Pavlin et al.[15] The authors noted that every subject who could perform a head lift or leg lift could successfully perform the tests of airway protection.

quires the use of a hand dynamometer. In supine healthy volunteers receiving slow administration (3-mg increments, then infusion) of *d*-tubocurarine, hand grip decreased to less than 40% of baseline when the MIP was 70% of baseline and the VC was above 90% of baseline;[15] hand grip was unobtainable when VC was still 40% of control[15] (approximately 2.0 L) and end-tidal CO_2 was normal (although the mandible may have been elevated by an investigator to maintain upper airway patency). After 12 mg of *d*-tubocurarine in healthy volunteers, hand grip decreased from 40 kg to 5 kg, while VC decreased only slightly (from 4.8 to 4.1 L).[33]

Leg lift, the ability to lift both legs off the table, is almost as difficult as head lift.[15] It is a helpful sign in infants, where it was associated with an MIP above −32 cm H_2O following reversal of paralysis at the conclusion of general anesthesia.[35]

Thus, head or leg lift and hand grip typically provide relatively sensitive indicators of the adequacy of neuromuscular function. However, although these are relatively conservative means of assessment in most settings, *head lift, leg lift, and hand grip occasionally "overestimate"* other indices; i.e., they do not always indicate sustained tetanus or a T_4/T_1 above 0.70,[29,36-40] and they do not always indicate adequate clinical function.[41,42] Head lift was less sensitive than tetanus at identifying a degree of block that was associated with a decreased VC and decreased maximum voluntary ventilation.[29] Despite well-sustained head lift following antagonism of pancuronium-induced block, 50% of patients reported diplopia and MEP was depressed by almost 40%.[41] In another study, seven of 21 patients with a T_4/T_1 ratio below 0.70 in the PACU nevertheless were able to sustain head lift.[40] It has been proposed that an arm lift test (maintaining the elbow elevated off the bed for >60 seconds) would be more discerning,[43] especially in patients with abdominal, neck, and chest pain. Hand grip was a less sensitive indicator of residual block than the swallowing reflex following pancuronium, 0.02 mg · kg^{-1}; this finding and associated electromyographic (EMG) results suggest that at least some of the upper airway muscles that are responsible for pharyngeal patency are more sensitive than hand muscles to NDRs.[42] Thus, one must remain aware of the potential for airway compromise.

It traditionally has been believed that *sustained tetanus*[29] or a T_4/T_1 >0.7[1,13,19] is associated with recovery of neuromuscular function that is adequate to allow *extubation of the trachea* in the absence of underlying disease. Awake volunteers who received low doses of *d*-tubocurarine until a T_4/T_1 ratio of 0.6 was reached had less than a 10% decrease in VC or peak expiratory flow rate (PEFR).[13] At T_4/T_1 ratios of 0.6, 0.7, 0.8, and 1.0, the VC was 55, 57, 60, and 59 mL · kg^{-1}, and the PEFR was 450, 445, 480, and 485 L · min^{-1},[13] respectively. Even after anesthesia, it has been reported that this "cutoff" typically is associated with a near-normal VT, a VC >15–20 mL · kg^{-1}, an MIP > –20 to –25 cm H$_2$O, ability to cough, and/or ability to maintain head lift.[1,12,19,30,44] In ASA class III patients recovering from major surgery, tracheal extubation when T_4/T_1 was above 0.80 was associated with "adequate" values for these parameters.[19] However, as noted above and elaborated on below, these values do not ensure airway patency and ventilatory adequacy.

◆ LIMITATIONS OF MONITORING AND ASSESSMENTS

Confidence in the above measurements may not always be totally justified for a number of reasons:

1. It may be difficult to compare data from different studies even if they all were obtained in nonsedated healthy volunteers. Such studies may differ with respect to type of relaxant, rate of infusion, patient position (e.g., supine vs. seated), the use of a mouthpiece for breathing tests, criteria for providing airway support, etc.
2. Although many patients have no clinical signs of weakness when T_4/T_1 = 0.7 at the adductor pollicis, others may exhibit neuromuscular weakness at ratios of 0.8–0.9[27,36]; e.g., in some patients, head lift may not be maintained unless T_4/T_1 is above 0.9.[36]
3. Alternatively, the T_4/T_1 ratio may be spuriously low in the presence of peripheral cooling, and clinical function may be adequate (Chap. 10).
4. Assessments of neuromuscular function are complicated by the fact that *mechanomyographic (MMG) and EMG indices may differ*. The MMG T_4/T_1 ratio at the adductor pollicis often is more sensitive to mild degrees of block than is the EMG T_4/T_1 ratio at the hypothenar eminence (Chap. 5). Following subparalyzing doses of vecuronium in conscious volunteers, the adductor pollicis MMG T_4/T_1 ratio associated with nor-

mal tests of ventilatory function was 0.50, while the EMG T_4/T_1 ratio at the hypothenar muscles was 0.90[44]

5. *A near-normal VT, VC, or PEFR does not ensure near-normal neuromuscular function.* Although VC and PEFR remained above 90% of control in volunteers receiving d-tubocurarine until a T_4/T_1 ratio of 0.6 was reached, MIP decreased to 69.3% ± 9.5% (SEM) of control at a T_4/T_1 of 0.6 and to 82.6% ± 9.6% at a T_4/T_1 of 0.7.[13] Furthermore, the ability to cough may be compromised at degrees of paralysis that cause virtually no change in flow rates.[22]

6. Even when established "cutoffs" are attained, the aforementioned *clinical criteria do not guarantee adequate ventilatory function or airway protection.* The criteria (for VC and MIP) that were established more than 25 years ago for "adequate respiratory function"[18] may not be wholly applicable to the patient with neuromuscular block. As noted in Table 6-1, a VC that is 33% of control and an MIP of −20 to −25 cm H_2O do not ensure effective ability to "protect one's airway" by being able to swallow, perform a Valsalva maneuver, or prevent airway obstruction.[15] Furthermore, it has been shown that a 20–25% decrease in MIP, VC, and MEP may be accompanied by a doubling of upper *airway resistance* (after 12 mg of d-tubocurarine administered to awake volunteers).[33] This may be attributable to effects on the *pharyngeal muscles* and tongue. Despite adequate diaphragmatic strength, neck and pharyngeal muscle weakness may be pronounced during recovery from tubocurarine-induced paralysis.[14,17,20,45] The masseter and neighboring upper airway muscles may be affected to the same or greater degree by NDRs as the adductor pollicis,[46] and the muscles required for effective swallowing may be even more sensitive.[42] Additionally, other respiratory muscles (e.g., intercostal, abdominal) may be more sensitive than the diaphragm[47] to muscle relaxants. These effects may combine to compromise airway integrity and ventilatory function in the partially relaxed subject.

Clearly, *a T_4/T_1 cutoff value* at which neuromuscular function is considered to be clinically adequate is arbitrary, and it does not hold true in all patients after all relaxants. The problems of using such a cutoff are compounded in the setting of general anesthesia and surgery. Anesthetized patients responded to as little as 0.5 mg of pancuronium with a decreased VT and an increased P_{CO_2}.[48] During *enflurane anesthesia,* after reversal of a long-acting NDR (pipecuronium) the T_4/T_1 ratio was 0.88, but T_1 had returned to only 75% of baseline.[49] This was attributed to enflurane-induced depression of muscle contractility.[49,50]

Residual effects of inhalational agents, as well as narcotics[51,52] and surgery itself, may compromise ventilation and airway protection even further. Postoperatively, the ventilatory function achieved at given levels of T_4/T_1

depression does not necessarily reach that noted in awake healthy volunteers.[19,48] Pharyngeal protective reflexes often are compromised for 2 or more hours after anesthesia even without relaxants.[53]

The aforementioned factors contribute to the *10–30% incidence of residual block* (clinical weakness and/or T_4/T_1 <0.70) noted on testing in the postanesthesia care unit, especially in patients who received long-acting relaxants.[36–40,54,55] The potential for morbidity is real. Ventilatory depression is an important cause of anesthesia-related mortality and morbidity; the presence of residual block is an important factor.[56,57] In a report of 32 deaths (attributable solely to anesthesia) within 6 days of surgery, 11 were attributed to postoperative ventilatory failure and, in 6 of the 11, neuromuscular block was considered a contributory factor.[58]

◆ MONITORING RELAXATION IN THE ICU

The adequacy of relaxation to facilitate mechanical ventilation in intensive care settings depends on the requirements (or perceived requirements) for a given case. Even within centers, opinions differ as to the degrees of paralysis that are required (or if any paralysis is required at all). Except in the most extreme circumstances, even partial paralysis should be accompanied by *sedation* and, if indicated, *analgesia*. Although not necessarily applicable to all situations, the following points should be borne in mind:

1. Relaxants should not be administered without appropriate monitoring (described below).
2. In many settings, it may be advisable to maintain some neuromuscular function. The desired degree of paralysis usually may be obtained without abolishing spontaneous inspiratory activity.[59,60] In addition to maintaining muscle training, this degree of relaxation should enable the patient to communicate pain, and it may provide a margin of safety (in case of a ventilator disconnect). Alternatively, there may be situations where spontaneous ventilation should be prevented, so as to optimize the effectiveness of mechanical ventilation, limit energy expenditure, or minimize ventilation-induced barotrauma and cardiopulmonary disturbances.[61–64] This degree of paralysis should be maintained for as brief a period as possible.
3. Repeated dosing adjustments may be required, especially for a drug with the potential for a cumulative effect.[65–67]
4. Long-term administration of NDRs may lead to accumulation of active metabolites, especially in patients with organ dysfunction (Chap. 11).
5. Long-term paralysis with NDRs has been associated with disuse atrophy and myopathies (Chap. 11).
6. High doses of certain relaxants may alter cardiovascular and respiratory

function and lead to accumulation of products with potential systemic effects (Chap. 11).

Careful monitoring of neuromuscular function and appropriate titration of relaxant are critical if one is to minimize the likelihood of excessively prolonged paralysis and/or development of a subsequent myopathy. Dosage should be tailored to clinical parameters (e.g., inspiratory pressures) and depth of block should be assessed periodically (at least hourly) with a nerve stimulator. The degree of block associated with 80–90% depression of the adductor pollicis twitch response typically is sufficient so long as adequate sedation and analgesia are provided. If a means of quantifying twitch depression is not available, this degree of relaxation may be approximated by maintaining one to three twitches in response to train-of-four stimulation[62,65–71] (Chaps. 3 through 5). When possible, lesser degrees of block should be maintained. If complete paralysis is attained, then it should be maintained for as brief a period as possible. One should seek to provide drug-free periods in order to allow (and document) appropriate recovery of neuromuscular function.

The risks of prolonged residual paralysis and/or subsequent myopathic changes are all too real. While individual drugs and underlying conditions have been implicated (Chap. 11), many feel "that the long-term use of excessive doses or irrational combinations of neuromuscular blocking agents—without even cursory monitoring—is probably the most likely cause of prolonged paralysis in critically ill patients. . . . Even cursory monitoring (presence/absence of twitch) allows titration to appropriate doses preventive of these applications."[62] Unfortunately, such monitoring is not employed routinely. In a 1991 report, only 34% of *anesthesia intensivists* reported that peripheral nerve stimulators were used routinely in ICU settings.[72] In another 1991 publication, ICU nurses reported that nerve stimulators were used in approximately 20% of ICUs, but in only 4% were they used routinely.[73] Written protocols for administration of relaxants were employed in only 6% of ICUs.[73]

Admittedly, there may be concern about repeatedly stimulating awake patients. Ideally, the patient will be sedated to a degree that is sufficient to minimize the discomfort associated with neurostimulation. However, if pain is evident, then one may stimulate with a reduced current intensity. Train-of-four and double-burst testing retain their accuracy at relatively low currents (Chap. 3, question d).

The criteria for *tracheal extubation in the ICU setting* often are comparable to those employed after surgery. In addition, patients often are assessed (e.g., with arterial blood gas measurements) after a period of spontaneous ventilation via the tracheal tube. It should be remembered that, in contrast to the progressive increase in strength that is anticipated during recovery from neuromuscular block at the end of surgery, a myriad of neuromuscular disorders may limit the progression of recovery in the ICU patient (Chap. 11, question m).

Discussion Questions ◆

a. If the T_4/T_1 *ratio* is 0.25 during a nitrous-narcotic-NDR anesthetic, is it likely that there will be *adequate relaxation* of the abdominal musculature for a laparotomy? Why or why not?

b. Why don't *"cutoffs" established* for neuromuscular monitoring in *healthy volunteers* necessarily ensure adequate airway protection and ventilatory function following anesthesia?

c. Does return of adequate spontaneous ventilation indicate return of adequate function of the *muscles responsible for protection of the airway*?

d. Does a $T_4/T_1 > 0.70$ that is documented mechanographically ensure that a patient will be able to *ventilate adequately* after a nondepolarizing relaxant?

e. Does a $T_4/T_1 > 0.90$ that is documented mechanographically ensure that a patient will be *asymptomatic*?

f. Does the ability to sustain *head lift*, generate a maximum inspiratory pressure in excess of -30 cm H_2O, sustain tetanus at 50 Hz, and maintain a $T_4/T_1 > 0.95$ indicate that there is no longer *receptor occlusion* by an NDR? Why or why not?

g. What is the significance of a *"curare cleft"* on the *end-tidal CO_2 tracing* of a patient who is suspected of having residual neuromuscular block?

h. Why is it particularly important to *titrate the depth of neuromuscular block* in patients receiving long-term administration of neuromuscular blocking agents in the ICU setting?

Answers ◆

a. A T_4/T_1 of 0.25 typically is noted with approximately 50% depression of T_1. This usually is not associated with adequate *abdominal relaxation* for a laparotomy, especially if a volatile inhalational anesthetic is not employed. For laparotomy, during nitrous-narcotic anesthesia, 85–100% depression of T_1 (or single twitch) generally is required.

b. Even in awake volunteers, cutoffs are arbitrary and do not necessarily apply to all subjects. In postsurgical patients, pain, residual anesthesia, analgesics, and other perioperative medications may decrease a patient's voluntary responses, strength, and respiratory function. In 10 ASA class III and IV patients recovering from major surgery,[19] at $T_4/T_1 > 0.70$ patients generated an MIP that was far less than the -69 cm H_2O averaged by awake volunteers[13] receiving tubocurarine to this degree of T_4/T_1 depression. The patients generated pressures as low as -22 cm H_2O.[19] As noted in Table 6-1, an MIP of -22 cm H_2O does not ensure protection against aspiration of oral secretions or ability to protect one's airway.[15] Additionally, *laryngeal incompetence* may persist for several hours following anesthesia even without relaxants.[33] It also has been shown that residual block may compound the respiratory depressant effects of *anesthetic and analgesic medications.*[51,52]

c. The return of an adequate *tidal volume* does not ensure the return of ability to protect the airway. It is a relatively insensitive indicator of persistent neuromuscular block, especially if upper airway integrity is artificially maintained with a tracheal tube, oronasal airway, or jaw lift. Pharyngeal muscles may still be depressed despite evidence of adequate ventilatory function and adequate neuromuscular function at other sites.[14,15,17,42] Airway reflexes and airway competence may remain depressed for several hours after general anesthesia.[53]

d. A T_4/T_1 >0.70 suggests that a patient will not develop significant *respiratory difficulty*. However, even a T_4/T_1 of 0.90 does not necessarily indicate recovery of full ventilatory capacity. The cutoff value of 0.70 is an arbitrary cutoff that may not hold true in all cases. A myriad of factors may interact in the perioperative setting to compromise ventilation. For example, agents (e.g., depolarizing agents) may decrease twitch height without fade, and agents that depress evoked muscle responses, such as dantrolene or inhalational agents (Chap. 9), certainly may compromise ventilation. Furthermore, there is evidence to suggest that the muscles of the upper airway that are responsible for its patency may be particularly sensitive to the effects of relaxants[14,15,33,43] and anesthetics.[53] Hence, despite adequate ventilation, neuromuscular function may not be sufficient to ensure protection against aspiration of oral contents or ability to maintain one's airway. Vigilance is essential.

e. As noted above, even a T_4/T_1 *of 0.90 does not guarantee full ventilatory capacity*. Additionally, even if the degree of neuromuscular depression is not of the magnitude that typically causes ventilatory compromise, this does not ensure that a patient will not have other symptoms due to block at more susceptible muscles. Eye divergence commonly results from weakness of the medial recti.[74,75] Weakness of the eyelids with diplopia, followed by weakness of the facial muscles and masseter, is noted at lesser levels of block than are difficulty swallowing and ventilatory compromise.[44] In a study where pretreatment with atracurium, 0.03 mg · kg^{-1}, only *decreased the* T_4/T_1 *ratio to 0.92*, a large number of subjects had ptosis, blurred vision, or a feeling of general discomfort.[76]

f. Neuromuscular and clinical monitoring may appear to be "normal" despite the *persistence of receptor occupancy* by an NDR. As many as 40–50% (and perhaps 60–70%) of receptors may remain occupied by relaxant in the context of normal T_4/T_1 and tetanic responses, an MIP >−40 cm H$_2$O, and sustained 5-second head lift. Clearly, the traditional cutoffs (T_4/T_1 >0.7[1,13,19] and an MIP >−20 to −30 cm H$_2$O[13,23,77]) do not ensure full restoration of the NMJ. The margin of safety may be greatly reduced, and the ability to maintain and protect the airway may be compromised.[15]

g. The "*curare cleft*" on the end-tidal CO_2 tracing indicates residual block. The patient's ability to maintain a deep inspiration is limited by inability to maintain contraction of the *ventilatory muscles*.

h. Although it is not common practice to do so routinely, it is critical to monitor the depth of neuromuscular block and titrate relaxant accordingly in patients receiving long-term administration of NDRs in the ICU. The effects of a given dose of relaxant vary among patients, especially in the context of the multiple disorders that may afflict ICU patients and the multiple medicines they may receive. In addition to seeking to attain an adequate depth of block, it is critical not to attain an excessive depth or duration of block. Long-term administration of relaxants may lead to accumulation of active metabolites (especially in patients with organ dysfunction). Long-term paralysis with NDRs has been associated with disuse atrophy and myopathies (Chap. 11). Furthermore, relaxants may be associated with dose-related systemic effects (most notably cardiovascular changes).

References ◆

1. Ali HH, Savarese JJ: Monitoring of neuromuscular function. Anesthesiology 45:216–249, 1976
2. Donlon JV, Ali HH, Savarese JJ: A new approach to the study of four nondepolarizing relaxants in man. Anesth Analg 53:934–939, 1974
3. Katz RL: Neuromuscular effects of *d*-tubocurarine, edrophonium and neostigmine in man. Anesthesiology 28:327–336, 1967
4. Katz RL: Comparison of electrical and mechanical recording of spontaneous and evoked muscle activity: the clinical value of continuous recording as an aid to the rational use of muscle relaxants during anesthesia. Anesthesiology 26:204–211, 1965
5. Katz RL: Clinical neuromuscular pharmacology of pancuronium. Anesthesiology 34:550–556, 1971
6. deJong RH: Controlled relaxation: I. Quantitation of EMG with abdominal relaxation. JAMA 197:393, 1966
7. deJong RH: Controlled relaxation: II. Clinical management of muscle relaxant administration. JAMA 198:1163, 1966
8. Lee CH: Some characteristics of neuromuscular block in the respiratory musculature in anaesthetized man. Can Anaesth Soc J 23:125–134, 1976
9. Usubiaga J, Moya F: The clinical use of a new nerve stimulator. Acta Anaesthesiol Scand 11:15, 1967
10. Ali HH, Savarese JJ, Lebowitz PW, Ramsey FM: Twitch, tetanus and train-of-four as indices of recovery from nondepolarizing neuromuscular blockade. Anesthesiology 54:294–297, 1981
11. Ali HH, Utting JE, Gray TC: Quantitative assessment of residual antidepolarizing block (Part I). Br J Anaesth 43:473–477, 1971
12. Ali HH, Utting JE, Gray TC: Quantitative assessment of residual antidepolarizing block (Part II). Br J Anaesth 43:478–485, 1971
13. Ali HH, Wilson RS, Savarese JJ, Kitz RJ: The effect of tubocurarine on indirectly elicited train-of-four muscle response and respiratory measurements in humans. Br J Anaesth 47:570–574, 1975

14. Gal TJ, Smith TC: Partial paralysis with d-tubocurarine and the ventilatory response to CO_2: an example of respiratory sparing? Anesthesiology 45:22–28, 1976
15. Pavlin EG, Holle RH, Schoene RB: Recovery of airway protection compared with ventilation in humans after paralysis with curare. Anesthesiology 70:381–385, 1989
16. Rigg JRA, Engel LA, Ritchie BC: Ventilatory response to carbon dioxide during partial paralysis with tubocurarine. Br J Anaesth 42:105–108, 1970
17. Gal TJ, Goldberg SK: Relationship between respiratory muscle strength and vital capacity during partial curarization in awake subjects. Anesthesiology 54:141–147, 1981
18. Pontoppidan H, Laver MB, Geffin B: Acute respiratory failure in the surgical patient. Adv Surg 4:163–254, 1970
19. Brand JB, Cullen DJ, Wilson NE, Ali HH: Spontaneous recovery from nondepolarizing neuromuscular blockade: correlation between clinical and evoked responses. Anesth Analg 56:55–58, 1977
20. Pavlin EG: Clinical tests of recovery from neuromuscular blocking agents. Anesthesiol Clin North Am 11:379–389, 1993
21. Sharpe MD, Lam AM, Nicholas FJ, Chung DC, Merchant R, Alyafi W, Beauchamp R: Correlation between integrated evoked EMG and respiratory function following atracurium administration in unanaesthetized humans. Can J Anaesth 37:307–312, 1990
22. Arora NS, Gal TJ: Cough dynamics during progressive expiratory muscle weakness in healthy curarized subjects. J Appl Physiol 51:494–498, 1981
23. Sahn SA, Lakshminarayan S: Bedside criteria for discontinuation of mechanical ventilation. Chest 63:1002–1005, 1973
24. Wescott DA, Bendixen HH: Neostigmine as a curare antagonist—a clinical study. Anesthesiology 23:324–332, 1962
25. Dam WH, Guldmann N: Inadequate postanesthetic ventilation: curare, anesthetic, narcotic, diffusion hypoxia. Anesthesiology 22:699–707, 1961
26. Miller RD: Antagonism of neuromuscular blockade. Anesthesiology 44:318–329, 1976
27. Engbaek J, Ostergaard D, Viby-Mogensen J: Clinical recovery and train-of-four ratio measured mechanically and electromyographically following atracurium. Anesthesiology 71:391–395, 1989
28. Viby-Mogensen J: Clinical assessment of neuromuscular transmission. Br J Anaesth 54:209–223, 1982
29. Walts LF, Levin N, Dillon JB: Assessment of recovery from curare. JAMA 213:1894–1986, 1970
30. Ali HH, Kitz RJ: Evaluation of recovery from nondepolarizing neuromuscular block, using a digital neuromuscular transmission analyzer: preliminary report. Anesth Analg 52:740–745, 1973
31. Johansen SH, Jorgensen M, Molbech S: Effect of tubocurarine on respiratory and nonrespiratory muscle power in man. J Appl Physiol 19:990–994, 1964
32. Gordon KL, Reilly CS: Recovery of neuromuscular function after infusion or intermittent bolus doses of atracurium or vecuronium. Br J Anaesth 62:269–273, 1989
33. Dodgson BG, Knill RL, Clement JL: Curare increases upper airway resistance while reducing ventilatory muscle strength (abstract). Can Anaesth Soc J 28:505–506, 1981
34. Gerber HR, Johansen SH, Mortimer JT, Yodlowski E: Frequency sweep electromyogram and voluntary effort in volunteers after d-tubocurarine. Anesthesiology 46:35–39, 1977
35. Mason LJ, Betts EK: Leg lift and maximum inspiratory force, clinical signs of neuromuscular blockade reversal in neonates and infants. Anesthesiology 52:441–442, 1980
36. Bevan DR, Smith CE, Donati F: Postoperative neuromuscular blockade: a comparison between atracurium, vecuronium, and pancuronium. Anesthesiology 69:272–276, 1988
37. Brull SJ, Ehrenwerth J, Connelly NR, Silverman DG: Assessment of residual curarization using low-current stimulation. Can J Anaesth 38:164–168, 1991
38. Pedersen T, Viby-Mogensen J, Bang U, Olsen NV, Jensen E, Engbaek J: Does perioperative tactile evaluation of the train-of-four response influence the frequency of postoperative residual neuromuscular blockade? Anesthesiology 73:835–839, 1990
39. Viby-Mogensen J, Jorgensen BC, Ording H: Residual curarization in the recovery room. Anesthesiology 50:539–541, 1979
40. Beemer GH, Rozental P: Postoperative neuromuscular function. Anaesth Intensive Care 14:41–45, 1986

41. Hutton P, Burchett KR, Madden AP: Comparison of recovery after neuromuscular blockade by atracurium or pancuronium. Br J Anaesth 60:36–42, 1988
42. Isono S, Ide T, Kochi T, Mizuguchi T, Nishino T: Effects of partial paralysis on the swallowing reflex in conscious humans. Anesthesiology 75:980–984, 1991
43. Bar ZG: The armlift test: an alternative to the headlift test for assessing recovery from neuromuscular blockade. Anaesthesia 40:630–633, 1985
44. Dupuis JY, Martin R, Tétrault JP: Clinical, electrical and mechanical correlations during recovery from neuromuscular blockade with vecuronium. Can J Anaesth 37:192–196, 1990
45. Donati F, Bevan DR: Not all muscles are the same (editorial I). Br J Anaesth 68:235, 1992
46. Smith CE, Donati F, Bevan DR: Differential effects of pancuronium on masseter and adductor pollicis muscle in humans. Anesthesiology 71:57–61, 1989
47. de Troyer A, Bastenier J, Delhez L: Function of respiratory muscles during partial curarization in humans. J Appl Physiol Respirat Environ Exercise Physiol 49:1049–1056, 1980
48. Nishino T, Yokokawa N, Hiraga K, et al: Breathing pattern of anaesthetized humans during pancuronium-induced partial paralysis. J Appl Physiol 64:78, 1988
49. Nguyen HD, Goldiner PL, Rabinowitz A, Nagashima H, Foldes FF: The neuromuscular effects of pipecuronium under enflurane anesthesia. Anesth Analg 66:S128, 1987
50. Ohta Y, Nagashima H, Lofrumento R, Foldes FF: Halothane-isoflurane-relaxant interactions *in vivo*. Anesthesiology 53:S265, 1980
51. Bellville JW, Cohen EN, Hamilton J: The interaction of morphine and *d*-tubocurarine on respiration and grip strength in man. Clin Pharmacol Ther 5:35–43, 1963
52. Lang DA, Kimura KK, Unna KR: The combination of skeletal muscle relaxing agents with various central nervous system depressants used in anesthesia. Arch Int Pharmacodyn Ther 85:257–272, 1951
53. Tomlin PJ, Howarth FH, Robinson JS: Postoperative atelectasis and laryngeal incompetence. Lancet 1:1402–1405, 1968
54. Andersen BN, Madsen JV, Schurizek BA, Juhl B: Residual curarization: a comparative study of atracurium and pancuronium. Acta Anaesthesiol Scand 32:79–81, 1988
55. Lennmarken C, Lofstrom JB: Partial curarization in the postoperative period. Acta Anaesthesiol Scand 28:260–262, 1984
56. Tiret L, Desmonts JM, Hatton F, et al: Complications associated with anaesthesia: a prospective study in France. Can Anaesth Soc J 33:336, 1986
57. Cooper AL, Leigh JM, Tring IC: Admissions to the intensive care unit after complication of anaesthetic techniques over 10 years: 1. The first 5 years. Anaesthesia 44:953, 1989
58. Lunn JN, Hunter AR, Scott DB: Anaesthesia-related surgical mortality. Anaesthesia 38:1090–1096, 1983
59. Braschi A, Lotti G: Partial ventilatory support in 1989. Intensive Care Med 15:488–490, 1989
60. Brochard L, Pluskwa F, Lemaire F: Improved efficacy of spontaneous breathing with inspiratory pressure support. Am Rev Respir Dis 136:411–416, 1987
61. Ward ME, Corbeil C, Gibbons W, et al: Optimization of respiratory muscle relaxation during mechanical ventilation. Anesthesiology 69:29–35, 1988
62. Agoston S, Seyr M, Khuenl-Brady KS, Henning RH: Use of neuromuscular blocking agents in the intensive care unit. Anesthesiol Clin North Am 11:345–359, 1993
63. Marini JJ, Capps JS, Culver BH: The inspiratory work of breathing during assisted mechanical ventilation. Chest 87:613–618, 1985
64. Marini JJ, Rodriguez RM, Lamb V: The inspiratory workload of patient initiated mechanical ventilation. Am Rev Respir Dis 134:902–909, 1986
65. Smith CL, Hunter JM, Jones RS: Vecuronium infusions in patients with renal failure in an ITU. Anaesthesia 42:387–393, 1987
66. Hunter JM: Infusions of atracurium and vecuronium in patients with multisystem organ failure in the intensive therapy unit. Insights Anaesthesiol 1:23–27, 1987
67. Segredo V, Caldwell JE, Matthay MA, Sharma ML, Gruenke LD, Miller RD: Persistent paralysis in critically ill patients after long-term administration of vecuronium. N Engl J Med 327:524–528, 1992
68. Darrah WC, Johnston JR, Mirakhur RK: Vecuronium infusions for prolonged muscle relaxation in the intensive care unit. Crit Care Med 17:1297–1300, 1987

69. Griffiths RB, Hunter JM, Jones RS: Atracurium infusion in patients with renal failure in an ITU. Anaesthesia 41:375–381, 1986
70. Kupfer Y, Namba T, Kaldawi E, Tessler S: Prolonged weakness after long-term infusion of vecuronium bromide. Ann Intern Med 117:484–486, 1992
71. Wadon AJ, Dogra S, Anand S: Atracurium infusion in the intensive care unit. Br J Anaesth 58:64S-67S, 1986
72. Klessig HT, Geiger HJ, Murray MJ, Coursin DB: A national survey on the practical patterns of anesthesiologists/intensivists in the use of muscle relaxants. Crit Care Med 20:1341–1345, 1992
73. Hansen-Flaschen JH, Brazinsky S, Basile C, Lanken PN: Use of sedating drugs and neuromuscular blocking agents in patients requiring mechanical ventilation for respiratory failure: a national survey. JAMA 266:2870–2875, 1991
74. Hannington-Kiff JG: Residual post-operative paralysis. Proc R Soc Med 63:73–76, 1970
75. Henegan C, McAuliffe R, Thomas D, Radford P: Morbidity after outpatient anaesthesia. Anaesthesia 36:4–9, 1981
76. Howardy-Hansen P, Moller J, Hansen B: Pretreatment with atracurium: the influence on neuromuscular transmission and pulmonary function. Acta Anaesthesiol Scand 31:642–4, 1987
77. Stanec A, Nuesa W, Akturk A, Pillon K, Capek K: Recovery of respiratory muscle function in surgical outpatients. Anesthesiology A:878, 1990

7

DAVID G. SILVERMAN | RICHARD R. BARTKOWSKI

Pharmacokinetics and Pharmacodynamics of Nondepolarizing Relaxants: Onset

Following *bolus* intravenous administration, the plasma concentration of a relaxant peaks virtually immediately. It then decreases rapidly as the drug is quickly distributed to various body tissues. Even for a long-acting agent such as *d*-tubocurarine, the distribution half-life is only 5 minutes.[1,2] With the possible exception of drugs with rapid metabolism (e.g., succinylcholine [SCh] and mivacurium), this rapid redistribution has a far greater impact than clearance on the initial plasma levels of drug.

Typically, a nondepolarizing relaxant (NDR) does not exhibit a clinically detectable effect for at least 30–60 seconds; and the *time to maximum block* (Time$_{max}$) after a subparalyzing dose of NDR typically is ≥5–7 minutes.[3] This is much greater than the Time$_{max}$ of 60–90 seconds for SCh, perhaps due to the high margin of safety[4] with respect to nondepolarizing block (Chap. 2). This "lag" is influenced by such factors as cardiac output, muscle blood flow, distance from the heart, volume of distribution, nonspecific binding, and the blood:tissue partition coefficient.[2,5–9]

Much of the "lag" occurs during a relaxant's passage through the biophase, the "extravascular effect compartment" that contains the neuromuscular junctions (NMJs).[5,6,10–14] An NDR's time in the *biophase* entails passage from the plasma to the extracellular space of the muscle, with repeated binding to nonspecific as well as specific receptors.[15] In vitro maneuvers (e.g., direct application of relaxant to the muscle) designed to lessen the impact of diffusional factors successfully accelerate onset and offset.[15] However, when drugs are applied directly to the end-plate by iontophoresis, diffusion to and from the receptors appears to be the rate-limiting process.[16]

It appears that NDR molecules bind rapidly and repeatedly to acetylcholine (ACh) receptors for brief intervals.[11,15–19] In order to achieve the high degree of receptor occupancy that is required for NDR-induced block, there must be a relatively large number of molecules available for binding. This large number of molecules has "difficulty entering and exiting" the narrow cleft of the NMJ and/or "getting past" nonspecific binding sites to reach the junctional cholinoceptors. The NDR concentration is "buffered," and the "macroscopic kinetics of inhibition are much slower than the molecular binding rates from the relaxant."[15]

Thus, the concept of *"buffered diffusion"* is often invoked to account for the relatively slow onset and offset of nondepolarizing block; i.e., changes in receptor occupancy lag significantly behind plasma concentration. Four factors have been cited as being inherent to *buffered diffusion* of the magnitude proposed for NDRs: (1) a *high density of receptor molecules,* (2) a *restricted space that forces repetitive interactions* between the transmitter and its receptors, (3) *high transmitter-receptor affinity,* and (4) the absence of other mechanisms more rapid than diffusion for removal of the transmitter.[15]

The *lag is more apparent when relatively few molecules are available* to the receptors in the NMJ (e.g., as a result of a low dose of relaxant or a relatively high degree of binding to plasma proteins and nonspecific binding sites). The limited number of free relaxant molecules may limit diffusion into the restricted space of the NMJ, since only unbound drug is free to move.[15] For a given dose of relaxant, the limitation is most marked for highly potent agents, since these are administered in relatively low doses; i.e., as receptor affinity (potency) increases, fewer molecules are administered. Thus, fewer molecules enter the NMJ, and it takes longer to achieve occupation of the requisite number of receptors to provide detectable block.[15,20-22] Whereas the time to maximum block for most NDRs is 5-7 minutes,[3] it is more than 10 minutes after doxacurium,[23] the most potent NDR in clinical use, and approximately 3-5 minutes for rocuronium,[24,25] an agent with very low potency (Chap. 14). Thus, while a more potent drug requires a lower concentration in the biophase to achieve a full-scale effect, its onset may be considerably slower. In addition to being observed in the clinical setting, the inverse relationship between drug potency and its rate of onset is also seen with iontophoretic application in an in vitro end-plate preparation.[22]

The *magnitude of a drug's effect* is determined by its availability to form drug-receptor complexes and by its efficacy (or intrinsic activity).[18] The latter may depend on the ability of a drug to bind to the receptors as well as its ability to induce a conformational change.[26] When *dose (x-axis)* is plotted vs. *receptor occupancy (y-axis),* a *rectangular hyperbola* is generated; this reflects the initial rapid rise in occupancy and the slower subsequent rise (plateau) (Fig. 7-1A). More commonly, one uses a *semilogarithmic plot,* with log-dose on the *x*-axis. This generates a sigmoidal curve, which accommodates a greater range of ligand (Fig. 7-1B).[12,18] At between 20% and 80% receptor occupancy, such a relationship is characterized by a linear increase in percent occupancy for a logarithmic increase in dose (or plasma concentration). *Linearity* at the extremes (encompassing 1-99% of the maximal response) can be obtained using a *probit or logit transformation*[18,27,28]; this

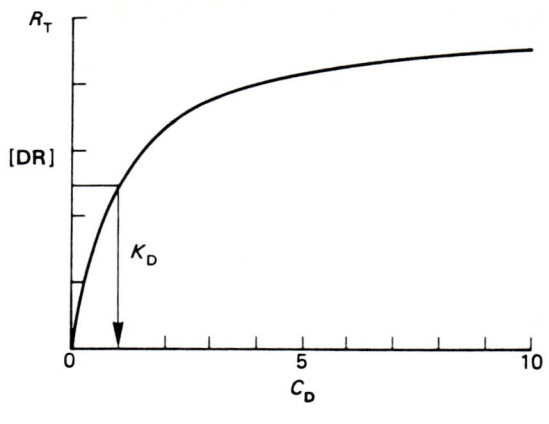

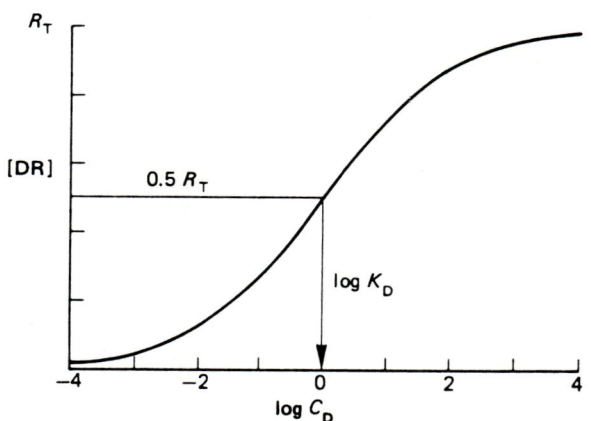

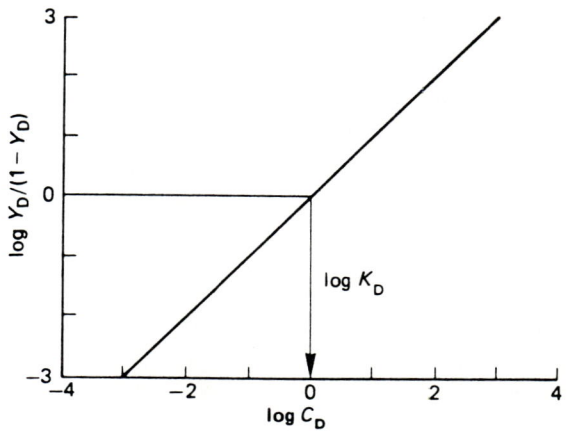

utilizes log-dose on the x-axis and the log of $Y_D/(1-Y_D)$ on the y-axis, with Y_D being the proportion of receptor sites that are occupied (Fig. 7-1C).

In light of the observation that the response to an NDR is not detected until a large percentage of receptors are blocked, some investigators have recommended that the pharmacodynamic model of NDRs include a "threshold term" that represents the steady-state plasma concentration that would just fail to evoke a detectable effect by exceeding the margin of safety in a sufficient number of endplates (Chap. 1).[29]

◆ DRUG SELECTION AND DOSAGES

The following dosage regimens are in good agreement with those derived from dose-response studies[12,30]:

Bolus Dose = Desired Concentration × Distribution Volume.
Infusion Rate = Desired Concentration × Total Clearance.

To achieve *intubating conditions* with an NDR, we commonly administer a dose that is twice the ED_{95} for the adductor pollicis muscle (question b). This increases the likelihood of paralysis of the airway musculature since, as described in Chapter 3, the ED_{95} of the airway musculature is 1.5–2 times that for the adductor pollicis muscle.

Increasing the dose to more than 2 times the ED_{95} offers the added benefit of accelerating the rate of onset.[31–43] For example, increasing the dose of vecuronium from 0.1 mg · kg^{-1} to 0.4 mg · kg^{-1} (from approximately 2 to 8 × ED_{95}) reduced the time to 95% twitch height depression at the abductor digiti quinti muscle of the hand from 208 to 106 seconds in adults[34] and from 83 to 39 seconds in children.[41] However, "high-dose" regimens do not consistently achieve the rapid onset of SCh[40,41,44]; even the rapid onset from "high-dose" vecuronium in children was markedly slower than the 24 seconds obtained after 2 mg · kg^{-1} of SCh.[41] Furthermore, there is *wide variability* among the responses of patients to a given dose of relaxant. Although administration of 0.4 mg · kg^{-1} of vecuronium provided a mean onset of 106 seconds, this was associated with a standard deviation of 36 seconds.[34] In another study, in five of 16 patients receiving more than 5 times the ED_{95} of an NDR, the time to 95% depression of twitch height at

---

FIGURE 7-1 The relationship between receptor binding (*DR*) and ligand concentration according to classical occupancy theory. **A,** linear relationship; **B,** semilogarithmic relationship; **C,** the means of linear transformation proposed by Hull. C_D = drug concentration, DR = concentration of bound receptors, R_T = total number of receptors, Y_D = proportion of receptor sites that are occupied, K_D = equilibrium dissociation constant (numerically equal to the free ligand concentration when half the receptor sites are occupied). In each case, a horizontal line corresponding to $Y_D = 0.5$ is dropped to the x-axis. In the linear plot this indicates K_D, and in the others, log K_D. (Reproduced with permission from Hull CJ: Pharmacodynamics of non-depolarizing neuromuscular blocking agents. Br J Anaesth 54:169–182, 1982.[18])

the adductor pollicis muscle was more than 120 seconds.[40] It is anticipated that the introduction of rocuronium will accelerate onset and thereby lessen the impact of such variability (Chap. 14). It has been reported that, for vecuronium, the major benefit of increasing dose is achieved by 3 times the ED_{95}.[31,37,44] However, above this, there still may be additional acceleration of onset and/or a more consistent effect.[32,34,38,41,43]

There are *limitations associated with increasing the dose* in order to accelerate onset. Factors other than dosage also play a significant role in "delaying" onset (e.g., circulation time, blood flow, local diffusion, and binding). Furthermore, the use of high doses of an NDR increases the likelihood and severity of side effects. A ceiling is not noted with respect to duration, and time to recovery typically increases with dose.[33,34,38,43] The increase in the dose of vecuronium from 0.10 to 0.40 mg · kg^{-1} was associated with an increase in the time to recovery of 25% twitch height (Dur_{25}) from 37 minutes to 138 minutes in adults[34] and from 24 minutes to 75 minutes in children.[41] As detailed in Chapters 13 and 14, such marked dose-related prolongation does not characterize *atracurium* or *mivacurium*. For mivacurium, the Dur_{95} only increased from 24.5 minutes after 0.1 mg · kg^{-1} to 30.4 minutes after 0.25 mg · kg^{-1}.[45] These agents undergo rapid metabolism, which is not dependent on organ elimination. However, these benzylisoquinolinium compounds cause dose-related histamine release if more than 2 times the ED_{95} is administered as a rapid bolus (Chap. 11).[39]

NDRs may potentiate one another,[46-57] perhaps by combining pre- and postsynaptic effects. The results of *combination therapy* appear to be inconsistent; *synergism* was not observed in all combinations.[48,54,55,58] *Combination therapy* has been recommended to accelerate onset of block,[59,60] but it has not always been more effective.[40,48,61] The data with respect to duration are somewhat confusing, with evidence that a combination of atracurium and vecuronium can be associated with a relative decrease as well as a relative increase in recovery time.[46,62,63] Pretreatment with pancuronium, 0.015 mg · kg^{-1}, accelerated the onset and prolonged the duration of block after mivacurium.[60]

◆ PRIMING TECHNIQUE

A *priming dose*[64] of an NDR may be administered 3–5 minutes prior to administration of the intubating dose in order to occupy a "subclinical" number of receptors and thereby accelerate onset of block. This has been shown to be of *variable efficacy*[40,65-85]; some workers have reported that this technique is of no significant value.[65,81,82] The general consensus is that priming tends to accelerate onset by 15–20% but still fails to ensure a rate of onset of complete paralysis equivalent to that provided by SCh (even in studies where the priming technique has been recommended as an acceptable alternative to SCh for rapid tracheal intubation[67,68]).[39,65,67,68,74] Perhaps the slight benefit provided by priming will be of significance for regimens that employ rocuronium, since its rate of onset approaches that of SCh (Chap. 14). As for most other agents, priming accelerated the onset of rocuronium by 20%.[85]

It has been shown in vitro that the *effectiveness* of priming is related to the concentration of drug achieved at the NMJ at the end of the priming interval.[86] In vivo, *individuals vary widely* in their response to priming doses (or equivalent defasciculating doses).[7,39,87–89] The efficacy and side effects of a given priming dose may be influenced by prior initiation of general anesthesia, the priming interval, and the size of the intubating dose. Consistent with the time required for an NDR to reach a maximum effect, a priming dose to intubating dose interval of 3–5 minutes appears to be most effective.[79]

Common symptoms after a *priming dose* that is 20% of the ED_{95} include heavy eyelids, diplopia, difficulty swallowing, weakness, and generalized discomfort.[84,90,91] Respiratory compromise and dyspnea are not common, but certainly may occur.[66,67,90,92–95] Pulmonary aspiration of gastric contents has been reported (in a patient who received a relatively large priming dose after receiving gentamicin).[96] However, other investigators have reported that the risk of acid reflux into the esophagus was not increased as a consequence of priming.[97,98] After a priming dose of atracurium, 0.06 mg · kg^{-1} (25–30% of the ED_{95}), four of 21 patients could not sustain head lift at 3.5 minutes after dosing, and maximum inspiratory force decreased by 38% in the 21 patients.[81] Similar results were noted after priming with 0.012 mg · kg^{-1} of vecuronium (20–30% of the ED_{95}).[82] The investigators concluded that priming is "complex, time-consuming, is not well tolerated, and may put patients at risk for aspiration."[81] One must assess the risks and benefits in each case and use a priming dose with caution. If significant contraindications exist (e.g., preexisting neuromuscular weakness, compromised ability to protect one's airway, severe respiratory insufficiency), it may be wise to avoid this technique.[71,82,83] If the priming technique is employed, the patient should be observed closely, especially if a dose more than 10% of the ED_{95} is administered.

The *"timing" principle* entails administering the intubating dose of relaxant prior to induction of general anesthesia. At 20 seconds after the relaxant[99] or at the onset of clinical weakness,[100,101] anesthesia is induced. However, the jury is still out; even its proponents have noted that "timing may not be appropriate for patients who cannot cooperate or understand."[101]

Discussion Questions ◆

a. Define *volume of distribution*. Why is it relatively small for muscle relaxants?
b. Define ED_{95}. What are its units?

- **c.** How do the *neonate's* relative amounts of *extracellular fluid* and *receptor immaturity* affect the ED_{95} for an initial dose of relaxant?
- **d.** Distinguish between the dose of NDR required for *50% receptor occupancy* and the dose required for *50% twitch height depression*.
- **e.** How would *increasing the dose* from the clinical ED_{25} to the ED_{75} affect (1) the *time to 25% twitch height* depression and (2) the time to maximum twitch height depression?
- **f.** How does *increasing the dose* from the ED_{100} to 3 times the ED_{100} affect the *time to maximum twitch height depression?*
- **g.** Does *increasing the dose above the clinical* ED_{100} increase the *depth of block?*
- **h.** How is the rate of equilibration of relaxants affected by their *tissue:blood partition coefficient?*
- **i.** What factors would make you hesitate to *increase the dose of an NDR* in order to *accelerate the onset* of relaxation?
- **j.** Why might you argue that a *priming dose* ideally should block approximately 50% of receptors?
- **k.** Does the likelihood of *symptoms* change markedly if the *priming dose* is increased from 10% to 20% of the ED_{95}?
- **l.** If a given *priming dose* has been shown to be *"safe"* in 20 of 20 consecutive patients, why would you still be concerned that it may be harmful to a subsequent patient?
- **m.** Discuss *dose selection and priming* with an NDR for the *parturient* undergoing a cesarean section.
- **n.** Why might the onset of *rocuronium be faster than the onset of an equivalent dose of vecuronium* and the onset of gallamine faster than the onset of tubocurarine or pancuronium?
- **o.** Why might it be easier to achieve *rapid-sequence* intubating conditions in *children* than in adults?
- **p.** What advantages and/or disadvantages theoretically might be noted if you administered a *combination* of 2 times the ED_{95} of *mivacurium* and 2 times the ED_{95} of *rocuronium,* as opposed to 4 times the ED_{95} of either agent alone?
- **q.** The following questions illustrate the potential *effects of potency* on distribution in the biophase, buffered diffusion, and rate of onset. Fill in the blanks and answer the questions:
    1. To achieve the same ultimate depth of block, a drug with 1/10th the potency of another typically is administered at _____ times the dose.
    2. This difference in potency is in large part attributable to differences in receptor affinity such that one may estimate that _____ times as many molecules of the low-potency drug must be free in the NMJ in order to attain the same degree of receptor occupancy.
    3. If the high-potency drug has a receptor:drug binding ratio of 300:1, then the drug with 1/10th potency has a ratio of 30:1. This theoreti-

cally indicates that within the NMJ, 1 of every _____ high-potency and 1 of every _____ low-potency drug molecules are free.
4. How many free molecules of the high-potency and low-potency drugs mentioned in question 3 must be in a theoretical NMJ where there is 50% occupancy of 1,800 receptors (i.e., 900 receptors are occupied)? How many total molecules of each drug (free plus bound) theoretically must be there?
5. How would equations 1 through 4 account for the faster onset of the lower-potency drug?

Answers ◆

a. The *volume of distribution* at steady state (V_{ss}) is a derived value that may be defined as the volume in which drug would have to be dissolved in order to provide the measured plasma concentration at equilibrium. Since *relaxants are polar molecules,* they do not readily cross lipid membranes and thus do not readily distribute to fat or enter cells. Hence, V_{ss} is approximately equivalent to the volume of extracellular fluid (0.2–0.6 L · kg^{-1}). V_{ss} tends to be greater for relaxants with increased lipid solubility (e.g., vecuronium).

b. There is some confusion as to the *definition of the ED_{95}* of neuromuscular relaxants. Many (including the authors) consider it to be the dose that produces an average of 95% peak depression of twitch in the population studied.[102] Others have referred to it as the dose that produces a median value of 95% peak twitch depression in the population studied.[103] These definitions are both in contrast to the definition that applies to most other drugs, that being the dose required to produce a specific effect in 95% of the population.

ED_{95} generally is determined on a *mg · kg^{-1} basis;* however, weight is not necessarily a good indication of volume of distribution.[104,105] It has been reported that, in adults, dosing according to lean tissue mass rather than total weight may minimize interpatient variability.[105] Dosing according to a *mg · m^{-2} basis* appears to be most reliable in infants, as it takes into account their increased V_{ss} (as a result of their increased extracellular fluid).

c. In *neonates,* two (or more) *offsetting factors* may alter the effectiveness of a given μg · kg^{-1} dose of an NDR^{107}:
  1. Infants have a relatively large percentage of *extracellular fluid* and thus a relatively greater central compartment and greater V_{ss}; a given dose is more widely distributed and hence is less effective than in adults.
  2. On the other hand, infants tend to be *more sensitive to an NDR;* they have underdeveloped NMJs,[108] contractile mechanisms, and elimination pathways.

When one selects a dose according to surface area, factor 1 is "overcome," while factor 2 remains.[109,110] For example, the ED_{50} for mivacurium on a $\mu g \cdot kg^{-1}$ basis is 46 $\mu g \cdot kg^{-1}$ in infants and 52 $\mu g \cdot kg^{-1}$ in children; corresponding values on a $\mu g \cdot m^{-2}$ basis are 870 $\mu g \cdot m^{-2}$ in infants and 1,400 $\mu g \cdot m^{-2}$ in children.[110] Likewise, on a $\mu g \cdot m^{-2}$ basis, infants need less atracurium than older children.[109] Unfortunately, all is not so simple: in neonates, there may be a persistence of fetal cholinoceptors with a relative "hyposensitivity" to a given dose of NDR (Chaps. 1 and 22). This would account for the finding that two of seven neonates had a shift of their "log concentration"–"response" curve for *d*-tubocurarine to the right (i.e., a larger dose was required for a given degree of block) (also see Chap. 10).[111]

d. The dose required for *50% receptor occupancy* is much less than that required for *50% twitch height depression*. In fact, 50% receptor occupancy causes virtually no twitch height depression. Twitch height depression is not noted until approximately 75% receptor occupancy; 50% depression is not noted until 80–85% receptor occupancy.

e. *Increasing the dose* from the ED_{25} to the ED_{75} logically will accelerate the time to 25% twitch height depression. It also may accelerate the time to maximum depression (25% and 75% depression for the ED_{25} and ED_{75}, respectively). For a potent agent such as doxacurium, the time to 75% depression after its ED_{75} may be less than the time to 25% depression after the ED_{25}.[23] Because of doxacurium's high potency, a relatively low dose is administered. This contains relatively few molecules with which to occupy the biophase and its nonspecific receptors and thereby rapidly achieve effective buffered diffusion. Increasing the number of molecules (by increasing the dose) accelerates the onset of block.[20]

f. *Increasing the dose* from the ED_{100} to 3 times the ED_{100} will *accelerate the time to 100% twitch depression;* i.e., when doses greater than the ED_{100} are administered, the degree of receptor occupancy required for 100% twitch height depression is reached more rapidly (regardless of drug potency). Thus, one may administer such a high dose to accelerate the onset of intubating conditions.

g. *Increasing the dose* above the clinical ED_{100} increases the *depth of block* even though 100% twitch depression is achieved at the lower dose. This is because 100% twitch depression does not require 100% receptor occupancy; it typically is noted at 90–95% receptor occupancy. At this degree of occupancy, one may still detect a response to tetanic stimulation and the presence of posttetanic counts (Chap. 5).

h. The relatively *low tissue:blood partition coefficient* (0.2–0.4) of neuromuscular blocking agents enables them to equilibrate rapidly in the extracellular fluid. Their partition coefficient is proportional to the ratio of extracellular fluid to total muscle volume.[9]

i. While *increasing the dose of NDR* accelerates onset of block, the benefit of progressively increasing the dose appears to lessen at above 3 times the ED_{95}. Unfortunately, the effect on duration persists, a feature that may limit the practicality of high-dose nondepolarizing block (except with a very short-acting or noncumulating agent). One also should hesitate to use high doses of agents that cause dose-related side effects such as ganglionic block, vagolysis, and histamine release.

j. The *priming dose* should occupy a relatively large number of receptors without eliciting significant clinical symptoms. Theoretically, this goal may be achieved when 20–50% of receptors are blocked. However, it should be noted that even doses less than or equal to 10% of the ED_{95} may cause blurred vision, heavy eyelids, and decreased respiratory function. Ideally, the priming dose should be sensitivity adjusted[87] (i.e., titrated so as to avoid significant block).

k. Although as much as 20% of the ED_{95} has been used as a *priming dose*,[72] doses above 10% of the ED_{95} may be associated with *depression of neuromuscular transmission and significant symptoms*.[67,69,90,92] Minor increases in the priming dose may cause significant changes in the degree of block; an increase from 0.007 mg · kg^{-1} to 0.008 mg · kg^{-1} caused a decrease in the T_4/T_1 ratio from 0.94 to 0.86.[91]

l. There is marked *variation in response* to NDRs.[7,40,87–89,95] Of 100 patients who received 0.1 mg · kg^{-1} of tubocurarine (20% of the ED_{95}), six had no twitch depression, while seven had 100% twitch depression.[88] Likewise, 40% of patients receiving 0.05 mg · kg^{-1} of tubocurarine after thiopental had less than a 10% reduction in T_1 height (on EMG), while 25% had more than 20%, and one had a 42% reduction.[89] This variability and the associated *risks of a priming* (or defasciculating) dose may be exacerbated by a patient's medical condition and concurrent medication.

m. The *parturient* poses unique problems with respect to *dose selection and priming* with an NDR. If one elects to avoid SCh, then high-dose vecuronium (or perhaps rocuronium) with or without a priming dose may be used. Although a priming dose of vecuronium, 0.01 mg · kg^{-1}, was well tolerated in a recent trial in 10 patients undergoing cesarean section,[112] special caution must be exercised in the context of the full stomach and decreased ventilatory reserve.

There is evidence of increased maternal sensitivity to NDRs.[113–117] Following vecuronium, 0.1 mg · kg^{-1}, the time to 90% depression of twitch height was 125 ± 66 seconds in patients undergoing cesarean section (vs. 288 ± 163 seconds in controls).[114] This increased sensitivity may be a consequence of relative "overdosing" when administering drug on a mg · kg^{-1} basis, increased cardiac output, and decreased protein binding (Chap. 10).

Increasing the intubating dose from 0.10 to 0.20 mg · kg^{-1} was accompanied by a 30% increase in *neonatal blood levels* that apparently caused some minor neuromuscular effects (Chap. 11).[112] Overall, neither a priming dose of 0.01 mg · kg^{-1} plus an intubating dose of 0.10 mg · kg^{-1} nor simply an intubating dose of 0.20 mg · kg^{-1} of vecuronium produced onset of block comparable to that which typifies SCh; the times to maximal twitch depression with the two nondepolarizing regimens were 177 and 175 seconds, respectively.[112]

n. The *onset of gallamine* is faster than the onset of its more potent counterparts pancuronium and tubocurarine,[118] and the *onset of rocuronium* (Org 9426) is faster than the onset of its more potent analogue vecuronium.[24,25] Because of their *low potency, more molecules* of gallamine and rocuronium are administered. This allows for more rapid occupation of a large number of receptors and nonspecific binding sites (i.e., faster entry through the biophase and more effective buffered diffusion). Additionally, the more rapid occupation is associated with a briefer distribution half-life, which allows less time for nonspecific binding and redistribution; hence, there is a greater peak effect in the biophase.[14] In light of a recent series of letters,[119–122] it is important to emphasize the importance of using the same definition for terms such as "onset" when comparing a new drug such as rocuronium to existing agents.

o. It may be easier to achieve *rapid-sequence intubating conditions using NDRs in children* than in adults, for several reasons: (1) Onset of paralysis typically is faster in children,[123–126] possibly a consequence of increased cardiac output and regional blood flow[40] (in contrast, onset may be slower in the child with congenital heart disease).[127] (2) Children are less prone to histamine release in response to high doses of benzylisoquinolinium compounds. (3) It is easier to overcome persistent muscle tone (i.e., inadequate relaxation) in a child. (4) The prolongation of clinical duration as a result of high doses of NDR is less marked in children.[41,123, 124,126,128,129] (This would not always be the case for neonates, however.[123,130]) It should be remembered that dose requirements are higher in children than in adults (Chap. 10).

p. The goal when using NDRs for *rapid-sequence intubation* is to attain intubating conditions rapidly and reliably without undue side effects. Theoretically, a *combination of mivacurium and rocuronium* may allow one to increase the size of the effective dose of relaxant while limiting the likelihood of marked prolongation of rocuronium-induced block or histamine release as a consequence of high-dose (>2 × ED$_{95}$) mivacurium. It remains to be confirmed whether this will optimize the benefits of rocuronium's rapid onset and mivacurium's brief duration (especially since some forms of combination therapy may result in prolonged duration).

q. The following answers about the theoretical example are derived from several sources[15,18,20,131] and are designed to emphasize the potential effect of potency.

1. The drug with 1/10th the potency of another should be administered at 10 times the dose to achieve the same depth of block.
2. Theoretically, 10 times as many molecules of the low-potency drug must be free in the NMJ.
3. Theoretically, one of every 300 molecules of the high-potency drug and 1 of every 30 molecules of the low-potency drug are free.
4. For a sample block of 1,800 receptors, 50% occupancy entails occupancy of 900 receptors. For the high-potency drug, this theoretically is accomplished with 903 molecules in the NMJ (3 free and 900 bound). For the low-potency drug, this theoretically requires 930 molecules (30 free and 900 bound). In other words, the need for 10 times more free drug in the NMJ actually necessitates the need for only 3% more total molecules (930 vs. 903).
5. Although the low-potency drug requires only 3% more molecules to achieve 50% occupancy in the NMJ, it typically is administered at 10 times the dose, and hence the requisite number of its molecules arrive much more quickly. Because receptors are so numerous in the junctional space and because both drugs must occupy the same number of receptors in order to achieve the same degree of block, the effects of buffered diffusion predominate and the onset of the low-potency drug is faster (as it provides a greater "molecular load"). However, once a steady state is achieved, the need for the higher concentrations (and doses) of the less potent relaxant is apparent.

References ◆

1. Kalow W: The distribution, destruction and elimination of muscle relaxants. Anesthesiology 20:505–518, 1959
2. Stanski DR, Sheiner LB: Pharmacokinetics and dynamics of muscle relaxants. Anesthesiology 51:103–105, 1979
3. Healy TEJ, Pugh ND, Kay B, Sivalingam T, Petts HV: Atracurium and vecuronium: effect of dose on the time of onset. Br J Anaesth 58:620–624, 1986
4. Paton WDM, Waud DR: The margin of safety of neuromuscular transmission. J Physiol 191:59–90, 1967
5. Donati F, Bevan DR: Role of circulation time in the modelling of the onset of atracurium neuromuscular blockade. Can J Anaesth 35:S125–126, 1988
6. Donati F: Onset of action of relaxants. Can J Anaesth 35:S52–S58, 1988
7. Donati F, Bevan DR: The influence of patient's sex, age and weight on pancuronium onset time. Can Anaesth Soc J 33:S86, 1986
8. Goat VA, Yeung ML, Blakeney C, Feldman SA: The effect of blood flow upon the activity of gallamine triethiodide. Br J Anaesth 48:69–73, 1976
9. Stanski DR, Ham J, Miller RD, Sheiner LB: Pharmacokinetics and pharmacodynamics of d-tubocurarine during nitrous oxide–narcotic and halothane anesthesia in man. Anesthesiology 51:235–241, 1979
10. Hull CJ, Van Beem HBH, McLeod K, Sibbald A, Watson MJ: A pharmacodynamic model for pancuronium. Br J Anaesth 50:1113–1122, 1978
11. Rang HP: The kinetics of action of acetylcholine antagonists in smooth muscle. Proc R Soc Lond [Biol] 164:488–510, 1966
12. Shanks CA: Pharmacokinetics of the nondepolarizing neuromuscular relaxants applied

to the calculation of bolus and infusion dosage regimens. Anesthesiology 64:72–86, 1986
13. Sheiner LB, Stanski DR, Vozeh S, Miller RD, Ham J: Simultaneous modeling of pharmacokinetics and pharmacodynamics: application to d-tubocurarine. Clin Pharmacol Ther 25:358–371, 1979
14. Stanski DR: Pharmacokinetics and pharmacodynamics for the clinician. Can J Anaesth 38:R48–R53, 1991
15. Armstrong DL, Lester HA: The kinetics of tubocurarine action and restricted diffusion within the synaptic cleft. J Physiol 294:365–386, 1979
16. Waud DR: The rate of action of competitive neuromuscular blocking agents. J Pharmacol Exp Ther 158:99–114, 1967
17. Colquhoun D, Sheridan RE: The effect of tubocurarine competition on the kinetics of agonist action on the nicotinic receptor. Br J Pharmacol 75:77–86, 1982
18. Hull CJ: Pharmacodynamics of nondepolarizing neuromuscular blocking agents. Br J Anaesth 54:169–182, 1982
19. Sheridan RE, Lester HA: Rates and equilibria at the acetylcholine receptor of *Electrophorus* electroplaques. J Gen Physiol 70:187–219, 1977
20. Bowman WC, Rodger IW, Houston J, Marshall RJ, McIndewar I: Structure:action relationships among some desacetoxy analogues of pancuronium and vecuronium in the anesthetized cat. Anesthesiology 69:57–62, 1988
21. Minsaas B, Stovner J: Artery-to-muscle onset time for neuromuscular blocking drugs. Br J Anaesth 52:403–407, 1980
22. Min JCL, Bekavac I, Glavinovic MI, Donati F, Bevan DR: Iontophoretic study of speed of action of various muscle relaxants. Anesthesiology 77:351–356, 1992
23. Murray DJ, Mehta MP, Choi WW, Forbes RB, Sokoll MD, Gergis SD, Rudd GD, Abou-Donia MM: The neuromuscular blocking and cardiovascular effects of doxacurium chloride in patients receiving nitrous oxide narcotic anesthesia. Anesthesiology 69:472–477, 1988
24. Bartkowski R, Witkowski T, Azad SS, Marr A, Lessin J: A comparison of onset and recovery of neuromuscular block after ORG9426 and vecuronium. Anesthesiology 75:A1071, 1991
25. Wierda JMKH, DeWit APM, Kuizenga K, Agoston S: Clinical observations on the neuromuscular blocking action of Org 9426, a new steroidal nondepolarizing agent. Br J Anaesth 64:521–523, 1990
26. Rang HP: Drug receptors and their function. Nature 231:91–96, 1971
27. Hill AV: The possible effect of the aggregation of the molecules of haemoglobin on its dissociation curves. J Physiol (Lond) 40:190, 1910
28. Harpley FW, Stewart GA, Young PA: Principles of biological assay. In Colton T, Grimm H, Harpley FW, Stewart GA, Weber E, Young PA (eds): Biostatistics in Pharmacology, Oxford, Pergamon Press, 1973, pp 971–1060
29. Parker CJR, Hunter JM: A new four-parameter threshold model for the plasma atracurium concentration-response relationship. Br J Anaesth 68:548–554, 1992
30. Mitenko PA, Ogilvie RI: Rapidly achieved plasma concentration plateaus, with observations on theophylline kinetics. Clin Pharmacol Ther 13:329–335, 1972
31. Casson WR, Jones RM: Vecuronium induced neuromuscular blockade: the effect of increasing dose on speed of onset. Anaesthesia 41:354–357, 1986
32. Fahey MR, Morris RB, Miller RD, Sohn YJ, Cronnelly R, Gencarelli P: Clinical pharmacology of ORG NC45 (Norcuron™): a new nondepolarizing muscle relaxant. Anesthesiology 55:6–11, 1981
33. Feldman SA, Liban JB: Vecuronium—a variable dose technique. Anaesthesia 42:199–201, 1987
34. Ginsberg B, Glass PS, Quill T, Shafron D, Ossey KD: Onset and duration of neuromuscular blockade following high-dose vecuronium administration. Anesthesiology 71:201–205, 1989
35. Kaufman J, Dubois M, Siegelman R, Chen J: Onset, intubation conditions and duration of action of vecuronium: high dose vs. low dose. Anesth Analg 67:S111, 1988
36. Lennon RL, Olson RA, Gronert GA: Atracurium or vecuronium for rapid sequence endotracheal intubation. Anesthesiology 64:510–513, 1986

37. Mirakhur RK, Ferres CJ, Clarke RSJ, Bali IM, Dundee JW: Clinical evaluation of ORG NC45. Br J Anaesth 55:119–124, 1983
38. Rorvik K, Husby P, Gramstad L, Vamnes JS, Bitsch-Larsen L, Koller M-E: Comparison of large dose of vecuronium with pancuronium for prolonged neuromuscular blockade. Br J Anaesth 61:180–185, 1988
39. Scott RPF, Savarese JJ, Basta SJ, Embree P, Ali HH, Sunder N, Hoaglin DC: Clinical pharmacology of atracurium given in high dose. Br J Anaesth 58:834–838, 1986
40. Silverman DG, Swift CA, Dubow HD, O'Connor TZ, Brull SJ: Variability of onset within and among relaxant regimens. J Clin Anesth 4:28–33, 1992
41. Sloan MH, Lerman J, Bissonnette B: Pharmacodynamics of high-dose vecuronium in children during balanced anesthesia. Anesthesiology 74:656–659, 1991
42. Savarese JJ, Ali HH, Basta SJ, Embree PB, Scott RPF, Sunder N, Weakly JN, Wastila WB, El-Sayad HA: The clinical neuromuscular pharmacology of mivacurium chloride (BW 1090U): a short-acting nondepolarizing ester neuromuscular blocking drug. Anesthesiology 68:723–732, 1988
43. Tullock WC, Diana P, Cook DR, Wilks DH, Brandom BW, Stiller RL, Beach CA: Neuromuscular and cardiovascular effects of high-dose vecuronium. Anesth Analg 70:86–90, 1990
44. Bencini A, Newton DEF: Rate of onset of good intubating conditions, respiratory depression and hand muscle paralysis after vecuronium. Br J Anaesth 56:959–965, 1984
45. Ali HH, Savarese JJ, Embree PB, Basta SJ, Stout RG, Bottros H, Weakly JN: Clinical pharmacology of mivacurium chloride (W B1090U) infusion: comparison with vecuronium and atracurium. Br J Anaesth 61:541–546, 1988
46. Black TE, Healy TEJ, Pugh ND, Kay B, Harper NJN, Petts HV, Sivalingham T: Neuromuscular block: atracurium and vecuronium compared and combined. Eur J Anaesthesiol 2:29–37, 1985
47. Foldes F, Aoki T, Ono K, Duncalf D, Nagashima H: Potentiation of pancurcnium, vecuronium and atracurium by d-tubocurarine and metocurine. Anesth Analg 63:A211, 1984
48. Ferres CJ, Mirakhur RK, Pandit SK, Clarke RS, Gibson FM: Dose-response studies with pancuronium, vecuronium and their combination. Br J Clin Pharmacol 18:947–950, 1984
49. Lebowitz PW, Ramsey FM, Savarese JJ, Ali HH: Potentiation of neuromuscular blockade in man produced by combinations of pancuronium and metocurine or pancuronium and d-tubocurarine. Anesth Analg 59:604–609, 1980
50. Lebowitz PW, Ramsey FM, Savarese JJ, Ali HH, deBros FM: Combination of pancuronium and metocurine: neuromuscular and hemodynamic advantages over pancuronium alone. Anesth Analg 60:12–17, 1981
51. Mirakhur RK, Pandit SK, Ferres CJ, Gibson FM: Time course of muscle relaxation with a combination of pancuronium and tubocurarine. Anesth Analg 63:437–440, 1984
52. Park WY, Balingit PE, MacNamara TE: Interactions of gallamine and pancuronium with tubocurarine under morphine-nitrous oxide-oxygen anesthesia in man. Anesth Analg 53:723–729, 1974
53. Wong KC, Jones JR: Some synergistic effects of d-tubocurarine and gallamine. Anesth Analg 50:285–290, 1971
54. Waud BE, Waud DR: Interaction among agents that block end-plate depolarization competitively. Anesthesiology 63:4–15, 1985
55. Waud BE, Waud DR: Quantitative examination of the interaction of competitive neuromuscular blocking agents on the indirectly elicited twitch. Anesthesiology 61:420–427, 1984
56. Watanabe K, Ohta Y, Tejeda J, Manabe N, Nagashima H, Foldes FF: Interaction of ORG9426 and other nondepolarizing relaxants in live rats. Anesthesiology 73:A888, 1990
57. Satwicz PR, Martyn JAJ, Szyfelbein SK, Firestone S: Potentiation of neuromuscular blockade using a combination of pancuronium and dimethyltubocurarine: studies in children following acute brain injury or during reconstructive surgery. Br J Anaesth 56:479–484, 1984
58. Donati F, Katz JM, Smith CE, Bevan DR: Atracurium-vecuronium combinations: lack of potentiating effects. Can J Anaesth 35:S126–127, 1988

59. Berman JA, Suh KK, Bleiweiss W, Seskin M: Evaluation of atracurium and vecuronium in combination to facilitate rapid tracheal intubation. Anesthesiology 63:A342, 1985
60. Brandom BW, Meretoja OA, Taivainen T, Wirtavuori K: Accelerated onset and delayed recovery of neuromuscular block induced by mivacurium preceded by pancuronium in children. Anesth Analg 76:998–1003, 1993
61. Pandit SK, Ferres CJ, Gibson FM, Mirakhur RK: Time course of action of combinations of vecuronium and pancuronium. Anaesthesia 41:151–154, 1986
62. Gibbs NM, Rung GW, Braunegg PW, et al: The onset and duration of neuromuscular blockade using combinations of atracurium and vecuronium. Anaesth Intensive Care 19:96, 1991
63. Stirt JA: Accelerated recovery from combined atracurium vecuronium neuromuscular block. Br J Anaesth 62:697, 1989
64. Foldes F: Rapid tracheal intubation with non-depolarizing neuromuscular blocking drugs: the priming principle (letter). Br J Anaesth 56:663, 1984
65. Brady MM, Mirakhur RK, Gibson FM: Influence of "priming" on the potency of non-depolarizing neuromuscular blocking agents. Br J Anaesth 59:1245–1249, 1987
66. Baumgarten RK, Reynolds WJ: The priming principle and the open eye-full stomach. Anesthesiology 63:561–562, 1985
67. Baumgarten RK, Carter CE, Reynolds WJ, Brown JL, DeVera HV: Priming with non-depolarizing relaxants for rapid tracheal intubation: a double blind-evaluation. Can J Anaesth 35:5–11, 1988
68. Boulanger A, Hardy J-F, Lepage Y: Rapid induction sequence with vecuronium: should we intubate after 60 or 90 seconds? Can J Anaesth 37:296–300, 1990
69. Donati F: The priming saga: where do we stand now? Can J Anaesth 35:1–4, 1988
70. Glass P, Wilson W, Mace J, Ossey K, Maroof M: Assessment of the optimal priming dose for atracurium, pancuronium and vecuronium to obtain rapid onset muscle relaxation. Anesth Analg 66:S67, 1987
71. Jones RM: The priming principle: how does it work and should we be using it? (editorial). Br J Anaesth 63:1–3, 1989
72. Kunjappan VE, Brown EM, Alexander GD: Rapid sequence induction using vecuronium. Anesth Analg 65:503–506, 1986
73. Mehta MP, Choi WW, Gergis SD, Sokoll MD, Adolphson AJ: Facilitation of rapid endotracheal intubations with divided doses of nondepolarizing neuromuscular blocking drugs. Anesthesiology 62:392–395, 1985
74. Martin C, Bonneru J-J, Brun J-P, Albanese J, Gouin F: Vecuronium or suxamethonium for rapid sequence intubation: which is better? Br J Anaesth 59:1240–1244, 1987
75. Miller RD: The priming principle. Anesthesiology 62:381–382, 1985
76. Mirakhur RK, Lavery GG, Gibson FM, Clarke RSJ: Intubating conditions after vecuronium and atracurium given in divided doses (the priming technique). Acta Anaesthesiol Scand 30:347–350, 1986
77. Naguib M, Gyasi HK, Abdulatif M, Absood GH: Rapid tracheal intubation with atracurium—a comparison of priming intervals. Can Anaesth Soc J 33:150–155, 1986
78. Naguib M, Abdulatif M, Absood GH: The optimal priming dose for atracurium. Can Anaesth Soc J 33:453–457, 1986
79. Rupp SM: The priming principle. Probl Anesth 3:436–445, 1989
80. Schwarz S, Ilias W, Lackner F, Mayrhofer O, Foldes FF: Rapid tracheal intubation with vecuronium: the priming principle. Anesthesiology 62:388–391, 1985
81. Sosis M, Larijani GE, Marr AT: Priming with atracurium. Anesth Analg 66:329–332, 1987
82. Sosis M, Stiner A, Larijani GE, Marr AT: An evaluation of priming with vecuronium. Br J Anaesth 59:1236–1239, 1987
83. Sosis M: On the efficacy of the priming principle with vecuronium (corresp). Anesthesiology 65:120–121, 1986
84. Taboada JA, Rupp SM, Miller RD: Refining the priming principle for vecuronium rapid-sequence induction of anesthesia. Anesthesiology 64:243–247, 1986
85. Foldes FF, Nagashima H, Nguyen HD, Schiller WS, Mason MM, Ohta Y: The neuromuscular effects of ORG9426 in patients receiving balanced anesthesia. Anesthesiology 75:191–196, 1991

86. Storella RJ, Jaffe J, Mehr E, Rosenberg H: *In vitro* investigation of the priming principle for rapid neuromuscular block. Br J Anaesth 62:476–480, 1989
87. Cheng M, Lee C, Katz RL, Nguyen NB: Sensitivity-adjusted priming consistently accelerates onset of vecuronium-induced neuromuscular block in cats. Anesth Analg 66:S26, 1987
88. Katz RL: Neuromuscular effects of *d*-tubocurarine, edrophonium and neostigmine in man. Anesthesiology 28:327–336, 1967
89. Sugioka K, Sebel PS, Kalayjian R, Ludgrove T, Speir A: The effect of pretreatment with curare on neuromuscular transmission. Anesth Analg 66:S173, 1987
90. Howardy-Hansen P, Moller J, Hansen B: Pretreatment with atracurium: the influence on neuromuscular transmission and pulmonary function. Acta Anaesthesiol Scand 31:642–644, 1987
91. Naguib M, Abdulatif M, Gyasi HK, Khawaji Y, Absood GH: The pattern of train-of-four fade after atracurium: influence of different priming doses. Anesth Analg 66:427–430, 1987
92. Engbaek J, Howardy-Hansen P, Ording H, Viby-Mogensen J: Precurarization with vecuronium and pancuronium in awake, healthy volunteers: the influence on neuromuscular transmission and pulmonary function. Acta Anaesthesiol Scand 29:117–120, 1985
93. Bruce DL, Downs JB, Kulkarni PS, et al: Precurarization inhibits maximal ventilatory effort. Anesthesiology 61:618–621, 1984
94. Sakuma K, Hashiba M, Shimoji K: Severe dyspnea caused by vecuronium bromide administration for priming and precurarization. Masui 40:483, 1991
95. Rao TLK, Jacobs HK: Pulmonary function following "pretreatment" dose of pancuronium in volunteers. Anesth Analg 59:659–661, 1980
96. Musich J, Walts LF: Pulmonary aspiration after a priming dose of vecuronium. Anesthesiology 64:517–519, 1986
97. Gorback MS, Graubert DA: Gastroesophageal reflux during anesthetic induction with thiopental and succinylcholine. J Clin Anesth 2:163, 1990
98. Martin C, Guillen JC, Dupin B, Ragni J, Aknin P, Gouin F: Lower oesophageal reflux during priming with vecuronium. Br J Anaesth 64:33–35, 1990
99. Cicala R, Westbrook L: An alternative method of paralysis for rapid-sequence induction. Anesthesiology 69:983–986, 1988
100. Culling RD, Middaugh RE, Menk EJ: Rapid tracheal intubation with vecuronium: the timing principle. J Clin Anesth 1:422–425, 1989
101. Silverman SM, Culling RD, Middaugh RE: Rapid-sequence orotracheal intubation: a comparison of three techniques. Anesthesiology 73:244–248, 1990
102. Ramsey FM: Basic pharmacology of neuromuscular blocking agents. Anesthesiol Clin North Am 11:219–235, 1993
103. Ducharme J, Donati F: Pharmacokinetics and pharmacodynamics of steroidal muscle relaxants. Anesthesiol Clin North Am 11:283–307, 1993
104. McLeod K, Hull J, Watson MJ: Effects of ageing on the pharmacokinetics of pancuronium. Br J Anaesth 51:435–438, 1979
105. Parker CJR, Hunter JM: Relationship between volume of distribution of atracurium and body weight. Br J Anaesth 70:443–445, 1993
106. Beemer GH, Bjorksten AR, Crankshaw DP: Optimizing dosing of atracurium to allow for variation in body somatotype. Anesthesiology 75:A778, 1991
107. Fisher DM, O'Keeffe C, Stanski DR, Cronnelly R, Miller RD, Gregory G: Pharmacokinetics and pharmacodynamics of *d*-tubocurarine in infants, children, and adults. Anesthesiology 57:203–208, 1982
108. Goudsouzian NG, Standaert FG: The infant and myoneural junction. Anesth Analg 65:1208–1217, 1986
109. Brandom BW, Woelfel SK, Cook DR, Fehr BL, Rudd GD: Clinical pharmacology of atracurium in infants. Anesth Analg 63:309–312, 1984
110. Woelfel SK, Brandom BW, McGowan FX Jr, Cook DR: Dose-response relationship of mivacurium chloride (Mivacron®) in infants during nitrous oxide–halothane anesthesia. Anesthesiology 75:A775, 1991
111. Matteo RS, Lieberman IG, Salantire E, et al: Distribution, elimination, and action of

d-tubocurarine in neonates, infants, children, and adults. Anesth Analg 63:799–804, 1984
112. Hawkins JL, Johnson TD, Kubicek MA, Skjonsky BS, Morrow DH, Joyce TH III: Vecuronium for rapid-sequence intubation for cesarean section. Anesth Analg 71:185–190, 1990
113. Baraka A, Noueihed R, Sinno H, Wakid N, Agoston S: Succinylcholine-vecuronium (Org NC 45) sequence for cesarean section. Anesth Analg 62:909–913, 1983
114. Baraka A, Jabbour S, Tabboush Z, et al: Onset of vecuronium neuromuscular block is more rapid in patients undergoing caesarean section. Can J Anaesth 39:135, 1992
115. Camp CE, Tessem J, Adenwala J, Joyce TH III: Vecuronium and prolonged neuromuscular blockade in post-partum patients. Anesthesiology 67:1006–1008, 1987
116. Cherala S, Eddie D, Halpern M, Shevde K: Priming with vecuronium in obstetrics (letter). Anaesthesia 42:1021, 1987
117. Rodrigue R, Durant NN, Nguyen N, et al: Comparison of vecuronium-induced neuromuscular blockade in pregnant and nonpregnant female rabbits. Anesthesiology 65: A401, 1986
118. Kopman AF: Pancuronium, gallamine, and d-tubocurarine compared: is speed of onset inversely related to drug potency? Anesthesiology 70:915–920, 1989
119. Ginsburg R, Lippmann M: ORG 9426, succinylcholine or vecuronium: which agent provides "overall superiority" for short outpatient procedures (letter). Anesth Analg 76:902–920, 1993
120. Puhringer FK, Khuenl-Brady KS, Koller J, Mitterschiffthaler G: ORG 9426, succinylcholine or vecuronium: which agent provides "overall superiority" for short outpatient procedures (letter in reply). Anesth Analg 76:904–905, 1993
121. Lippmann M, Ginsburg R: Neuromuscular blockers in day-case surgery: is speed of onset more important than duration of action? (letter). Br J Anaesth 70:235, 1993
122. Mirakhur RK, Cooper RA, Clarke RSJ, Boules Z: In reply: Lippmann M, Ginsburg R: Neuromuscular blockers in day-case surgery: is speed of onset more important than duration of action? (letter). Br J Anaesth 70:235, 1993
123. Bevan JC, Donati F, Bevan DR: Attempted acceleration of the onset of action of pancuronium: effects of divided doses in infants and children. Br J Anaesth 57:1204–1208, 1985
124. Fisher DM, Miller RD: Neuromuscular effects of vecuronium (ORG NC45) in infants and children during N_2O, halothane anesthesia. Anesthesiology 58:519–523, 1983
125. Meretoja OA, Wirtavuori K, Neuvonen PJ: Age-dependence of the dose-response curve of vecuronium in pediatric patients during balanced anesthesia. Anesth Analg 67:21, 1988
126. O'Kelly B, Frossard J, Meistelman C, Ecoffey C: Neuromuscular blockade following Org 9426 in children during N2O-halothane anesthesia. Anesthesiology 75:A787, 1991
127. Lucero VM, Lerman J, Burrows FA: Onset of neuromuscular blockade with pancuronium in children with cyanotic and acyanotic disease. Anesth Analg 66:S108, 1987
128. Meistelman C, Loose JP, Saint-Maurice C, et al: Clinical pharmacology of vecuronium in children: studies during nitrous oxide and halothane in oxygen anaesthesia. Br J Anaesth 58:996, 1986
129. Woelfel SK, Dong ML, Brandom BW, et al: Vecuronium infusion requirements in children during halothane-narcotic-nitrous oxide, isoflurane-narcotic-nitrous oxide, and narcotic-nitrous oxide anesthesia. Anesth Analg 73:33, 1991
130. Meretoja OA: Is vecuronium a long-acting neuromuscular blocking agent in neonates and infants? Br J Anaesth 62:184–187, 1989
131. Hull CJ: The rate of onset of nondepolarizing muscle relaxants. Presented at the 4th International Neuromuscular Meeting, Montreal, May 1992

8

DAVID G. SILVERMAN | RICHARD R. BARTKOWSKI

Pharmacokinetics and Pharmacodynamics of Nondepolarizing Relaxants: Maintenance and Recovery

◆ DOSAGES FOR INFUSION AND MAINTENANCE

During *infusion* of any drug, the plasma concentration increases to approximately 50%, 75%, 88%, and 94% of its *steady-state concentration* (C_{ss}) in *one, two, three, and four elimination half-lives* ($t_{1/2elim}$), respectively. It virtually has reached its steady-state (C_{ss}) in five half-lives (96.9%).[1,2] The infusion rate that will achieve a *desired steady-state concentration* is: C_{ss} times clearance. As for log-dose, plotting log-C_{ss} vs. pharmacological response typically generates a *sigmoidal curve*; the 20–80% response range can be approximated with a straight line.[3] It should be remembered that the infusion rate may have to be lowered during long-term infusion as redistribution sites become saturated; this is more likely with a long-acting agent (e.g., pancuronium) than with a rapidly metabolized agent (e.g., atracurium or mivacurium).

In light of their faster clearance, we tend to infuse short-acting compounds at a faster rate. For mivacurium, the hourly infusion rate (mg · kg^{-1} · hr^{-1}) typically is 450–600% of the ED$_{95}$. For atracurium and vecuronium, the typical *hourly infusion rate* is 75–200% of the ED$_{95}$. An even slower rate would be indicated for pancuronium. Logically, the longer the duration of block after a bolus dose in a given patient, the lower the subsequent infusion requirements.[4]

In a recent study, the *steady-state infusion rates* necessary to maintain 95% twitch height depression during general anesthesia with thiopental, fentanyl, and nitrous oxide were: *mivacurium*—8.3 ± 0.7, *atracurium*—7.9 ± 0.4, and *vecuronium*—1.2 ± 0.3 μg · kg^{-1} · min^{-1},[5] or 0.49, 0.47, and 0.07 mg · kg^{-1} · hr^{-1}, respectively. This translates to approximately 6 times the ED$_{95}$ for mivacurium and 1.5 times the ED$_{95}$ for atracurium and vecuronium. Unfortunately, data from different studies are often difficult to compare because of such variables as different depths of block, different loading doses, different anesthetic techniques, and different patient ages. For example, infusion requirements may be decreased markedly in the presence of inhalational anesthetics.[6]

Infusion of succinylcholine (SCh) at 90 µg · kg^{-1} · min^{-1} (>10 × ED$_{95}$) provides a comparable depth of block to that obtained with the above infusions.[7] However, long-term infusion of SCh may be complicated by bradyphylaxis, by tachyphylaxis, or by a dual block that may delay (and complicate) recovery (Chap. 16).

The *incremental dose* required to restore the depth of block from 25% twitch height depression back to 95% depression for nondepolarizing relaxants (NDRs) is approximately 20% of the ED$_{95}$. Supplementation may be indicated when the single twitch height has returned to between 5% and 20% of its baseline. Prompt supplementation is especially important for short-acting agents. To maintain a desired level of paralysis, intermittent bolus administration must be more frequent for a drug with a brief $t_{1/2elim}$.

◆ RECOVERY KINETICS

For most relaxants, the *initial phase of recovery* is almost exclusively due to redistribution of the drug from the neuromuscular junction (NMJ) to less well-perfused compartments. The two most prominent exceptions are SCh and mivacurium; their rapid metabolism by pseudocholinesterase contributes to early recovery.

Following the redistribution phase, neuromuscular recovery is predominantly due to *elimination*.[8] This consists of a slow transfer of drug from the tissue compartment to plasma (as drug is cleared from the blood). The rate of recovery of neuromuscular function is proportional to the rate of decline of the plasma concentration of relaxant.[3] The *elimination constant*, K_{el}, is the slope of the terminal portion of the line representing the relationship between the log-concentration vs. time (Fig. 8-1). The time required for a 50% decrease in plasma concentration during the elimination phase, the *half-time of elimination*, may be determined as follows: $t_{1/2elim} = 0.693/K_{el}$ (with 0.693 being the natural log of 2). As detailed in Chapters 12 through 14, $t_{1/2elim}$ ranges from approximately 2 minutes for the active isomers of mivacurium and 20 minutes for atracurium to well beyond 100 minutes for agents such as d-tubocurarine and metocurine.[2]

Clearance, defined as the volume of blood (or plasma) that is cleared of drug per unit time (regardless of drug concentration), is proportional to V_{ss} and K_{el}. It ranges from 1–2 mL · kg^{-1} · min^{-1} for long-acting agents like tubocurarine to 3–4 mL · kg^{-1} · min^{-1} for vecuronium, 5–6 mL · kg^{-1} · min^{-1} for atracurium, and even faster (as much as 50–100 mL · kg^{-1} · min^{-1}) for mivacurium.

The *recovery time following a continuous infusion* of a muscle relaxant will be influenced by the duration of infusion. Agents that undergo rapid

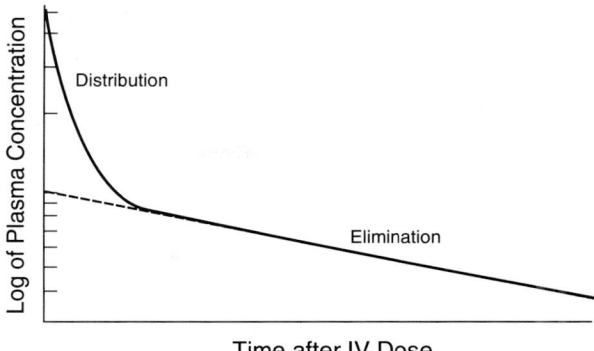

FIGURE 8-1 Graph illustrating decline in plasma concentration of a drug after IV bolus administration. Initial rapid decline is predominantly due to distribution from blood to tissues. Subsequent decline is primarily due to elimination. In a two-compartment model, the elimination (or beta) phase is represented by the elimination constant, K_{el}, which is a straight line on this log-linear graph.

metabolism (e.g., *mivacurium*) tend to show less prolongation than longer-acting agents. Those that depend almost exclusively on redistribution for their short duration will tend to show some prolongation.[5]

Following therapy with a combination of muscle relaxants, recovery has a varied time course; acceleration as well as delay of recovery have been reported (Chap. 7). When an *intermediate-acting relaxant* is given to prolong neuromuscular block after partial recovery from a long-acting relaxant, the recovery profile more closely resembles that of the longer-acting agent until several doses of the shorter-acting agent have been administered (Chap. 9).

◆ MONITORING

As expected, a relationship exists between plasma levels of relaxant and twitch height depression[9–11] such that the return of twitch height toward baseline follows the decline in plasma (and hence junctional) levels. Following 0.05–0.1 mg · kg^{-1} of pancuronium, a response at the adductor pollicis first became evident at 0.21 ± 0.03 µg · mL^{-1}, and 25%, 50%, and 75% recovery appeared at 0.13 ± 0.01, 0.11 ± 0.01, and 0.10 ± 0.1 µg · mL^{-1} (±SEM), respectively.[9]

The time until 10% recovery of *single* twitch height (Dur$_{10}$) is clinically useful for the following reasons[12–14]:

1. The twitch responses usually become detectable by visual or tactile means at this stage.

2. This degree of block generally is associated with adequate surgical relaxation.
3. Subsequent recovery usually occurs more rapidly than recovery until this point.
4. A repeat bolus or a continuous infusion of a relaxant typically is administered when 10–25% recovery of twitch height has been achieved.
5. Effective reversal of the neuromuscular block becomes increasingly likely between 10% and 25% recovery.

The time to 25% recovery of neuromuscular function (Dur_{25}), referred to as the *"clinical duration,"* identifies the time at which reinforcement of a block often is necessary and when reversal is readily accomplished. After a typical intubating dose ($2 \times ED_{95}$), the average Dur_{25} is 15–20 minutes for mivacurium, 30–60 minutes for atracurium and vecuronium, and 90–120 minutes for pancuronium, *d*-tubocurarine, gallamine, and metocurine (Table 12-1).

The interval between *25% and 75%* recovery of twitch height (RI_{25-75}) provides a standard of comparison that is, for the most part, independent of drug dosage and is inversely proportional to K_{el} (i.e., to the rate of drug elimination).[2] Typical values for this *"recovery index"* are 5–10 minutes for mivacurium, 10–15 minutes for atracurium, 10–15 minutes for vecuronium, and 25–50 minutes for tubocurarine (Table 12-1). There generally is a consistent linear relationship between log-plasma concentration and drug effect in the 25–75% range.[2] Ideally, such an index *should be independent of drug dose*. However, for agents where redistribution plays a major role in recovery, the RI_{25-75} may be increased after large doses, serial doses, or a continuous infusion.[15–19] For example, as the dose of vecuronium was increased from 0.1 to 0.4 mg · kg^{-1}, the RI was prolonged linearly.[18] Such prolongation of action is even more prominent after a large dose of relaxant is administered to an obese patient.[20] When large enough doses are administered, a cumulative effect has been reported even for *mivacurium*,[21] but it was of relatively small magnitude.

Beyond 75% recovery of twitch height, the relationship between the declining log-plasma concentration and the increasing twitch height is no longer linear; twitch height slowly approaches its baseline magnitude as the plasma concentration continues to decrease. The Dur_{95} *(time to return of twitch height to 95% of baseline)* generally approximates twice the Dur_{25}. After a typical intubating dose (approximately $2 \times ED_{95}$), the Dur_{95} is approximately 25 minutes after mivacurium, 70 minutes after atracurium, 80 minutes after vecuronium, and ≥150 minutes after most long-lasting agents (Table 12-1).

As noted in Chapter 4, *we typically assess recovery in terms of fade* in response to tetanic or train-of-four stimulation. T_4 generally becomes detectable when T_1 has returned to 20–30% of its baseline height (Dur_{25}). The subsequent return of T_4 tends to roughly parallel that of T_1 (Table 6-1), such that when T_1 reaches 95–100% of baseline, T_4 typically is 70% of baseline ($T_4/T_1 \cong 0.70$). Subsequent *recovery of T_4* requires more than 20 minutes for long-lasting agents, 5–15 minutes for intermediate-acting agents, and less than 5 minutes for mivacurium (the lone short-acting agent).[22,23] As detailed in Chapters 14 and 15, this permits one to extubate the trachea with more confidence after mivacurium, even if a "reversal dose" of anticholinesterase has not been administered.

Discussion Questions ◆

a. How do the different time courses of recovery and onset affect monitoring of the T_4/T_1 ratio?
b. Given that the *plasma concentration of pancuronium* associated with 50% depression of twitch height is 0.14 µg · mL^{-1} during a *continuous infusion*, what would you expect it to be during recovery from a *bolus injection* or after a tourniquet is removed from an *isolated arm* (into which pancuronium had been infused)?
c. Do the *clinical durations* of relaxants differ by the magnitude of the differences in their clearance?
d. Estimate the *times to 95% recovery* (Dur$_{95}$) of twitch height and the *25–75% recovery index* (RI$_{25-75}$) after a dose of atracurium (or vecuronium) that resulted in 25% recovery of twitch height at 22 minutes after loss of twitch height.
e. Why does *doubling the dose* of *mivacurium* within clinical dosing ranges typically have relatively little impact on its *duration?*
f. If twitch height has returned to 95% of baseline, how long would you wait before being confident that the T_4/T_1 ratio has returned to >0.70?
g. What is meant by the following statement? After a relatively low dose, the reduction in the clinical effect of *vecuronium* is primarily due to *redistribution*; after a very high dose, the reduction becomes more dependent on *elimination.*
h. Why do the *kidneys* play a relatively large role in the *clearance* of most NDRs?
i. How is the *duration* of a block affected when an *intermediate-acting NDR* is administered *after partial recovery from a long-acting NDR*? Why?

Answers ◆

a. During recovery, there generally is ample time to distinguish between the return of T_4 and T_1 during train-of-four stimulation and thereby monitor the resolution of fade. Following paralysis with a 2 × ED$_{95}$ dose of a short, intermediate or long-acting agent, the time from the initial detection of T_4 to a T_4/T_1 ratio >0.70 typically is more than 15, 40, and 70 minutes, respectively. The slow changes in junctional concentrations of an NDR allow for differential binding to (or "unbinding" from) sites with different tendencies to elicit fate (e.g., they may selectively remain effective at presynaptic sites). In contrast, after bolus administration of these doses, there is complete ablation of all twitches within 5 minutes. Such a rapid time course precludes clinically significant differential binding, especially after high doses[24,26] (or intra-arterial injection[27]).

b. The relationship between the *concentration of relaxant at the NMJ and in the plasma* depends on the means of drug delivery and/or the conditions under which it is removed. During a continuous infusion, the concentration of relaxant in the plasma is greater than or equal to that at the NMJ.[1,2] During recovery, there is an NMJ to plasma gradient. This gradient would be largest in a limb that had been isolated by an arterial tourniquet for relaxant infusion and underwent washout after tourniquet release. At 50% recovery of twitch height, the systemic plasma concentration of pancuronium was 0.05 μg · mL^{-1} after tourniquet release, 0.10 μg · mL^{-1} during recovery from a systemic bolus, and 0.14 μg · mL^{-1} during continuous systemic infusion.[28] Most agree that, in the context of recovery from a continuous infusion (or bolus), the rate-limiting factor is the speed of removal of drug from the NMJ.[29] Recovery of twitch height correlates well with the decrease in log-plasma concentration.[3,9,10,30] However, when there is a large NMJ to plasma gradient (as occurs after tourniquet release), then dissociation from the receptor may play a significant role.[28,31]

c. The *duration* of action of nondepolarizing agents does not typically differ by the magnitude of the differences in their clearance rates, because the *rapid alpha phase (redistribution)* plays a major role in terminating the clinically evident drug effect. Drug subsequently returns slowly to the central compartment, and clearance is responsible for the subsequent removal of relaxant from the plasma (and NMJs).

Redistribution is especially critical for the relatively short duration of *vecuronium* (and probably *rocuronium*). Vecuronium's $t_{1/2elim}$ is 2–3 times longer than that of atracurium. Redistribution is most effective in reducing the effect of a relaxant after a single bolus. The impact of redistribution decreases as the drug accumulates (e.g., multiple doses, long-term infusion, large doses in obese patients) and the sites of redistribution become saturated.

d. Given that the Dur_{25} after a dose of atracurium is 22 minutes, we can anticipate Dur_{95} to be 44 minutes.[32] *Typically, Dur_{25} is approximately 1/2 of Dur_{95}*. The RI_{25-75} is consistent for a single dose of vecuronium and for virtually all doses of atracurium that are employed clinically: 12–14 minutes.[32] Thus, consistent with the sigmoidal relationship, the first 25% of recovery requires 22 minutes, 25–75% recovery requires only 12–14 minutes, and the next 20% of recovery (75–95% recovery) requires approximately 10–12 minutes.

e. Because of its rapid metabolism,[33] *mivacurium does not typically dem-*

onstrate a marked prolongation of duration when its dose is doubled. The prolongation of effect may be approximated by its $t_{1/2}$ (which has been reported to be as low as 2–4 minutes[33]), similar to the way doubling the dose of SCh causes a prolongation of action that is proportional to its $t_{1/2}$.[34]

f. After T_1 has returned to 95% of its baseline height, T_4 typically requires in excess of 20 minutes to reach 70% of its baseline height ($T_4/T_1 \geq 0.70$) after a *long-acting NDR*. It thus is not uncommon to detect residual weakness in the postanesthesia care unit (Chap. 6). Following an agent of intermediate duration, T_4 typically recovers within 15 minutes of T_1. This is true for virtually all clinical doses of *atracurium* but is not necessarily true for high doses of *vecuronium*, since the latter is eliminated rather slowly and typically depends on redistribution for termination of its effect. The lone short-acting NDR, *mivacurium*, commonly requires less than 5 minutes for recovery of T_4/T_1 after recovery of T_1.

g. After a relatively *low dose of vecuronium*, redistribution away from the NMJ is primarily responsible for the return of neuromuscular function. Drug concentrations in the blood and NMJs decrease below the effective drug concentrations. Metabolism and elimination do not exert a predominant role until after drug concentrations are below clinically effective levels.

Alternatively, after a very *large dose*, multiple doses, or continuous infusion, sites for *redistribution* become saturated. Thus, the body must rely on metabolism and elimination to lower the drug level below the effective concentration. Clearance is relatively slow, as the $t_{1/2elim}$ of vecuronium is 2–5 times that of atracurium. Hence, there is prolongation of block and an increase in recovery indices.

h. Nondepolarizing relaxants are charged molecules. As such, they do not readily cross the hepatocyte membranes for metabolism by the liver. Alternatively, their polarity promotes their excretion via the kidney, as it prevents reabsorption across the cells of the renal tubule. Some drugs (e.g., vecuronium) are more lipid soluble and, as such, are more likely to undergo hepatic metabolism.

i. When an *intermediate-duration NDR* is administered *during recovery* from a long-acting NDR, the duration of block more closely resembles that of the long-acting agent.[35–39] Although prior occupation of redistribution sites and clearance pathways should be considered, the most likely explanation is that, despite considerable return of twitch height toward baseline, *most receptors are still occupied by the original NDR*, and thus the block predominantly has the characteristics of the original agent administered.

References ◆

1. Stanski DR, Sheiner LB: Pharmacokinetics and dynamics of muscle relaxants. Anesthesiology 51:103–105, 1979

2. Shanks CA: Pharmacokinetics of the nondepolarizing neuromuscular relaxants applied to the calculation of bolus and infusion dosage regimens. Anesthesiology 64:72–86, 1986
3. Shanks CA, Somogyi AA, Triggs EJ: Dose-response and plasma concentration-response relationships of pancuronium in man. Anesthesiology 51:111–118, 1979
4. Meretoja OA: Vecuronium infusion requirements in pediatric patients during fentanyl-N_2O/O_2 anesthesia. Anesth Analg 68:20–24, 1989
5. Ali HH, Savarese JJ, Embree PB, Basta SJ, Stout RG, Bottros H, Weakly JN: Clinical pharmacology of mivacurium chloride (W B1090U) infusion: comparison with vecuronium and atracurium. Br J Anaesth 61:541–546, 1988
6. Cannon JE, Fahey MR, Castognoli KP, Furuta T, Canfell PC, Sharma M, Miller RD: Continuous infusion of vecuronium: the effect of anesthetic agents. Anesthesiology 67:503–506, 1974
7. Brandom BW, Woelfel SK, Cook DR, Weber S, Powers DM, Weakly JN: Comparison of mivacurium and suxamethonium administered by bolus and infusion. Br J Anaesth 62:488–493, 1989
8. Greenblatt DJ, Koch-Weser J: Clinical pharmacokinetics. N Engl J Med 293:702–705, 1975
9. Agoston S, Crul J, Kersten UW, Scaf AHJ: Relationship of the serum concentration of pancuronium to its neuromuscular activity in man. Anesthesiology 47:509–512, 1977
10. Matteo RS, Spector S, Horowitz PE: Relation of serum d-tubocurarine concentration to neuromuscular blockade in man. Anesthesiology 41:440, 1974
11. Waud BE: Serum d-tubocurarine concentration and twitch height. Anesthesiology 43:381–382, 1975
12. Caldwell JE, Heier T, Kitts JB, Lynam DP, Fahey MR, Miller RD: Comparison of the neuromuscular block induced by mivacurium, suxamethonium or atracurium during nitrous oxide–fentanyl anaesthesia. Br J Anaesth 63:393–399, 1989
13. Kopman AF: Tactile evaluation of train-of-four count as an indicator of reliability of antagonism of vecuronium- or atracurium-induced neuromuscular blockade. Anesthesiology 75:588–593, 1991
14. Viby-Mogensen J: Clinical assessment of neuromuscular transmission. Br J Anaesth 54:209–223, 1982
15. Brull SJ, Silverman DG: Tetanus-induced changes in apparent recovery following bolus doses of atracurium or vecuronium. Anesthesiology (in press)
16. Fisher DM, Rosen JI: A pharmacokinetic explanation for increasing recovery time following larger or repeated doses of nondepolarizing muscle relaxants. Anesthesiology 65:286–291, 1986
17. Feldman SA, Liban JB: Vecuronium—a variable dose technique. Anaesthesia 42:199–201, 1987
18. Ginsberg B, Glass PS, Shafron D, Ossey KD: Onset and duration of neuromuscular blockade following high-dose vecuronium administration. Anesthesiology 71:201–205, 1989
19. Kopman AF: Recovery times following edrophonium and neostigmine reversal of pancuronium, atracurium, and vecuronium steady-state infusions. Anesthesiology 65:572–578, 1986
20. Weinstein JA, Matteo RS, Ornstein E, Schwartz AE, Goldstoff M, Thal G: Pharmacodynamics of vecuronium and atracurium in the obese surgical patient. Anesth Analg 67:1149–1153, 1988
21. Shanks CA, Fragen RJ, Pemberton D, Katz JA, Risner ME: Mivacurium-induced neuromuscular blockade following single bolus doses and with continuous infusion during either balanced or enflurane anesthesia. Anesthesiology 71:362–366, 1989
22. Savarese JJ, Ali HH, Basta SJ, Embree PB, Scott RPF, Sunder N, Weakly JN, Wastila WB, El-Sayad HA: The clinical neuromuscular pharmacology of mivacurium chloride (BW B1090U): a short-acting nondepolarizing ester neuromuscular blocking drug. Anesthesiology 68:723–732, 1988
23. Sarner JB, Brandom BW, Woelfel SK, Dong M-L, Horn MC, Cook DR, McNulty BF, Foster VJ: Clinical pharmacology of mivacurium chloride (BW B1090U) in children during nitrous oxide–halothane and nitrous oxide–narcotic anesthesia. Anesth Analg 68:116–121, 1989
24. Power SJ, Jones RM: Relationship between single twitch depression and train-of-four

fade: influence of relaxant dose during onset and spontaneous offset of neuromuscular blockade. Anesth Analg 66:633–636, 1987
25. Turner GA, Williams JD, Baker DJ: Train-of-four fade during onset and recovery of neuromuscular block: a study in non-anaesthetized subjects. Br J Anaesth 62:279–286, 1989
26. Pearce AC, Casson WR, Jones RM: Factors affecting train-of-four fade. Br J Anaesth 57:602–606, 1985
27. Bowman WC, Webb SN: Tetanic fade during partial transmission failure produced by non-depolarizing neuromuscular blocking drugs in the cat. Clin Exp Pharmacol Physiol 3:545–555, 1976
28. Agoston S, Feldman SA, Miller RD: Plasma concentrations of pancuronium and neuromuscular blockade after injection into the isolated arm, bolus injection, and continuous infusion. Anesthesiology 51:119–122, 1979
29. Hull CJ: Pharmacodynamics of nondepolarizing neuromuscular blocking agents. Br J Anaesth 54:169–182, 1982
30. Hull CJ, Van Beem HBH, McLeod K, Sibbald A, Watson MJ: A pharmacodynamic model for pancuronium. Br J Anaesth 50:1113–1122, 1978
31. Feldman SA, Tyrrell MF: A new theory on the termination of action of the muscle relaxants. Proc R Soc Med 63:692–695, 1970
32. Basta SJ, Ali HH, Savarese JJ, Sunder N, Gionfriddo M, Cloutier G, Lineberry C, Cato AE: Clinical pharmacology of atracurium besylate (BW 33A): a new non-depolarizing muscle relaxant. Anesth Analg 61:723–729, 1982
33. Cook DR, Stiller RL, Weakly NJ, Chakravorti S, Brandom BW, Welch RM: In vitro metabolism of mivacurium chloride (BW 1090U) and succinylcholine. Anesth Analg 68:452–456, 1989
34. Levy G: Kinetics of pharmacologic activity of succinylcholine in man. J Pharmacol Sci 56:1687–1688, 1967
35. Janda A, Muhlsteiger B, Schwarz S: Atracurium increased duration of its effect following alcuronium. Anasth Intensivther Notfallmed 25:303, 1990
36. Kay B, Chestnut RJ, Sum Ping JST, Healy TEJ: Economy in the use of muscle relaxants: vecuronium after pancuronium. Anaesthesia 42:277–280, 1987
37. Middleton CM, Pollard BJ, Healy TE, et al: Use of atracurium or vecuronium to prolong the action of tubocurarine. Br J Anaesth 62:659, 1989
38. Rashkovsky OM, Agoston S, Ket JM: Interaction between pancuronium bromide and vecuronium bromide. Br J Anaesth 57:1063–1066, 1985
39. Smith I, White PF: Pipecuronium-induced prolongation of vecuronium neuromuscular block. Br J Anaesth 70:446–448, 1993

9

DAVID G. SILVERMAN | RAJINDER K. MIRAKHUR

Effects of Other Agents on Nondepolarizing Relaxants

Many of the medications that are used in perioperative and intensive care settings may alter the pharmacodynamics and pharmacokinetics of nondepolarizing relaxants (NDRs). Nondepolarizing block may be increased or decreased by the effects of other drugs on regional perfusion, plasma proteins, nerve terminals, junctional binding sites, junctional enzymes, muscle fibers, and sites of elimination. The interactions that may be encountered most commonly in the clinical setting, and their effects on nondepolarizing neuromuscular block, are outlined in Table 9-1. When effects are specific for an individual relaxant, they are discussed with that relaxant (Chaps. 12, 13, or 14). Likewise, if a perioperative drug has an impact on a particular feature of neuromuscular block, then it is also discussed with that feature (e.g., Reversal, Chap. 15). Please note, however, that results are not always clear-cut, as they are influenced by a myriad of study conditions. This chapter highlights the most salient features.

TABLE 9-1
Effects of Other Agents on Nondepolarizing Relaxants

Agent	Δ	Mechanism, Evidence, and Comments
AMINOPYRIDINES (e.g., 4-aminopyridine, guanidine)	D	Oppose K^+ efflux from the nerve, causing prolongation of the nerve action potential and increased release of acetylcholine (ACh).[1-3] This may partially restore transmission and may augment reversal,[4,5] but it also may elicit central nervous system (CNS) and autonomic excitation. Thus, aminopyridines are not routinely used in clinical practice. They may be particularly helpful in the presence of antibiotic-induced exacerbation of NDR-induced block[4,5] and for treatment of the Eaton-Lambert (myasthenic) syndrome.[6-8]

(Continued)

I = increases effect of block; D = decreases effect of block; i = minor or theoretical increase; d = minor or theoretical decrease.

Effects of Other Agents on Nondepolarizing Relaxants

TABLE 9-1
(Continued)

Agent	Δ	Mechanism, Evidence, and Comments
ANTIBIOTICS	I	Exert their neuromuscular blocking effects by a variety of different potential mechanisms. In their presence, the depth of neuromuscular block may be increased, and reversal is inconsistent.[9-27] The most notable effects occur with polymyxins and aminoglycosides. In many cases, no appreciable effect is noted.[27] Short- and intermediate-duration agents may be less affected than most other NDRs[22,28] (questions a and b).
▪ Polymixins	I	Cause the most depression of neuromuscular function.[14,18,21] They may depress postsynaptic sensitivity to ACh (with channel block),[19] muscle sensitivity to direct stimulation,[21] and possibly quantal release of ACh (a local anesthetic-like effect). Effects are not readily reversible.
▪ Aminoglycosides (e.g., gentamicin, kanamycin, neomycin, streptomycin, tobramycin)	I	Used commonly and therefore of concern.[9,13,19,22,27] Effects often resemble those of Mg^{2+} and/or local anesthetics[9,21]; they may decrease ACh release (like Mg^{2+} and/or local anesthetics), cause channel block, decrease postsynaptic sensitivity,[19,22,27] or decrease muscle contractility.[22] The effects sometimes may be reversible with Ca^{2+}, but this is not routinely recommended. Anticholinesterases are not usually effective antagonists. Aminopyridines may be partially effective for reversing the effects of these (and other) antibiotics.[4,5]
▪ Vancomycin	i	Implicated in a case of prolonged block after vecuronium.[24]
▪ Lincomycin and clindamycin	I	Among other effects, they may cause channel block and have a direct effect on muscle contractility.[19,29] They may be partially offset with 4-aminopyridine.[28]
▪ Tetracycline	i	Produces less profound block. Since tetracycline presumably decreases ACh release by chelation of Ca^{2+}, it may be reversed with calcium (but not anticholinesterases).[19] Again, reversal of effects is inconsistent at best.[12,15] Also, tetracycline may decrease receptor sensitivity.[21]
▪ Penicillins	—	Negligible effect.
▪ Metronidazole	i	Contradictory reports. Metronidizole prolongs the effect of vecuronium but not pancuronium in animals[17] and possibly humans,[30] but not consistently[31,32]; and it has actually been reported to facilitate neuromuscular transmission in the presence of vecuronium.[31]
ANTICHOLINESTERASES	D	Increase the availability of ACh, which can then compete more effectively with NDRs. Excesses may result in poisoning (Chap. 15).
ANTICONVULSANTS		
▪ Acute	I	Intravenous (IV) dose of diphenylhydantoin may acutely enhance block, probably by membrane stabilization and decreased ACh release.[33,34]

(Continued)

I = increases effect of block; D = decreases effect of block; i = minor or theoretical increase; d = minor or theoretical decrease.

TABLE 9-1
(Continued)

Agent	Δ	Mechanism, Evidence, and Comments
■ Chronic	D	Requirements for NDRs are doubled and recovery times halved in patients receiving chronic diphenylhydantoin (phenytoin) or carbamazepine therapy.[35-48] Potential mechanisms include: (1) a drug-induced increase in *alpha$_1$-acid glycoprotein*, which then increases NDR protein binding (from 26% in control rats to 33% in phenytoin-treated rats) and decreases its free fraction[38,49]; and (2) a compensatory *upgrading of postsynaptic receptors*[38-40,50] as a consequence of prolonged depression of neuromuscular transmission (with decreased ACh release).[33,50-52] (3) Phenytoin may also cause neuromuscular disorders.[9,53] (4) An increase in *cytochrome P450* in the liver plays a minor role, since clearance of unbound drug is relatively unchanged. Effects may be less evident for atracurium than for vecuronium or long-lasting NDRs[42]; however, atracurium exhibited no "sparing" when exposed to carbamazepine plus phenytoin or valproic acid[46] (question c).
ANTIEMETICS		
■ Droperidol	i	May prolong recovery, attributable to a decrease in nerve action potential and to postsynaptic block.[54] Of relatively little clinical significance.
■ Metoclopramide	—	Prolongs SCh-induced block (Chap. 17) but not NDR-induced block.
■ Ondansetron	—	No effect on atracurium-induced neuromuscular block in the clinical setting.[55]
ANTINEOPLASTICS	I	Intraperitoneal thiotepa (triethylene thiophosphoramide) increased NDR-induced block in a patient with myasthenia gravis,[56] perhaps because this tertiary ammonium compound is transformed to a quaternary ammonium derivative.[56] It is also possible that these drugs, which are similar in structure to ACh, may cause weakness due to prolonged depolarization. Of note, several cancer drugs compete for pseudocholinesterase[57] and thus may prolong the action of mivacurium (as well as succinylcholine).
ANTIRHEUMATIC DRUGS	I	*d-Penicillamine* treatment of rheumatoid arthritis may cause an immunologic disorder similar to myasthenia gravis.[9,58,59] *Chloroquine* may be associated with postoperative neuromuscular block, especially if introduced intraperitoneally (IP) during surgery, perhaps by presynaptic local anesthetic-like and postsynaptic NDR-like actions.[9,60]
CARDIOVASCULAR DRUGS	i	May alter regional perfusion and exert direct neuromuscular effects.

(Continued)

I = increases effect of block; D = decreases effect of block; i = minor or theoretical increase; d = minor or theoretical decrease.

TABLE 9-1

(Continued)

Agent	Δ	Mechanism, Evidence, and Comments
■ Beta blockers	i	May increase depth and duration,[61] perhaps by depressing excitable tissue.[62]
■ Other antiarrhythmics	i	Mild potentiation has been noted after bretylium,[63] disopyramide,[64,65] quinidine,[66] lidocaine, and procaine (see Local anesthetics).
■ Vasodilators	i	Nitroglycerin decreases the ED_{95} of pancuronium,[67,68] perhaps by increasing muscle blood flow. Nitroglycerin and adenosine triphosphate (ATP) potentiated atracurium-induced block.[69]
■ Ca^{2+} channel blockers	i	Affect slow Ca^{2+} channels (Chap. 1) with possible pre- and/or postjunctional effects, including channel block.[70-82] Possible interference with excitation-contraction coupling in certain muscles.[81] Verapamil exerts greater effect than nifedipine.[78] May compromise reversal[79]; even if NDR potency is increased, recovery often may not be significantly prolonged.[83] In many cases, an effect is not detectable in humans.[84,85] The effects of calcium channel blocking are of less consequence to skeletal muscle than to smooth (e.g., vascular) muscle.
■ Epinephrine	d/i	Mixed effects[86,87]: may increase presynaptic release of ACh (perhaps by an alpha-mediated increase in Ca^{2+} entry via slow channels) but decrease electrical excitability of muscle fibers (by $beta_2$ alteration of the Na^+/K^+ pump and/or shortening of contraction).[88,89]
■ $Beta_2$ agonists	I	Salbutamol (a $beta_2$ agonist used to treat bronchospasm), 125 μg IV, caused an additional decrease in twitch height after pancuronium, from 55% of baseline to 34% of baseline.[90]
■ Ganglionic blockers	i	Compete with ACh and may augment or prolong block.[91,92] In addition, *trimethaphan* theoretically may limit metabolism of mivacurium by competing for plasma pseudocholinesterase.
DANTROLENE	I	Causes direct muscle depression,[93,94] but muscle action potential (MAP) is normal; hence the electromyogram (EMG) is normal. A dosage of 0.4 mg · kg^{-1} decreased grip strength; dosages of 0.6, 1.0, and 2.5 mg · kg^{-1} decreased mechanomyographic (MMG) twitch by 50%, 65%, and 75%, respectively[94] (Chap. 20).
DOXAPRAM	I	Causes an increase in NDR block in vitro.[95] Delays recovery from and impairs neostigmine reversal of vecuronium-induced block,[96,97] delaying it by 40%.[96,98]

(Continued)

I = increases effect of block; D = decreases effect of block; i = minor or theoretical increase; d = minor or theoretical decrease.

TABLE 9-1
(Continued)

Agent	Δ	Mechanism, Evidence, and Comments
H$_2$ ANTAGONISTS	I/D	The effects, which are not clear-cut, depend on the dose, route, timing, and nature of the H$_2$ antagonist as well as the nature of the NDR. In some studies, *pretreatment with a single dose* had no effect on NDR-induced block.[99,100] Others noted that a moderately *large dose of cimetidine* (400 mg), but not ranitidine, was associated with prolongation of vecuronium-induced block[101]; e.g., Dur$_{25}$ and RI$_{25-75}$ were prolonged by approximately 13 minutes and 6 minutes, respectively.[101] This may be due to decreased hepatic clearance as a result of decreased hepatic blood flow and competition for metabolic pathways (e.g., cytochrome P450). In addition, there is evidence to suggest that *high doses of cimetidine and ranitidine can produce neuromuscular block*,[102] with a reduced response to ACh and development of fade. Alternatively, IV administration of high doses of ranitidine and, to a lesser degree, cimetidine *partially "reversed" NDR-induced block* in animals and laboratory models; the effect was seen almost immediately and lasted for several minutes.[103-105] It appears to be due to *anticholinesterase properties*. As is the case for traditional reversal agents, ranitidine and cimetidine preferentially affect acetylcholinesterase of the NMJ (as opposed to pseudocholinesterase, which metabolizes SCh in the plasma)[102,106,107] (Chap. 17). An appreciable effect typically is not seen with the relatively low plasma concentration attained with the doses of H$_2$ antagonist used for aspiration prophylaxis prior to induction of anesthesia. However, levels sufficient to affect anticholinesterase may be approached with ranitidine.[108] The plasma concentration of ranitidine peaked at >10 μg · ml^{-1} immediately after IV injection of 150 mg,[108] and that of cimetidine was >5 μg · ml^{-1} at 15 minutes after 300 mg IV.[109] This may lead to increased *cholinergic activity* at muscarinic as well as nicotinic sites.[102,108,110-112] Potential muscarinic effects include bradycardia[111,112] and increased gastroesophageal tone.[110]
IMMUNOSUPPRESSIVES	i/d	Mixed effects, which depend on length of use (and thus time for ACh receptor proliferation). *Cyclosporine* potentiated atracurium and vecuronium[113] and was associated with an increased incidence of postoperative respiratory failure.[114] *Azathioprine* (Imuran) has caused mixed effects, which appear to be influenced by the study model.[115] It caused resistance to NDRs,[115,116] presumably by causing motor axons to fire repetitively (due to phosphodiesterase inhibition—see Theophylline) and causing a dose-related increase in the force of contraction[116]; this effect appears to be short-lived under steady-state conditions.[115] In contrast, azathioprine also has been reported to prolong nondepolarizing block.[117]

(Continued)

I = increases effect of block; D = decreases effect of block; i = minor or theoretical increase; d = minor or theoretical decrease.

TABLE 9-1

(Continued)

Agent	Δ	Mechanism, Evidence, and Comments
INDUCTION AGENTS	i	There may be slight dose-related potentiation by most induction agents.[17,118]
▪ Thiopental	i	May alter amplitude, latency, and duration of MAPs.[119] A dosage of 5 mg · kg^{-1} had no effect, while 10 mg · kg^{-1} increased the effect of vecuronium by 30%.[17] This has little clinical implication.
▪ Propofol	i	Shifts the dose-response curve of atracurium and vecuronium slightly to the left,[120] but the effect appears to be minimal.[121] Overall, propofol's effects on SCh, atracurium, and vecuronium are similar to those of thiopental.[122] Propofol may decrease twitch tension at far greater concentrations than are encountered clinically.[123]
▪ Ketamine	i	May cause a slight increase in block,[124-127] perhaps by decreasing the release of ACh[124] or decreasing end plate sensitivity; alternatively, it may increase baseline twitch height.[124]
INHALATIONAL ANESTHETICS	I	Cause a decrease in twitch height, T_4/T_1 ratio, peak tetanic contraction, and especially the ability to sustain tetanus in the presence of NDRs.[17,128-157] Also suppress motor evoked potentials in response to spinal cord[158] and transcranial[159-161] stimulation. The *effect on tetanus* may be more pronounced than on the train-of-four response,[129,131,133,137,153] perhaps because of altered muscle contractility.[139,152,153,162] Facilitation of posttetanic twitch height (considered to be a presynaptic effect) was not affected.[163] Effects are *dose and time dependent*.[147,150] Inhalational agents cause a *delay in reversal*,[133-136,164] especially if they are maintained after administration of the reversing agent. *The effects of inhalational anesthetics are greater for long-lasting relaxants* and during infusions.[132,145-148,149,165,166] Enflurane is associated with a 30% decrease in mivacurium infusion requirements[148] (despite mivacurium's lack of dependence on organ elimination). The effects of other agents are related in the following fashion: diethyl ether[151] > enflurane[128,134,147,151,157] > isoflurane[128,140,142,151,167] = desflurane[131] > halothane.[128,140,142]
▪ Nitrous oxide	i	Causes a slight increase in block within 5–10 minutes.[168]
LITHIUM	I	Competes with Na$^+$ and may cause decreased ACh release[169]; may increase and prolong block.[170,171]
LOCAL ANESTHETICS	i	May block nerve action potential, block ACh release, cause channel block, and/or reduce propagation from the endplate.[61,172-175] Augmented block produced by lidocaine-pancuronium in cats[71] effectively was reversed with anticholinesterases. May cause denervation-like changes, attributable to blocking axonal transmission.[176]

(Continued)

I = increases effect of block; D = decreases effect of block; i = minor or theoretical increase; d = minor or theoretical decrease.

TABLE 9-1
(Continued)

Agent	Δ	Mechanism, Evidence, and Comments
MANNITOL	—	No effect on relaxant elimination, since that depends on the rate of glomerular filtration, not secretion.[177]
NARCOTICS	i	Tend to increase block[17,178,179] but generally to a minimal degree.[17] The onset of neuromuscular block is faster if anesthesia is induced with N_2O, fentanyl, and thiopental than with thiopental alone.[179]
■ Morphine	i	Possible presynaptic action,[178] but generally minimal.[17] Original implication was with high doses that led to respiratory depression in mice.[180]
NDR's (prior)		
■ Long term	D	May decrease the response to subsequent NDR due to up-regulation of postsynaptic receptors[39,181-183] (Chap. 22). Alternatively, long-term infusions may affect muscle integrity and result in persistent weakness and myopathies (Chap. 11).
■ Previous Intraop.	I	Previous administration of pancuronium with 25% recovery markedly increased the RI of a subsequent 0.05 mg · kg^{-1} dose of vecuronium[184] (perhaps because approximately 85% of *receptor occupancy* still was by pancuronium, and/or because pancuronium occupied some of the sites of vecuronium redistribution and/or elimination). Similarly, long durations were noted in other assessments of long-short or long-intermediate relaxant sequences.[185-189] As expected, the effect of the long-lasting NDR dissipated on serial dosing with the shorter-acting agent.[186,187] Likewise, the effect of vecuronium predominated when it was given before pancuronium.[188] One also should consider the potential for *synergism* when combinations of certain NDRs are used. The prolongation of *mivacurium after pancuronium*[190] may be attributable in part to pancuronium's inhibition of pseudocholinesterase activity.
PHYSOSTIGMINE	d	Inhibits phosphodiesterase[32,191] (see Theophylline). This *tertiary amine* does not produce the increase in ACh that results from anticholinesterases with a quaternary nitrogen.
SEDATIVES/ANXIOLYTICS		
■ Benzodiazepines	i	Enhance binding of gamma-aminobutyric acid to GABA receptors, thus enhancing GABA's action as an inhibitory transmitter, primarily in brain but also in peripheral nerves; hence, benzodiazepines tend to relieve spasticity. High doses of diazepam potentiated pancuronium in vitro,[192] but 0.14–0.2 mg · kg^{-1} of diazepam was without effect on pancuronium[193] or vecuronium.[17] An induction dose of midazolam had an effect equal to that of thiopental.[194]

(Continued)

I = increases effect of block; D = decreases effect of block; i = minor or theoretical increase; d = minor or theoretical decrease.

Effects of Other Agents on Nondepolarizing Relaxants

TABLE 9-1
(Continued)

Agent	Δ	Mechanism, Evidence, and Comments
■ Chlorpromazine	I	Causes muscle weakness, perhaps by internuncial neuronal depression and/or membrane stabilization.[195]
STEROIDS	D/I	Contradictory. Most likely decrease neuromuscular block, but also may increase block or exert no effect.[195–203] *Factors leading to decreased block* include increased Ach release[204–206] (perhaps by increased cyclic nucleotides[32]), increased neural excitability with autoexcitability,[202,208] and/or augmented muscle contraction. *Factors leading to increased block* include decreased receptor sensitivity at the end-plate with large doses,[205] steroid-induced muscle weakness and myopathy, and decreased clearance of NDR.[207] Testosterone therapy was associated with resistance to nondepolarizing and depolarizing block.[201] Of note, *high-dose steroids* (as may be used to treat status asthmaticus) may cause *severe myopathies* in the presence of prolonged infusions of NDRs (Chap. 11).
SUCCINYLCHOLINE		
■ Prior to NDR	I	May increase the depth of subsequent NDR block and possibly prolong block,[209–215] but not always.[216] Most recently shown to not affect rocuronium[216] or mivacurium.[217] The effect was even more pronounced after recovery from a neuromuscular block induced by *decamethonium*, 0.1 mg · kg^{-1}.[218] Potential mechanisms include: (1) prolonged channel block and desensitization, (2) alteration of the postsynaptic Na$^+$/K$^+$ pump, and (3) ACh depletion,[219–221] possibly the sequela of SCh's presynaptic activation with altered intracellular Ca^{2+} transients[222] and membrane hyperpolarization[220] (Chap.16).
■ After NDR	D/I	Opposes NDR block by competing at cholinoceptors; but large dose may deepen overall block by causing depolarizing block (Chap. 16).
THEOPHYLLINE	d	Phosphodiesterase inhibitors *allow an epinephrine-induced increase in cAMP*, which increases Ca^{2+} entry via slow channels and thus increases ACh release and antagonizes the block.[115,223–225]
TOXINS		May decrease nerve action potential, presynaptic release of ACh (or its breakdown), postsynaptic binding, and/or muscle contraction.[226–233]

(Continued)

I = increases effect of block; D = decreases effect of block; i = minor or theoretical increase; d = minor or theoretical decrease.

TABLE 9-1
(Continued)

Agent	Δ	Mechanism, Evidence, and Comments
▪ *Clostridium botulinum*	I/D	Blocks ACh release, causes weakness and paralysis, and thereby increases block.[227,228,234] The amplitude of the response increased with rapid stimulation,[234] resembling Eaton-Lambert myasthenic syndrome (Chap. 21). Long-term functional denervation may lead to receptor proliferation and hence hyposensitivity to NDRs[39] as well as hypersensitivity to ACh and SCh.[229,230]
▪ *Clostridium tetani*	I/D	Blocks ACh release; however, as opposed to *C. botulinum*, it primarily affects central synapses and thereby leads to spasticity and convulsions.[228,231]
▪ Tetrodotoxin	I	Blocks nerve action potential.
▪ Snake alpha-bungarotoxin	I	Binds to postsynaptic receptors.[232] The effect may resemble acute muscle denervation,[233] which may lead to postsynaptic cholinoceptor proliferation.

I = increases effect of block; D = decreases effect of block; i = minor or theoretical increase; d = minor or theoretical decrease.

Discussion Questions ◆

a. Are the neuromuscular effects of *antibiotics* consistently opposed by *neostigmine*? Explain.
b. Are the neuromuscular effects of *antibiotics* consistently opposed by *calcium*? Explain.
c. Why are nondepolarizing agents affected by *chronic anticonvulsant* therapy? To what degree?
d. What is the effect of increased binding to *plasma proteins* on drug availability for activity at *effector sites* and for *clearance*?

Answers ◆

a. There is variation among *antibiotics* with respect to whether their neuromuscular effects are reversible.[10,12,15,18–20] There is evidence that neither anticholinesterases nor calcium are effective.[10,18,20] Anticholinesterases (Chap. 15) and aminopyridines[4,5] may be worth considering in the context of aminoglycosides. Alternatively, it has also been suggested that anticholinesterases may augment the block associated with polymyxin.[16]
b. *Calcium* is most successful at reversing the neuromuscular effects of *aminoglycosides*[16] and *tetracyclines*. However, it is not effective against all agents. In addition, high doses of calcium theoretically may oppose antibacterial actions and thus may be contraindicated.
c. In the context of chronic *phenytoin* (diphenylhydantoin, Dilantin) or

carbamazepine (Tegretol) therapy, the requirements for NDRs are increased by approximately 80%, and their duration is comparably decreased.[35-46] A *pharmacodynamic effect* is suggested by the finding that the plasma levels required for a given depth of block are increased.[41] It has long been appreciated that phenytoin *depresses synaptic transmission.*[50,52,53] It thus is reasonable that acute phenytoin administration may augment an NDR block. As noted in a recent review,[39] long-term (>2 weeks) use of phenytoin or carbamazepine may be comparable to relaxant infusion and immobilization of moderate duration (Chap. 22); i.e., it may result in *proliferation of postsynaptic ACh receptors*[39,40] (which probably remain within the end-plate). This proliferation is of a nature and degree such that it leads to NDR "resistance" but not to extrajunctional receptor proliferation and succinylcholine-induced hyperkalemia (which would typify the response to denervation injury).

A *pharmacokinetic mechanism* may be attributable to the finding that chronic use of anticonvulsants may lead to a systemic increase in *alpha$_1$-acid glycoprotein,*[38,40] an acute-phase protein that binds NDRs. The increase in this protein is very prominent after burns, and it contributes to the increased NDR requirements in burned patients (Chap. 22). Other pharmacokinetic mechanisms appear to be unlikely. Even though anticonvulsants induce hepatic enzymes, they do not change plasma decay curves for free drug to a degree that could account for the increased NDR requirements.

d. *Drug that is bound to plasma proteins* is not "free" to exert an effect at an effector site such as the neuromuscular junction (NMJ). Only free drug is capable of leaving the plasma and equilibrating in the biophase. This may account for the decreased effectiveness of NDRs in patients receiving chronic anticonvulsant therapy; such therapy increases levels of *alpha$_1$-acid glycoprotein,* which binds relaxant in the blood. Likewise, bound drug is not available for passage across the membranes of hepatocytes or across the renal glomeruli for subsequent excretion.

References ◆

1. Katz B, Miledi R: Estimates of quantal content during "chemical potentiation" of transmitter release. Proc R Soc Lond 205:369–378, 1979
2. Beaufort TM, Wierda JMKH, Kruyswijk JE, Agoston S: 2,4-Diaminopyridine: clinical evaluation of a recently synthesized 4-aminopyridine derivative for reversal of competitive neuromuscular blockade. Eur J Anaesthesiol 7:453–457, 1990
3. Thesleff S: Aminopyridines and synaptic transmission. Neuroscience 5:1413, 1980
4. Booij LHDJ, Miller RD, Crul JF: Neostigmine and 4-aminopyridine antagonism of lincomycin-pancuronium neuromuscular blockade in man. Anesth Analg 57:316–321, 1978
5. Singh YN, Marshall IG, Harvey AL: Reversal of antibiotic induced muscle paralysis by 3,4 diaminopyridine. J Pharm Pharmacol 30:249–250, 1978
6. Agoston S, van Weerden T, Westra P, Broekert A: Effects of 4-aminopyridine in Eaton Lambert syndrome. Br J Anaesth 50:383–385, 1978

7. Oh SJ, Kim KW: Guanidine hydrochloride in the Eaton-Lambert syndrome (electrophysiologic improvement). Neurology 23:1084–1090, 1973
8. Telford RJ, Hollway TE: The myasthenic syndrome: anaesthesia in a patient treated with 3 • 4 diaminopyridine. Br J Anaesth 64:363–366, 1990
9. Argov Z, Mastaglia FL: Disorders of neuromuscular transmission caused by drugs. N Engl J Med 301:409–413, 1979
10. Adamson RH, Marshall FN, Long JP: Neuromuscular blocking properties of various polypeptide antibiotics. Proc Soc Exp Biol Med 105:494–497, 1960
11. Burkett L, Bilkhazi GM, Thamas KC, et al: Mutual potentiation of the neuromuscular effects of antibiotics and relaxants. Anesth Analg 58:107–115, 1979
12. Bezzi G, Gessa GL: Influence of antibiotics on the neuromuscular transmission in mammals. Antibiot Chemother 11:710–714, 1961
13. Hall DR, McGibbon DH, Evans LL, et al: Gentamicin, tubocurarine, lignocaine and neuromuscular blockade: a case report. Br J Anaesth 44:1329–1332, 1972
14. Kronenfeld MA, Thomas SJ, Turndorf H: Recurrence of neuromuscular blockade after reversal of pancuronium in a patient receiving polymyxin/amikacin sternal irrigation. Anesthesiology 65:93–94, 1986
15. Kubikowski P, Szreniawaski Z: The mechanism of the neuromuscular blockade by antibiotics. Arch Int Pharmacodyn Ther 146:549–560, 1963
16. Miller RD: Antagonism of neuromuscular blockade. Anesthesiology 44:318–329, 1976
17. McIndewar IC, Marshall RJ: Interactions between the neuromuscular blocking drug ORG NC45 and some anesthetic, analgesic and antimicrobial agents. Br J Anaesth 53:785–791, 1981
18. Naiman JG, Martin JD: Some aspects of neuromuscular blockade by polymyxin B. J Surg Res 7:199–206, 1967
19. Singh YN, Marshall IG, Harvey PL: Pre- and postjunctional blocking effects of aminoglycoside, polymyxin, tetracycline and lincosamide antibiotics. Br J Anaesth 54:1295–1306, 1982
20. Timmerman JC, Long JP, Pittinger CB: Neuromuscular blocking properties of various antibiotic agents. Toxicol Appl Pharmacol 1:299–304, 1959
21. Wright JM, Collier B: The site of neuromuscular block produced by polymyxin B and rolitetetracycline. Can J Physiol Pharmacol 54:926–936, 1976
22. Dupuis JY, Martin R, Tétrault J-P: Atracurium and vecuronium interaction with gentamicin and tobramycin. Can J Anaesth 36:407–411, 1989
23. Rawlins MD: Drug interactions and anaesthesia. Br J Anaesth 50:689–693, 1978
24. Huang KC, Heise A, Shrader AK, et al: Vancomycin enhances the neuromuscular blockade of vecuronium. Anesth Analg 71:194, 1990
25. Jeideikin R, Dolgunski E, Kaplan R, Hoffman S: Prolongation of neuromuscular blocking effect of vecuronium by antibiotics. Anaesthesia 42:858–860, 1987
26. Sokoll MD, Gergis SD: Antibiotics and neuromuscular function. Anesthesiology 55:148, 1981
27. Lippmann M, Yang E, Au E, et al: Neuromuscular blocking effects of tobramycin, gentamicin, and cefazolin. Anesth Analg 61:767, 1982
28. Cooper R, Maddineni VR, Mirakhur RK: Clinical study of the interaction of rocuronium with commonly used antimicrobial agents. Eur J Anaesthesiol 10:331–335, 1993
29. Wright JM, Collier B: The site of neuromuscular block produced by clindamycin and lincomycin. Can J Physiol Pharmacol 54:937–944, 1976
30. Smith CL, Hunter JM, Jones RS: Vecuronium infusions in patients with renal failure in an ITU. Anaesthesia 42:387–393, 1987
31. Anagnostou JM, Bell GC: Effects of metronidazole on neuromuscular transmission in rabbits. Anesth Analg 68:S10, 1989
32. d'Hollander A, Agoston S, Capouet V: Failure of metronidazole to alter a vecuronium neuromuscular blockade in humans. Anesthesiology 63:99–102, 1985
33. Yaari P, Pincus JH, Argov Z: Depression of synaptic transmission by diphenylhydantoin. Ann Neurol 1:334–338, 1977
34. Gray HSJ, Slater RM, Pollard BJ: The effect of acutely administered phenytoin on vecuronium-induced neuromuscular blockade. Anaesthesia 44:379–381, 1989
35. Bulkley R, Ebrahim Z, Roth S, DeBoer G, Run S: Resistance to vecuronium in patients receiving carbamazepine. Anesthesiology 67:A345, 1987

36. Chen J, Kim YD, Dubois M, et al: The increased requirement of pancuronium in neurosurgical patients receiving dilantin chronically. Anesthesiology 59:A288, 1983
37. Kumar CM, Lawler PG: Phenytoin induced resistance to vecuronium. Anaesthesia 44:263–264, 1989
38. Kim CS, Arnold FJ, Itani MS, Martyn JAJ: Decreased sensitivity to metocurine during long-term phenytoin therapy may be attributable to protein binding and acetylcholine receptor changes. Anesthesiology 77:500–506, 1992
39. Martyn JAJ, White DA, Gronert GA, Jaffe RS, Ward JM: Up-and-down regulation of skeletal muscle acetylcholine receptors: effects on neuromuscular blockers. Anesthesiology 76:822–843, 1992
40. Martyn JAJ, Kim CS: Decreased sensitivity to metocurine during chronic phenytoin may be due to protein binding and receptor changes. Anesthesiology 75:A640, 1991
41. Ornstein E, Matteo RS, Young WL, Diaz J: Resistance to metocurine-induced neuromuscular blockade in patients receiving phenytoin. Anesthesiology 63:294–298, 1985
42. Ornstein E, Matteo RS, Schwartz AE, et al: The effect of phenytoin on the magnitude and duration of neuromuscular block following atracurium or vecuronium. Anesthesiology 67:191–196, 1987
43. Ornstein E, Matteo R, Weinstein J, Halevy J, Young W, Abou-Donia M: Accelerated recovery from doxacurium-induced neuromuscular blockade in patients receiving chronic anticonvulsant therapy. J Clin Anesth 3:108–111, 1991
44. Plotkin CN, Ornstein E: Resistance to pancuronium: adult respiratory distress syndrome or phenytoin. Anesth Analg 65:820, 1986
45. Roth S, Ebrahim ZY: Resistance to pancuronium in patients receiving carbamazepine. Anesthesiology 66:691–693, 1987
46. Tempelhoff R, Modica PA, Jellish WS, Spitznragel EL: Resistance to atracurium-induced neuromuscular blockade in patients with intractable seizure disorders treated with anticonvulsants. Anesth Analg 71:665–669, 1990
47. Ebrahim ZY, Bulkley R, Roth S: Carbamazepine therapy and neuromuscular blockade with atracurium and vecuronium. Anesth Analg 67:S55, 1988
48. Modica P, Templehoff R, Jellish W, Williams EL: Accelerated recovery from pipecuronium in neurosurgical patients treated with chronic carbamazepine therapy. Anesthesiology 75:A187, 1991
49. Abramson FP, Lutz MP: The effects of phenytoin dosage on the induction of α_1-acid glycoprotein and antipyrine clearance in the dog. Eur J Drug Metab Pharmacokinet 11:135–143, 1986
50. Alderice MT, Trommer BA: Differential effects of the anticonvulsant phenobarbital, ethosuximide and carbamazepine on neuromuscular transmission. J Pharmacol Exp Ther 215:92–96, 1980
51. Gordon AS, Miljay D, Diamond I: Phosphorylation of the membrane-bound acetylcholine receptor: inhibition by diphenylhydantoin. Ann Neurol 5:201–203, 1974
52. Raines A, Standaert FG: Pre and postjunctional effects of diphenylhydantoin at the cat soleus neuromuscular junction. J Pharmacol Exp Ther 153:361–366, 1966
53. So EL, Penry JK: Adverse effects of phenytoin on peripheral nerves and neuromuscular junction: a review. Epilepsia 22:467–473, 1981
54. Sokoll MD, Gergis SD, Post EL, Cronnelly R, Long JP: Effects of droperidol on neuromuscular transmission and muscle membrane. Eur J Pharmacol 28:209–213, 1974
55. Lien CA, Gadalla F, Kudlak TT, Embree PB, Sharp GJ, Savarese JJ: The effect of ondansetron on atracurium-induced neuromuscular blockade. J Clin Anesth 5:399–403, 1993
56. Bennett EJ, Schmidt GB, Patel KP, Grundy EM: Muscle relaxants, myasthenia, and mustards? Anesthesiology 46:220–221, 1977
57. Zsigmond EK, Robins G: The effect of a series of anti-cancer drugs on plasma cholinesterase activity. Can Anaesth Soc J 19:75–82, 1972
58. Bucknall RC: Myasthenia associated with D-penicillamine therapy in rheumatoid arthritis. Proc R Soc Med 70(suppl 3):114–117, 1977
59. Masters CL, Dawkins RL, Zilko PJ, et al: Penicillamine-associated myasthenia gravis, antiacetylcholine receptor and antistriational antibodies. Am J Med 63:639–694, 1977
60. Jui-Yen T: Clinical and experimental studies on mechanism of neuromuscular blockade by chloroquine diorotate. Jpn J Anesthesiol 20:491–503, 1971

61. Harrah MD, Way WL, Katzung BG: The interaction of *d*-tubocurarine with antiarrhythmic drugs. Anesthesiology 33:406–410, 1970
62. Werman R, Wislicki L: Propranolol, a curariform and cholinomimetic agent at the frog neuromuscular junction. Comp Gen Pharmacol 2:69–81, 1971
63. Welch GW, Waud BE: Effect of bretylium on neuromuscular transmission. Anesth Analg 61:442–444, 1982
64. Baurain M, Barvais L, d'Hollander A, Hennart D: Impairment of the antagonism of vecuronium-induced paralysis and intraoperative disopyramide administration. Anaesthesia 44:34–36, 1989
65. Healey TEJ, O'Shea M, Massey J: Disopyramide and neuromuscular transmission. Br J Anaesth 53:495–498, 1981
66. Miller RD, Way WL, Katzung BG: The potentiation of neuromuscular blocking agents by quinidine. Anesthesiology 28:1036–1041, 1967
67. Glisson SN, El-Atr AA, Lim R: Prolongation of pancuronium-induced neuromuscular blockade by intravenous infusion of nitroglycerin. Anesthesiology 51:47, 1979
68. Koyama T, Amaki Y, Kobayashi K: Nitroglycerin reduces requirement of pancuronium in surgical patients. Jpn J Anesthesiol 40:1242–1244, 1991
69. Chan KH, Mui WC, Yang MW, et al: Influence of controlled hypotension by adenosine triphosphate or nitroglycerin on the neuromuscular blocking effect of atracurium in dogs. Neurosci Lett 123:226, 1991
70. Bikhazi GB, Leung I, Foldes FF: Ca-channel blockers increase potency of neuromuscular blocking agents *in vivo*. Anesthesiology 59:A269, 1983
71. Carpenter RL, Mulroy MF: Edrophonium antagonizes combined lidocaine-pancuronium and verapamil-pancuronium neuromuscular blockade in cats. Anesthesiology 65:506–510, 1986
72. Durant NN, Nguyen N, Katz RL: Potentiation of neuromuscular blockade by verapamil. Anesthesiology 60:298–303, 1984
73. Kraynack BJ, Lawson NW, Gintantas J, et al: Effects of verapamil on indirect muscle twitch responses. Anesth Analg 62:827–830, 1983
74. Salvatore A, Del Pozo E, Carlos R, Baeyens JM: Differential effects of calcium channel blocking agents on pancuronium- and suxamethonium-induced neuromuscular blockade. Br J Anaesth 60:495–499, 1988
75. van Poorten JF, Dhasmana KM, Kuypers RSM, Erdmann W: Verapamil and reversal of vecuronium neuromuscular blockade. Anesth Analg 63:155–157, 1984
76. Chang CC, Lin SO, Hong SJ, et al: Neuromuscular block by verapamil and diltiazem and inhibition of acetylcholine release. Brain Res 454:332, 1988
77. Chang CC, Chiou LC, Hwang LL, et al: Mechanisms of the synergistic interactions between organic calcium channel antagonists and various neuromuscular blocking agents. Jpn J Pharmacol 53:285, 1990
78. Gomez-Iglesias E, Garcia E, Suarez E, et al: *In vivo* potentiation of atracurium neuromuscular blockade by nimodipine in rabbits. Acta Anaesthesiol Scand 36:67, 1992
79. Jones RM, Cashman JN, Casson WR, et al: Verapamil potentiation of neuromuscular blockade: failure of reversal with neostigmine but prompt reversal with edrophonium. Anesth Analg 64:1021, 1985
80. Jelen-Esselborn S, Blobner M: Potentiation of nondepolarizing muscle relaxants by nifedipine iv in inhalation anesthesia. Anaesthesist 39:173, 1990
81. Kawagoe R, Mino H, Takeuchi A: Effects of organic Ca antagonist, diltiazem, on neuromuscular transmission. Jpn J Physiol 40:325, 1990
82. del Pozo E, Baeyens JM: Neuromuscular blockade induced by flunarizine alone and in combination with pancuronium, suxamethonium or neomycin: studies in isolated rat phrenic-hemidiaphragm preparations. Acta Anaesthesiol Scand 33:582, 1989
83. Bikhazi GB, Leung I, Flores C, Mikati HMJ, Foldes FF: Potentiation of neuromuscular blocking agents by calcium channel blockers in rats. Anesth Analg 67:1–8, 1988
84. Bell PF, Mirakhur RK, Elliott P: Onset and duration of clinical relaxation of atracurium and vecuronium in patients on chronic nifedipine therapy. Eur J Anaesthesiol 6:343, 1989
85. Kanaya N, Sato Y, Tsuchida H, et al: The effects of nicardipine and verapamil on the recovery time of vecuronium-induced neuromuscular blockade. Masui 40:246, 1991

86. Krnjevic K, Miledi R: Some effects produced by adrenalin upon neuromuscular propagation in rats. J Physiol 141:291–304, 1958
87. Kuba K: Effects of catecholamines on the neuromuscular junction in the rat diaphragm. J Physiol 211:551–570, 1970
88. Bowman WC, Nott MW: Actions of some sympathomimetic bronchodilator and beta-adrenoceptor blocking drugs on contractions of the cat soleus muscle. Br J Pharmacol 38:37–49, 1970
89. Clausen T, Flatman JA: The effect of catecholamines on Na-K transport and membrane potential in rat soleus muscle. J Physiol 270:383–414, 1977
90. Salib Y, Donati Y: Potentiation of pancuronium and vecuronium neuromuscular blockade by intravenous salbutamol. Can J Anaesth 40:50–53, 1993
91. Deacock AR, Hargrove RL: The influence of certain ganglion blocking agents on neuromuscular transmission. Br J Anaesth 34:357, 1962
92. Wilson SL, Miller RN, Wright C, et al: Prolonged neuromuscular blockade associated with trimethaphan: a case report. Anesth Analg 55:353–356, 1976
93. Driessen JJ, Wuis EW, Gielen MJM: Prolonged vecuronium neuromuscular blockade in a patient receiving orally administered dantrolene. Anesthesiology 62:523–524, 1985
94. Flewellen EH, Nelson TE, Jones WP, Arens JF, Wagner DL: Dantrolene dose-response in awake man: implications for management of malignant hyperthermia. Anesthesiology 59:275–280, 1983
95. Pollard BJ, Randall NPC, Pleuvry BJ: Doxapram and the neuromuscular junction. Br J Anaesth 62:664–668, 1989
96. Orlowski M, Pollard BJ: Effect of doxapram on neostigmine evoked antagonism of vecuronium neuromuscular block. Br J Anaesth 68:418–419, 1992
97. Pollard BJ, Orlowski M: Doxapram- and neostigmine-evoked antagonism of vecuronium neuromuscular block. Br J Anaesth 65:586P, 1990
98. Cooper R, McCarthy G, Mirakhur RK, Maddenini VR: Effect of doxapram and the rate of recovery of atracurium and vecuronium neuromuscular block. Br J Anaesth 68:527–528, 1992
99. Hawkins JL, Adenwala J, Camp C, Joyce TH III: The effect of H_2-receptor antagonist premedication on the duration of vecuronium-induced neuromuscular blockade in postpartum patients. Anesthesiology 71:175–177, 1989
100. Sato Y, Tsuchida H, Harada Y, et al: Effect of cimetidine on neuromuscular blockade by succinylcholine and pancuronium. Masui 39:168, 1990
101. McCarthy G, Mirakhur RK, Elliott P, Wright J: Effect of H_2-receptor antagonist pretreatment on vecuronium- and atracurium-induced neuromuscular block. Br J Anaesth 66:713, 1991
102. Gwee MCE, Cheah LS: Actions of cimetidine and ranitidine at some cholinergic sites: implications in toxicology and anesthesia. Life Sci 39:383–388, 1986
103. Law SC, Ramzan IM, Brandom BW, et al: Intravenous ranitidine antagonizes intense atracurium-induced neuromuscular blockade in rats. Anesth Analg 69:611–613, 1989
104. Lee HS, Cheah LS, Gwee MCE: Inhibition of acetylcholinesterase by histamine agonists and antagonists. Clin Exp Pharmacol Physiol 12:613–620, 1985
105. Mishra Y, Ramzan I: Ranitidine reverses gallamine paralysis in rats. Anesth Analg 76:627–630, 1993
106. Hansen WE, Bertl S: Inhibition of cholinesterases by ranitidine. Lancet 1:235, 1983
107. Mishra Y, Ramzan I: Interaction between succinylcholine and ranitidine in rats. Can J Anaesth 40:32–37, 1993
108. Van Hecken AM, Tjandramaga TB, Mullie A, Verbesselt R, De Schepper PJ: Ranitidine: single dose pharmacokinetics and absolute bioavailability in man. Br J Clin Pharmacol 14:195–200, 1982
109. Walkenstein SS, Dubb JW, Randolph WC, Westlake WJ, Stote RM, Intoccia AP: Bioavailability of cimetidine in man. Gastroenterology 74:360–365, 1978
110. Brock-Utne JG, Downing JW, Humphrey D: Effect of ranitidine given before atropine sulphate on lower oesophageal sphincter tone. Anaesth Intensive Care 12:140–142, 1984
111. Camarri E, Chirone E, Fanteria G, Zocchi M: Ranitidine induced bradycardia (letter). Lancet 2:160, 1982

112. Shah RR: Symptomatic bradycardia in association with H_2-receptor antagonists (letter). Lancet 2:1108, 1982
113. Gramstad L, Gjerlow JA, Hysing ES, et al: Interaction of cyclosporin and its solvent, cremophor, with atracurium and vecuronium. Br J Anaesth 58:1149–1155, 1986
114. Sidi A, Kaplan RF, Davis RF: Prolonged neuromuscular blockade and ventilatory failure after renal transplantation and cyclosporine. Can J Anaesth 37:543–548, 1990
115. Gramstad L: Atracurium, vecuronium and pancuronium in end-stage renal failure: dose-response properties and interactions with azathioprine. Br J Anaesth 59:995–1003, 1987
116. Dretchen KL, Morgenroth VH III, Standaert FG, Walts LF: Azathioprine: effects on neuromuscular transmission. Anesthesiology 45:604–609, 1976
117. Vetten KB: Immunosuppressive therapy and anaesthesia. S Afr Med J 47:767–770, 1973
118. Torda TA, Murphy EC: Presynaptic effect of I.V. anaesthetic agents at the neuromuscular junction. Br J Anaesth 51:353–356, 1979
119. Quilliam JP: The action of thiopentone sodium on skeletal muscle. Br J Pharmacol 10:141–146, 1955
120. Robertson EN, Fragen RJ, Booij LHDJ, et al: Some effects of disopropyl phenol (ICI 35868) on the pharmacodynamics of atracurium and vecuronium in anaesthetized man. Br J Anaesth 55:723–728, 1983
121. McCarthy G, Mirakhur RK, Pandit SK: Lack of interaction between propofol and vecuronium. Anesth Analg 75:536–538, 1992
122. Nightingale P, Petts NV, Healy TEJ, Kay B, McGuiness K: Induction of anaesthesia with propofol ("Diprivan") or thiopentone and interactions with suxamethonium, atracurium and vecuronium. Postgrad Med J 61(suppl 3):31–34, 1985
123. Lebeda MD, Wegrzynowicz ES, Wachtel RE: Propofol potentiates both pre- and post-synaptic effects of vecuronium in the rat hemidiaphragm. Br J Anaesth 68:282, 1992
124. Amaki Y, Nagashima H, Radnay PA, Foldes FF: Ketamine interaction with neuromuscular blocking agents in the phrenic nerve-hemidiaphragm preparation of the rat. Anesth Analg 57:238–243, 1978
125. Cronnelly R, Dretchen KL, Sokoll MD, et al: Ketamine myoneural activity and interaction with neuromuscular blocking agents. Eur J Pharmacol 22:17–22, 1973
126. Johnston RR, Miller RD, Way WL: The interaction of ketamine with d-tubocurarine, pancuronium, and succinylcholine in man. Anesth Analg 53:496, 1974
127. Toft P, Helbo-Hansen S: Interaction of ketamine with atracurium. Br J Anaesth 62:319–320, 1989
128. Ali HH, Savarese JJ: Monitoring of neuromuscular function. Anesthesiology 45:216–249, 1976
129. Baurain MJ, d'Hollander AA, Melot C, Dernovoi BS, Barvais L: Effects of residual concentrations of isoflurane on the reversal of vecuronium-induced neuromuscular blockade. Anesthesiology 74:474–478, 1991
130. Brett RS, Dilger JP, Yland KF: Isoflurane causes "flickering" of the acetylcholine receptor channel: observations using the patch clamp. Anesthesiology 69:161–170, 1988
131. Caldwell JE, Laster MJ, Magorian T, Heier T, Yasuda N, Lynam DP, Eger EI II, Weiskopf RB: The neuromuscular effects of desflurane, alone and combined with pancuronium or succinylcholine in humans. Anesthesiology 74:412–418, 1991
132. Cannon JE, Fahey MR, Castognoli KP, Furuta T, Canfell PC, Sharma M, Miller RD: Continuous infusion of vecuronium: the effect of anesthetic agents. Anesthesiology 67:503–506, 1974
133. Dernovoi B, Agoston S, Barvais L, Baurain M, Lefebvre R, d'Hollander A: Neostigmine antagonism of vecuronium paralysis during fentanyl, halothane, isoflurane, and enflurane anesthesia. Anesthesiology 66:698–701, 1987
134. Delisle S, Bevan DR: Impaired antagonism of pancuronium during enflurane anaesthesia in man. Br J Anaesth 54:441–445, 1982
135. Gill SS, Bevan DR, Donati F: Edrophonium antagonism of atracurium during enflurane anaesthesia. Br J Anaesth 64:300–305, 1990
136. Gencarelli PJ, Miller RD, Eger II EI, Newfield P: Decreasing enflurane concentrations and d-tubocurarine neuromuscular blockade. Anesthesiology 56:192–194, 1982
137. Hughes R, Payne JP: Interaction of halothane with non-depolarizing neuromuscular blocking drugs in man. Br J Clin Pharmacol 7:485–490, 1979

138. Kennedy RD, Galindo AD: Comparative site of action of various anaesthetic agents at the mammalian myoneural junction. Br J Anaesth 47:533–540, 1975
139. Katz JA, Fragen RJ, Shanks CA, Dunn K, McNulty B, Rudd GD: Dose-response relationships of doxacurium chloride in humans during anesthesia with nitrous oxide and fentanyl, enflurane, isoflurane, or halothane. Anesthesiology 70:432–436, 1989
140. Miller RD, Way WL, Dolan WM, Stevens WC, Eger EI II: The dependence of pancuronium and d-tubocurarine-induced neuromuscular blockades on alveolar concentrations of halothane and forane. Anesthesiology 37:573–581, 1972
141. Miller RD, Way WL, Dolan WM, et al.: Comparative neuromuscular effects of pancuronium, gallamine, and succinylcholine during forane and halothane anesthesia in man. Anesthesiology 35:509–514, 1971
142. Ohta Y, Nagashima H, Lofrumento R, Foldes FF: Halothane-isoflurane-relaxant interactions *in vivo*. Anesthesiology 53:S265, 1980
143. Rupp SM, Fahey MR, Miller RD: Neuromuscular and cardiovascular effects of atracurium during nitrous oxide–fentanyl and nitrous oxide–isoflurane anaesthesia. Br J Anaesth 55:67S–70S, 1983
144. Rupp SM, McChristian JW, Miller RD: Neuromuscular effects of atracurium during halothane–nitrous oxide and enflurane–nitrous oxide anesthesia in humans. Anesthesiology 63:16–19, 1985
145. Rupp SM, Miller RD, Gencarelli PJ: Vecuronium-induced neuromuscular blockade during enflurane, isoflurane, and halothane anesthesia in humans. Anesthesiology 60:102–105, 1984
146. Swen J, Gencarelli PJ, Koot HWJ: Vecuronium infusion dose requirements during fentanyl and halothane anesthesia in humans. Anesth Analg 64:411–414, 1985
147. Stanski DR, Ham J, Miller RD, Sheiner LB: Pharmacokinetics and pharmacodynamics of d-tubocurarine during nitrous oxide–narcotic and halothane anesthesia in man. Anesthesiology 51:235–241, 1979
148. Shanks CA, Fragen RJ, Pemberton D, Katz JA, Risner ME: Mivacurium-induced neuromuscular blockade following single bolus doses and with continuous infusion during either balanced or enflurane anesthesia. Anesthesiology 71:362–366, 1989
149. Shanks CA, Fragen RJ, Ling D, Pemberton D, Dunn K, Howard K: Infusion requirements of ORG 9426 in patients receiving balanced, enflurane or isoflurane anesthesia. Anesthesiology 75:A1068, 1991
150. Withington DE, Donati F, Bevan DR, Varin F: Potentiation of atracurium neuromuscular blockade by enflurane: time-course of effect. Anesth Analg 72:469–473, 1991
151. Waud BE, Waud DR: The effects of diethyl ether, enflurane and isoflurane at the neuromuscular junction. Anesthesiology 42:275–280, 1975
152. Waud BE: Decrease in dose requirement of d-tubocurarine by volatile anesthetics. Anesthesiology 51:298–302, 1979
153. Waud BE, Waud DR: Effects of volatile anesthetics on directly and indirectly stimulated skeletal muscle. Anesthesiology 50:103, 1979
154. Waud BE, Waud DR: Comparison of the effects of general anesthetics on the endplate of skeletal muscle. Anesthesiology 43:540, 1975
155. Weber S, Brandom BW, Powers DM, Sarner JB, Woelfel SK, Cook DR, Foster VJ, McNulty BF, Weakly JN: Mivacurium chloride (BW B1090U)-induced neuromuscular blockade during nitrous oxide–isoflurane and nitrous oxide–narcotic anesthesia in adult surgical patients. Anesth Analg 67:495–499, 1988
156. Woloszczuk-Gebicka B: Influence of halothane on the train-of-four face after atracurium in children. Br J Anaesth 65:540–541, 1990
157. Fogdall RP, Miller RD: Neuromuscular effects of enflurane alone and in combination with d-tubocurarine, pancuronium and succinylcholine in man. Anesthesiology 42:173, 1975
158. Adams DC, Emerson RG, Heyer EJ, McCormick PC, Carmel PW, Stein BM, Farcy JP, Gallo EJ: Monitoring of intraoperative motor-evoked potentials under conditions of controlled neuromuscular blockade. Anesth Analg 77:913–918, 1993
159. Calancie B, Klose KJ, Baier S, Green BA: Isoflurane-induced attenuation of motor evoked potentials caused by electrical motor cortex stimulation during surgery. J Neurosurg 74:897–904, 1991

160. Kalkman CJ, Drummond JC, Kennely NA, et al: Intraoperative monitoring of tibialis anterior muscle motor evoked responses to transcranial electrical stimulation during partial neuromuscular blockade. Anesth Analg 73:584–589, 1992
161. Zentner J, Albrech T, Heuser D: Influence of halothane, enflurane, and isoflurane on motor evoked potentials. Neurosurgery 31:298–305, 1992
162. Kennedy R, Galindo A: Neuromuscular transmission in a mammalian preparation during exposure to enflurane. Anesthesiology 42:432–442, 1975
163. Saitoh Y, Toyooka H, Amaha K: Recoveries of post-tetanic twitch and train-of-four responses after administration of vecuronium with different inhalation anaesthetics and neuroleptanaesthesia. Br J Anaesth 70:402–404, 1993
164. Gyermek L: Halogenated vapor anesthetics adversely influence edrophonium reversal. Int J Clin Pharmacol Ther Toxicol 26:75, 1988
165. Miller RD, Rupp SM, Fisher DM, Cronnelly R, Fahey MR, Sohn YF: Clinical pharmacology of vecuronium and atracurium. Anesthesiology 61:444–453, 1984
166. Swen J, Rashkovsky OM, Ket JM, et al: Interaction between nondepolarizing neuromuscular blocking agents and inhalational anesthetics. Anesth Analg 69:752, 1989
167. Woelfel SK, Dong ML, Brandom BW, et al: Vecuronium infusion requirements in children during halothane-narcotic-nitrous oxide, isoflurane-narcotic-nitrous oxide, and narcotic-nitrous oxide anesthesia. Anesth Analg 73:33, 1991
168. Fiset P, Balendran P, Bevan DR, Donati F: Nitrous oxide potentiates vecuronium neuromuscular blockade in humans. Can J Anaesth 38:866–869 1991
169. Vizi ES, Illes P, Ronai A, Knoll J: The effect of lithium on acetylcholine release and synthesis. Neuropharmacology 11:521–530, 1972
170. Borden H, Clarke MT, Katz H: The use of pancuronium bromide in patients receiving lithium carbonate. Can Anaesth Soc J 21:79–82, 1974
171. Hill GE, Wong KC, Hodges MR: Lithium carbonate and neuromuscular blocking agents. Anesthesiology 46:122, 1977
172. Matsuo S, Rao DBS, Chaudry I, et al: Interaction of muscle relaxants and local anesthetics at the neuromuscular junction. Anesth Analg 57:580–587, 1978
173. Morita K, Matsuo S, Nagashima H, et al: *In vivo* muscle relaxant-local anesthetic interaction. Anesthesiology 51:S282, 1979
174. Telivuo L, Katz RL: The effects of modern intravenous local analgesics on respiration during partial neuromuscular block in man. Anaesthesia 25:30–35, 1970
175. Zukaitis MG, Hoech GP: Train of four measurement of potentiation of curare by lidocaine. Anesthesiology 51:S288, 1979
176. Libelius R, Sonesson B, Stamenovic BA, et al: Denervation-like changes in skeletal muscle after treatment with a local anesthetic (Marcaine). J Anat 106:297–309, 1970
177. Matteo RS, Nishitateno K, Pua EK, et al: Pharmacokinetics of d-tubocurarine in man: effect of an osmotic diuretic on urinary excretion. Anesthesiology 52:335, 1980
178. Duke PC, Johns CH, Pinsky C, Goertzen P: The effect of morphine on human neuromuscular transmission. Can Anaesth Soc J 26:201–205, 1979
179. Scott RPF, Savarese JJ, Basta SJ, Embree P, Ali HH, Sunder N, Hoaglin DC: Clinical pharmacology of atracurium given in high dose. Br J Anaesth 58:834–838, 1986
180. Lang DA, Kimura KK, Unna KR: The combination of skeletal muscle relaxing agents with various central nervous system depressants used in anesthesia. Arch Int Pharmacodyn Ther 85:257–272, 1951
181. Berg DK, Hall ZW: Increased extrajunctional acetylcholine sensitivity produced by chronic post-synaptic neuromuscular blockade. J Physiol 244:659–676, 1975
182. Chang CC, Chuang ST, Huang MC: Effects of chronic treatment with various neuromuscular blocking agents on the number and distribution of acetylcholine receptors in the rat diaphragm. J Physiol (Lond) 250:161–173, 1975
183. Hogue CW, Ward JM, Itani MS, Martyn JAJ: Tolerance and up-regulation of acetylcholine receptors follows chronic infusion of d-tubocurarine. J Appl Physiol 72:1326–1331, 1992
184. Lin ML, Tsai SK, Mok MS: Pancuronium pretreatment prolonged recovery index of vecuronium in children. Anesth Analg 74:S188, 1992
185. Janda A, Muhlsteiger B, Schwarz S: Atracurium increased duration of its effect following alcuronium. Anasth Intensivther Notfallmed 25:303, 1990

186. Kay B, Chestnut RJ, Sum Ping JST, Healy TEJ: Economy in the use of muscle relaxants: vecuronium after pancuronium. Anaesthesia 42:277–280, 1987
187. Middleton CM, Pollard BJ, Healy TE, et al: Use of atracurium or vecuronium to prolong the action of tubocurarine. Br J Anaesth 62:659, 1989
188. Rashkovsky OM, Agoston S, Ket JM: Interaction between pancuronium bromide and vecuronium bromide. Br J Anaesth 57:1063–1066, 1985
189. Smith I, White PF: Pipecuronium-induced prolongation of vecuronium neuromuscular block. Br J Anaesth 70:446–448, 1993
190. Brandom BW, Meretoja OA, Taivainen T, Wirtavuori K: Accelerated onset and delayed recovery of neuromuscular block induced by mivacurium preceded by pancuronium in children. Anesth Analg 76:998–1003, 1993
191. Curley WH, Dretchen KL, Standaert FG: Inhibition by physostigmine of neural phosphodiesterase. Fed Proc 39:410, 1980
192. Driessen JJ, Vree TB, van Egmond J, Booij LHDJ, Crul JF: In vitro interaction of diazepam and oxazepam with pancuronium and suxamethonium. Br J Anaesth 56:1131–1138, 1984
193. Asbury AJ, Henderson PD, Brown BH, Turner DJ, Linkens DA: Effect of diazepam on pancuronium-induced neuromuscular blockade maintained by a feedback system. Br J Anaesth 53:859–863, 1981
194. Cronnelly R, Morris RB, Miller RD: Comparison of thiopental and midazolam on the neuromuscular responses to succinylcholine or pancuronium in humans. Anesth Analg 62:75–77, 1983
195. Argov Z, Yaari Y: The action of chlorpromazine at an isolated cholinergic synapse. Brain Res 164:227–236, 1979
196. Durant NN, Briscoe JR, Katz RL: The effect of acute and chronic hydrocortisone treatment on neuromuscular blockade in the anesthetized cat. Anesthesiology 51:144, 1984
197. Laflin MJ: Interaction of pancuronium and corticosteroids. Anesthesiology 47:471–472, 1977
198. Meyers EF: Partial recovery from pancuronium neuromuscular blockade following hydrocortisone administration. Anesthesiology 46:148–150, 1977
199. Parr SM, Robinson BJ, Rees D, Galletly DC: Interaction between betamethasone and vecuronium. Br J Anaesth 67:447–451, 1991
200. Parr SM, Galletly DC, Robinson BJ: Betamethasone-induced resistance to vecuronium: a potential problem in neurosurgery? Anaesth Intensive Care 19:103–105, 1991
201. Reddy P, Guzman A, Robalino J, Shevde K: Resistance to muscle relaxants in a patient receiving prolonged testosterone therapy. Anesthesiology 70:871–873, 1989
202. Riker WF Jr, Baker T, Okamoto M: Glucocorticoids and mammalian motor nerve excitability. Arch Neurol 32:688–694, 1975
203. Schwartz AE, Matteo RS, Ornstein E, Silverberg PA: Acute steroid therapy does not alter nondepolarizing muscle relaxant effects in humans. Anesthesiology 65:326–327, 1986
204. Veldsema-Currie RD, Van Wilenburg H, Labruyere WT, Langemeijer MWE: Presynaptic, facilitatory effects of the corticosteroid dexamethasone in rat diaphragm: modulation by beta-bungarotoxin. Brain Res 294:315–325, 1984
205. Wilson RW, Ward MD, Johns TR: Corticosteroids: a direct effect at the neuromuscular junction. Neurology 24:1091–1095, 1974
206. Van Wilenburg H, Njio KD, Belling GAC, Van Den Hoven S: Effects of corticosteroids on the myoneural junction: a morphometric and electrophysiological study. Eur J Pharmacol 84:129–137, 1982
207. Shima H: The effect of corticosteroids on the recovery from vecuronium induced block. Masui 39:619, 1990
208. Hall ED: Glucocorticoid effects on the electrical properties of spinal motor neurons. Brain Res 240:109–116, 1982
209. Donati F, Gill SS, Bevan DR, Ducharme J, Theoret Y, Varin F: Pharmacokinetics and pharmacodynamics of atracurium with and without previous suxamethonium administration. Br J Anaesth 66:557–561, 1991
210. d'Hollander AA, Agoston S, DeVille A, et al: Clinical and pharmacological actions of a bolus injection of suxamethonium: two phenomena of distinct duration. Br J Anaesth 55:131–134, 1983

211. Katz RL: Modification of the action of pancuronium by succinylcholine and halothane. Anesthesiology 35:602–606, 1971
212. Krieg N, Hendrickx HHL, Crul JF: Influence of suxamethonium on the potency of ORG NC 45 in anaesthetized patients. Br J Anaesth 53:259–262, 1981
213. Ono K, Manabe N, Ohta Y, Morita K, Kosaka F: Influence of suxamethonium on the action of subsequently administered vecuronium or pancuronium. Br J Anaesth 62:324–326, 1989
214. Ollkoke KT, Schwilden H: Quantitation of the interaction between atracurium and succinylcholine using closed-loop feedback control of infusion of atracurium. Anesthesiology 73:614–618, 1990
215. Swen J, Koot HWJ, Bencini A, Ket JM, Hermans J, Agostson S: The interaction between suxamethonium and the succeeding non-depolarizing neuromuscular blocking agents. Eur J Anaesthesiol 7:203–209, 1990
216. Cooper R, Mirakhur RK, Clarke RSJ, Boules Z: Comparison of intubating conditions after administration of ORG 9426 (rocuronium) and suxamethonium. Br J Anaesth 69:269–273, 1992
217. Maddenini VR, Mirakhur RK, McCoy EP, Fee JPH, Clarke RSJ: Neuromuscular effects and intubating conditions following mivacurium: a comparison with suxamethonium. Anaesthesia 48:940–945, 1993
218. Feldman S, Fauvel N: Potentiation and antagonism of vecuronium by decamethonium. Anesth Analg 76:631–634, 1993
219. Creese R, Head SD, Jenkinson D: Prolonged action of depolarizing drugs in guinea pig muscle. Br J Pharmacol 77:413P, 1982
220. Hartman GS, Fiamengo SA, Riker WF: Succinylcholine: mechanism of fasciculations and their prevention by d-tubocurarine or diphenylhydantoin. Anesthesiology 65:405–413, 1986
221. Standaert FG, Adams JE: The actions of succinylcholine on the mammalian motor nerve terminal. J Pharmacol Exp Ther 149:113–123, 1965
222. Kimura I, Kondoh T, Kimura M: Changes in intracellular Ca^{2+} produced in the mouse diaphragm by neuromuscular blocking drugs. J Pharm Pharmacol 42:626–631, 1990
223. Azar I, Kumar D, Betcher AM: Resistance to pancuronium in an asthmatic patient treated with aminophylline and steroids. Can Anaesth Soc J 29:280–282, 1982
224. Wilson DF: The effects of dibutyryl cyclic AMP, theophylline and aminophylline on neuromuscular transmission in the rat. J Pharmacol Exp Ther 188:447–452, 1974
225. Standaert FG, Dretchen KL: Cyclic nucleotides in neuromuscular transmission. Anesth Analg 60:91–99, 1981
226. Whittaker VP: The contribution of drugs and toxins to understanding cholinergic function. Trends Pharmacol Sci 11:8–13, 1990
227. Gundersen CB: The effects of botulinum toxin on the synthesis, storage and release of acetylcholine. Prog Neurobiol 14:99, 1980
228. Simpson LL: Molecular pharmacology of botulinum toxin and tetanus toxin. Ann Rev Pharmacol Toxicol 26:427–453, 1986
229. Roth F, Wuthrich H: The clinical importance of hyperkalemia following suxamethonium administration. Br J Anaesth 41:311–316, 1969
230. Thesleff S: Supersensitivity of skeletal muscle produced by botulinum toxin. J Physiol 151:598, 1960
231. Orko R, Rosenberg PH, Himberg JJ: Intravenous infusion of midazolam, propofol and vecuronium in a patient with severe tetanus. Acta Anaesthesiol Scand 32:590–592, 1988
232. Lee CY: Chemistry and pharmacology of polypeptide toxins in snake venom. Ann Rev Pharmacol 12:265, 1972
233. Abe T, Jimbrick AR, Miledi R: Acute muscle denervation induced by B-bungarotoxin. Proc R Soc Lond (Biol) 194:545–553, 1976
234. Mayer RF: The neuro-muscular defect in human botulism (abstract). Electroencephalogr Clin Neurophysiol 25:397, 1968

10

DAVID G. SILVERMAN | RAJINDER K. MIRAKHUR

Effects of Patient Status and Conditions on Nondepolarizing Relaxants

In our role as clinical pharmacologists, we often find ourselves administering medications to patients with a wide range of physiological and pathological disturbances. These may increase or decrease the rate of onset, overall effectiveness, and duration of neuromuscular relaxants. As noted in Table 10-1, many patient conditions share common features and thus affect neuromuscular blocking agents similarly. These typically affect the number, location, and even type of cholinoceptors, the volume of steady-state distribution (V_{ss}), and/or organ function. The general descriptions provided in Table 10-1 are detailed for the individual nondepolarizing relaxants (NDRs) in Chapters 12 through 14 and for specific nerve and muscle disorders in Chapters 21 through 23.

TABLE 10-1
Effects of Patient Condition on Nondeplorizing Relaxants

Status or Condition	Δ	Mechanism, Evidence, and Comments
ACIDOSIS/ALKALOSIS		See Acid-Base/Lytes at end of this table.
ALBUMIN AND OTHER PROTEINS		
■ Hypoalbuminemia	I/D	Less drug is bound, hence more drug is free for action but also for distribution and clearance.[1,2] Relaxants are less dependent on binding to albumin (i.e., they typically are <50% bound) than are drugs like thiopental, diazepam, and midazolam.[3,4] The percent binding of pancuronium is approximately 10% and is not significantly altered by age, sex, oral contraceptive use, pregnancy, or renal disease.[3] The relative binding of atracurium may be higher.[5]

(Continued)

I = increases effect of block; D = decreases effect of block; i = minor or theoretical increase; d = minor or theoretical decrease.

TABLE 10-1
(Continued)

Status or Condition	Δ	Mechanism, Evidence, and Comments
■ Increased alpha$_1$-acid glycoprotein	D	Plasma levels of alpha$_1$-acid glycoprotein are elevated as a result of burns, injury, stress, cancer, and diphenylhydantoin therapy.[2,6–11] It binds relaxants with greater affinity than albumin,[7,9] causing decreased drug distribution to tissues.[12,13] This leads to hyposensitivity or "resistance" to NDRs[14] (discussed for anticonvulsants in Chap. 9 and for neuromuscular injury in Chap. 22).
CALCIUM		See Acid-Base/Lytes at end of this table.
CARDIOPULMONARY BYPASS	I	Associated with hypothermia (see below) and decreased elimination[15–17] vs. a transient increase in the volume of distribution (V_{ss}). Hypothermic bypass may decrease the spontaneous breakdown of atracurium by spontaneous Hofmann degradation.[18]
CEREBRAL PALSY	D	Time to 25% recovery (Dur_{25}) after vecuronium, 0.1 mg · kg^{-1}, decreased from 44 min (controls) to 19 min,[19] probably due to acetylcholine (ACh) receptor proliferation with "resistance" to NDRs (Chap. 22).
CRITICAL ILLNESS NEUROPATHY	I/D	There is a high incidence of neural damage (with primary axonal degeneration) in ICU patients with sepsis and multiple organ failure (Chap. 11).[20–31]
DISUSE ATROPHY	I/D	Progressive muscle weakness with ACh receptor proliferation (Chap. 22).
GEOGRAPHY	i/d	There are differences among populations; e.g., vecuronium is "more potent in Montreal than in Paris,"[32] and tubocurarine was more potent in New York than in London.[33]
HYPO-/HYPERCARBIA		See Acid-Base/Lytes at end of this table.
HYPERPARATHYROIDISM	D	Decreases effectiveness[34] and/or shortens duration[35] (see Calcium at end of this table).
HYPOPERFUSION	I/D	May lessen delivery and/or removal of relaxant. Hypotension and peripheral vascular disease have been implicated in motor and sensory deficits in ICU patients.[36–38]
HYPOTHERMIA	I	Decreases removal and metabolism of relaxants, decreases nerve conduction, and decreases muscle contraction. At a skin temperature <32 °C, there is progressive twitch height decline and fade.[39–50] Hypothermia has been implicated as a cause of T_4/T_1 fade in patients after anesthesia.[39,41,42,48,51] Effects vary with the degree of hypothermia and the nature of the study model (question a).[52]

(Continued)

I = increases effect of block; D = decreases effect of block; i = minor or theoretical increase; d = minor or theoretical decrease.

TABLE 10-1
(Continued)

Status or Condition	Δ	Mechanism, Evidence, and Comments
INJURIES		
▪ Burns	D	Tend to decrease response to NDRs (Chap. 22).
▪ Lower motor nerve injuries	D	Tend to decrease response to NDRs, but effects are not clear-cut (Chap. 22).
▪ Upper motor nerve injuries	D	Tend to decrease response to NDRs, but effects are not clear-cut (Chap. 22).
LIVER FAILURE		
▪ Overall effect	I	*Cellular damage* leads to decreased metabolism, especially of hepatic-dependent NDRs such as vecuronium[53–56]; however, cellular damage also decreases the clearance and elimination of pancuronium (which is not highly dependent on liver metabolism)[57,58] and rocuronium,[59] and there was even a case of prolonged atracurium-induced block.[60] *Decreased albumin* has little impact; V_{ss} may be increased as a result of *increased extracellular fluid*, but not always.[55,58] *Decreased production of esterases* may affect the breakdown of atracurium or mivacurium. *Biliary obstruction* opposes hepatic clearance of drugs[55] even if they are not markedly metabolized[61,62]; there are exceptions (e.g., gallamine,[62] atracurium[63]). The clinical impact of liver failure depends on the dose of drug administered,[54] since redistribution plays a major role in decreasing a drug's effects until distribution sites are occupied (after which metabolism plays a more prominent role).
▪ Initial effect	D	The initial effect of a small bolus dose of NDR may be decreased, presumably as a consequence of increased V_{ss}.[57,64–67]
MAGNESIUM		See Acid-Base/Lytes at end of this table.
MALIGNANT HYPERTHERMIA	—	See Chapters 19 and 20.
MALNUTRITION	I	Decreased muscle strength and decreased maximum ventilatory ability.[68]
MYASTHENIA GRAVIS	I	See Chapter 21.
MYASTHENIC SYNDROME	I	See Chapter 21.
OBESITY	I	NDRs are relatively insoluble in lipids and thus are less affected by obesity than are more lipid-soluble compounds. Obesity increases the duration of vecuronium[69] but not of atracurium (which is less lipid soluble and relatively independent of organ elimination) (Chap. 13).[69] Potential for prolongation of any agent when drug is administered on the basis of body weight.

(Continued)

I = increases effect of block; D = decreases effect of block; i = minor or theoretical increase; d = minor or theoretical decrease.

TABLE 10-1
(Continued)

Status or Condition	Δ	Mechanism, Evidence, and Comments
OBSTETRICS		
■ Pregnancy	I/D	Pregnancy is associated with an increase in weight that is disproportionate to the increase in the volume of distribution. There is evidence that clearance is greater and $t_{1/2elim}$ is shorter (for pancuronium and vecuronium) in patients undergoing cesarean section,[70–72] perhaps due to progesterone-induced enzyme stimulation and delivery-induced fluid shifts.[73] One study noted that, after administration of vecuronium (dosed according to body weight), onset was faster and recovery was slower in pregnant women undergoing cesarean section than in nonpregnant counterparts; following 0.1 mg · kg⁻¹, the time to 90% depression of twitch height was 125 ± 66 sec in pregnant women and 288 ± 163 sec in controls, and the time to 20% recovery was 46 ± 10 and 28 ± 10 min, respectively.[72] The investigators noted that these features may be due to relative overdosing because of increased maternal weight as well as being a consequence of the increased cardiac output,[74] decreased peripheral resistance,[75] and decreased protein concentrations[76] associated with pregnancy. In rabbits, pregnancy likewise was associated with increased sensitivity (lower ED_{50}) to vecuronium and a 67% slower recovery time.[77] In contrast, another study noted that $t_{1/2elim}$ of vecuronium was shortened in pregnant humans (Chap. 7, answer m).[71] Since *pseudocholinesterase activity* is decreased during pregnancy (Chap. 17), the duration of *mivacurium* may be slightly prolonged (Chap. 14). Remember that doses may need to be limited so as not to affect the newborn (Chap.11).
■ Post partum	I	Increase in the duration of vecuronium but not of atracurium.[78,79] The duration of vecuronium, 0.1 mg · kg⁻¹, was increased to 60 min (vs. 35 min) in postpartum patients.[79] The increase was attributed to changed liver blood flow and/or competition for liver uptake by hormones.
OLD AGE	I	Aging is associated with progressive decreases in extracellular fluid (V_{ss} of water-soluble drugs), albumin, splanchnic blood flow, and glomerular filtration. *Pharmacodynamics* remain essentially unchanged; e.g., the dose-response (or plasma concentration-response) relationship is essentially unchanged for pancuronium,[80–81] vecuronium,[80,82] or atracurium.[80] *Pharmacokinetic effects* (e.g., delayed elimination) are of lesser magnitude for atracurium[83–87] (which is metabolized in peripheral as well as central compartments) than for *d-tubocurarine*,[88] metocurine,[88] *pancuronium*,[81,89,90] *vecuronium*,[90–93] or *doxacurium*.[94] However, the data are not always clear-cut. Although some studies have noted no significant prolongation of

(Continued)

I = increases effect of block; D = decreases effect of block; i = minor or theoretical increase; d = minor or theoretical decrease.

TABLE 10-1
(Continued)

Status or Condition	Δ	Mechanism, Evidence, and Comments
OLD AGE (cont.)	I	vecuronium, others have noted significant prolongation of Dur_{25} and RI_{25-75}.[90,92,93,95,96] Further, it was noted that the clearance of vecuronium decreased significantly, even though $t_{1/2elim}$ and RI_{25-75} were similar; this was attributed to the declines in clearance and V_{ss} offsetting each other.[90] Another study identified a decrease in the clearance and an increase in $t_{1/2elim}$ of vecuronium with no change in V_{ss}.[92] Despite a 30–50% decrease in effective renal plasma flow by 70–80 years of age (1% per year), the elimination of renally excreted drugs such as *pancuronium*[90] or *pipecuronium*[97] was not altered significantly (perhaps because differences are masked by wide intersubject variability). *Onset of block* in the elderly may be slightly slower, owing to an overall 1% decrease in cardiac output per year. *Reversal* may also be delayed[98,99] but generally is not markedly affected.[100] Delays in reversal and the need for a higher dose of neostigmine[101] may be attributable to slower spontaneous recovery from the NDR in the elderly.
PEDIATRICS		See Chapters 12 through 14 on specific agents, 7 and 8 on pharmacodynamics and pharmacokinetics, 15 on reversal, and Chapter 2 question l on receptor types.
▪ Children	D	Children (but not necessarily neonates) *require more drug* on a mg · kg^{-1} basis (due to increased extracellular fluid), and they *recover faster*[102–115] (Chaps. 12 through 14). *Reversal* occurs more rapidly and the needed dose of reversal agent is less in children and most infants.[116–118] Residual postoperative block appears to be less likely (question b, this chapter). When equivalent doses are administered, onset is faster in children than in adults, perhaps as a consequence of increased regional cardiac output.[103,110]
▪ Premature neonate (and perhaps newborn)	I	Receptor immaturity and decreased clearance cause *increased sensitivity*, which is offset, in part, by an increase in V_{ss}.[103–105,112–115,117,119–129] The steady-state plasma concentration of *d*-tubocurarine needed to produce 50% depression of twitch height in neonates is one-third that of adults for humans[104] and rats,[130] and doses were required at longer and more variable intervals in infants than in children ≥ 1 year of age.[104] Onset is more rapid in infants, presumably owing to increased sensitivity and increased cardiac output. Increased V_{ss} and decreased organ function combine to *decrease clearance*, leading to prolongation, as noted for *d*-tubocurarine,[104] *pancuronium*,[109,110] and *vecuronium*.[103,105,109,131] *Atracurium*, though often prolonged,[102,132] tends to be less affected.[112] Mivacurium metabolism may be compromised by decreased pseudocholinesterase activity in newborns.[133]

(Continued)

I = increases effect of block; D = decreases effect of block; i = minor or theoretical increase; d = minor or theoretical decrease.

TABLE 10-1
(Continued)

Status or Condition	Δ	Mechanism, Evidence, and Comments
PHOSPHATE		See Acid-Base/Lytes at end of this table.
POTASSIUM (hypo-, hyper-)		See Acid-Base/Lytes at end of this table.
RENAL FAILURE		
■ Overall effect	I	Associated with *abnormal electrolytes* and *decreased elimination* of relaxants (both treatable with dialysis), and *generalized weakness*. *Clearance* of some agents (e.g., gallamine, doxacurium, metocurine, pancuronium) is markedly compromised, and these agents are particularly difficult to reverse.[134–143] Renal failure has less effect on agents with primarily hepatic elimination (e.g., vecuronium[144]) but still may decrease clearance and prolong the effects of the parent drug or its metabolites.[145–153] Clearance of rocuronium also decreases in renal failure, resulting in greater individual variability.[154] Of potential concern, renal failure has been associated with prolonged weakness after long-term infusions of vecuronium and pancuronium in ICU patients (Chap. 11).[152] Even mivacurium may be affected,[155] possibly because of decreased pseudocholinesterase. Atracurium is relatively unaffected,[63,156–158] but there is the potential for accumulation of its metabolite *laudanosine* during long-term infusions in ICU patients with organ failure (Chap. 14). *Recurarization* is highly unlikely,[136,159,160] since the clearances of pyridostigmine,[159] edrophonium,[161,162] and neostigmine[161] also are decreased (Chap. 15). However, it is best to avoid large doses of NDRs that depend almost solely on renal elimination (e.g., gallamine, doxacurium, metocurine, pancuronium). Prolongation is greatest after large doses, repeated doses, and continuous infusions,[163] as sites for redistribution become occupied in these settings. Infusion requirements for vecuronium and pancuronium decreased by 23% and 62%, respectively, while that for atracurium was essentially unchanged[164] (questions c and d, this chapter).
■ Initial effect	D	An increased V_{ss} may increase the initial dose requirements[137,143,144,164]; however, no significant difference in onset was noted after atracurium, 0.5 mg • kg^{-1}.[156]
SEPSIS	i	Prolonged sepsis leads to muscle weakness, catabolism, multiple organ failure, electrolyte abnormalities, polyneuropathy, and myositis.[29–31]
ACID-BASE/LYTES		*Results often appear contradictory!* Multiple factors interact as changes in acid-base status and electrolytes affect the NMJ, muscles, NDR ionization, protein binding, drug metabolism, and clearance. These changes also affect each other (e.g., alkalosis promotes entry of K$^+$ into cells, causing hypokalemia, acidosis promotes exit of K$^+$ and hence hyperkalemia). Results are influenced by the acuteness of change, by the study model, and by the presence of anesthetic agents.

(Continued)

I = increases effect of block; D = decreases effect of block; i = minor or theoretical increase; d = minor or theoretical decrease.

TABLE 10-1
(Continued)

Status or Condition	Δ	Mechanism, Evidence, and Comments
■ Decreased Ca^{2+}	I	Decreases ACh release, MAP, and muscle contraction (Chap. 1).[165–167] The effect is relatively small for ionized Ca^{2+} between 0.8 and 1.6 mM.[168]
■ Increased Ca^{2+}	D	Increased Ca^{2+} in bath over the physiological range of concentrations increased the ED_{50} of *d*-tubocurarine and pancuronium by 27%.[167] ED_{95} was higher and duration was decreased in the setting of increased Ca^{2+} (e.g., ionized 3.2 mEq · L^{-1}) due to primary *hyperparathyroidism*.[34,35]
■ Increased Mg^{2+}	I	Competes with Ca^{2+} and thus causes decrease in ACh release; decreased end-plate sensitivity is also noted.[165,166,169–171] May compromise weaning from prolonged mechanical ventilation.[151]
■ Decreased phosphate	I	Levels < 2 mg · dL^{-1} and especially < 1 mg · dL^{-1} cause muscle weakness and possible respiratory failure.[172–178] May also affect CNS and hematopoietic systems.
■ Potassium	i	Marked hyper- as well as hypokalemia can produce a clinical picture of flaccid paralysis.[179–182]
decreased serum K^+	i	A relative decrease in extracellular K^+ causes hyperpolarization of the end-plate with resistance to ACh. A relative fall in both intra- and extracellular K^+ tends not to alter the *resting membrane potential.* Extremely low values (<2.5) may potentiate block.[165,167,183,184]
increased serum K^+	d	A relative increase in extracellular K^+ lowers the resting membrane potential (partially depolarizes and thus increases sensitivity to ACh. This promotes depolarization and theoretically opposes an NDR.[165,167,184] An increase in K^+ over the physiological range in a abath increased the dose requirements for d-dubocurarine and pancuronium by 36%.[167]
■ Increased $Paco_2$	I	Most commonly potentiates NDR-induced block, but the effects are not clear-cut: a decrease in twitch height[185–191] and an increase in block by tubocurarine[189–192] stand in contrast to reports of nonsignificant effects[187,193,194] and even decreased block by certain agents.[190,191] Investigations have identified the following effects of increased $Paco_2$: a. A decrease in twitch height during partial block by vecuronium or pancuronium,[186,187] but maximum depression and recovery indices were not affected when hypercarbia was initiated prior to NDR administration.[187] b. Slowed return to normal twitch height after pancuronium in one study[187] but not in another.[193] c. Increased the block by atracurium,[188] by pancuronium,[185] and by vecuronium infusion.[186]

(Continued)

I = increases effect of block; D = decreases effect of block; i = minor or theoretical increase; d = minor or theoretical decrease.

TABLE 10-1
(Continued)

Status or Condition	Δ	Mechanism, Evidence, and Comments
■ Increased $Paco_2$ (cont.)	I	d. In a rat hemidiaphragm preparation, increased the block by tubocurarine or vecuronium but reduced the block by metocurine, pancuronium, or alcuronium.[190,191] These differences may be attributable to the mixed mono- and bisquaternary configurations of tubocurarine and vecuronium vs. the bisquaternary structures of metocurine, pancuronium, and alcuronium (Fig. 2-1).[190] In the context of acidosis, tubocurarine's tertiary ammonium group would be more likely to combine with an H^+ ion and perhaps have a greater affinity for the anionic ACh receptors.[190,195,196] Acidosis has less effect on bisquaternary compounds, and the effect of acidosis on the other aspects of neuromuscular activity (e.g., protein binding, receptor affinity) may predominate in the presence of bisquaternary compounds.[190] e. Increased resistance to reversal[194,197–199]: e.g., with pH of 7.13 and Pco_2 of 66, neostigmine requirements to reverse tubocurarine at the cat anterior tibial muscle more than doubled.[194] f. An increase in $Paco_2$ to 53.6 mm Hg in humans was associated with slower reversal of 90% pancuronium-induced twitch depression (8 min vs. 14 min for recovery to 90% of baseline MMG twitch height).[200] Since there was no increase in train-of-four fade nor alteration in EMG "twitch height," the authors postulated that the twitch suppression was a consequence of decreased contractility of muscle fibers.[200] Another investigation likewise showed that twitch tension is affected more than the compound MAP, suggesting depressed contractility.[199]
■ Decreased $Paco_2$	d	May decrease block or exert no effect; effects are not clear-cut. Investigations have identified the following effects of decreased $Paco_2$: a. Tended to increase the twitch height in the absence of an NDR.[190,191] b. No significant effect on infusion requirements for tubocurarine or its reversal with neostigmine at the cat anterior tibialis muscle was noted.[194] c. Decrease in block by atracurium.[188] d. Increased the twitch height during partial block by vecuronium or pancuronium infusion but did not affect maximum depression or recovery if the decrease in $Paco_2$ occurred before a bolus.[187]

(Continued)

I = increases effect of block; D = decreases effect of block; i = minor or theoretical increase; d = minor or theoretical decrease.

TABLE 10–1
(Continued)

Status or Condition	Δ	Mechanism, Evidence, and Comments
■ Decreased PaCO_2 (cont.)	d	e. In a rat hemidiaphragm preparation, decreased the block by tubocurarine or vecuronium but increased the block by metocurine, pancuronium, or alcuronium.[190] f. Decreased block by vecuronium.[186] g. Decreased recovery after gallamine.[201]
■ Metabolic acidosis	I	Confusing data: tends to decrease twitch height,[201] but also increased by 27.7% the infusion rate of tubocurarine required to maintain 90% depression of cat anterior tibial muscle.[194] No difficulty reversing in an animal model,[194] but there are reports of difficult reversal in the clinical setting,[202] possibly due to concurrent cellular hypoxia.[194] Increased the block by atracurium,[188] vecuronium,[186] and pancuronium.[185] In the rat hemidiaphragm preparation, it increased the block by tubocurarine or vecuronium but decreased the block by pancuronium or metocurine.[191]
■ Metabolic alkalosis	I	Confusing data: may increase the twitch height,[189,191,203] but was also found to enhance tubocurarine-induced block[194,204] and pancuronium-induced block.[205] May cause resistance to reversal, possibly due to decreased Ca^{2+} and K^+.[197,198] Metabolic alkalosis decreased by 32.5% the infusion rate of tubocurarine required to maintain 90% depression of the cat anterior tibial muscle[194] and more than doubled neostigmine requirements for reversal.[194] Decreased block by atracurium[188] and by vecuronium infusion.[186] In a rat hemidiaphragm preparation it decreased the block by tubocurarine or vecuronium but increased the block by pancuronium or metocurine.[191] May complicate weaning after prolonged ventilation.[151]

I = increases effect of block; D = decreases effect of block; i = minor or theoretical increase; d = minor or theoretical decrease.

Discussion Questions ◆

a. How might *hypothermia* affect relaxant usage?
b. How does *onset of nondepolarizing block* differ in the *neonate* and *adult* when relaxant is administered at (1) equal mg · kg^{-1} doses and (2) equal mg · m^{-2} doses? Why?
c. Would you anticipate major changes in t$_{½elim}$ and in clearance for metocurine, pancuronium, doxacurium, and/or gallamine in the patient with *renal failure*?
d. Is the effect of *renal failure* greater on the early (alpha) or late (beta) phase of the decline in plasma concentration (and hence clinical effect) of a drug that is highly dependent on renal clearance?

Answers ◆

a. *Hypothermia* results in several factors that *decrease twitch height* and *promote fade*. Systemically, it causes a decrease in metabolism and clearance. Locally, it decreases regional blood flow, relaxant washout, nerve conduction, muscle contraction, and skin conductance. A direct effect on muscle is suggested by the more prominent effect on tension (mechanomyogram; MMG) than on the compound action potential (electromyogram; EMG).[41,46]

Recent findings include the following:

1. Mild hypothermia (35.4 °C) during intraoperative relaxation after vecuronium, 0.1 mg · kg^{-1}, prolonged the *time of recovery* of T_1 to 10% of baseline from 28 minutes (control) to 63 minutes, and of subsequent recovery of T_4/T_1 to 0.75 from 37 minutes to 80 minutes.[43]
2. A core temperature 36 °C may be associated with muscle temperatures 35 °C[45]; below this level, twitch height decreases by 10–15%·°C^{-1} decrease in muscle temperature.[45]
3. A decrease in muscle temperature to 31 °C caused a 20% decrease in twitch tension and a 10% decrease in the MMG T_4/T_1 ratio.[42]
4. In the absence of an NDR, cooling the skin from 32.7 °C to 27 °C (with ice packs) caused a decrease in muscle temperature from 35.1 °C to 30.8 °C, a 0.1 decrease in the T_4/T_1 ratio, and a 20% decrease in twitch height.[39]
5. A linear relationship existed between peripheral skin temperature and the T_4/T_1 ratio.[39,48]
6. In two patients who had received NDRs, a 3 °C difference between arms was associated with interarm T_4/T_1 differences of 0.39 and 0.36.[49] Likewise, a difference in temperature between a peripheral muscle (of a limb) and a central muscle (e.g., diaphragm) may contribute to more pronounced twitch depression in the former.[206]
7. Cooling one arm to 27 °C prolonged vecuronium's apparent effect by 60% on that side and distorted the relationship between posttetanic count and the subsequent return of response to train-of-four stimulation.[40]

b. Two opposing sets of factors interact to affect dose-response relationships in the *infant, child, and adult* and lead to different relative mg · kg^{-1} and mg · m^{-2} requirements[104,113,115,120,122,124,128]:

1. The *extracellular (ECF) volume* is 40% of body weight at birth, 25–30% at 1 year, and 20% in the adult. If drugs are given on a *per-weight basis*, then, because of the increased V_{ss}, dose requirements will be increased and onset will be slower in children. Dosing based on *surface area* more closely reflects ECF: since the ECF volume varies with age but not with surface area throughout life, use of mg · m^{-2}

TABLE 10-2
Dose-Response Relationships for Atracurium in the Pediatric Population

Age	ED_{95} (µg · kg−1)	ED_{95} (µg · m−2)
Infants[114]	156	3,330
Children[115]	260	6,628
Adolescents[115]	157	6,302

    corrects for marked differences in V_{ss} in patients of disparate age and size.[104,115,121,129]

2. When *surface area–adjusted doses* (e.g., mg · m^{-2}) are administered, the requirements are clearly less in neonates than in older children. This is primarily due to the increased susceptibility of the neonatal NMJ to NDRs. The nerve terminal and junction are less developed, with less margin of safety. This contributes to a faster onset, as does the infant's high cardiac output. In addition, clearance may be reduced due, owing to immature organ function. The resulting dose-response relationships for atracurium are illustrated in Table 10-2.

c. Gallamine, doxacurium, and, to a lesser extent, metocurine and pancuronium are largely dependent on renal elimination. In the patient with *renal failure*, the clearance of gallamine decreases (and its t½ increases) 6-fold. The other agents exhibit 2- to 3-fold changes.[134,135,137–142,153]

d. The impact of *renal failure* on drug clearance often is not noticeable immediately following bolus administration of a routine dose of an NDR. The alpha phase primarily entails redistribution. The subsequent beta phase (or beta plus gamma phases) is dependent on elimination; thus, the t½elim of a drug that is renally excreted would be increased in the presence of renal failure. For relaxants dependent on renal filtration (i.e., on the glomerular filtration rate, which typically is 120 mL · min^{-1}), drug normally is cleared at approximately 0.5–1%/min such that the half-life is between 60 and 180 minutes. As renal function deteriorates, the time required for elimination increases.

References ◆

1. Wood M: Plasma binding and limitation of drug access to site of action. Anesthesiology 75:721–723, 1991
2. Wood M: Plasma drug binding: implications for anesthesiologists. Anesth Analg 65:786–804, 1986
3. Wood M, Stone WJ, Wood AJ: Plasma binding of pancuronium: effects of age, sex, and disease. Anesth Analg 62:29–32, 1983

4. Duvaldestin P, Henzel D: Binding of tubocurarine, fazadinium, pancuronium and Org NC 45 to serum proteins in normal man and in patients with cirrhosis. Br J Anaesth 54:513, 1982
5. Hunter FM: Resistance to non-depolarizing neuromuscular blocking agents. Br J Anaesth 67:511–513, 1991
6. Kim CS, Arnold FJ, Itani MS, Martyn JAJ: Decreased sensitivity to metocurine during long-term phenytoin therapy may be attributable to protein binding and acetylcholine receptor changes. Anesthesiology 77:500–506, 1992
7. Piafsky KM: Disease-induced changes in the plasma binding of basic drugs. Clin Pharmacokinet 5:246–262, 1980
8. Martyn JAJ, White DA, Gronert GA, Jaffe RS, Ward JM: Up-and-down regulation of skeletal muscle acetylcholine receptors. Effects on neuromuscular blockers. Anesthesiology. 76:822–843, 1992
9. Piafsky KM, Borga O, Odar-Cederlof I, Johansson C, Sjoqvist F: Increased plasma protein binding of propranolol and chlorpromazine mediated by disease induced elevation of plasma α_1-acid glycoprotein. N Engl J Med 299:1435–1439, 1978
10. Routledge PA: The plasma protein binding of basic drugs. Br J Clin Pharmacol 22:499–506, 1986
11. Abramson FP, Lutz MP: The effects of phenytoin dosage on the induction of α_1-acid glycoprotein and antipyrine clearance in the dog. Eur J Drug Metab Pharmacokinet 11:135–143, 1986
12. Evans GH, Neis AS, Shand DG: The disposition of propranolol III: decreased half-time and volume of distribution as a result of plasma binding in man, monkey, dog and rat. J Pharmacol Exp Ther 186:114–122, 1973
13. Wilkinson GR, Shand DG: A physiological approach to hepatic drug clearance. Clin Pharmacol Ther 18:377–390, 1975
14. Tatman AJ, Wrigley SR, Jones RM: Resistance to atracurium in a patient with an increase in plasma alpha$_1$ globulins. Br J Anaesth 67:623–625, 1991
15. Buzello W, Pollmaecher T, Schluermann D, et al: The influence of hypothermic cardiopulmonary bypass on neuromuscular transmission in the absence of muscle relaxants. Anesthesiology 64:279, 1986
16. Buzello W, Schluermann D, Pollmacher T, et al: Unequal effects of cardiopulmonary bypass-induced hypothermia on neuromuscular blockade from constant infusion of alcuronium, d-tubocurarine, pancuronium, and vecuronium. Anesthesiology 66:842, 1987
17. Walker JS, Shanks CA, Brown KF: Altered d-tubocurarine disposition during cardiopulmonary bypass surgery. Clin Pharmacol Ther 35:686–694, 1984
18. Flynn PJ, Hughes R, Walton B: Use of atracurium in cardiac surgery involving cardiopulmonary bypass with induced hypothermia. Br J Anaesth 56:967, 1984
19. Moorthy SS, Krishna G, Dierdorf SF: Resistance to vecuronium in patients with cerebral palsy. Anesth Analg 73:275–277, 1991
20. Bolton CF, Gilbert JJ, Hahn AF, Sibbald WJ: Polyneuropathy critically ill patients. J Neurol Neurosurg Psychiatry 47:1223–1231, 1984
21. Coakley JH, Nagendran K, Honavar M, Hinds CJ: Preliminary observations on the neuromuscular abnormalities in patients with organ failure and sepsis. Intensive Care Med 19:323–328, 1993
22. Coronel B, Meracatello A, Couturiere J-C, et al: Polyneuropathy: potential cause of difficult weaning. Crit Care Med 18:486–489, 1990
23. Harrison P, Feldman SA: Intubating conditions with ORG NC 45; a preliminary study. Anaesthesia 36:874–877, 1981
24. Hunter JM, Jones RS, Utting JE: Use of atracurium during general surgery monitored by the train-of-four stimuli. Br J Anaesth 54:1243–1250, 1982
25. Witt NJ, Zochodne DW, Bolton CF, Grand'Maison F, Wells G, Young B, Sibbald WJ: Peripheral nerve function in sepsis and multiple organ failure. Chest 99:176–184, 1991
26. Wokke JHJ, Jennekens FGI, van den Dord CJM, et al: Histological investigations of muscle atrophy and end plates in two critically ill patients with generalized weakness. J Neurol Sci 88:95–106, 1988
27. Witt NJ, Bolton CF, Sibbald WJ: The incidence and early features of the polyneuropathy of critical illness. Neurology 35:74, 1985

28. Zochodne DW, Bolton CF, Wells GA, Gilbert J, Hahn A, Brown J, et al: Critical illness polyneuropathy, a complication of sepsis and multiple organ failure. Brain 110:819–842, 1987
29. Roelofs RI, Cerra F, Beilka N, et al: Prolonged respiratory insufficiency due to acute motor neuropathy: a new syndrome? Neurology 33(suppl 2):240, 1983
30. Bolton CF: Neuromuscular abnormalities in critically ill patients. Intensive Care Med 19:309–310, 1993
31. Bolton CF, Laverty DA, Brown JD, Witt NJ, Hahn AF, Sibbald WJ: Critically ill polyneuropathy: electrophysiological studies and differentiation from Guillain-Barré syndrome. J Neurol Neurosurg Psychiatry 49:563–573, 1986
32. Fiset P, Donati F, Balendran P, Meistelman C, Lira E, Bevan DR: Vecuronium is more potent in Montreal than in Paris. Can J Anaesth 38:717–721, 1991
33. Katz R, Norman J, Seed RF, Conrad L: A comparison of the effects of suxamethonium and tubocurarine in patients in London and New York. Br J Anaesth 41:1041–1047, 1969
34. Roland E, Roupie E, Wierda JMKH, Sarfati E, Villiers S, Dubost C, Eurin B: Effects of hyperparathyroidism on the vecuronium-induced neuromuscular blockade. Anesthesiology 73:A901, 1990
35. Caldwell JE, Heier T: Hyperparathyroidism and vecuronium-induced neuromuscular blockade. Anesthesiology 71:A814, 1989
36. Coakley JH, Edwards RHT, McClelland P, et al: Occult ischaemic necrosis of skeletal muscle associated with renal failure. Br Med J 301:370, 1990
37. Fiamengo SA, Savarese JJ: In reply to H814: Muscle relaxants in intensive care patients (letter). Crit Care Med 21:1404–1405, 1993
38. Rivner MH, Kim S, Greenberg M, et al: Reversible generalized paresis following hypotension: a new neurological entity (abstract). Neurology 33(suppl 2):1664, 1983
39. Eriksson LI, Jensen E, Viby-Mogensen J, Lennmarken C: Train-of-four (TOF) response following prolonged neuromuscular monitoring: influence of peripheral temperature. Anesthesiology 71:A827, 1989
40. Eriksson LI, Viby-Mogensen J, Lennmarken C: The effect of peripheral hypothermia on a vecuronium-induced neuromuscular block. Acta Anaesthesiol Scand 35:387–392, 1991
41. Engbaek J, Skovgaard LT, Friis B, Kann T: The effect of temperature on the evoked EMG response. Anesthesiology 70:A810, 1989
42. Eriksson LI, Jensen E, Viby-Mogensen J, Lennmarken C: Influence of peripheral hypothermia on the train-of-four response in the absence of neuromuscular blockade (abstract). Acta Anaesthesiol Scand 33:157, 1989
43. Heier T, Caldwell JE, Sessler D, Miller RD: Mild intraoperative hypothermia increases duration of action and spontaneous recovery of vecuronium blockade during nitrous oxide–isoflurane anesthesia in humans. Anesthesiology 74:815–819, 1991
44. Heier T, Caldwell JE, Sessler DI, Miller RD: The effect of local surface and central cooling on adductor pollicis twitch tension during nitrous oxide/isoflurane and nitrous oxide/fentanyl anesthesia in humans. Anesthesiology 72:807–811, 1990
45. Heier T, Caldwell JE, Sessler DI, Kitts JB, Miller RD: The relationship between adductor pollicis twitch tension and core, skin and muscle temperature during nitrous oxide–isoflurane anesthesia in humans. Anesthesiology 71:381–384, 1989
46. Hopf HC, Maurer K: Temperature dependence of the electrical and mechanical responses of the adductor pollicis muscle in humans. Muscle Nerve 13:259–262, 1990
47. Miller RD, Agoston S, Van der Pol F, et al: Hypothermia and pharmacokinetics and pharmacodynamics of pancuronium in the cat. J Pharmacol Exp Ther 207:532, 1978
48. Pedersen T, Viby-Mogensen J, Bang U, Olsen NV, Jensen E, Engbaek J: Does perioperative tactile evaluation of the train-of-four response influence the frequency of postoperative residual neuromuscular blockade? Anesthesiology 73:835–839, 1990
49. Pedersen T, Bang U, Olsen NV, Jensen E, Engbaek J, Viby-Mogensen J: Reply: Nerve stimulation and residual neuromuscular block. Anesthesiology 74:957–958, 1991
50. Thornberry EA, Mazumdar B: The effects of changes in arm temperature on neuromuscular monitoring in the presence of atracurium blockade. Anaesthesia 43:447, 1988
51. Ali HH, Shorten G: Nerve stimulation and residual neuromuscular block (letter). Anesthesiology 74:956–957, 1991

52. Foldes FF: Factors which alter the effects of muscle relaxants. Anesthesiology 20:464–504, 1959
53. Duvaldestin P, Berger JL, Videcoq M, Desmonts JM: Pharmacokinetics and pharmacodynamics of Org NC 45 in patients with cirrhosis. Anesthesiology 57:A238, 1982
54. Hunter JM, Parker CJR, Bell CF, Jones RS, Utting JE: The use of different doses of vecuronium in patients with liver dysfunction. Br J Anaesth 57:758–764, 1985
55. Lebrault C, Duvaldestin P, Henzel D, Chauvin M, Guesnon P: Pharmacokinetics and pharmacodynamics of vecuronium in patients with cholestasis. Br J Anaesth 58:983–987, 1986
56. Lebrault C, Berger JL, D'Hollander AA, et al: Pharmacokinetics and pharmacodynamics of vecuronium (ORG NC45) in patients with cirrhosis. Anesthesiology 62:601, 1985
57. Duvaldestin P, Agoston S, Henzel D, Kersten UW, Desmonts JM: Pancuronium pharmacokinetics in patients with liver cirrhosis. Br J Anaesth 50:1131–1135, 1978
58. Ward S, Judge S, Corall I: Pharmacokinetics of pancuronium bromide in liver failure. Br J Anaesth 54:227P, 1982
59. Magorian T, Wood P, Caldwell JE, Szenohradszky J, Segredo V, Sharma H, Gruenke LD, Miller RD: Pharmacokinetics, onset, and duration of action of rocuronium in humans: normal vs. hepatic dysfunction. Anesthesiology 75:A1069, 1991
60. Gyasi HK, Naguib M: Atracurium and severe hepatic disease: a case report. Can Anaesth Soc J 32:161, 1985
61. Westra P, Keulemans GTP, Houwertjes MC, Hardonk MJ, Meijer DKF: Mechanisms underlying the prolonged duration of action of muscle relaxants caused by extra hepatic cholestasis. Br J Anaesth 53:217, 1981
62. Westra P, Vermeer GA, de Lange AR, Scaf AHJ, Meijer DKF, Wesseling H: Hepatic and renal disposition of pancuronium and gallamine in patients with extra hepatic cholestasis. Br J Anaesth 53:331, 1981
63. Ward S, Weatherley BC: Pharmacokinetics of atracurium and its metabolites. Br J Anaesth 58:6S-1010S, 1986
64. Bell CF, Hunter JM, Jones RS, Utting JE: Use of atracurium and vecuronium in patients with oesophageal varices. Br J Anaesth 57:160–168, 1985
65. Dundee JW, Gray TC: Resistance to d-tubocurarine chloride in the presence of liver damage. Lancet 2:16–17, 1953
66. Nana A, Cardan E, Leitersdorfer T: Pancuronium bromide: its use in asthmatics and patients with liver disease. Anaesthesia 27:154–158, 1972
67. Parker CJR, Hunter JM: Pharmacokinetics of atracurium and laudanosine in patients with hepatic cirrhosis. Br J Anaesth 62:177–183, 1989
68. Arora NS, Rochester DF: Respiratory muscle strength and maximal voluntary ventilation in undernourished patients. Am Rev Respir Dis 126:5, 1982
69. Weinstein JA, Matteo RS, Ornstein E, Schwartz AE, Goldstoff M, Thal G: Pharmacodynamics of vecuronium and atracurium in the obese surgical patient. Anesth Analg 67:1149–1153, 1988
70. Duvaldestin P, Demetriou M, Henzel D, Desmonts JM: The placental transfer of pancuronium and its pharmacokinetics during caesarean section. Acta Anaesthesiol Scand 22:327–333, 1978
71. Dailey PA, Fisher DM, Shnider SM, Baysinger CL, Shinohara Y, Miller RD, Abboud TK, Kim KC: Pharmacokinetics, placental transfer, and neonatal effects of vecuronium and pancuronium administered during cesarean section. Anesthesiology 60:569–574, 1984
72. Baraka A, Jabbour S, Tabboush Z, et al: Onset of vecuronium neuromuscular block is more rapid in patients undergoing caesarean section. Can J Anaesth 39:135, 1992
73. Pritchard JA: Changes in blood volume during pregnancy and delivery. Anesthesiology 26:393, 1965
74. Lees MM, Taylor SH, Scott DB, Kerr MG: A study of cardiac output at rest throughout pregnancy. J Obstet Gynaecol Br Commonw 74:319–328, 1967
75. Ginsburg J, Duncan S: Peripheral blood flow in normal pregnancy. Cardiovasc Res 1:132–137, 1967
76. Ganrot PO: Variation of the concentrations of some plasma proteins in normal adults, in pregnant women and in newborns. Scand J Clin Lab Invest 29:83–88, 1972
77. Rodrigue R, Durant NN, Nguyen N, et al: Comparison of vecuronium-induced neuro-

muscular blockade in pregnant and nonpregnant female rabbits. Anesthesiology 65:A401, 1986
78. Khuenl-Brady KS, Koller J, Mair P, Puhringer F: Comparison of vecuronium- and atracurium-induced neuromuscular blockade in postpartum and nonpregnant patients. Anesth Analg 72:110–113, 1991
79. Hawkins JL, Adenwala J, Camp C, Joyce TH III: The effect of H_2-receptor antagonist premedication on the duration of vecuronium-induced neuromuscular blockade in postpartum patients. Anesthesiology 71:175–177, 1989
80. Bell PF, Mirakhur RK, Clarke RSJ: Dose-response studies of atracurium, vecuronium and pancuronium in the elderly. Anaesthesia 44:925–927, 1989
81. Duvaldestin P, Saada J, Berger JL, et al: Pharmacokinetics, pharmacodynamics, and dose-response relationships of pancuronium in control and elderly subjects. Anesthesiology 56:36–40, 1982
82. Rupp SM, Fisher DM, Miller RD, Castagnoli K: Pharmacokinetics and pharmacodynamics of vecuronium in the elderly. Anesthesiology 59:A270, 1983
83. deBros F, Okutani R, Lai A, Lawrence KW, Basta S: Pharmacokinetics and pharmacodynamics of atracurium in the elderly. Anesthesiology 72:272–275, 1990
84. d'Hollander AA, Luyckx C, Barvais L, De Ville A: Clinical evaluation of atracurium beseylate requirement for a stable muscle relaxation during surgery: Lack of age-related effects. Anesthesiology 59:237–240, 1983
85. Kent AP, Parker CJR, Hunter JM: Pharmacokinetics of atracurium and laudanosine in the elderly. Br J Anaesth 63:661–666, 1989
86. Kitts JB, Fisher DM, Canfell PC, Spellman MJ, Caldwell JE, Heier T, Fahey MR, Miller RD: Pharmacokinetics and pharmacodynamics of atracurium in the elderly. Anesthesiology 72:272–275, 1990
87. Parker CJR, Hunter JM, Snowdon SL: Effect of age, sex and anaesthetic technique on the pharmacokinetics of atracurium. Br J Anaesth 69:439–443, 1992
88. Matteo RS, Backus WW, McDaniel DD, Brotherton WP, Abraham R, Diaz J: Pharmacokinetics and pharmacodynamics of d-tubocurarine and metocurine in the elderly. Anesth Analg 64:23–29, 1985
89. McLeod K, Hull J, Watson MJ: Effects of ageing on the pharmacokinetics of pancuronium. Br J Anaesth 51:435–438, 1979
90. Rupp SM, Castagnoli KD, Fisher DM, Miller RD: Pancuronium and vecuronium pharmacokinetics and pharmacodynamics in younger and elderly patients. Anesthesiology 67:45–49, 1987
91. d'Hollander AA, Massaux F, Nevelsteen M, Agoston S: Age-dependent dose-response relationship of ORG NC 45 in anaesthetized patients. Br J Anaesth 54:653–658, 1982
92. Lien CA, Matteo RS, Ornstein E, Schwartz AE, Diaz J: Distribution, elimination, and action of vecuronium in the elderly. Anesth Analg 73:39–42, 1991
93. McCarthy G, Elliott P, Mirakhur RK, Cooper R, Sharpe TDE, Clarke RSJ: Onset and duration of action of vecuronium in the elderly: comparison with adults. Acta Anaesthesiol Scand 36:383–386, 1992
94. Dresner DL, Basta SJL, Ali HH, Schwartz AF, Embree PB, Wargin WA, Lai A, Brady KA, Savarese JJ: Pharmacokinetics and pharmacodynamics of doxacurium in young and elderly patients during isoflurane anesthesia. Anesth Analg 71:498–502, 1990
95. Lowry KG, Mirakhur RK, Lavery GG, Clarke RSJ: Vecuronium and atracurium in the elderly: a clinical comparison with pancuronium. Acta Anaesthesiol Scand 29:405–408, 1985
96. O'Hara DA, Fragen RJ, Shanks CA: The effects of age on the dose-response curves for vecuronium in adults. Anesthesiology 63:542, 1985
97. Ornstein E, Matteo RS, Schwartz AE, Jamdar SC, Diaz J: Pharmacokinetics and pharmacodynamics of pipecuronium bromide (Arduan) in elderly surgical patients. Anesth Analg 74:841–844, 1992
98. Marsh RHK, Chjmielewski AT, Goat VA: Recovery from pancuronium: a comparison between old and young patients. Anaesthesia 35:1193–1196, 1980
99. Young WL, Matteo RS, Ornstein E: Duration of action of neostigmine and pyridostigmine in the elderly. Anesth Analg 67:775–778, 1988
100. Bevan DR, Donati F, Kopman AF: Reversal of neuromuscular blockade. Anesthesiology 77:785–805, 1992

101. McCarthy GJ, Cooper R, Stanley JC, Mirakhur RK: Dose-response relationships for neostigmine antagonism of vecuronium-induced neuromuscular block in adults and the elderly. Br J Anaesth 69:281–283, 1992
102. Fisher DM, Canfell PC, Spellman MJ, Miller RD: Pharmacokinetics and pharmacodynamics of atracurium in infants and children. Anesthesiology 73:33–37, 1990
103. Fisher DM, Miller RD: Neuromuscular effects of vecuronium (Org NC45) in infants and children during N_2O, halothane anesthesia. Anesthesiology 58:519–523, 1983
104. Fisher DM, O'Keefe C, Stanski DR, et al: Pharmacokinetics and pharmacodynamics of d-tubocurarine in infants, children, and adults. Anesthesiology 57:203–208, 1982
105. Fisher DM, Castanoli K, Miller RD: Vecuronium kinetics and dynamics in anesthetized infants and children. Clin Pharmacol Ther 37:402–406, 1985
106. Goudsouzian NG, Alifimoff JK, Liu LMP, Foster V, McNulty B, Savarese JJ: Neuromuscular and cardiovascular effects of doxacurium in children anesthetized with halothane. Br J Anaesth 62:263–268, 1989
107. Pittet JF, Tassonyi E, Morel DR, Gemperle G, Rouge JC: Neuromuscular effect of pipecuronium bromide in infants and children during nitrous oxide–alfentanil anesthesia. Anesthesiology 72:432–435, 1990
108. Sarner JB, Brandom BW, Cook DR, Dong ML, Horn MC, Woelfel SK, Davis PJ, Rudd D, Foster VJ, McNulty BF: Clinical pharmacology of doxacurium chloride (BW A938U) in children. Anesth Analg 67:303–306, 1988
109. Meistelman C, Agoston S, Kersten UW, Saint-Maurice C, Bencini AF, Loose J-P: Pharmacokinetics and pharmacodynamics of vecuronium and pancuronium in anesthetized children. Anesth Analg 65:1319–1323, 1986
110. Bevan JC, Donati F, Bevan DR: Attempted acceleration of the onset of action of pancuronium: effects of divided doses in infants and children. Br J Anaesth 57:1204–1208, 1985
111. Woelfel SK, Dong ML, Brandom BW, et al: Vecuronium infusion requirements in children during halothane-narcotic-nitrous oxide, isoflurane-narcotic-nitrous oxide, and narcotic-nitrous oxide anesthesia. Anesth Analg 73:33, 1991
112. Meakin G, Shaw EA, Baker RD, Morris P: Comparison of atracurium-induced neuromuscular blockade in neonates, infants and children. Br J Anaesth 60:171–175, 1988
113. Meistelman C, Debaene B, Saint-Maurice C, Nebout T, Bargy F, Loose JP: Potency of atracurium in infants during halothane anesthesia. Anesthesiology 65:A290, 1986
114. Brandom BW, Woelfel SK, Cook DR, Fehr BL, Rudd GD: Clinical pharmacology of atracurium in infants. Anesth Analg 63:309–312, 1984
115. Brandom BW, Rudd GD, Cook DR: Clinical pharmacology of atracurium in pediatric patients. Br J Anaesth 55:117S–121S, 1983
116. Debaene B, Meistelman C, d'Hollander A: Recovery from vecuronium neuromuscular blockade following neostigmine administration in infants, children, and adults during halothane anesthesia. Anesthesiology 71:840–844, 1989
117. Fisher DM, Cronnelly R, Miller RD, Sharma M: The neuromuscular pharmacology of neostigmine in infants and children. Anesthesiology 59:220, 1983
118. Meakin G, Sweet PT, Bevan JC, Bevan DR: Neostigmine and edrophonium as antagonists of pancuronium in infants and children. Anesthesiology 59:316–321, 1983
119. Bush GH, Stead AL: The use of d-tubocurarine in neonatal anaesthesia. Br J Anaesth 34:721, 1962
120. Crumrine RS, Yodlowski EH: Assessment of neuromuscular function in infants. Anesthesiology 54:29–32, 1981
121. Cook DR: Sensitivity of the newborn to tubocurarine. Br J Anaesth 53:319, 1981
122. Matteo RS, Lieberman IG, Salantire E, et al: Distribution, elimination, and action of d-tubocurarine in neonates, infants, children, and adults. Anesth Analg 63:799–804, 1984
123. Nightingale DA, Bush GH: Atracurium in paediatric anaesthesia. Br J Anaesth 55:115S, 1983
124. Schippers HC, Bell B, Erdmann W, Jackson Rees G: Dose response curve of vecuronium bromide in anesthetized neonates, infants and children. Anesthesiology 69:A761, 1988
125. Woelfel SK, Brandom BW, McGowan FX Jr, Cook DR: Dose-response relationship of mivacurium chloride (Mivacron®) in infants during nitrous oxide–halothane anesthesia. Anesthesiology 75:A775, 1991

126. Fitzpatrick KTJ, Black GW, Crean PM, Mirakhur RK: Continuous vecuronium infusion for prolonged muscle relaxation in children. Can J Anaesth 38:169–174, 1991
127. Meretoja OA: Vecuronium infusion requirements in pediatric patients during fentanyl-N_2O-O_2 anesthesia. Anesth Analg 68:20–24, 1989
128. Walts LF, Dillon JB: The response of newborns to succinylcholine and d-tubocurarine. Anesthesiology 31:35–38, 1969
129. Cook DR: Muscle relaxants in infants and children. Anesth Analg 60:335–343, 1981
130. Meakin G, Morton RH, Wareham AC: Age-dependent variation in response to tubocurarine in the isolated rat diaphragm. Br J Anaesth 68:161–163, 1992
131. Meretoja OA: Is vecuronium a long-acting neuromuscular blocking agent in neonates and infants? Br J Anaesth 62:184–187, 1989
132. Meretoja OA, Kalli I: Spontaneous recovery of neuromuscular function after atracurium in pediatric patients. Anesth Analg 65:1042–1046, 1986
133. Zsigmond EK, Downs JR: Plasma cholinesterase activity in newborn and infants. Can Anaesth Soc J 18:278–285, 1971
134. Agoston S, Vermeer GA, Kersten UW, et al: The fate of pancuronium bromide in man. Acta Anaesthesiol Scand 17:267, 1973
135. Agoston S, Vermeer GA, Kersten UW, et al: A preliminary investigation of the renal and hepatic excretion of gallamine triethiodide in man. Br J Anaesth 50:345, 1978
136. Bevan DR, Archer D, Donati F, Ferguson A, Higgs BD: Antagonism of pancuronium in renal failure: no recurarization. Br J Anaesth 54:63–68, 1982
137. Brotherton WP, Matteo RS: Pharmacokinetics and pharmacodynamics of metocurine in humans with and without renal failure. Anesthesiology 55:273–276, 1981
138. Cook DR, Freeman JA, Lai AA, Robertson KA, Kang Y, Stiller RL, Aggarwal S, Abou-Donia MM, Welch RM: Pharmacokinetics and pharmacodynamics of doxacurium in normal patients and in those with hepatic or renal failure. Anesth Analg 72:145–150, 1991
139. Cashman JN, Luke J, Marshall CA, Jones RM: Pharmacodynamics of doxacurium in patients with renal failure. Anesthesiology 71:A829, 1989
140. Matteo RS, Brotherton WP, Nishitateno K, et al: Pharmacokinetics and pharmacodynamics of metocurine in humans: comparison to d-tubocurarine. Anesthesiology 57:183, 1982
141. Miller RD, Stevens WC, Way WL: The effect of renal failure and hyperkalemia on the duration of pancuronium neuromuscular blockade in man. Anesth Analg 52:661–666, 1972
142. McLeod K, Watson MJ, Rawlins MD: Pharmacokinetics of pancuronium in patients with normal and impaired renal function. Br J Anaesth 48:341, 1976
143. Somogyi AA, Shanks CA, Triggs EJ: The effect of renal failure on the disposition and neuromuscular blocking action of pancuronium bromide. Eur J Clin Pharmacol 12:23–29, 1977
144. Fahey MR, Morris RB, Miller RD, Nguyen TL, Upton RA: Pharmacokinetics of Org NC45 (Norcuron) in patients with and without renal failure. Br J Anaesth 53:1049–1053, 1981
145. Cody MW, Dormon FM: Recurarisation after vecuronium in a patient with renal failure. Anaesthesia 42:993–995, 1987
146. Hunter JM, Jones RS, Utting JE: Comparison of vecuronium, atracurium and tubocurarine in normal patients and in patients with no renal function. Br J Anaesth 56:941, 1984
147. Lynam DP, Cronnelly R, Castagnoli KP, Canfell C, Caldwell J, Arden J, Miller RD: The pharmacokinetics and pharmacodynamics of vecuronium in patients anesthetized with isoflurane with normal renal function or with renal failure. Anesthesiology 69:227–231, 1988
148. Peschaud JL, Kienlen J, Rey G, Marres F, Momas I, d'Athis F, du Cailar J: Pharmacodynamics of vecuronium in patients with and without renal failure. Anesthesiology 73:A916, 1990
149. Smith CL, Hunter JM, Jones RS: Vecuronium infusions in patients with renal failure in an ITU. Anaesthesia 42:387–393, 1987
150. Slater RM, Polard BJ, Doran BRH: Prolonged neuromuscular blockade with vecuronium in renal failure. Anaesthesia 43:250, 1988

151. Segredo V, Matthay MA, Sharma ML, Gruenke LD, Caldwell JE, Miller RD: Prolonged neuromuscular blockade after long-term administration of vecuronium in two critically ill patients. Anesthesiology 72:566–570, 1990
152. Segredo V, Caldwell JE, Matthay MA, Sharma ML, Gruenke LD, Miller RD: Persistent paralysis in critically ill patients after long-term administration of vecuronium. N Engl J Med 327:524–528, 1992
153. Churchill-Davidson HC, Way WL, De Jong RH: The muscle relaxants and renal excretion. Anesthesiology 28:540, 1967
154. Cooper R, Maddineni VR, Mirakhur RK, Wierda JMKH, Brady M, Fitzpatrick KTJ: Time course of neuromuscular effect and pharmacokinetics of rocuronium bromide (ORG 9426) during isoflurane anesthesia in patients with and without renal failure. Br J Anaesth 71:222–226, 1993
155. Phillips BJ, Hunter JM: The use of mivacurium chloride by constant infusion in the anephric patient. Br J Anaesth 68:492–498, 1992
156. Fahey MR, Rupp SM, Fisher DM, et al: The pharmacokinetics and pharmacodynamics of atracurium in patients with and without renal failure. Anesthesiology 61:699–702, 1984
157. Hunter JM, Jones RS, Utting JE: Use of atracurium in patients with no renal function. Br J Anaesth 54:1251–1258, 1982
158. Ward S, Boheimer N, Weatherley BC, et al: Pharmacokinetics of atracurium and its metabolites in patients with normal renal function and in patients in renal failure. Br J Anaesth 59:697–706, 1987
159. Cronnelly R, Morris RB: Antagonism of neuromuscular blockade. Br J Anaesth 54:183–194, 1982
160. Miller RD, Cullen DJ: Renal failure and postoperative respiratory failure: recurarization? Br J Anaesth 48:253–256, 1976
161. Morris RB, Cronnelly R, Miller RD, et al: Pharmacokinetics of edrophonium and neostigmine when antagonizing d-tubocurarine neuromuscular block in man. Anesthesiology 54:399–402, 1981
162. Morris RB, Cronnelly R, Miller RD, et al: Pharmacokinetics of edrophonium in anephric and renal transplant patients. Br J Anaesth 53:1311–1314, 1981
163. Gibaldi M, Levy G, Hayton WL: Tubocurarine and renal failure. Br J Anaesth 44:163, 1972
164. Gramstad L: Atracurium, vecuronium and pancuronium in end-stage renal failure: dose-response properties and interactions with azathioprine. Br J Anaesth 59:995–1003, 1987
165. Feldman SA: Effect of changes in electrolytes, hydration and pH upon the reactions to muscle relaxants. Br J Anaesth 35:546–551, 1963
166. Fatt P, Katz B: An analysis of the endplate potential recorded with an intracellular electrode. J Physiol 115:320–370, 1951
167. Waud BE, Waud DR: Interaction of calcium and potassium with neuromuscular blocking agents. Br J Anaesth 52:863–866, 1980
168. Gramstad L, Hysing ES: Effect of ionized calcium on the neuromuscular blocking actions of atracurium and vecuronium in the cat. Br J Anaesth 64:199–206, 1990
169. Del Castillo J, Katz B: The effect of magnesium on the activity of nerve endings. J Physiol (Lond) 124:553–559, 1954
170. Engbaek L: The pharmacological actions of magnesium ions with particular reference to the neuromuscular and cardiovascular systems. Pharmacol Rev 4:396–410, 1954
171. Ghoneim MM, Long JP: The interaction between magnesium and other neuromuscular blocking agents. Anesthesiology 32:23–27, 1970
172. Varsano S, Shapiro M, Taragan R, Bruderman I: Hypophosphataemia as a reversible cause of refractory ventilatory failure. Crit Care Med 11:908, 1983
173. Brown EL, Jenkins BA: A case of respiratory failure complicated by acute hypophosphatemia. Anaesthesia 35:42, 1980
174. Newman JH, Neff TA, Ziporin P: Acute respiratory failure associated with hypophosphatemia. N Engl J Med 296:1101, 1977
175. Furlan AJ, Hanson M, Cooperman A, et al: Acute areflexic paralysis, association with hyperalimentation and hypophosphatemia. Arch Neurol 32:706, 1975

176. Fitzgerald F: Clinical hypophosphatemia. Annu Rev Med 29:177, 1978
177. Knochel JP: The pathophysiology and clinical characteristics of severe hypophosphatemia. Arch Intern Med 137:203, 1977
178. Lotz M, Zisman E, Bartter FC: Evidence for a phosphorus-depletion syndrome in man. N Engl J Med 278:409, 1968
179. Barker GL: Hyperkalaemia presenting as ventilatory failure. Anaesthesia 35:885–886, 1980
180. Freeman SJ, Fale AD: Muscular paralysis and ventilatory failure caused by hyperkalaemia. Br J Anaesth 70:226–227, 1993
181. Livingstone IR, Cumming WJK: Hyperkalaemic paralysis resembling Guillain-Barré syndrome. Lancet 2:963–964, 1979
182. Udezue EO, Harrold BP: Hyperkalaemic paralysis due to spironolactone. Postgrad Med J 56:254–255, 1980
183. Miller RD, Roderick LL: Diuretic-induced hypokalaemia, pancuronium neuromuscular blockade and its antagonism by neostigmine. Br J Anaesth 50:541–544, 1978
184. Vaughan RS, Lunn JN: Potassium and the anaesthetist. Anaesthesia 28:1181–31, 1973
185. Crul-Sluijter EJ, Crul JF: Acidosis and neuromuscular blockade. Acta Anaesthesiol Scand 18:224, 1974
186. Funk DI, Crul JF, Pol FM: Effects of changes in acid-base balance on neuromuscular blockade produced by ORG-NC 45. Acta Anaesthesiol Scand 24:119–124, 1980
187. Gencarelli PJ, Swen J, Koot HWJ, Miller RD: The effects of hypercarbia and hypocarbia on pancuronium and vecuronium neuromuscular blockades in anesthetized humans. Anesthesiology 59:376–380, 1983
188. Hughes R, Chapple DJ: The pharmacology of atracurium: a new competitive neuromuscular blocking agent. Br J Anaesth 53:31–44, 1981
189. Katz RL, Wolf CE: Neuromuscular and electromyographic studies in man: effects of hyperventilation, carbon dioxide inhalation and d-tubocurarine. Anesthesiology 25:781–787, 1964
190. Ono K, Ohta Y, Morita K, Kosaka F: The influence of respiratory-induced acid-base changes on the action of non-depolarizing muscle relaxants in rats. Anesthesiology 68:357–362, 1988
191. Ono K, Nagano O, Ohta Y, Kosaka F: Neuromuscular effects of respiratory and metabolic acid-base changes *in vitro* with and without nondepolarizing muscle relaxants. Anesthesiology 73:710–716, 1990
192. Baraka A: The influence of carbon dioxide on the neuromuscular block caused by tubocurarine chloride in the human subject. Br J Anaesth 36:272, 1964
193. Dann WL: The effects of different levels of ventilation on the action of pancuronium in man. Br J Anaesth 43:959–962, 1971
194. Miller RD, Van Nyhuis LS, Eger EI II, Vitez TS, Way WL: The effect of acid-base balance on neostigmine antagonism of d-tubocurarine-induced neuromuscular blockade. Anesthesiology 42:377–383, 1975
195. Durant NN, Bowman WC, Marshall LG: A comparison of neuromuscular and autonomic blocking activities of (+)-tubocurarine and its O, O, N-trimethyl analogues. Eur J Pharmacol 46:297–302, 1977
196. Feldman SA: Effect of blood flow, temperature, pH and age on action of muscle relaxants. In Feldman SA (ed): Muscle Relaxants. Philadelphia, WB Saunders, 1979, pp 146–150
197. Miller RD, Roderick LL: The influence of acid-base changes on neostigmine antagonism of pancuronium neuromuscular blockade. Br J Anaesth 50:317–324, 1978
198. Miller RD, Sohn YJ, Matteo RS: Enhancement of d-tubocurarine neuromuscular blockade by diuretics in man. Anesthesiology 45:442, 1976
199. Wirtavouri K, Salmenpera M, Tauristo T: Effect of hypocarbia and hypercarbia on the antagonism of pancuronium-induced neuromuscular blockade with neostigmine in man. Br J Anaesth 54:57–61, 1982
200. Tammisto T, Wirtavouri K, Salmenpera M: Effect of hypo- or hypercarbia on the neostigmine antagonism of pancuronium-induced neuromuscular blockade in man. Br J Anaesth 53:116P, 1981
201. Walts LF, Dillon JB: Durations of action of d-tubocurarine and gallamine. Anesthesiology 29:499–504, 1968

202. Brooks DK, Feldman SA: Metabolic acidosis: a new approach to "neostigmine resistant curarization." Anaesthesia 17:161–169, 1962
203. Creese R: Bicarbonate ion and striated muscle. J Physiol 110:450, 1949
204. Payne JP: The influence of changes in blood pH on the neuromuscular blocking properties of tubocurarine and dimethyltubocurarine in the cat. Acta Anaesthesiol Scand 4:83–90, 1960
205. Miller RD, Roderick LL: Acid-base balance and neostigmine antagonism of pancuronium neuromuscular blockade. Br J Anaesth 50:317–324, 1978
206. Alderson AM, MacLagan J: The action of decamethonium and tubocurarine on the respiratory and limb muscles of the cat. J Physiol (Lond) 173:38–56, 1964

11

DAVID G. SILVERMAN | RICHARD R. BARTKOWSKI

Systemic and Long-Term Effects of Nondepolarizing Relaxants

This chapter focuses on the effects of families or groups of nondepolarizing relaxants (NDRs). The effects of specific agents are discussed where deemed appropriate; they are addressed in more detail in Chapters 12 through 14.

◆ CARDIOVASCULAR CHANGES

Nondepolarizing relaxants may directly *alter cardiovascular function* by (1) exerting a vagolytic (atropine-like) effect, (2) blocking reuptake of norepinephrine, (3) blocking preganglionic nicotinic receptors, and/or (4) causing histamine release. The NDRs vary in these tendencies[1]; vagolytic effects characterize certain steroidal derivatives, while histamine release characterizes benzylisoquinolinium compounds (Table 11-1). The most widespread effects tend to be noted after *d-tubocurarine* (Curare). It blocks ganglionic nicotinic receptors and produces parasympathetic and sympathetic ganglion block.[1-3] In clinical doses, it also induces histamine release (see below). The sympathetic block contributes to tubocurarine's effects of reducing blood pressure, blunting autonomic reflexes, and blunting compensatory responses.[1,4-7]

Gallamine, pancuronium, alcuronium, and fazadinium have *vagolytic and/or sympathomimetic effects*[1,7-11] which may lead to tachycardia, arrhythmias, hypertension, and ischemia.[12,13] Gallamine[14] and, to a lesser extent, pancuronium[15] block muscarinic receptors in the heart but otherwise are generally without significant atropine-like activity. *Gallamine* and, to a lesser extent, *pancuronium* may also cause noradrenaline release.[16-18] The effects of even a defasciculating dose of gallamine may be significant,[19] especially in the context of labile hemodynamics (e.g., severe pre-eclampsia[19]). Pancuronium in particular also blocks noradrenaline reuptake.[17,20-22] *Rocuronium*, a new steroidal derivative, also appears to have the potential to induce tachycardia; however, it remains to be determined if this will have

TABLE 11-1
Comparative Cardiovascular Effects of Nondepolarizing Relaxants
(1 = none or minimal, 2 = slight to moderate, 3 = marked)

Effects	Cur	Meto	Gal	Pan	Vec	Atr	Miv	Dox	Pip	Roc	Alc
Ganglionic block	3	1	1	1	1	1	1	1	1	1	2
Vagal block	2	1	3	2	1	1	1	1	1	1–2	2
Increased catechol effects	1	1	2	2	1	1	1	1	1	1	1
Histamine release	3	2	2	1	1	2	2	1–2	1	1	1

Cur = *d*-tubocurarine, Meto = metocurine, Gal = gallamine, Pan = pancuronium, Vec = vecuronium, Atr = atracurium, Miv = mivacurium, Dox = doxacurium, Pip = pipecuronium, Roc = rocuronium, Alc = alcuronium.

an impact on its clinical utility. The ratio of rocuronium's ED_{50} for vagal block to its ED_{50} for neuromuscular block was 7.2 in cats and 4.4 in pigs.[23]

Some NDRs have little, if any, effect on *autonomic activity*. The first of these to gain clinical acceptance was *dimethyltubocurarine* (metocurine)[1,24–26]; however, it elicits dose-related histamine release (see below). *Atracurium* and mivacurium exhibit similar properties.[27,28] *Vecuronium* is essentially devoid of autonomic effects, and also lacks histamine release.[29–31] The bradycardia associated with vecuronium[32–38] most likely is due to lack of the vagolytic effect that characterized its predecessor (pancuronium)[29,30]; the absence of vagolytic effect allows unopposed lowering of heart rate by high doses of narcotics and procedures that cause vagal stimulation.[39] Comparable bradycardia may also be seen with atracurium,[40] pipecuronium,[41] and doxacurium.[42] The potential advantages of two new long-lasting NDRs that lack autonomic effects, *doxacurium* and *pipecuronium*, were shown in recent comparisons of bolus dosing in patients undergoing *coronary bypass surgery: pancuronium* produced small but significant increases in blood pressure, heart rate, and cardiac index; *doxacurium*[42] and pipecuronium[43,44] caused fewer changes.

◆ HISTAMINE RELEASE

Histamine, a chemical effector of the inflammatory response, dilates vascular smooth muscle, exerts positive inotropic and chronotropic influences on the heart, and permits movement of phagocytic cells.[45–49] In low concentrations, it commonly causes skin erythema; in high concentrations, it may cause systemic *vasodilation* (with hypotension) and increased *bronchomotor tone*.[24,50–55] Responses may be limited to specific tissues,[54,56] most commonly the skin.[56] When vasodilation occurs, it may be attributable to histamine stimulation of H_1 receptors of the vascular endothelium and the subsequent release of vasodilating prostaglandins (e.g., $PGF_{1\alpha}$).

Histamine release, a dose-related feature of benzylisoquinolinium derivatives and related organic compounds,[48,56-76] appears to be due to displacement of histamine from mast cells. This release is nonimmunologic and does not require prior exposure. It is most prominent with *tubocurarine*.[50,51,56,57,62] When administered in comparable fashion, *metocurine*,[24-26,57] *atracurium*,[56,57,63-68] and *mivacurium*[69,70] respectively elicit 50%, 40%, and 30-40% of the histamine release associated with tubocurarine. A benzylisoquinolinium compound, *doxacurium* also has the potential to elicit significant histamine release but generally does not do so in clinical doses.[71,72] Histamine release may also accompany the administration of *succinylcholine* (SCh) and *decamethonium*. It is rare after steroidal relaxants. It should be noted that relaxants may also impede the degradation of histamine by *histamine N-methyl transferase:* vecuronium > pancuronium > gallamine > *d*-tubocurarine > metocurine > atracurium > pipecuronium.[73]

The effects of *histamine release* tend to be more prominent in adults than in children.[65,74,77] Release is increased in *adults with low plasma IgE* levels, perhaps related to less IgE on mast cells.[56,78] (IgE tends to be low in atopic individuals, as they have a high degree of IgE binding.)

The *release of histamine may be blunted* by slow drug administration, infusion, or divided dosing. These mechanisms minimize peak plasma levels of drug.[69,72,75,76,79,80] Generally, slow infusion over 60-75 seconds of a clinical dose of atracurium or mivacurium does not elicit detectable release of histamine,[72,75,76] but individual responses may vary.[69,80,81] As noted in Table 11-2, infusion over 75 seconds eliminated the increase in histamine after atracurium administration.[80] Likewise, whereas four of eight patients experienced a greater than 20% decline in mean arterial pressure after a 0.25 mg · kg^{-1} bolus dose of mivacurium, none of nine patients experienced this change or even cutaneous flushing after a 60-second infusion (Table 11-3).[70] Infusion

TABLE 11-2
Effect of Atracurium, 0.6 mg · kg^{-1}, on Mean Arterial Pressure and Heart Rate

Rate of Administration	n	Plasma Histamine (pg · mL^{-1})		Mean Arterial Pressure (% of Baseline)	Heart Rate (% of Baseline)
		Baseline	2 Min		
Injection within 5 sec	9	715.3 ± 93.6	1415.1 ± 203.5	82.1 ± 6.4	108.6 ± 4.6
Injection over 75 sec	9	951.4 ± 131.7	949.9 ± 154.1	95.7 ± 2.6	97.7 ± 2.3

SOURCE: Data derived from Scott RPF, et al: Atracurium: clinical strategies for preventing histamine release and attenuating the haemodynamic response. Br J Anaesth 57:550-553, 1985.

TABLE 11-3
Effect of Mivacurium Dose and Injection Time on Histamine-Mediated Effects

Dose $(mg \cdot kg^{-1})$	Injection Time (sec)	Incidence of Flushing	Incidence of Decline of MAP Below 80% of Control
0.15	10–15	1/9	0/9
0.20	10–15	2/9	4/9
0.25	10–15	6/9	4/8
0.25	30	3/9	3/9
0.25	60	0/9	0/9

SOURCE: Data derived from Savarese JJ, et al: The cardiovascular effects of mivacurium chloride (BW B1090U) in patients receiving nitrous oxide-opiate-barbiturate anesthesia. Anesthesiology 70:386–394,1989.

over 30 seconds offered relatively little benefit.[70,75] However, mivacurium administered in divided doses (0.15 mg · kg⁻¹, then 0.10 mg · kg⁻¹) 30 seconds apart elicited no apparent cardiovascular changes.[82] Alternatively, it should be noted that, because of mivacurium's rapid metabolism (Chap. 14), the neuromuscular blocking effect of a divided dose was less than that of a rapid bolus dose.[83]

Histamine's effects, many of which are mediated by prostaglandins,[84] may also be *mitigated by H_1 and H_2 antagonists*[59,76,85–89] and *aspirin*.[84] Pretreatment with diphenhydramine, 1 mg · kg⁻¹, and cimetidine, 4 mg · kg⁻¹, 30 minutes prior to administration of atracurium, 1.5 mg · kg⁻¹, prevents the hemodynamic consequences of a 10- to 19-fold increase in histamine.[86,90] However, it does not prevent, and actually may augment, the increase in plasma histamine levels.[75,86,90,91] Also of note, a lesser time interval between pretreatment and challenge may not afford comparable protection.[75,86]

In the relatively rare case of an *allergic (anaphylactic) reaction,* the release of histamine and related mediators (and their consequences) may be particularly severe.[55,92–96] True anaphylaxis (type 1 hypersensitivity) has been reported.[92,94,97–104] It entails an IgE-mediated response in an individual with prior exposure to a drug or to a substance of similar structure. There is cross-sensitivity among relaxants.[55,94,97,98] The *ammonium* group appears to be the responsible allergen, and thus anaphylaxis may occur with steroidal as well as benzylisoquinolinium compounds (although the incidence appears to be lower with the former). Similar severe responses may occur if a relaxant is mixed with thiopental in the same syringe or unflushed intravenous (IV) tubing.[95,105]

The occurrence of life-threatening anaphylaxis does not appear to be related to the ability of drugs to release histamine.[94] At times it may be difficult to distinguish between anaphylactic and anaphylactoid reactions; the latter may be quite severe, especially in patients with underlying disorders (e.g., asthma).[106] The potential for IgE-mediated anaphylaxis may be determined by intradermal testing or radioimmunoassay. Of note, the antibodies to the quaternary ammonium group of neuromuscular blockers can recognize the lecithin present within the lipid solvent of propofol; thus there may be cross-reactivity.[107–109]

◆ EFFECTS ON NONSTRIATED MUSCLE

Except for effects mediated by altered autonomic activity, NDRs spare *nonstriated muscle*. They affect the *cricopharyngeal muscle* (striated muscle) but do not affect the lower esophagus or *esophagogastric junction* (smooth muscle). Likewise, they do not exert direct effects on smooth muscle of the urinary tract and do not affect uterine contractions.

◆ OBSTETRICAL IMPLICATIONS

The use of NDRs in obstetrical patients is of concern primarily because of the potential for maternal and neonatal weakness. Relaxants have a low potential for causing developmental toxicity during organogenesis.[110] A drug-induced abnormality would be even less likely in the term or near-term fetus. The altered pharmacodynamics and pharmacokinetics of NDRs during pregnancy are discussed in Chapter 10.

Except for *gallamine*, NDRs typically do not *cross the placenta* in large amounts. They are highly ionized and lack the lipophilicity required for rapid equilibration across this lipid membrane. However, the *amount of transfer* may be substantial in the presence of a very high maternal plasma level, as may occur after bolus administration of a very large dose.[111] Likewise, because fetal levels approach maternal levels over time,[112,113] maintaining maternal drug levels (as by repeated injections) when the time from initial drug administration to delivery is prolonged may lead to myoneural block in the infant.[114] Even relatively small amounts have the potential to affect the newborn,[115] especially in the setting of hypoxia and acid-base disturbances.

The average *fetal:maternal ratios* have been reported as 0.12 after tubocurarine,[112] 0.19–0.26 after pancuronium (a range of 0.1–0.4 was reported in one study[109]),[112,116–119] 0.07–0.12 after atracurium,[115,120,121] 0.26 after alcuronium,[122] and 0.11 after vecuronium.[118,123]

Clearly, one must take into account the dose of relaxant and the *dose-to-delivery interval*. Table 11-4 summarizes the levels of radioactivity following the injection of 0.005 mg · kg^{-1} of ^{14}C-labeled dimethyl tubocurarine to women undergoing cesarean section. The data[113] indicate that umbilical vein concentrations are appreciable by 2 minutes and peak within 6 minutes, that umbilical artery concentrations continue to increase for more than 10

TABLE 11-4
Radioactivity (nCi · mL^{-1}) After Administration of 0.005 mg · kg^{-1} of ^{14}C-Dimethyltubocurarine to Women Undergoing Cesarean Section

Time (min)	Maternal Vein	Umbilical Vein	Umbilical Artery
2	4.4	0.04	0.01
4	2.1	0.07	0.03
6	1.9	0.12	0.06
10	1.7	0.12	0.07

SOURCE: Data derived from Kivalo I, et al: Placental transfer of ^{14}C-labeled dimethyltubocurarine during Caesarean section. Br J Anaesth 48:239–241, 1976.

minutes, and that *fetal uptake* (as evidenced by the umbilical vein–umbilical artery gradient) continues despite a marked decrease in maternal vein (and even umbilical vein) values.

Many studies have focused on the effects of *pancuronium in doses required for surgical muscle relaxation* for cesarean section. As for tubocurarine, pancuronium was detected in the umbilical vein within 2–3 minutes following IV administration to the mother.[112,116] There is little evidence to suggest that doses in the range of 0.04–0.10 mg · kg^{-1} significantly affect the neonate.[116,118,124,125] The fetal concentration often reaches 0.04–0.12 µg · mL^{-1}.[112,116] Although this concentration approaches the concentrations associated with neuromuscular block in adults,[126,127] it is highly unlikely that the fetal neuromuscular junctions (NMJs) will acquire a significant amount of drug during the relatively brief period of fetal exposure in most cases.

Vecuronium likewise is relatively safe in comparable doses.[118,123,128,129] Although it is more lipid soluble than pancuronium, vecuronium does not accumulate in the fetal plasma, since much is taken up as one half of umbilical vein blood passes through the fetal liver. *Increasing the intubating dose of vecuronium from 0.10 to 0.20 mg · kg^{-1} increased neonatal levels by 30%* and apparently caused some minor neuromuscular effects.[129]

Atracurium has also been used successfully.[130] Its fetal:maternal ratio is 0.07–0.12,[115,120,131] and the levels typically are well below those associated with neuromuscular block in infants.[132] Although some studies demonstrated that atracurium did not cross the placenta in amounts likely to be of clinical significance,[120,131] others found a lower modal score for active extension of the neck by the newborn at 15 minutes[115] (the significance of this finding is unclear). The fetal:maternal ratio for the atracurium metabolite *laudanosine* was 0.14–0.19. Although the resulting levels of laudanosine would not be considered clinically significant (Chap. 13),[115,121] "the toxic concentration of laudanosine in the human neonate is unknown."[121]

◆ CENTRAL NERVOUS SYSTEM EFFECTS

Whereas *depolarizing agents* tend to increase *cerebral blood flow* by causing cerebral stimulation as a result of input into the reticular activating system via afferents from muscle spindles (Chap. 18), *NDRs have no effect on or tend to decrease* spindle activity and overall cerebral activity (as evidenced by *EEG synchronization*[133]).[134-136] It has been proposed that this results in decreased anesthetic requirements,[137] but this has not been confirmed.[138] A recent study in awake, healthy volunteers noted no change in mental status as a consequence of vecuronium-induced paralysis.[139] Although SCh may decrease the *lidocaine seizure threshold,* gallamine, pancuronium, vecuronium, and atracurium increase it.[140]

The beneficial effects are noted even though many NDRs release histamine, which may increase cerebral blood flow.[141] The effects of *laudanosine, a cerebral stimulant* that is generated by Hofmann elimination of *atracurium,* may be noted after high doses of this NDR (especially with long-term infusions in patients with organ failure). (Because laudanosine production is limited to atracurium, it is discussed with this relaxant in Chapter 13.)

◆ CHOLINESTERASE INHIBITION

By virtue of their chemical similarities to acetylcholine (ACh), all neuromuscular blocking drugs have the potential to interact with cholinesterases. Hexafluorenium interacts with *pseudocholinesterase* (anti-acetylcholine acylhydrolase or plasma cholinesterase or butyryl cholinesterase) such that it significantly slows the disappearance of ^{14}C-labeled SCh from the plasma.[142] Benzoquinonium affects acetylcholinesterase in the NMJ[143,144]; it thus is not readily reversible by traditional anticholinesterases and is not commonly used.

Of the commonly used relaxants, only *pancuronium* causes significant cholinesterase inhibition. At less than 10% of the concentration of other NDRs it inhibits *pseudocholinesterase*[145-148] and thus may lead to prolongation of the effect of SCh[146,149-153] or mivacurium.[154] High doses (0.2 mg · kg^{-1}) of vecuronium may cause up to a 16% reduction in pseudocholinesterase activity,[147] but this effect is not clinically significant.

◆ POTENTIALLY HARMFUL METABOLITES

We are concerned about the potential for generation of metabolites with neuromuscular blocking activity, cardiovascular and nervous system effects, or long-term sequelae.

Whereas most relaxants are excreted unchanged or undergo standard biotransformation processes in the liver, *atracurium* undergoes *Hofmann elimination,* giving rise to *laudanosine* and *acrylates.* The former is a potential stimulant (Chap. 13). The latter may disturb cellular membranes, but this effect appears unlikely to occur in the amounts generated by routine clinical use (Chap. 13). Alternatively, it has been proposed that the active metabolite of certain steroidal relaxants (e.g., pancuronium and vecuronium) may be associated with prolonged paralysis (discussed below). This possibility has led some to recommend the use of other agents. However, as stated previously, they may be accompanied by unwanted hemodynamic effects. With respect to atracurium, although laudanosine has not proved to be problematic in humans, published experiences with prolonged infusions in the ICU setting are limited.

◆ LONG-TERM PARALYSIS OR MYOPATHY IN ICU PATIENTS

A distressingly large number of patients—well in excess of 60 reported cases[155]—have developed *prolonged weakness or myopathy* after long-term administration of NDRs to facilitate mechanical ventilation in the ICU. Weakness and even paralysis may persist well beyond the anticipated time for recovery after discontinuing relaxant administration. These symptoms are most commonly noted in patients who were not carefully monitored to assess depth of neuromuscular block. They are also more likely to occur in patients who are receiving other drugs (e.g., high-dose steroids and antibiotics), in patients with renal, hepatic, or multiple organ failure (and hence compromised elimination), and in patients who are septic (with the potential for circulating peptides that may induce muscle proteolysis[156]). Thus, the problem appears to be multifactorial and may cross multiple specialties. An appreciation and working knowledge of ventilatory requirements, neuromuscular pharmacology, and neuromuscular monitoring—and how they interact with a patient's condition and concomitant medications—are necessary to limit the likelihood of these sequelae.

The most severe sequela, *postparalysis myopathy,* is characterized by diffuse weakness and diffuse muscle *fiber necrosis* without accompanying sensory deficits. It may be associated with marked elevation of *creatine kinase (CK)* levels and release of *myoglobin. Muscle biopsies* have been described as showing histological alteration consistent with pharmacological denervation and disuse atrophy,[157–159] with targetoid atrophy[160,161] and widespread necrosis of Type I and II muscle fibers (described in Chap. 1).[159–168] *Electrophysiological studies* show normal sensory and motor conduction, but motor-evoked responses and compound action potentials are decreased in duration and amplitude, with rapid fatigue and scattered fibrillation potentials.[155,160,167] These features differ from those of the typical polyneuropathy of critical illness, which is a neuronal disorder with a sensory component as well as a motor component.[159,169–173] Disuse atrophy may contribute to muscle weakness[174–177] and muscle necrosis[178–180]; however, it typically is not associated with the total or near-total paralysis seen with a necrotizing myopathy.

Although the differential diagnosis of the prolonged weakness includes a number of factors that would not implicate neuromuscular blocking agents (question m), certain *features of long-term paralysis* with nondepolarizing agents are causes for potential concern:

1. Long-term paralysis may cause a denervation-like pattern with up-regulation of postsynaptic receptors and the potential for subsequent muscle atrophy (Chap. 22).
2. Long-term administration of NDRs in ICU settings may lead to marked accumulation of the parent compound and its metabolites (Chaps. 10, 12 through 14).
3. Long-term administration of NDRs to patients receiving other medications may lead to untoward drug interactions and the potentiation of neuromuscular effects (Chap. 9). The effects of antibiotics and steroids generally are appreciated. However, the potential consequences of other agents that may affect neuromuscular transmission and neuromuscular block (e.g., H_2 antagonists, anticonvulsants, and local anesthetics/antiarrhythmics [Chap. 9]) are less well-known.

Most *assessments of relaxant toxicity* were performed with the expectation that the drugs would be used intraoperatively, i.e., that high doses would be used for relatively short periods of time. Hence, NDRs have not been adequately assessed for long-term use in ICU settings. Not uncommonly, *doses* greater than 100 times those typically used intraoperatively are administered over the course of several days to an ICU patient. For example, in a 1992 report, the mean dose of vecuronium was 1,352 mg (administered over a median of 7.2 days) in a group of ICU patients who subsequently developed neuromuscular dysfunction, as compared to 527 mg (administered over 3.8 days) in patients who did not develop sequelae.[181]

The vast majority of cases have been reported after administration of *pancuronium*[*] or *vecuronium*.[†] This may be due to a variety of factors, which may or may not be attributable to specific features of these agents. It may be argued that the high incidence of weakness or paralysis after pancuronium and vecuronium is primarily a result of the *disproportionate use of these agents* in ICU settings.[207,208] As detailed earlier in this chapter and in Chapter 13, vecuronium is particularly attractive because it is relatively short-acting and it lacks (1) significant autonomic ganglion blocking activity (vs. tubocurarine), (2) antimuscarinic and sympathomimetic effects (vs. gallamine and pancuronium), (3) histamine release (vs. tubocurarine, metocurine, atracurium, and mivacurium), and (4) metabolites with poten-

*References 155, 169, 157, 161, 164, 166, and 182–196.
†References 155, 158, 161–165, 173, 181, 187, 192, and 197–206.

tial cerebral excitatory effects (vs. atracurium). In a recent survey of anesthesiologist-intensivists, 52% reported that vecuronium was the primary NDR used in their ICUs; pancuronium, metubine, and atracurium were the main drugs for 28%, 5%, and 3% of respondents, respectively.[207] In 1991, head nurses reported that pancuronium, vecuronium, and atracurium were the NDRs of choice in 47%, 22%, and 4% of ICUs, respectively.[208]

Some features of *vecuronium* and *pancuronium* may be a cause for concern in certain settings. The *3-OH metabolites* of these agents (but not of their new analogue, rocuronium) are highly active. Significant concentrations may accumulate during prolonged infusions, especially in the presence of organ dysfunction (question 1).[155,200,201] Of potentially greater concern, there are scores of reported cases of prolonged paralysis and myopathy after *high-dose corticosteroids* and long-term neuromuscular block with a steroidal relaxant.* In contrast to pancuronium and vecuronium, *atracurium* does not have a steroidal structure, and its breakdown is relatively independent of organ function. Although it has been used effectively in some series,[210,211] atracurium has been associated with prolonged weakness in two ICU patients.[212] In addition, there is a theoretical concern that atracurium's metabolites (laudanosine and acrylates) may be associated with disturbing systemic effects (Chap. 13),[155,211] and its safety remains to be confirmed in large series.[155] The utility of mivacurium and rocuronium remains to be explored (Chap. 14).

Authors defending the use of pancuronium and vecuronium in ICU settings have cited the disproportionate use of these agents (discussed above) as well as reports that *postventilation weakness and myopathies may be noted in the absence of NDRs*.[178–180,213–219] One should be concerned about *high-dose steroid* administration regardless of whether steroid-based relaxants are administered.[194,216,218] Glucocorticoid receptors in the rat gastrocnemius muscle increased to 3 times control values within 3 weeks after surgical interruption of the sciatic nerve, suggesting that denervated muscle may be hypersensitive to treatment with corticosteroids and perhaps that "atrophy of an individual muscle is the result of increased glucocorticoid sensitivity."[219] The depletion of myosin in surgically denervated rat muscle fibers was greater in animals that were treated with therapeutic doses of steroids[220]; dexamethasone-treated, denervated rat muscle showed a severe, preferential depletion of thick (myosin) filaments.[220] An increase in glucocorticoid receptors also was noted with disuse atrophy,[221] consistent with a report that the catabolic effects of cortisone are more pronounced in less active muscles, perhaps because "in mobilizing body protein for gluconeogenesis the hormone spares those muscles physiologically most ac-

---

*References 155, 157, 162, 164–166, 173, 182, 183, 187, 188, 191, 193, 194, 198, 199, 204–206, and 209.

tive."[222] The atrophy reverses over several weeks if innervation of the muscle is restored.[187] It remains to be determined whether the steroidal structures of pancuronium and vecuronium can exacerbate these changes.

Myopathic changes may be noted in the absence of any drug therapy. *Trauma and sepsis* may in themselves cause accelerated proteolysis (perhaps to satisfy the requirements for immunologic defense and healing), with release of circulating proteolytic peptide.[156] Renal failure, a major risk factor associated with postrelaxant myopathy,[155,200,201] may actually be a consequence of the rhabdomyolysis and myoglobinuria that may result from occult myopathic changes[223,224]; i.e., the myopathic processes may have preceded relaxant administration in some reported cases of apparent relaxant-induced myopathy.

Those hesitant to incriminate specific relaxants or relaxants in general have concluded the following:

1. There was no statistical relationship between the neuromuscular abnormalities and the administration of muscle relaxants.[171]
2. "Studies implicating toxicity of these drugs as a cause of the neuromuscular condition have been based on small, unsystematic retrospective studies or single case reports."[225]
3. "There is an understandable tendency to apply *post hoc ergo propter hoc* logic to suspected adverse drug effects, but in intensive care medicine, with the vast array of agents administered, it is difficult to pin down any particular culprit."[215]
4. Their recent experience[213, 214,217,226] and that of others[170,171,227,228] suggest that attributing the problem to steroidal relaxants may be an overly simplistic view.[215]
5. Neuromuscular abnormalities are almost invariable in long-stay ICU patients, and their origin is multifactorial, with "no obvious etiological factors."[213]
6. The long-term use of excessive doses of irrational combinations of neuromuscular blocking agents, without even cursory monitoring, is probably the most likely cause of prolonged paralysis in critically ill patients.[229]

As noted in Chapter 6, the likelihood of excessive block and of subsequent weakness and paralysis is much lower when the depth of the block is monitored. Several reports have demonstrated the value of monitoring neuromuscular function.* Unfortunately, such monitoring has not been routinely employed.[207,208] Leading teams in neuromuscular research have decried its absence. In a recent editorial and subsequent letter, Fiamengo and Savarese emphasized a "treatable and preventable cause of muscle weakness: the injudicious administration of nondepolarizing neuromuscular re-

*References 155, 158, 164, 184, 188, 199, and 229–232.

laxant. . . . ."[184,233] Agoston et al. concluded that "It is evident that careful monitoring of neuromuscular blockade may eliminate at least that part of the neuromuscular complications that might be attributable to long-term administration of high doses of muscle relaxants."[229]

In light of the above, *we recommend* the following:

1. Determine whether a patient has an underlying condition that will predispose to neuromuscular dysfunction or an exaggerated response to an NDR (Chap. 10). Select and titrate relaxants accordingly.
2. Document concomitant medication use (Chap. 9); attempt to minimize the use of agents that compromise neuromuscular function or prolong the effects of NDRs. Select and titrate relaxants accordingly.
3. Administer appropriate sedation and analgesia to address the patient's needs for these agents as well as to minimize the need for relaxants.
4. Titrate NDR administration to maintain the least degree of block that is necessary to achieve the requisite degree of clinical relaxation (Chap. 6).
5. Monitor for potential systemic effects of the parent compounds and metabolites (e.g., cardiovascular changes, evidence of histamine release, cerebral excitation).
6. Unless absolutely necessary, avoid total paralysis for longer than 48 hours.
7. Especially if total paralysis or near-total paralysis has been attained, attempt to provide drug-free periods (at least once every 48 hours) during which return of function can be documented and the absence of unacceptable systemic effects assured.
8. If paralysis of more than 48 hours' duration is required, consider changing relaxants and preferably changing the family of relaxants (e.g., steroidal derivatives, benzylisoquinolinium derivatives). The need for persistent paralysis may be obviated by temporarily increasing the dose of sedative medication.
9. Be aware of particularly "high-risk" settings. For example, in the patient who has renal insufficiency and who is also receiving high-dose steroids, seek to avoid continuous administration of any relaxant (and particularly a steroid-based relaxant) for longer than 48 hours and attempt to rapidly taper steroids. Even if the patient has normal renal function, continuous administration of steroid-based relaxants for more than 48 hours might best be avoided in the patient receiving high-dose steroids. Admittedly, this approach may constitute overcautiousness, in view of the lack of clear data and the disagreement among investigators. It is tempting to argue that even if one strongly prefers a drug such as vecuronium because of its clean cardiovascular profile and lack of systemically active metabolites, brief respites from this agent (possibly with a brief trial of another agent) would not be harmful. However, this cannot be guaranteed, since the nonsteroidal relaxants (benzylisoquino-

lonium derivatives) have a tendency to cause histamine release. The patient's care team must weigh the pros and cons of each approach and closely monitor neuromuscular and pulmonary function.
10. Periodically sample serum chemistries to identify electrolyte disturbances. Monitor plasma CK concentrations and urine myoglobin levels, as they may identify the onset of myopathic changes.
11. Allow for deliberate muscle activity (active movement, isometric exercise) or otherwise provide some "passive" movement to minimize disuse atrophy.
12. Be cognizant that long-term paralysis or myopathic changes may predispose to severe hyperkalemia in response to a depolarizing relaxant such as SCh, especially in the patient with severe trauma or sepsis (Chap. 18).

Discussion Questions ◆

a. Why might the *decrease in venous return* during nondepolarizing block be greatest with *d-tubocurarine?*
b. Arrange the following with respect to their propensity to cause *vagal block*, from least likely to most likely: *d*-tubocurarine, dimethyl tubocurarine (metocurine), atracurium, pancuronium, gallamine.
c. Are the effects of pancuronium and gallamine on *heart rate* more pronounced when the resting heart is low? Why or why not?
d. How does *diphenhydramine* (Benadryl) affect the *histamine release* elicited by a benzylisoquinolinium compound such as *d*-tubocurarine?
e. Why might you be more inclined to administer an H_1 *blocker* prior to rapidly administering a large dose of a histamine-releasing relaxant to a patient on *chronic cimetidine therapy?*
f. Why is a *precipitate of thiopental and relaxant* potentially harmful?
g. Why are *skin tests* more effective in detecting a sensitivity (i.e., an allergy) to relaxants than a sensitivity to thiopental?
h. Why does *pretreatment with aspirin* blunt the hemodynamic response to tubocurarine?
i. Why is it difficult to compare the plasma levels of relaxant attained in the *fetus* with those associated with detectable block during infusion of a relaxant in adults?
j. What accounts for *umbilical vein–umbilical artery* gradient that is typically noted for relaxant?
k. What features of the different relaxants would influence your choice of an NDR for *rapid-sequence induction for a cesarean section* (in a patient in whom you have elected not to use SCh)?
l. Is it likely that *metabolites* will contribute to *prolonged paralysis* after long-term administration of NDRs to ICU patients?

m. List at least ten potential disorders in *ICU patients* that may lead to *neuromuscular dysfunction* and myopathies.
n. What is the potential effect of *high-dose steroid* administration on *neuromuscular function*?

Answers ◆

a. *Tubocurarine* may cause *peripheral vasodilation* and venous pooling because of its tendency to cause (1) histamine release and (2) decreased sympathetic tone due to ganglionic block at doses similar to those that produce neuromuscular block[1,5,31] (the latter mechanism has been disputed[51]). As with all NDRs, tubocurarine may also cause a decrease in pressure because of decreased extremity muscle tone (with decreased pumping effect on venous return) and the need for positive pressure ventilation.

b.

Agents	Vagal ED_{50}/Neuromuscular ED_{50}[27]
Dimethyl tubocurarine	24.6
Atracurium	24.4
Pancuronium	5.2
Tubocurarine*	1.5
Gallamine	0.7

c. The vagolytic effects of *pancuronium* and *gallamine* are proportionally greater when the resting heart rate is low (high vagal tone).[10] However, their sympathomimetic effects are also noticeable in the context of sympathetic stimulation (even after atropine). This effect is probably a consequence of interference with the reuptake of norepinephrine, the release of which is increased in response to stimulation.

d. *Diphenhydramine* (Benadryl) decreases hemodynamic and respiratory symptoms of *histamine release* by competing at the H_1 receptors, but it does not lower plasma histamine levels. Antihistamines actually may increase plasma levels by (1) blocking H_1-receptor binding sites, (2) inhibiting H_3 receptors, which autoregulate histamine release,[91] and (3) inhibiting (competing at) histamine N-methyltransferase, the principal route of histamine metabolism. Nevertheless, diphenhydramine's overall effect appears to be beneficial. Note that several minutes may be required for histamine antagonists to afford adequate protection.

e. Some *H_2-receptor blockers,* such as cimetidine, can also block H_3 receptors[91] and inhibit histamine N-methyltransferase. In this context, a histamine-releasing agent may elicit greater histamine release and/or in-

---

*Although tubocurarine causes vagal block, this effect tends to be offset by tubocurarine-induced block of sympathetic ganglia.

hibit its breakdown. Moreover, the histamine will bind preferentially to H_1 receptors (which mediate such responses as bronchospasm and the immediate component of the vasodilatory response), since the H_2 receptors would be blocked.[59,86] This has led to the statement that "histamine-releasing agents may be contraindicated in patients subject to chronic H_2 receptor block."[86]

f. It has been proposed that, if the IV line is not flushed between *thiopental* administration and relaxant administration, then the resulting *precipitate* may cause an *aggregate reaction* and elicit severe bronchospasm when it passes through the lung.[68] One report noted that following thiopental and atracurium administration, an "inflammatory rash" spread along the arm, followed by small airway obstruction that responded to aminophylline.[68] Anaphylactic responses were reported when thiopental plus pancuronium[95] or thiopental plus SCh were given in rapid succession.[95] It is probably best to separate their administration by several seconds of a fast-flowing infusion.[105] Remember, anaphylaxis certainly can occur when relaxants are given "alone."

g. Prick tests and intradermal tests are based on *histamine release from mast cells,* induced by di- or multivalent antigens that bridge two IgE molecules. Because they are divalent molecules, neuromuscular blockers induce positive skin tests with high specificity and sensitivity (>95%) in individuals who are allergic to them. Other drugs used in anesthesia, including thiopental, behave as univalent haptens, and skin tests have a low sensitivity, so that a negative skin test does not exclude sensitization. However, positive tests are specific.[95,104] One additional note: it has recently been reported that anaphylaxis to neuromuscular blocking drugs can be demonstrated at the time of the reaction by detecting *relaxant-specific IgE* and/or *tryptase,* a mast cell component, in the plasma[99] rather than several days to weeks later with in vitro[103] testing.

h. A large part of the *hypotension caused by tubocurarine* results from its histamine-releasing properties after rapid high-dose administration. The effects of histamine on vascular tone are mediated through H_1 receptors. These have been shown to activate prostacyclin synthesis, which leads to vasodilation. Thus, blocking cyclo-oxygenase by aspirin is effective in blocking the vasodilatory action of tubocurarine.[84]

i. It may be tempting to compare *fetal blood levels* to those associated with *known responses in adults.* However, the *duration for which a given level is maintained* must be taken into account:

1. During recovery from pancuronium (i.e., when levels in the NMJ are greater than those in plasma), 50% block occurred in adults at a plasma pancuronium concentration (bound plus unbound drug) of $0.11\ \mu g \cdot mL^{-1}$.[126] Infants typically have umbilical artery concentrations of $0.04–0.12\ \mu g \cdot mL^{-1}$ after maternal doses of approximately

0.06–0.10 mg · kg^{-1}.^{112,116} These levels are achieved very briefly, however, and the levels in the NMJ have not equilibrated with their plasma counterparts.

2. During a steady infusion of 1.6 µg · kg^{-1} · min^{-1}, a plasma level of 0.25 µg · mL^{-1} was associated with 50% block; however, this degree of block was not attained until approximately 40 minutes (60 µg · kg^{-1}) of infusion,^{127} by which time the concentration in the NMJ was approaching that in plasma. Hence, it is not likely that such degrees of fetal paralysis would be achieved unless fetal arterial levels (and thus myoneural delivery) were maintained for many minutes more than is typically encountered during a cesarean delivery.

3. After 0.3 mg · kg^{-1} of atracurium, umbilical artery levels transiently reached 55 ± 34 ng · mL^{-1}.^{121} The plasma concentration required to produce 50% neuromuscular block in infants is 363 ± 118 ng · mL^{-1}.^{132} In addition to the difficulty extrapolating because of different durations of exposure to a given concentration, data may be compromised by the varying sensitivities of assays.^{118}

j. The *arteriovenous concentration difference in the cord vessels* suggests an extensive uptake of relaxant by the fetal liver, which receives 50% of umbilical blood flow and decreases the effects of placental transfer. Umbilical artery levels, which more accurately reflect the concentration delivered to the muscle end-plates, gradually approach umbilical vein levels.

k. For a rapid-sequence induction in a patient in whom one wishes to avoid SCh, one would administer an "intubating dose" of a short- or intermediate-duration NDR. The *parturient* and her passenger pose unique problems with respect to *dose selection and priming*. One must be prepared to treat the undesirable consequences.

High-dose vecuronium, with or without a priming dose, has been evaluated in this setting.^{129} Although a *priming dose* of 0.01 mg · kg^{-1} was well tolerated in a recent trial in ten patients undergoing cesarean section,^{129} special caution must be exercised in the context of the full stomach and decreased ventilatory reserve. Increasing the intubating dose from 0.10 to 0.20 mg · kg^{-1} caused a 30% increase in *neonatal blood levels* and apparently some minor neuromuscular effects.^{129} The times to maximal twitch depression were 177 and 175 seconds after the 0.01 + 0.10 mg · kg^{-1} and 0.20 mg · kg^{-1} regimens.^{129}

Other agents likewise pose potential problems. *Atracurium* would evidence less prolongation but, in high doses, may elicit significant histamine release,^{57,63,79} and atracurium (or its metabolite) may transiently alter some neonatal neurological assessments.^{115} *Mivacurium* is relatively untested in this setting. Its rapid metabolism may prove to be a distinct advantage; however, again we must be aware of possible histamine release. The rapid onset of *rocuronium* may prove to be helpful; like vecuronium, its duration is prolonged in proportion to dose.

l. There is evidence that the accumulation of breakdown products (e.g., the 3-desacetyl [3-OH] *derivatives of vecuronium and pancuronium*) may contribute to excessive block after long-term (unmonitored) relaxant administration in the presence of compromised organ function. The 3-hydroxy derivative of pancuronium, as well as the parent molecule, remained in substantial plasma and muscle concentrations for more than 4 days after a pancuronium infusion was discontinued in a patient who had respiratory and renal failure.[196] In two ICU patients with *renal failure*,[200] vecuronium's desacetyl metabolite (*3-desacetyl vecuronium*) remained in high concentrations and apparently accumulated in a "storage compartment" that equilibrated slowly with the plasma.[200] This metabolite is approximately 50–70% as potent as vecuronium[234,235]; the 3-OH levels in the two patients (244–586 ng · mL^{-1}) were higher than the corresponding vecuronium concentration (165 ng · mL^{-1}) that is required for 90% twitch depression.[200,236] In a more extensive study, neuromuscular block was prolonged as much as 7 days in 7 of 16 critically ill patients who were studied prospectively after receiving vecuronium for longer than 2 days; each of the affected patients had renal failure and was found to have pharmacologically active plasma concentrations of 3-desacetyl vecuronium.[201]

The above results are somewhat confusing. Although it appeared that renal clearance contributes significantly to elimination of 3-desacetyl vecuronium[237] and that renal failure predisposes to accumulation of 3-desacetyl vecuronium in humans,[200,201] animal studies suggest that its disposition is affected by hepatic, not renal, failure.[238–241] Of note, the 3,17-OH derivative of vecuronium actually may decrease the effectiveness of vecuronium-induced block by competing with the more potent parent molecule.[242] This may lead to increasing dose requirements during long-term administration.[243]

m. Patients in the ICU often have a number of problems that may lead to *neuromuscular dysfunction and myopathic changes* (Chap. 10). These include:
   1. Disuse atrophy
   2. Nutritional deficiency
   3. Prolonged sepsis
   4. Hyperpyrexia or hypothermia
   5. Hypotension and peripheral vascular disease
   6. Renal failure
   7. Hepatic failure
   8. Endocrine dysfunction
   9. Multiple organ failure

10. Denervation injury
11. Chemical denervation with relaxant, toxin, etc. (Chaps. 9 and 22)
12. Critical illness neuropathy (typically associated with multiple organ failure and sepsis with decreased albumin and increased glucose)
13. Necrotizing myopathy
14. Other non-relaxant-induced nerve and muscle changes
15. Acidosis
16. Hypophosphatemia
17. Hypocalcemia
18. Hypermagnesemia
19. Hypo-/hyperkalemia

n. *High-dose steroid administration* (as in the treatment of status asthmaticus) has been associated with several cases of subsequent weakness and paralysis diagnosed as *myopathy*.* In most cases (but not necessarily always[194,216,218]), the patient also received long-term infusion of a steroid-based NDR (vecuronium or pancuronium) to facilitate *mechanical ventilation*. It should also be noted that very high doses of aminophylline might augment the myopathic effects of steroids by themselves, promoting rhabdomyolysis.[244] The beta agonists used to treat asthma also may alter neuromuscular function (Chap. 9). The three patients who developed myopathies in one series received high-dose *steroids* and *pancuronium or vecuronium* and subsequently each developed (1) muscle weakness of both *proximal and distal muscle groups* that improved over weeks to months, (2) *elevated CK levels,* (3) *diffuse necrosis* and degeneration of *Type I and II muscle fibers* on muscle biopsy, and (4) *reduced motor-evoked potentials* with normal velocity and latency on electrophysiological testing.[164] Even though these changes do not typify all cases, one should be alerted to the possibility of myopathic changes by an increase in serum CK levels.[163,164] These features differ from those of the classic Cushing's (steroid) myopathy, which is characterized by Type II fiber atrophy of proximal muscle and usually normal to slightly elevated CK levels.[245]

These findings have led to conclusions such as "corticosteroids should not be administered for uncertain or unproved indications during prolonged neuromuscular block."[155] Likewise, it has been recommended that, in asthmatics with a history of myopathy or neuropathy, one should try to avoid IV corticosteroids entirely if possible, especially when treatment will include relaxant-induced (e.g., pancuronium) paralysis and mechanical ventilation.[186] Our recommendations for administration in this context are given in this chapter's text.

---

*References 157, 161–166, 173, 181–183, 187, 188, 191, 194, 197, 199, 204, and 206.

References ◆

1. Hughes R, Chapple DJ: Effect of non-depolarizing neuromuscular blocking agents on peripheral autonomic mechanisms in cats. Br J Anaesth 48:59–68, 1976
2. Guyton AC, Reeder RC: Quantitative studies on autonomic actions of curare. J Pharmacol Exp Ther 98:188–193, 1950
3. Savarese JJ: The autonomic margin of safety of metocurine and d-tubocurarine in the cat. Anesthesiology 5:40–46, 1979
4. Burstein CL, Jackson A, Bishop HF, Rovenstine EA: Curare in the management of autonomic reflexes. Anesthesiology 11:409, 1950
5. Longnecker DE, Stoelting RK, Morrow AG: Cardiac and peripheral vascular effects of d-tubocurarine in man. Anesth Analg 49:660, 1970
6. McDowell SA, Clarke RSJ: A clinical comparison of pancuronium with d-tubocurarine. Anaesthesia 24:581, 1969
7. Stoelting RK: The hemodynamic effects of pancuronium and d-tubocurarine in anesthetized patients. Anesthesiology 36:612–615, 1972
8. Eisele JH, Marta JA, Davis HS: Quantitative aspects of the chronotropic and neuromuscular effects of gallamine in anesthetized men. Anesthesiology 35:630–633, 1971
9. Lee Son S, Waud DR: Effects of non-depolarizing neuromuscular blocking agents on the cardiac vagus nerve in the guinea pig. Br J Anaesth 52:981, 1980
10. Miller RD, Eger EI II, Stevens WC, Gibbons R: Pancuronium induced tachycardia in relation to alveolar halothane, dose of pancuronium, and prior atropine. Anesthesiology 42:352, 1975
11. Stoelting RK: Hemodynamic effects of gallamine during halothane–nitrous oxide anesthesia. Anesthesiology 39:645–647, 1973
12. Gilbert M, Anderson EA, Brondbo A, Bjertnaes LJ: Muscle relaxants change myocardial metabolism in patients with ischaemic heart disease during high-dose fentanyl anaesthesia. Acta Anaesthesiol Scand 34:47–54, 1990
13. Thomson IR, Putnins CL: Adverse effects of pancuronium during high-dose fentanyl anesthesia for coronary artery bypass grafting. Anesthesiology 62:708–713, 1985
14. Riker WF, Wescoe WC: The pharmacology of flaxedil with observations on certain analogs. Ann NY Acad Sci 54:373, 1951
15. Saxena PR, Bonta IL: Mechanism of selective cardiac vagolytic action of pancuronium bromide: specific blockade of cardiac muscarinic receptors. Eur J Pharmacol 11:332–341, 1970
16. Brown BR, Crout JR: The sympathomimetic effect of gallamine on the heart. J Pharmacol Exp Ther 172:266, 1970
17. Marshall RJ, Ojewole JAO: Comparison of the autonomic effects of some currently-used neuromuscular blocking agents. Br J Pharmacol 66:77P, 1979
18. Nana A, Cardan E, Domokos M: Blood catecholamine changes after pancuronium. Acta Anaesthesiol Scand 17:83, 1973
19. Kingsley BP, Vaughan MS, Vaughan RW: Cardiovascular effects of nondepolarizing relaxants employed for pretreatment prior to succinylcholine. Can Anaesth Soc J 31:13–19, 1984
20. Docherty JR, McGrath JC: Sympathomimetic effects of pancuronium bromide on the cardiovascular system of the pithed rat: a comparison with the effects of drugs blocking the neuronal uptake of noradrenaline. Br J Pharmacol 64:589, 1978
21. Ivankovich AD, Miletich DJ, Albrecht RF, Zahed B: The effect of pancuronium on myocardial contraction and catecholamine metabolism. J Pharm Pharmacol 27:837, 1975
22. Salt PJ, Barnes PK, Conway CM: Inhibition of neuronal uptake of noradrenaline in the isolated perfused rat heart by pancuronium and its homologues, Org 6368, Org 7268 and Org NC 45. Br J Anaesth 52:313, 1980
23. Muir AW, Houston J, Green KL, Marshall RJ, Bowman WC, Marshall IG: Effects of a new neuromuscular blocking agent (Org 9426) in anaesthetized cats and pigs and in isolated nerve-muscle preparations. Br J Anaesth 63:400–410, 1989
24. McCullogh LS, Stone WA, Delaunis AL, et al: The effects of dimethyltubocurarine iodide on cardiovascular parameters, postganglionic sympathetic activity and histamine release. Anesth Analg 51:554–559, 1972

25. Savarese JJ, Ali HH, Antonio RP: The clinical pharmacology of metocurine: dimethyltubocurarine revisited. Anesthesiology 47:277–284, 1977
26. Stoelting RK: Hemodynamic effects of dimethyltubocurarine during nitrous oxide–halothane anesthesia. Anesth Analg 53:513–515, 1974
27. Hughes R, Chapple DJ: The pharmacology of atracurium: a new competitive neuromuscular blocking agent. Br J Anaesth 53:31–44, 1981
28. Maehr RB, Belmont MR, Wray DW, et al: Autonomic and neuromuscular effects of mivacurium and isomers in cats. Anesthesiology 75:A772, 1991
29. Marshall RJ, McGrath JC, Miller RD, Docherty JR, Lamar JC: Comparison of the cardiovascular actions of Org NC 45 with those produced by other non-depolarising neuromuscular blocking agents in experimental animals. Br J Anaesth 52:21S-29S, 1980
30. Salmenpera M, Peltola K, Takkunen O, Heinonen J: Cardiovascular effects of pancuronium and vecuronium during high-dose fentanyl anesthesia. Anesth Analg 62:1059–1064, 1983
31. Saxena FR, Dhasmana KM, Prakash O: A comparison of systemic and regional hemodynamic effects of d-tubocurarine, pancuronium, and vecuronium. Anesthesiology 59:102–108, 1983
32. Dhamee MS, Olund T, Reynolds AC, Entrees J, Kalbfleich J: Cardiovascular effects of pancuronium, vecuronium and atracurium during induction of anaesthesia with sufentanil and lorazepam for myocardial revascularization. J Cardiothorac Anesth 4:336–339, 1990
33. Inoue K, El-Banayosy A, Stolarski L, Reichelt W: Vecuronium induced bradycardia following induction of anaesthesia with etomidate or thiopentone, with or without fentanyl. Br J Anaesth 60:10–17, 1988
34. Janik R, Dick W: Sufentanil: the effect on cardiocirculatory parameters and intubation conditions of administration of pancuronium or vecuronium. Anaesthesist 38:673–680, 1989
35. Milligan KR, Beers HT: Vecuronium-associated cardiac arrest. Anaesthesia 40:385, 1985
36. May JR: Vecuronium and bradycardia. Anaesthesia 40:710, 1985
37. Starr NJ, Sethna DH, Estafanous FG: Bradycardia and asystole following the rapid administration of sufentanil with vecuronium. Anesthesiology 64:521–523, 1986
38. Cozanitis DA, Pouttu J, Rosenberg PH: Bradycardia associated with the use of vecuronium: a comparative study with pancuronium with and without glycopyrronium. Anaesthesia 42:192–194, 1987
39. Lavery GG, Mirakhur RK, Clarke RSJ, Gibson FM: The effect of atracurium, vecuronium and pancuronium on heart rate and arterial pressure in normal individuals. Eur J Anaesthesiol 3:459–468, 1986
40. Carter ML: Bradycardia after the use of atracurium. Br Med J 287:247–248, 1983
41. Wittek L, Gecsenyi M, Barna B, Hargitay Z, Adorjan K: Report on clinical test of pipecuronium bromide. Arzneimittelforsch 30:379–383, 1980
42. Emmott RS, Bracey BJ, Goldhill DR, Yate PM, Flynn PJ: Cardiovascular effects of doxacurium, pancuronium and vecuronium in anaesthetized patients presenting for coronary artery bypass surgery. Br J Anaesth 65:480–486, 1990
43. Stanley JC, Carson IW, Gibson FM, McMurray TJ, Elliott P, Lyons SM, Mirakhur RK: Comparison of the haemodynamic effects of pipecuronium and pancuronium during fentanyl anaesthesia. Acta Anaesthesiol Scand 35:262–266, 1991
44. Tassonyi E, Neidhart P, Pittet JF, Morel DR, Gemperle M: Cardiovascular effects of pipecuronium and pancuronium in patients undergoing coronary artery bypass grafting. Anesthesiology 69:793–796, 1988
45. Douglas WW: Histamine and 5-hydroxytryptamine (serotonin) and their antagonists. In Gilman AG, Goodman LS, Rall TW, Murad F (eds): Goodman and Gilman's The Pharmacological Basis of Therapeutics. New York, Macmillan, 1985, p 22
46. Lorenz W, Doenicke A, Schoning B, Ohmann C, Grote B, Neugebauer E: Definition and classification of the histamine-release response to drugs in anaesthesia and surgery: studies in the conscious human subject. Klin Wochenschr 60:896, 1982
47. Lorenz W, Roher HD, Doenicke A, et al: Histamine release in anesthesia and surgery: a new method to evaluate its clinical significance with several types of causal relationships. Clin Anesthesiol 2:403–406, 1984

48. Moss J, Rosow CE: Histamine release by narcotics and muscle relaxants in humans. Anesthesiology 59:330–339, 1983
49. Vigorito C, Russo P, Picotti GB, et al: Cardiovascular effects of histamine infusion in man. J Cardiovasc Pharmacol 5:53–537, 1983
50. Harrison GA: The cardiovascular effects and some relaxant properties of four relaxants in patients about to undergo cardiac surgery. Br J Anaesth 44:485–494, 1972
51. Moss J, Rosow CE, Savarese JJ, Philbin DM, Kniffen KJ: Role of histamine in the hypotensive action of d-tubocurarine in humans. Anesthesiology 55:19–25, 1981
52. Owen DAA: Physiology and pharmacology of histamine: cardiovascular studies in man. Clin Anesthesiol 2:383–402, 1984
53. Mehr EH, Lindeman KS, Hirshman CA: Airway constriction following atracurium is due to histamine release. Anesthesiology 75:A974, 1991
54. Smith DA, Wright DJ, Hammond JE: Influence of tubocurarine, pancuronium and atracurium on bronchomotor tone. Br J Anaesth 57:753–757, 1985
55. Fisher MM, Munro I: Life-threatening anaphylactoid reactions to muscle relaxants. Anesth Analg 62:559–564, 1983
56. Lavery GG, Clarke RSJ, Watkins J: Histaminoid response after intradermal and intravenous administration of atracurium, vecuronium and tubocurarine: a comparative study. Eur J Anaesthesiol 3:439–447, 1986
57. Basta SJ, Savarese JJ, Ali HH, Moss J, Gionfriddo M: Histamine-releasing properties of atracurium, dimethyl tubocurarine and tubocurarine. Br J Anaesth 55:105S–106S, 1983
58. Basta SJ, Moss J, Savarese JJ, Ali HH, Sunder N, Gionfriddo M, Lineberry CG: Cardiovascular effects of BWA444U: correlation with plasma histamine levels. Anesthesiology 55:A198, 1981
59. Basta SJ: Release of histamine by nondepolarizing neuromuscular blocking agents. Anesthesiol Rev 16:19–23, 1989
60. Clarke RSJ, Lavery GG, Mirakhur RK, Gibson FM: Histaminoid changes and dosage of atracurium. Ir J Med Sci 153:407, 1984
61. Mirakhur RK, Lavery GG, Clarke RSJ, Gibson FM, McAteer E: Atracurium in clinical anaesthesia: effect of dosage on onset, duration and conditions for tracheal intubation. Anaesthesia 40:801–805, 1985
62. Naguib M, Abdulatif M, Absood GH: Comparative effects of pipecuronium and tubocurarine and plasma concentrations of histamine in humans. Br J Anaesth 67:320–322, 1991
63. Basta SJ, Ali HH, Savarese JJ, Sunder N, Gionfriddo M, Cloutier G, Lineberry C, Cato AE: Clinical pharmacology of atracurium besylate (BW 33A): a new non-depolarizing muscle relaxant. Anesth Analg 61:723–729, 1982
64. Fox MA: Atracurium in normal doses may release histamine (letter). Anesthesiology 60:386, 1984
65. Goudsouzian NG, Young ET, Moss J, Liu MP: Histamine release during the administration of atracurium or vecuronium in children. Br J Anaesth 58:1229–1233, 1986
66. Lavery GG, Boyle MM, Mirakhur RK: Probable histamine liberation with atracurium: a case report. Br J Anaesth 57:811–813, 1985
67. Moyers JR, Carter JG, Fehr BL, Lineberry CC, Sokoll MD, Shimosato S: Circulatory effects of atracurium in patients with cardiovascular disease. Br J Anaesth 58:83S–88S, 1986
68. Watkins J: Histamine release and atracurium. Br J Anaesth 58:19S–22S, 1986
69. Choi WW, Mehta MP, Murray DJ, Sokoll MD, Forbes RB, Gergis SD, Abou-Donia M, Kirchner J: Neuromuscular and cardiovascular effects of mivacurium chloride in surgical patients receiving nitrous oxide–narcotic or nitrous oxide–isoflurane anaesthesia. Can J Anaesth 36:641–650, 1989
70. Savarese JJ, Ali HH, Basta SJ, Scott RPF, Embree PB, Wastila WB, Abou-Donia MM, Gelb C: The cardiovascular effects of mivacurium chloride (BW B1090U) in patients receiving nitrous oxide-opiate-barbiturate anesthesia. Anesthesiology 70:386–394, 1989
71. Basta SJ, Savarese JJ, Ali HH, Embree PB, Schwartz AF, Rudd GD, Wastila WB: Clinical pharmacology of doxacurium chloride (BW A938U): a new long-acting nondepolarizing muscle relaxant. Anesthesiology 69:478–486, 1988
72. Savarese JJ, Wastila WB, Rudd GD, Welch RE, Samara B: Pharmacodynamics and pharmacokinetics of doxacurium chloride (BW A938U): background and overview. J Cardiothorac Anesth 4:14–19, 1990

73. Futo J, Kupferberg JP, Moss J: Inhibition of histamine n-methyltransferase (HNMT) in vitro by neuromuscular relaxants. Biochem Pharm 39:415–420, 1990
74. Brandom BW, Woelfel SK, Cook DR, Fehr BL, Rudd GD: Clinical pharmacology of atracurium in infants. Anesth Analg 63:309–312, 1984
75. Scott RPF, Savarese JJ, Basta SJ, Embree P, Ali HH, Sunder N, Hoaglin DC: Clinical pharmacology of atracurium given in high dose. Br J Anaesth 58:834–838, 1986
76. Scott RPF, Savarese JJ, Basta SJ, Sunder N, Ali HH, Gargarian M, Gionfriddo M, Batson AG: Atracurium: clinical strategies for preventing histamine release and attenuating the haemodynamic response. Br J Anaesth 57:550–553, 1985
77. Marone G, Poto S, Columbo M, Quattrin S, Condorelli M: Histamine release from human basophils *in vitro:* effects of age of cell donor. Monogr Allergy 18:139, 1983
78. Lavery GG, Clarke RSJ, Mirakhur RK: Atracurium and vecuronium: relationship between plasma IgE levels, intradermal testing and clinical evidence of histamine liberation. Anesthesiology 63:A333, 1985
79. Beaven MA: Anaphylactoid reactions to anesthetic drugs (editorial). Anesthesiology 55:3–5, 1981
80. Cheng M, Lee C, Yang E, Cantley E: Comparison of fast and slow bolus injections of mivacurium chloride under narcotic–nitrous oxide anesthesia. Anesthesiology 69:A877, 1988
81. Philbin DM, Machaj VR, Tomickek RC, Schneider RC, Allan JC, Lowenstein E, Lineberry CC: Haemodynamic effects of bolus injection of atracurium in patients with coronary artery disease. Br J Anaesth 55:131S, 1983
82. Ali HH, Brull SJ, Witkowski T, Kopman A, Silverman DG, Goudsouzian NG, Bartkowski R, Weakly N: Efficacy and safety of divided dose administration of mivacurium for rapid tracheal intubation. Anesthesiology 79:A934, 1993
83. Silverman DG, Brull SJ: Depth of block after divided doses of mivacurium spaced 60 seconds apart. Anesth Analg 77:164–167, 1993
84. Hatano Y, Arai T, Noda J, et al: Contribution of prostacyclin to *d*-tubocurarine-induced hypotension in humans. Anesthesiology 72:28–32, 1990
85. Adt M, Baumert J-H, Reimann H-J: The role of histamine in the cardiovascular effects of atracurium. Br J Anaesth 68:155–160, 1992
86. Hosking MP, Lennon RL, Gronert GA: Combined H_1- and H_2-receptor blockade attenuates the cardiovascular effects of high dose atracurium for rapid sequence endotracheal intubation. Anesth Analg 67:1089–1092, 1988
87. Lorenz W, Doenicke A, Schoning B, Mamorski J, Weber D, Hinterlang E, Schwartz B, Neugebauer E: H_1 + H_2 receptor antagonists for premedication in anaesthesia and surgery: a critical view based on randomized clinical trials with Haemaccel and various anti-allergic drugs. Agents Actions 10:114–124, 1980
88. Tryba M, Zevounou F, Zenz M: Prevention of histamine-induced cardiovascular reactions during the induction of anaesthesia following premedication with H_1 and H_2 receptor antagonists i.m. Br J Anaesth 58:478–482, 1986
89. Doenicke A, Mayer M, Nebauer AE, Lorenz W, Moss J, Peter K: Mivacurium and histamine levels: oral premedication with H_1/H_2 antagonists prevents side effects. Anesthesiology 79:A931, 1993
90. Rosow CE, Basta SJ, Savarese JJ, Ali HH, Kniffen KJ, Moss J: BW 785U: correlation of cardiovascular effects with increases in plasma histamine. Anesthesiology 53:S270, 1980
91. Arrang JM, Garbarg M, Schwartz JC: Auto-inhibition of brain histamine release mediated by a novel class (H_3) of histamine receptor. Nature 327:117–123, 1983
92. Fisher MMcD, More DG: The epidemiology and clinical features of anaphylactic reactions in anaesthesia. Anaesth Intensive Care 9:226–234, 1981
93. Evans PJ, McKinnon I: An anaphylactoid reaction to gallamine triethiodide. Anaesth Intensive Care 5:239–243, 1977
94. Fisher MMcD, Baldo BA: Anaphylactoid reactions during anaesthesia. Clin Anesthesiol 2:677–692, 1984
95. Moneret-Vautrin DA, Widmer S, Guéant J-L, Kamel L, Laxenaire MC, Mouton C, Gerard H: Simultaneous anaphylaxis to thiopentone and a neuromuscular blocker: a study of two cases. Br J Anaesth 64:743–745, 1990
96. Patriarca G, Nucera A, Schiavino D, Romano A, DiRienzo V, Pellegrino S, Fais G: Pancuronium allergy: a case report. Br J Anaesth 62:210–212, 1989

97. Harle DG, Baldo BA, Fisher MM: Cross-reactivity of metocurine, atracurium, vecuronium and fazadinium with IgE antibodies from patients unexposed to these drugs but allergic to other myoneural blocking drugs. Br J Anaesth 57:1073–1076, 1985
98. Moneret-Vautrin DA, Guéant J-L, Kamel L, et al: Anaphylaxis to muscle relaxants: cross-sensitivity studied by radio-immuno-assays compared to intradermal tests in 34 cases. J Allergy Clin Immunol 82:745, 1988
99. Laroche D, Lefrancois C, Gérard J-L, Dubois F, Vergnaud M-C, Guéant J-L, Bricard H: Early diagnosis of anaphylactic reactions to neuromuscular blocking drugs. Br J Anaesth 69:611–614, 1992
100. Laxenaire MC, Moneret-Vautrin DA, Widmer S, Mouton C, Guéant J-L Anaesthetic drugs responsible for anaphylactic shock: French multi-center study. Ann Fr Anesth Reanim 9:501–506, 1990
101. Baldo BA, Fisher MM: Substituted ammonium ions as allergenic determinant in drug allergy. Nature (Lond) 306:262–264, 1983
102. Didier A, Benzarti M, Senft M, Charpin D, Lagier F, Charpin J, Vervloet D: Allergy to suxamethonium: persisting abnormalities in skin tests, specific IgE antibodies and leukocyte histamine release. Clin Allergy 17:385–392, 1987
103. Weiss ME, Adkinson NF, Hirshman CA: Evaluation of allergic drug reactions in the perioperative period. Anesthesiology 71:483–486, 1989
104. Fisher MMcD: The diagnosis of acute anaphylactoid reactions to anaesthetic drugs. Anaesth Intensive Care 8:454–459, 1981
105. Hughes R: Local reactions and histamine release by atracurium (letter). Anaesthesia 40:593–594, 1985
106. Oh TE, Horton J: Adverse reactions to atracurium. Br J Anaesth 62:467–468, 1989
107. Doenicke A: Atracurium is contraindicated in patients with a known allergy to drugs (letter). Anesthesiology 76:607, 1993
108. Laxenaire M-C, Mata-Bermejo E, Moneret-Vautrin DA, Guéant J-L: Life-threatening anaphylactoid reactions to propofol (Diprivan®). Anesthesiology 77:275–280, 1992
109. Laxenaire M-C, Moneret-Vautin D-A, Guéant J-L: In reply: Atracurium is contraindicated in patients with a known allergy to drugs (letter). Anesthesiology 78:607–609, 1993
110. Fujinaga M, Baden JM, Mazze RI: Developmental toxicity of nondepolarizing muscle relaxants in cultured rat embryos. Anesthesiology 76:999–1003, 1992
111. Thomas J, Climie CR, Mather LE: The placental transfer of alcuronium: a preliminary report. Br J Anaesth 41:297–302, 1969
112. Booth PN, Watson MJ, McLeod K: Pancuronium and the placental barrier. Anaesthesia 32:320–323, 1977
113. Kivalo I, Saarikoski S: Placental transfer of ^{14}C-dimethyltubocurarine during Caesarean section. Br J Anaesth 48:239–241, 1976
114. Older PO, Harris JM: Placental transfer of tubocurarine: case report. Br J Anaesth 40:459–463, 1968
115. Perreault C, Guay J, Gaudreault P, Cyrenne L, Varin F: Residual curarization in the neonate after caesarean section. Can J Anaesth 38:587–591, 1991
116. Abouleish E, Wingard LB Jr, De La Vega S, Uy N: Pancuronium in caesarean section and its placental transfer. Br J Anaesth 52:531–536, 1980
117. Duvaldestin P, Demetriou M, Henzel D, Desmonts JM: The placental transfer of pancuronium and its pharmacokinetics during caesarian section. Acta Anaesthesiol Scand 22:327–333, 1978
118. Dailey PA, Fisher DM, Shnider SM, Baysinger CL, Shinohara Y, Miller RD, Abboud TK, Kim KC: Pharmacokinetics, placental transfer, and neonatal effects of vecuronium and pancuronium administered during cesarean section. Anesthesiology 60:569–574, 1984
119. Wingard LB Jr, Abouleish E, West DC, Goehl TJ: Modified fluorometric quantitation of pancuronium bromide and metabolites in human maternal and umbilical serums. J Pharmacol Sci 68:914–916, 1979
120. Flynn PJ, Frank M, Hughes R: Use of atracurium in caesarean section. Br J Anaesth 56:599–605, 1984
121. Shearer ES, Fahy LT, O'Sullivan EP, Hunter JM: Transplacental distribution of atracurium, laudanosine and monoquaternary alcohol during elective caesarean section. Br J Anaesth 66:551–556, 1991

122. Ho PC, Stephens ID, Triggs EJ: Caesarean section and placental transfer of alcuronium. Anaesth Intensive Care 9:113–118, 1981
123. Demetriou M, Depoix J-P, Diakite B, Fromentin M, Duvaldestin P: Placental transfer of Org NC 45 in women undergoing caesarean section. Br J Anaesth 54:643–645, 1982
124. Neeld JB Jr, Seabrook PD Jr, Chastain GM, Frederickson EL: A clinical comparison of pancuronium and tubocurarine for cesarean section anesthesia. Anesth Analg 53:7–11, 1974
125. Spiers I, Sim AW: The placental transfer of pancuronium bromide. Br J Anaesth 44:370–373, 1972
126. Agoston S, Crul J, Kersten UW, Scaf AHJ: Relationship of the serum concentration of pancuronium to its neuromuscular activity in man. Anesthesiology 47:509–512, 1977
127. Shanks CA, Somogyi AA, Triggs EJ: Dose-response and plasma concentration-response relationships of pancuronium in man. Anesthesiology 51:111–118, 1979
128. Baraka A, Noueihed R, Sinno H, Wakid N, Agoston S: Succinylcholine-vecuronium (Org NC 45) sequence for cesarean section. Anesth Analg 62:909–913, 1983
129. Hawkins JL, Johnson TD, Kubicek MA, Skjonsky BS, Morrow DH, Joyce TH III: Vecuronium for rapid-sequence intubation for cesarean section. Anesth Analg 71:185–190, 1990
130. Frank M, Flynn PJ, Hughes R: Atracurium in obstetric anaesthesia: a preliminary report. Br J Anaesth 55(suppl 1):113S–114S, 1983
131. Skarpa M, Dayan AD, Follenfant M, James DA, Moore WB, Thomson PM, Lucke JN, Morgan M, Lovell R, Medd R: Toxicity testing of atracurium. Br J Anaesth 55:27S–29S, 1982
132. Fisher DM, Canfell PC, Spellman MJ, Miller RD: Pharmacokinetics and pharmacodynamics of atracurium in infants and children. Anesthesiology 73:33–37, 1990
133. Hodes R: Electrocortical synchronization resulting from reduced proprioceptive drive caused by neuromuscular blocking agents. Electroencephalogr Clin Neurophysiol 14:220–232, 1962
134. Minton MD, Stirt JA, Bedford RF, Haworth C: Intracranial pressure after atracurium in neurosurgical patients. Anesth Analg 64:1113–1116, 1985
135. Rosa G, Orfei P, Sanfilippo M, Vilardi V, Gasparetto A: The effects of atracurium besylate (Tracrium®) on intracranial pressure and cerebral perfusion pressure. Anesth Analg 65:381–384, 1986
136. Rosa G, Sanfilippo M, Vilardi V, Orfei P, Gasparetto A: Effects of vecuronium bromide on intracranial pressure and cerebral perfusion pressure. Br J Anaesth 58:437–440, 1986
137. Forbes AR, Cohen NH, Eger EI II: Pancuronium reduces halothane requirements in man. Anesth Analg 58:497–499, 1979
138. Gibbs NM, Larach DR, Schuler HG: The effect of neuromuscular blockade with vecuronium on hemodynamic responses to noxious stimuli in the rat. Anesthesiology 71:214–217, 1989
139. Topulos GP, Lansing RW, Banzett RB: The experience of complete neuromuscular blockade in awake humans. J Clin Anesth 5:369–374, 1993
140. Lanier WL, Sharbrough FW, Michenfelder JD: Effects of atracurium, vecuronium or pancuronium pretreatment on lignocaine seizure thresholds in cats. Br J Anaesth 60:74–80, 1988
141. Tindall GT, Greenfield JC Jr: The effects of intra-arterial histamine on blood flow in the internal and external carotid artery in man. Stroke 4:46–49, 1973
142. Dal Santo G: Kinetics of distribution of radioactive labeled muscle relaxants: III. Investigations with ^{14}C-succinyldicholine and ^{14}C-succinylmonocholine during controlled conditions. Anesthesiology 29:435–443, 1969
143. Bowman WC: The neuromuscular blocking action of benzoquinonium chloride in the cat and the hen. Br J Pharmacol 13:521, 1958
144. Hoppe JO: A new series of synthetic curare-like compounds. Ann NY Acad Sci 54:395, 1951
145. Bowman WC: Non-relaxant properties of neuromuscular blocking drugs. Br J Anaesth 54:147–160, 1982
146. Ivankovich AD, Sidell N, Cairoli VJ, Dietz AA, Albrecht RF: Dual action of pancuronium on succinylcholine block. Can Anaesth Soc J 24:228–241, 1977

147. Mirakhur RK, Ferres CJ, Lavery TD: Plasma cholinesterase levels following pancuronium and vecuronium. Acta Anaesthesiol Scand 27:451–453, 1983
148. Stovner J, Oftedal N, Holmboe J: The inhibition of cholinesterases by pancuronium. Br J Anaesth 47:949–954, 1975
149. Bennett EJ, Montgomery SJ, Dalal FY, Raj PP: Pancuronium and the fasciculations of succinylcholine. Anesth Analg 52:892–896, 1973
150. Erkola O, Salmenpera A, Kuoppamaki R: Five nondepolarizing muscle relaxants in precurarization. Acta Anaesthesiol Scand 27:427–432, 1983
151. Ferguson A, Bevan DR: Mixed neuromuscular block: the effect of precurarization. Anaesthesia 36:661–666, 1981
152. Nishizawa M: Influence of small doses of vecuronium and pancuronium on succinylcholine-induced neuromuscular blockade. Masui 39:1188–1197, 1990
153. Ostergaard D, Viby-Mogensen J, Hanel HK, Skovgaard LT: Pretreatment with pancuronium before suxamethonium administration in patients heterozygous for the usual and the atypical plasma cholinesterase gene. Acta Anaesthesiol Scand 35:502–507, 1991
154. Brandom BW, Meretoja OA, Taivainen T, Wirtavuori K: Accelerated onset and delayed recovery of neuromuscular block induced by mivacurium preceded by pancuronium in children. Anesth Analg 76:998–1003, 1993
155. Hansen-Flaschen J, Cowen J, Raps EC: Neuromuscular blockade in the intensive care unit: more than we bargained for. Am Rev Respir Dis 147:234–236, 1993
156. Clowes GHA, George BC, Villee CA, Saravis CA: Muscle proteolysis induced by a circulating peptide in patients with sepsis or trauma. N Engl J Med 308:545–552, 1983
157. Kupfer Y, Okrent DG, Twersky RA, Tessler S: Disuse atrophy in a ventilated patient with status asthmaticus receiving neuromuscular blockade. Crit Care Med 15:795–796, 1987
158. Partridge BL, Abrams JH, Bazemore C, Rubin R: Prolonged neuromuscular blockade after long-term infusion of vecuronium bromide in the intensive care unit. Crit Care Med 18:1177–1179, 1990
159. Wokke JHJ, Jennekens FGI, van den Dord CJM, et al: Histological investigations of muscle atrophy and end plates in two critically ill patients with generalized weakness. J Neurol Sci 88:95, 1988
160. Benzing G, Iannaccone ST, Bove KE, et al: Prolonged myasthenic syndrome after one week of muscle relaxants. Pediatr Neurol 6:190, 1990
161. Gooch JL, Suchyta MR, Balbierz JM, Petajan JH, Clemmer TP: Prolonged paralysis after treatment with neuromuscular junction blocking agents. Crit Care Med 19:1125–1131, 1991
162. Danon MJ, Carpenter S: Myopathy with thick filament (myosin) loss following prolonged paralysis with vecuronium during steroid treatment. Muscle Nerve 14:1131–1139, 1991
163. Douglass JA, Tuxen DV, Horne M, et al: Myopathy in severe asthma. Am Rev Respir Dis 146:517–519, 1992
164. Griffin D, Fairman N, Coursin D, Rawsthorne L, Grossman JE: Acute myopathy during treatment of status asthmaticus with corticosteroids and steroidal muscle relaxants. Chest 102:510–514, 1992
165. Hirano M, Ott B, Raps E, et al: Acute quadriplegic myopathy: a complication of treatment with steroids, nondepolarizing blocking agents, or both. Neurology 42:2082–2087, 1992
166. Kaplan P, Rocha W, Saunders D, D'Souza B, Spock A: Acute steroid tetraplegia following status asthmaticus. Pediatrics 78:121–123, 1986
167. Subramony SH, Carpenter DE, Raju S, Pride M, Evans OB: Myopathy and prolonged neuromuscular blockade after lung transplant. Crit Care Med 19:1580–1582, 1991
168. Grossman JE: Acute myopathy during treatment of status asthmaticus with corticosteroids and steroidal muscle relaxants. Chest 102:110–114, 1992
169. Bolton CF, Gilbert JJ, Hahn AF, Sibbald WJ: Polyneuropathy in critically ill patients. J Neurol Neurosurg Psychiatry 47:1223–1231, 1984
170. Coronel B, Meracatello A, Couturiere J-C, et al: Polyneuropathy: potential cause of difficult weaning. Crit Care Med 18:486–489, 1990

171. Witt NJ, Zochodne DW, Bolton CF, et al: Peripheral nerve function in sepsis and multiple organ failure. Chest 99:176–184, 1991
172. Witt NJ, Bolton CF, Sibbald WJ: The incidence and early features of the polyneuropathy of critical illness. Neurology 35:74, 1985
173. Zochodne DW, Bolton CF, Wells GA, Gilbert J, Hahn A, Brown J, et al: Critical illness polyneuropathy, a complication of sepsis and multiple organ failure. Brain 110:819–842, 1987
174. Duchateau J, Hainaut K: Electrical and mechanical changes in immobilized human muscle. J Appl Physiol 62:2168, 1987
175. Gogia P, Schneider VS, LeBlanc AD, et al: Bed rest effect on extremity muscle torque in healthy men. Arch Phys Med Rehabil 69:1030, 1988
176. Lieber RL, Friden JO, Hargens AR, et al: Differential response of the dog quadriceps muscle to external skeletal fixation of the knee. Muscle Nerve 11:193, 1988
177. Muller EA: Influence of training and of inactivity on muscle strength. Arch Phys Med Rehabil 51:449, 1970
178. Cooper RR: Alterations during immobilization and regeneration of skeletal muscle in cats. J Bone Joint Surg 54A:919–952, 1972
179. Hikida RS, Gollnick PD, Dudley GA, Convertino VA, Buchanan P: Structural and metabolic characteristics of human skeletal muscle following 30 days of simulated microgravity. Aviat Space Environ Med 60:664–670, 1989
180. Sargeant AJ, Davies CTM, Edwards RHT, Maunder C, Young A: Functional and structural changes after disuse of human muscle. Clin Sci Mol Med 52:337–342, 1977
181. Kupfer Y, Namba T, Kaldawi E, Tessler S: Prolonged weakness after long-term infusion of vecuronium bromide. Ann Intern Med 117:484–486, 1992
182. Bachmann P, Gaussorgues P, Piperno D, et al: Hydrocortisone and pancuronium bromide: acute myopathy during status asthmaticus. Crit Care Med 16:731, 1988
183. Brun-Buisson C, Gherardi R: Letter. Crit Care Med 16:731, 1988
184. Fiamengo SA, Savarese JJ: Use of muscle relaxants in intensive care units. Crit Care Med 19:1457–1459, 1991
185. Haas JL, Shaefer MS, Miwa LJ, et al: Prolonged paralysis associated with long-term pancuronium use. Pharmacotherapy 9:154–157, 1989
186. Lacomis D, Smith TW, Chad DA: Acute myopathy and neuropathy in status asthmaticus: case report and literature review. Muscle Nerve 16:84–90, 1993
187. MacFarlane I, Rosenthal F: Severe myopathy after status asthmaticus. Lancet 2:615, 1977
188. Op-de-Coul AA, Lambregts PC, Koeman J, van Ruyenbrock MJ, Ter Laak HJ, Gabreels-Festen AA: Neuromuscular complications in patients given Pavulon (pancuronium bromide) during artificial ventilation. Clin Neurol Neurosurg 87:17–22, 1985
189. Panacek EA, Sherman B: Disuse atrophy in a ventilated patient with status asthmaticus receiving neuromuscular blockade (letter). Crit Care Med 16:732, 1988
190. Rossiter A, Souney PF, McGowan S, Carvajal P: Pancuronium-induced prolonged neuromuscular blockade. Crit Care Med 19:1583–1587, 1991
191. Sitwell L, Weinshenker B, Monpetit V, Reid D: Complete ophthalmoplegia as a complication of acute corticosteroid- and pancuronium-associated myopathy. Neurology 41:921–922, 1991
192. Tanigaki T, Kondo T, Ohta Y, Yamabayashi H: Transient neuromuscular impairment resulting from prolonged inhalation of halothane and enflurane. Chest 98:1012–1013, 1990
193. Torres CF, Maniscalco WM, Agostinelli T: Muscle weakness and atrophy following prolonged paralysis with pancuronium bromide in neonates. Ann Neurol 18:403, 1985
194. Williams T, O'Heir R, Czarny D, Horne M, Bowes G: Acute myopathy in severe acute asthma with intravenously administered corticosteroids. Am Rev Respir Dis 137:460–463, 1988
195. Kupfer Y, Tessler S: In reply: Disuse atrophy in a ventilated patient with status asthmaticus receiving neuromuscular blockade (letter). Crit Care Med 16:732, 1988
196. Vandenbrom RHG, Wierda MKH: Pancuronium bromide in the intensive care unit: a case of overdose. Anesthesiology 69:996–997, 1988

197. Douglass J, Tuxen M, Horne C, Scheinkestel D, Czarny M, Bowes G: Acute myopathy following treatment of severe life threatening asthma. Am Rev Respir Dis 141:A397, 1990
198. Lacomis D, Samuels MA: Adverse neurologic effects of glucocorticosteroids. J Gen Intern Med 6:367–377, 1991
199. Margolis BD, Khachikian D, Friedman Y, Garrard C: Prolonged reversible quadriparesis in mechanically ventilated patients who received long-term infusions of vecuronium. Chest 100:877–878, 1991
200. Segredo V, Matthay MA, Sharma ML, Gruenke LD, Caldwell JE, Miller RD: Prolonged neuromuscular blockade after long-term administration of vecuronium in two critically ill patients. Anesthesiology 72:566–570, 1990
201. Segredo V, Caldwell JE, Matthay MA, Sharma ML, Gruenke LD, Miller RD: Persistent paralysis in critically ill patients after long-term administration of vecuronium. N Engl J Med 327:524–528, 1992
202. Slater RM, Polard BJ, Doran BRH: Prolonged neuromuscular blockade with vecuronium in renal failure. Anaesthesia 43:250, 1988
203. Vanderheyden BA, Reynolds UN, Gerold KB, Emanuele T: Prolonged paralysis after long-term vecuronium infusion. Crit Care Med 20:304–307, 1992
204. Waclawik AC, Sufit RL, Beinlich BR, Schutta HS: Acute myopathy with selective degradation of myosin filaments following status asthmaticus. J Neurol Sci 98(suppl):470, 1990
205. Sury MRJ, Russel GN, Heaf DP: Hydrocortisone myopathy (letter). Lancet 2:515, 1988
206. Shee CD: Risk factors for hydrocortisone myopathy in acute severe asthma. Respir Med 84:229–233, 1990
207. Klessig HT, Geiger HJ, Murray MJ, Coursin DB: A national survey on the practical patterns of anesthesiologists/intensivists in the use of muscle relaxants. Crit Care Med 20:1341–1345, 1992
208. Hansen-Flaschen JH, Brazinsky S, Basile C, Lanken PN: Use of sedating drugs and neuromuscular blocking agents in patients requiring mechanical ventilation for respiratory failure: a national survey. JAMA 266:2870–2875, 1991
209. De Smet Y, Jaminet M, Jaeger U, Jacob J, Neurav H, Haus G, Ledesch-Camaus D, Meyers R: Myopathie aigue cortisonique de l'asthmatique. Rev Neurol 147:682–685, 1991
210. Hunter JM: Infusions of atracurium and vecuronium in patients with multisystem organ failure in the intensive therapy unit. Insights Anaesthesiol 1:23–27, 1987
211. Griffiths RB, Hunter JM, Jones RS: Atracurium infusion in patients with renal failure on an I.T.U. Anaesthesia 41:375–381, 1986
212. Meyer KC, Prielipp RC, Grossman JE, Coursin DB: Prolonged weakness after infusion of atracurium in two intensive care unit patients. Anesth Analg 78:772–774, 1994
213. Coakley JH, Nagendran K, Honavar M, et al: Preliminary observations on the neuromuscular abnormalities in patients with organ failure. Intensive Care Med 19:323–328, 1993
214. Helliwell TR, Coakley JH, Wagenmakers AJM, Griffiths RD, Campbell IT, Green C, McClelland P, Williams PS, Bone JM: Necrotizing myopathy in critically ill patients. J Pathol 164:307–314, 1991
215. Hinds CJ, Nagendran K, Honauar M, Coakley JH: Muscle relaxants in intensive care patients (letter). Crit Care Med 21:1403–1404, 1993
216. Knox AJ, Mascie-Taylor BH, Muers MF: Acute hydrocortisone myopathy in acute severe asthma. Thorax 41:411–412, 1986
217. Coakley JH, Edwards RHT, McClelland P, Bone JM, Helliwell TR: Occult ischaemic necrosis of skeletal muscle associated with renal failure. Br Med J 301:370, 1990
218. Van Marle W, Woods KL: Acute hydrocortisone myopathy. Br Med J 281:271–272, 1980
219. Dubois DC, Almon RA: A possible role for glucocorticoids in denervation atrophy. Muscle Nerve 4:370–373, 1981
220. Rouleau G, Karpati G, Carpenter S, Soza M, Prescott S, Holland P: Glucocorticoid excess induces preferential depletion of myosin in denervated skeletal muscle fibers. Muscle Nerve 10:428–438, 1987

221. DuBois DC, Almon RR: Disuse atrophy of skeletal muscle is associated with an increase in number of glucocorticoid receptors. Endocrinology 107:1649–1651, 1980
222. Goldberg AL, Goodman HM: Relationship between cortisone and muscle work in determining muscle size. J Physiol (Lond) 200:667–675, 1969
223. Bywaters EGL, Beall D: Crush injuries with impairment of renal function. Br Med J 1:427–432, 1941
224. Garcia G, Snider T, Feldman C, et al: Nephrotoxicity of myoglobin in the rat: relative importance of urine pH and prior dehydration. Kidney Int 19:200, 1981
225. Bolton CF: Neuromuscular abnormalities in critically ill patients. Intensive Care Med 19:309–310, 1993
226. Coakley JH, Ferguson C, Walker R, et al: Prolonged weakness in patients receiving mechanical ventilation for exacerbations of airflow limitation. Chest 101:1413–1416, 1992
227. Rivner MH, Kim S, Greenberg M, et al: Reversible generalized paresis following hypotension: a new neurological entity (abstract). Neurology 33(suppl 2):1664, 1983
228. Roelofs RI, Cerra F, Beilka N, et al: Prolonged respiratory insufficiency due to acute motor neuropathy: a new syndrome? Neurology 33(suppl 2):240, 1983
229. Agoston S, Seyr M, Khuenl-Brady KS, Henning RH: Use of neuromuscular blocking agents in the intensive care unit. Anesthesiol Clin North Am 11:345–359, 1993
230. Darrah WC, Johnston JR, Mirakhur RK: Vecuronium infusions for prolonged muscle relaxation in the intensive care unit. Crit Care Med 17:1297–1300, 1987
231. Smith CL, Hunter JM, Jones RS: Vecuronium infusions in patients with renal failure in an ITU. Anaesthesia 42:387–393, 1987
232. Fitzpatrick KTJ, Black GW, Crean PM, Mirakhur RK: Continuous vecuronium infusion for prolonged muscle relaxation in children. Can J Anaesth 38:169–174, 1991
233. Fiamengo SA, Savarese JJ: Muscle relaxants in intensive care patients (letter). Crit Care Med 21:1404–1405, 1993
234. Bencini AF, Houwertjes MC, Agoston S: Effects of hepatic uptake of vecuronium bromide and its putative metabolites on their neuromuscular blocking actions in the cat. Br J Anaesth 57:789–795, 1985
235. Marshall IG, Gibb AJ, Durant NN: Neuromuscular and vagal blocking actions of pancuronium bromide, its metabolites, and vecuronium bromide (ORG NC45) and its potential metabolism in the anesthetized cat. Br J Anaesth 55:703–714, 1983
236. Cannon JE, Fahey MR, Castognoli KP, Furuta T, Canfell PC, Sharma M, Miller RD: Continuous infusion of vecuronium: the effect of anesthetic agents. Anesthesiology 67:503–506, 1987
237. Castagnoli KP, Caldwell JE, Canfell PC, Lynam DP, Arden JR, Miller RD: Does the independent measurement of 3-desacetyl vecuronium influence the pharmacokinetics of vecuronium? Anesthesiology 69:A479, 1988
238. Bencini AF, Scaf AHJ, Agoston S, Houwertjes MC, Kersten UW: Disposition of vecuronium bromide in the cat. Br J Anaesth 57:782–788, 1985
239. Segredo V, Shin YS, Sharma ML, et al: Pharmacokinetics, neuromuscular effects, and biodisposition of 3-desacetylvecuronium (Org 7268) in cats. Anesthesiology 74:1052–1059, 1991
240. Upton RA, Nguyen T, Miller RD, Castagnoli N Jr: Renal and biliary elimination of vecuronium (org NC 45) and pancuronium in rats. Anesth Analg 61:313–316, 1982
241. Waser PG, Wiederkehr H, Sin-Ren AC, Kaiser-Schonenberger E: Distribution and kinetics of ^{14}C-vecuronium in rats and mice. Br J Anaesth 59:1044–1051, 1987
242. Khuenl-Brady KS, Mair P, Koller J: Antagonism of vecuronium by one of its metabolites in vitro. Eur J Pharmacol 222:153–156, 1992
243. Coursin DB, Klasek G, Goelzer SL: Increased requirements for continuously infused vecuronium in critically ill patients. Anesth Analg 69:518–521, 1989
244. MacDonald JB, Jones HM, Cowan RA: Rhabdomyolysis and acute renal failure after theophylline overdose. Lancet 1:932–933, 1985
245. Lane RJM, Mastaglia FL: Drug-induced myopathies in man. Lancet 2:562, 1978

12

DAVID G. SILVERMAN / RAJINDER K. MIRAKHUR

Nondepolarizing Relaxants of Long Duration

This chapter and the following two chapters describe the features specific to individual nondepolarizing relaxants (NDRs). Characteristics that apply to multiple relaxants were detailed in earlier chapters. Structures are illustrated in Figure 2-1.

Agents of long duration typically have a half-time of elimination ($t_{1/2elim}$) that is greater than 100 minutes and a clearance that is less than 2–3 mL · kg^{-1} · min^{-1}. Their clinically effective block time (Dur$_{25}$) averages 45–60 minutes after an ED$_{95}$ dose and 90–120 minutes after 2 times the ED$_{95}$ (Table 12-1). When a dose that is 25% of the ED$_{95}$ is administered at the time of 25% recovery of single twitch amplitude, its effect lasts approximately 40–60 minutes.

◆ d-TUBOCURARINE

d-Tubocurarine (or *curare*) is the prototypic NDR, having been used clinically for approximately 50 years.[1] Classically viewed as a bisquaternary structure (see Fig. 2-1), *d*-tubocurarine may also have a monoquaternary monotertiary configuration.[2] It is associated with a relatively large degree of *fade,* presumably the result of binding to presynaptic cholinoceptors (Chap. 2).[3-5] As discussed in Chapter 11, it typically elicits a greater *decrease in blood pressure* than other commonly employed relaxants (see Table 11-1).[6-14] After bolus administration of a typical intubating dose of 0.5 mg · kg^{-1}, it tends to cause a relatively high degree of *histamine release,*[7,15-17] especially if given rapidly and a relatively high degree of block at *autonomic ganglia.*[8,18] These features occur at or near the clinical dosing range.

d-Tubocurarine undergoes relatively little metabolism, being excreted in both urine and bile, primarily the former.[19-22] As is the case for most relaxants, its $t_{1/2elim}$ is prolonged in renal failure[20] and in the setting of decreased glomerular filtration, as in the elderly.[21]

TABLE 12-1
Dosages and Durations

	ED_{95} (mg·kg^{-1})	$1 \times ED_{95}$			$2 \times ED_{95}$		
		Dur_{25}	RI_{25-75}	Dur_{95}	Dur_{25}	Dur_{95}	$t_{\frac{1}{2}elim}$
LONG-ACTING							
■ *d*-Tubocurarine	0.45–0.50	45–60	35	90	90–120	≥150	80–150
■ Pancuronium	0.05–0.07	45–60	35	90	90–120	≥150	80–150
■ Metocurine	0.25–0.30	45–60	35	90	90–120	≥150	80–150
■ Pipecuronium	0.04–0.05	45–60	35	≥90	100–120	≥150	80–150
■ Doxacurium	0.015–0.03	50–60	45	>90	100–120	≥150	80–150
■ Gallamine	2.5–3.0	45–60	35	80	90–120	≥130	80–150
■ Alcuronium	0.20–0.25	45–60	35	90	90–120	>150	80–150
INTERMEDIATE-ACTING							
■ Atracurium	0.20–0.25	20–30	13	45	30–55	70	20–25
■ Vecuronium	0.04–0.06	20–30	13	40	30–60	80	55–80
■ Rocuronium	0.25–0.30	20–30	13	40	30–60	80	60–100
SHORT-ACTING							
■ Mivacurium	0.06–0.08	10–15	7	23	15–20	27	2–4

Note: The doses and times (in minutes) are estimates based on extrapolations from the literature. There is marked intersubject variability, especially in the context of differing ages, organ function, and perioperative agents. This variability is illustrated for the Dur_{25} values.

◆ DIMETHYLTUBOCURARINE

Dimethyltubocurarine, or metocurine (Metubine), was created by methylation of two hydroxy groups of *d*-tubocurarine. It is devoid of autonomic effects and causes *fewer cardiovascular effects* than its parent compound.[8,12,13,23–25] A benzylisoquinolinium compound, it causes *histamine release* (but to a lesser degree than tubocurarine).[15,23,24] It thus may produce hypotension, usually after bolus doses $\geq$ 0.4 mg $\cdot$ kg^{-1}.[24] Its elimination is predominantly renal,[22,26] and its clearance tends to be more prolonged than that of *d*-tubocurarine in renal failure[27] and in the elderly.[21]

◆ GALLAMINE

Gallamine (Flaxedil) is a synthetic NDR with a unique structure: it has three quaternary ammonium groups. It is now rarely used, primarily because it is associated with marked tachycardia. It is *vagolytic*[8,28–31] and somewhat *sympathomimetic*[32] even in doses below those required for complete paralysis (Chap. 11). It blocks muscarinic receptors in the heart,[30] and it may cause release of noradrenaline.[11,32] In susceptible patients, even a defasciculating dose may have significant effects on heart rate.[33] The onset of action of gallamine is slightly faster than that of tubocurarine or pancuronium[34] (perhaps because more molecules are administered in view of its lower potency; Chap. 7), and it has a greater tendency to cause channel block. Gallamine is *contraindicated* in patients with tachycardia/hypovolemia (or in situations where tachycardia should be avoided); in patients with renal failure, because it is virtually 100% renally excreted[35–37]; in pregnant women, because it crosses the placenta more readily than other NDRs; and in patients with iodine allergy, because it contains iodine.

◆ PANCURONIUM

Pancuronium bromide (Pavulon), an aminosteroid, is basically two acetylcholine (ACh)-like fragments on a rigid steroid nucleus which maintains a fixed distance between its two charged nitrogen atoms.[38] It was introduced in 1967 as an agent which lacked the histamine-releasing properties and pronounced cardiovascular effects of *d*-tubocurarine.[10] However, it has *vagolytic and sympathomimetic effects* at doses necessary for complete paralysis.[8,11,14,29,39–46] It thus tends to accelerate atrioventricular conduction and to increase heart rate and arterial pressure; and it may lead to arrhythmias. These effects are exacerbated by hypercarbia, other sympathomimetic agents, and tricyclic antidepressants[47]; they may contribute to ischemia in susceptible patients.[48,49]

The *duration* of pancuronium-induced block is similar to that of tubocurarine.[50] As for all NDRs, there is wide intersubject variability: although the mean Dur_{25} after 0.08 mg · kg^{-1} (slightly less than 1.5 × ED_{95}) averaged 86 minutes in one study, the range was 43–133 minutes.[50]

The kidney is ordinarily responsible for up to 80% of *pancuronium elimination,* with more than 50% excreted unchanged in the urine.[51–53] Pancuronium's $t_{1/2elim}$ increased from 132 ± 25 minutes in normal subjects to 257 ± 128 minutes in patients with *kidney failure,*[54] and by as much as 500% in other studies of renal failure and anephric patients.[55–57] Its clinical duration is prolonged in these contexts.[54,56,58] In patients with renal failure, the infusion rate required to maintain 90% depression decreased by 62%, while that for vecuronium decreased by 23% and that for atracurium was essentially unaffected.[59]

In view of the decline in renal function with age, the clearance of pancuronium is *reduced in the elderly,*[60] and its duration may be increased.[60–62] Overall, RI_{25-75} increased from 39 ± 13 minutes to 62 ± 30 minutes in patients over 75 years of age.[61] Others have reported statistically insignificant prolongation in healthy elderly patients.[63] The dose needed to attain a given level of block (i.e., potency) is not changed in the elderly.[64]

Pancuronium is metabolized to some extent in the *liver,* and its plasma clearance is reduced in patients with hepatic disease.[51,53,65–67] The only detectable *metabolite is a 3-hydroxy compound* that has approximately 50% of the activity of the parent compound. Pancuronium's $t_{1/2elim}$ increased from 94 to 303 minutes in *liver failure*[66] and from 114 to 208 minutes in patients with cirrhosis.[67] Recovery from pancuronium-induced block may be slowed further in this context because of an increased volume of distribution; this leads to the need for a relatively high initial dose in order to attain a desired depth of block.[67]

◆ ALCURONIUM

Alcuronium (Alloferin) has been used more commonly in Europe. It is a synthetic derivative of tubocurarine, with a lesser tendency toward hypotension and tachycardia. However, *cardiovascular changes* (e.g., hypotension) still may occur,[7,68–70] primarily as a result of block of autonomic ganglia. Of 1,425 patients receiving routine clinical doses of alcuronium intraoperatively, a 20% or greater decline in blood pressure was noted in 195 (13.7%).[68] Alcuronium occasionally causes a moderate increase in heart rate due to vagolysis.[7,68,71] It is twice as potent[69,72,73] as tubocurarine and has a slightly shorter duration of action.[74] It depends on the *kidney* for 60–90% of its *elimination,* and its duration may be prolonged in the elderly.[75]

◆ PIPECURONIUM

Pipecuronium bromide (Arduan), an analogue of pancuronium, is approximately 20% more potent than pancuronium (ED_{95} between 0.04 and 0.05 mg · kg^{-1}).[76] Its *duration* has been reported to range from slightly shorter to 210% longer than pancuronium's duration.[77-85] Although the volume of distribution for pipecuronium is greater, its clearance is also greater and hence its $t_{1/2elim}$ is similar (1.4 mL · kg^{-1} · min^{-1} with a $t_{1/2elim}$ of 115 minutes for pancuronium, 2.5 mL · kg^{-1} · min^{-1} with a $t_{1/2elim}$ of 137 minutes for pipecuronium).[80] The effect of increasing the dose of pipecuronium on its time course is similar to that of other long-acting agents.[83]

Pipecuronium's main advantage is that it is virtually *devoid of cardiovascular effects*. It lacks the autonomic effects of pancuronium[82,83,86-89] and does not elicit histamine release.[90] Doses 1–3 times the ED_{95} caused no significant changes in heart rate or blood pressure in patients undergoing coronary artery bypass grafting,[87,88] although mild bradycardia has been reported.[91]

Like pancuronium, pipecuronium's *clearance* is highly dependent on the *kidney*.[83,85,92-95] More than 75% is excreted unchanged in the urine.[92] Its clearance is decreased by 33% (and its $t_{1/2elim}$ doubled to 263 minutes) in *renal failure*,[92] and there is a wide range of durations in patients with renal failure.[92] The duration of action of pipecuronium was not significantly prolonged in *elderly patients* with normal renal function.[96] The liver may participate to a limited degree in the elimination of pipecuronium[93,94]; infusion requirements were markedly decreased after clamping the hepatic vessels of pigs.[93] Among pipecuronium's metabolites is a *3-deacetyl derivative* that has 40–50% the potency of the parent drug. Pipecuronium is approximately 32% bound to plasma protein.

As for other NDRs, a given mg · kg^{-1} dose of pipecuronium exerts a greater effect in adults and infants than in children (i.e., the ED_{95} is highest in children aged 2–10 years).[97-99] Its ED_{95} is reduced in the presence of enflurane and isoflurane.[85,100] In respect to reversibility with anticholinesterases and the effects of inhalational agents on recovery, pipecuronium is comparable to other long-acting relaxants.[83,101,102] Edrophonium is relatively ineffective against pipecuronium-induced block[85,101] even when considerable recovery has taken place.[101]

Lyophilized pipecuronium can be dissolved in a variety of solvents. After reconstitution with bacteriostatic water, it can remain stable for 5 days under refrigeration (2–8 °C) or at room temperature (<30 °C). After reconstitution with 0.9% NaCl, 5% glucose in water, lactated Ringer's solution, it can be stored for 24 hours under refrigeration.[103]

◆ DOXACURIUM

Doxacurium chloride (Nuromax) is a long-acting, potent benzylisoquinolinium compound; it has a high potency (2–3 times that of pancuronium), with an ED_{95} in adults between 0.015 and 0.035 mg · kg^{-1}.[104-114] Like pipecuronium, it was introduced to provide relaxation for long procedures without the autonomic effects that accompany pancuronium. At doses of 0.025, 0.05, and 0.08 mg · kg^{-1} (approximately 1, 2, and 3 × ED_{95}), its clinically effective block times (Dur_{25}) averaged 55–60, 100–107, and 160 minutes respectively.[104,106]

Recovery after doxacurium tends to be slower than after pancuronium.[104,108,113] Doxacurium is largely *cleared unchanged primarily in the urine* and to a lesser degree in the bile.[115,116] In contrast to pancuronium's and pipecuronium's metabolism to an active metabolite, doxacurium is not metabolized. Although there is wide interpatient variation with respect to doxacurium's time course,[109,111] the time course appears to remain consistent for any given patient.[104] Doxacurium's clearance typically decreases by 50% and its $t_{1/2elim}$ doubles in severe *renal disease*.[104,115,117] Whereas the normal $t_{1/2elim}$ after an ED_{95} dose is 99 minutes, it is markedly increased to 221 minutes in renal failure[115] and slightly increased to 115 minutes in hepatic failure[115]; the Dur_{25} increased by 120% and 40%, respectively.[115] Doxacurium's duration may be increased in the *elderly*, but its kinetics (e.g., $t_{1/2elim}$) typically are not changed markedly in the elderly patient with adequate renal function.[113,118] Its $t_{1/2elim}$ increased from 86 minutes to 96 minutes[118] and its ED_{95} was also essentially unchanged in elderly patients.[118,119]

Doses of doxacurium within the typical clinical range are essentially devoid of *cardiovascular effects*.[104,108,110,114,115,120-124] It lacks significant autonomic effects. Its high potency allows it to be used in doses that do not elicit significant *histamine release*; it typically does not release significant histamine unless a dose more than 3 times the ED_{95} is administered as a rapid bolus injection.[104] Rapid bolus injection of 0.03, 0.04, 0.05, and 0.08 mg · kg^{-1} resulted in histamine levels that were 119% ± 21%, 120% ± 18%, 90% ± 19%, and 107% ± 19% of baseline.[104] In a recent comparison of bolus dosing in patients undergoing coronary artery bypass surgery, pancuronium produced small but significant increases in blood pressure, heart rate, and cardiac index; vecuronium was associated with slight bradycardia; and doxacurium caused the fewest changes.[120] A case of flushing and hypotension has been reported after rapid bolus injection of 0.05 mg · kg^{-1} (1.7 × ED_{95}).[125] A dose of 0.04 mg · kg^{-1} was associated with a 5 mm Hg decline in mean arterial pressure over a 5-minute postinjection period, but this had no clinical significance.[110] In patients with *cardiac disease*, doxacurium was associated with occasional hypotension which the authors did not feel were attributable to histamine release (as the changes did not have the acute time course)[122]; overall, changes were small and not considered clinically significant.[122] The likelihood of histamine release can be decreased even further by slow injection or divided dosing (Chap. 11). In high doses (e.g., 3 × ED_{95}), doxacurium may be associated with a decrease in heart rate[120,126,127] similar to (but slightly less pronounced than) that noted with vecuronium.

The ED_{95} of doxacurium is slightly greater in *children* (0.027–0.032 mg · kg^{-1}), and its onset is faster.[128,129] Bolus doses of 0.028 and 0.05 mg · kg^{-1} in children were not associated with significant changes in blood pressure or heart rate, and no cases of cutaneous flushing were observed.[128,129] The ED_{95} of doxacurium is decreased in the presence of inhalational anesthetics.[106,111] As for other NDRs, its block is reversible with anticholinesterases; antagonism of deep block may be slow and incomplete.[104,108–110,114,119]

Discussion Questions ◆

a. After complete atropinization, does pancuronium cause further cardiovascular alteration?

b. Although it is a benzylisoquinolonium compound, doxacurium typically does not elicit significant histamine release. Why?

Answers ◆

a. After atropine, *pancuronium* still may result in further cardiovascular stimulation.[43] It may stimulate *adrenergic activity*, by causing increased release of catecholamines and blocking norepinephrine reuptake.[39,40,44,46,130]

b. In clinical doses, we typically do not see *histamine release after doxacurium* because of the drug's relatively high "safety" ratio. It is very potent, and thus relatively few molecules are required to achieve a desired effect. After routine clinical doses, peak plasma levels of drug are below those that typically elicit significant histamine release.

References ◆

1. Griffith HR, Johnson GE: The use of curare in general anesthesia. Anesthesiology 3:412–420, 1942
2. Everett AJ, Lowe LA, Wilkinson S: Revision of structure of (+)− tubocurarine chloride and chondracurine. J Chem Soc (Chem Commun) 1:1020–1021, 1970
3. Bowman WC: Prejunctional and postjunctional cholinoceptors at the neuromuscular junction. Anesth Analg 59:935–943, 1980
4. Gibson FM, Mirakhur RK: Train-of-four fade during onset of neuromuscular block with nondepolarising neuromuscular blocking agents. Acta Anaesthesiol Scand 33:204–206, 1989

5. Galindo A: The role of pre-junctional effects in myoneural transmission. Anesthesiology 36:598–608, 1972
6. Burstein CL, Jackson A, Bishop HF, Rovenstine EA: Curare in the management of autonomic reflexes. Anesthesiology 11:409, 1950
7. Harrison GA: The cardiovascular effects and some relaxant properties of four relaxants in patients about to undergo cardiac surgery. Br J Anaesth 44:485–494, 1972
8. Hughes R, Chapple DJ: Effect of non-depolarizing neuromuscular blocking agents on peripheral autonomic mechanisms in cats. Br J Anaesth 48:59–68, 1976
9. Longnecker DE, Stoelting RK, Morrow AG: Cardiac and peripheral vascular effects of d-tubocurarine in man. Anesth Analg 49:660, 1970
10. McDowell SA, Clarke RSJ: A clinical comparison of pancuronium with d-tubocurarine. Anaesthesia 24:581–590, 1969
11. Marshall RJ, Ojewole JAO: Comparison of the autonomic effects of some currently-used neuromuscular blocking agents. Br J Pharmacol 66:77P, 1979
12. Savarese JJ: The autonomic margin of safety of metocurine and d-tubocurarine in the cat. Anesthesiology 5:40–46, 1979
13. Stoelting RK: Hemodynamic effects of dimethyltubocurarine during nitrous oxide–halothane anesthesia. Anesth Analg 53:513–515, 1974
14. Stoelting RK: The hemodynamic effects of pancuronium and d-tubocurarine in anesthetized patients. Anesthesiology 36:612–615, 1972
15. Basta SJ, Savarese JJ, Ali HH, Moss J, Gionfriddo M: Histamine-releasing properties of atracurium, dimethyl tubocurarine and tubocurarine. Br J Anaesth 55:105S–106S, 1983
16. Lavery GG, Clarke RSJ, Watkins J: Histaminoid response after intradermal and intravenous administration of atracurium, vecuronium and tubocurarine: a comparative study. Eur J Anaesthesiol 3:439–447, 1986
17. Moss J, Roscow CE, Savarese JJ, et al: Role of histamine in the hypotensive action of d-tubocurarine in humans. Anesthesiology 55:19–25, 1981
18. Guyton AC, Reeder RC: Quantitative studies on autonomic actions of curare. J Pharmacol Exp Ther 98:188–193, 1950
19. Cohen EN, Corbascio A, Fleischli G: The distribution and fate of d-tubocurarine. J Pharmacol Exp Ther 147:120–129, 1965
20. Miller RD, Matteo RS, Benet LZ, et al: The pharmacokinetics of d-tubocurarine in man with and without renal failure. J Pharmacol Exp Ther 202:1–7, 1977
21. Matteo RS, Backus WW, McDaniel DD, Brotherton WP, Abraham R, Diaz J: Pharmacokinetics and pharmacodynamics of d-tubocurarine and metocurine in the elderly. Anesth Analg 64:23–29, 1985
22. Matteo RS, Brotherton WP, Nishitateno K, et al: Pharmacokinetics and pharmacodynamics of metocurine in humans: comparison to d-tubocurarine. Anesthesiology 57:183–190, 1982
23. McCullogh LS, Stone WA, Delaunis AL, et al: The effects of dimethyltubocurarine iodide on cardiovascular parameters, postganglionic sympathetic activity and histamine release. Anesth Analg 51:554–559, 1972
24. Savarese JJ, Ali HH, Antonio RP: The clinical pharmacology of metocurine: dimethyltubocurarine revisited. Anesthesiology 47:277–84, 1977
25. Durant NN, Bowman WC, Marshall LG: A comparison of neuromuscular and autonomic blocking activities of (+)-tubocurarine and its O, O, N-trimethyl analogues. Eur J Pharmacol 46:297–302, 1977
26. Meijer DKF, Weitering JG, Vermeer GA, et al: Comparative pharmacokinetics of d-tubocurarine and metocurine in man. Anesthesiology 51:402, 1979
27. Brotherton WP, Matteo RS: Pharmacokinetics and pharmacodynamics of metocurine in humans with and without renal failure. Anesthesiology 55:273, 1981
28. Eisele JH, Marta JA, Davis HS: Quantitative aspects of the chronotropic and neuromuscular effects of gallamine in anesthetized men. Anesthesiology 35:630–633, 1971
29. Lee Son S, Waud DR: Effects of non-depolarizing neuromuscular blocking agents on the cardiac vagus nerve in the guinea pig. Br J Anaesth 52:981, 1980
30. Riker WF, Wescoe WC: The pharmacology of flaxedil with observations on certain analogs. Ann NY Acad Sci 54:373, 1951

31. Stoelting RK: Hemodynamic effects of gallamine during halothane–nitrous oxide anesthesia. Anesthesiology 39:645–647, 1973
32. Brown BR, Crout JR: The sympathomimetic effect of gallamine on the heart. J Pharmacol Exp Ther 172:266, 1970
33. Kingsley BP, Vaughan MS, Vaughan RW: Cardiovascular effects of nondepolarizing relaxants employed for pretreatment prior to succinylcholine. Can Anaesth Soc J 31:13–19, 1984
34. Kopman AF: Pancuronium, gallamine, and d-tubocurarine compared: is speed of onset inversely related to drug potency? Anesthesiology 70:915–920, 1989
35. Agoston S, Vermeer GA, Kersten UW, et al: A preliminary investigation of the renal and hepatic excretion of gallamine triethiodide in man. Br J Anaesth 50:345, 1978
36. Churchill-Davidson HC, Way WL, de Jong RH: The muscle relaxants and renal excretion. Anesthesiology 28:540–546, 1967
37. Ramzan MI, Shanks CA, Triggs EJ: Gallamine disposition in surgical patients with chronic renal failure. Br J Clin Pharmacol 12:141, 1981
38. Buckett WR, Hewitt CL, Savage DS: Pancuronium bromide and other steroidal neuromuscular blocking agents containing acetylcholine fragments. J Med Chem 16:1116, 1973
39. Docherty JR, McGrath JC: Sympathomimetic effects of pancuronium bromide on the cardiovascular system of the pithed rat: a comparison with the effects of drugs blocking the neuronal uptake of noradrenaline. Br J Pharmacol 64:589–599, 1978
40. Ivankovich AD, Miletich DJ, Albrecht RF, Zahed B: The effect of pancuronium on myocardial contraction and catecholamine metabolism. J Pharm Pharmacol 27:837, 1975
41. Janik R, Dick W: Sufentanil: the effect on cardiocirculatory parameters and intubation conditions of administration of pancuronium or vecuronium. Anaesthesist 38:673–680, 1989
42. Kelman GR, Kennedy BR: Cardiovascular effects of pancuronium in man. Br J Anaesth 43:335–338, 1971
43. Miller RD, Eger EI II, Stevens WC, Gibbons R: Pancuronium induced tachycardia in relation to alveolar halothane, dose of pancuronium, and prior atropine. Anesthesiology 42:352, 1975
44. Salt PJ, Barnes PK, Conway CM: Inhibition of neuronal uptake of noradrenaline in the isolated perfused rat heart by pancuronium and its homologues, Org 6358, Org 7268 and Org NC45. Br J Anaesth 52:313, 1980
45. Saxena PR, Bonta IL: Mechanism of selective cardiac vagolytic action of pancuronium bromide: specific blockade of cardiac muscarinic receptors. Eur J Pharmacol 11:332–341, 1970
46. Segarra Domenech J, Carlos Garcia R, Rodriquez Sasiain JM, et al: Pancuronium bromide: an indirect sympathomimetic agent. Br J Anaesth 48:1143–1148, 1976
47. Edwards RP, Miller RD, Roizen MF, et al: Cardiac responses to imipramine and pancuronium during anesthesia with halothane or enflurane. Anesthesiology 50:421–425, 1979
48. Gilbert M, Anderson EA, Brondbo A, Bjertnaes LJ: Muscle relaxants change myocardial metabolism in patients with ischaemic heart disease during high-dose fentanyl anaesthesia. Acta Anaesthesiol Scand 34:47–54, 1990
49. Thomson IR, Putnins CL: Adverse effects of pancuronium during high-dose fentanyl anesthesia for coronary artery bypass grafting. Anesthesiology 62:708–713, 1985
50. Katz RL: Clinical neuromuscular pharmacology of pancuronium. Anesthesiology 34:550–556, 1971
51. Agoston S, Vermeer GA, Kersten UW, et al: The fate of pancuronium bromide in man. Acta Anaesthesiol Scand 17:267, 1973
52. Duvaldestin P, Demetriou M, D'Hollander A: Pharmacokinetics of pancuronium in man: a linear system. Eur J Clin Pharmacol 23:L369, 1982
53. Westra P, Vermeer GA, de Lange AR, Scaf AHJ, Meijer DKF, Wesseling H: Hepatic and renal disposition of pancuronium and gallamine in patients with extra hepatic cholestasis. Br J Anaesth 53:331, 1981
54. Somogyi AA, Shanks CA, Triggs EJ: The effect of renal failure on the disposition and neuromuscular blocking action of pancuronium bromide. Eur J Clin Pharmacol 12:23–29, 1977

55. McLeod K, Watson MJ, Rawlins MD: Pharmacokinetics of pancuronium in patients with normal and impaired renal function. Br J Anaesth 48:341, 1976
56. Miller RD, Stevens WC, Way WL: The effect of renal failure and hyperkalemia on the duration of pancuronium neuromuscular blockade in man. Anesth Analg 52:661–666, 1972
57. Buzello W, Agoston S: Pharmacokinetics of pancuronium in patients with normal and impaired renal function. Anaesthesist 27:291, 1978
58. Berntman L, Rosberg B, Shweikh I, Yousef H: Atracurium and pancuronium in renal insufficiency. Acta Anaesthesiol Scand 33:48, 1989
59. Gramstad L: Atracurium, vecuronium and pancuronium in end-stage renal failure: dose-response properties and interactions with azathioprine. Br J Anaesth 59:995–1003, 1987
60. McLeod K, Hull J, Watson MJ: Effects of ageing on the pharmacokinetics of pancuronium. Br J Anaesth 51:435–438, 1979
61. Duvaldestin P, Saada J, Berger JL, D'Hollander AA, Desmonts JM: Pharmacokinetics, pharmacodynamics, and dose-response relationships of pancuronium in control and elderly subjects. Anesthesiology 56:36–40, 1982
62. Lowry KG, Mirakhur RK, Lavery GG, Clarke RSJ: Vecuronium and atracurium in the elderly: a clinical comparison with pancuronium. Acta Anaesthesiol Scand 29:405–408, 1985
63. Rupp SM, Castagnoli KD, Fisher DM, Miller RD: Pancuronium and vecuronium pharmacokinetics and pharmacodynamics in younger and elderly patients. Anesthesiology 67:45–49, 1987
64. Bell PF, Mirakhur RK, Clarke RSJ: Dose-response studies of atracurium, vecuronium and pancuronium in the elderly. Anaesthesia 44:925–927, 1989
65. Somogyi AA, Shanks CA, Triggs EJ: Disposition kinetics of pancuronium bromide in patients with total biliary obstruction. Br J Anaesth 49:1103, 1977
66. Ward S, Judge S, Corall I: Pharmacokinetics of pancuronium bromide in liver failure. Br J Anaesth 54:227P, 1982
67. Duvaldestin P, Agoston S, Henzel D, Kersten UW, Desmonts JM: Pancuronium pharmacokinetics in patients with liver cirrhosis. Br J Anaesth 50:1131–1135, 1978
68. Beemer GH, Dennis WL, Platt PR, Bjorksten AR, Carr AB: Adverse reactions to atracurium and alcuronium. Br J Anaesth 1:680–684, 1988
69. Hunter AR: Diallyltoxiferine. Br J Anaesth 36:466, 1964
70. Tammisto T, Welling I: The effect of alcuronium and tubocurarine on blood pressure and heart rate: a clinical comparison. Br J Anaesth 41:317, 1979
71. Kennedy BR, Kelman GR: Cardiovascular effects of alcuronium in man. Br J Anaesth 42:625, 1970
72. Krieg N, Crul JF, Booij LHDJ: Relative potency of ORG NC45, pancuronium, alcuronium and tubocurarine in anaesthetized man. Br J Anaesth 52:783–788, 1980
73. Foldes FF, Brown IM, Lunn JN, et al: The neuromuscular effects of diallylnortoxiferine in anesthetized subjects. Anesthesiology 42:117, 1963
74. Walker JS, Shanks CA, Triggs EJ: Clinical pharmacokinetics of alcuronium chloride in man. Eur J Clin Pharmacol 17:449–457, 1980
75. Stephens ID, Ho PC, Holloway AM, Bourne DWA, Triggs EJ: Pharmacokinetics of alcuronium in elderly patients undergoing total hip replacement or aortic reconstructive surgery. Br J Anaesth 56:465, 1984
76. Stanley JC, Mirakhur RK: Comparative potency of pipecuronium bromide and pancuronium bromide. Br J Anaesth 63:754–755, 1989
77. Azad S, Goldberg ME, Larijani GE, et al: A dose-response evaluation of pipecuronium bromide in elderly patients under balanced anesthesia. J Clin Pharmacol 29:657–659, 1989
78. Agoston S, Richardson FJ: Pipecuronium bromide (Arduan)--a new long-acting non-depolarizing neuromuscular blocking drug. Clin Anesthesiol 3:361–369, 1985
79. Boros M, Szenohradszky J, Kertiesz A, Morosi G, Tutsek L: Clinical experiences with pipecuronium bromide. Acta Chir Hung 24:207–214, 1983
80. Caldwell JE, Castagnoli KP, Canfell PC, Fahey MR, Lynam DP, Fisher DM, Miller RD: Pipecuronium and pancuronium: comparison of pharmacokinetics and duration of action. Br J Anaesth 61:693–697, 1988
81. Tassonyi E, Pittet J-F, Schopfer C, Gemperle G, Rouge JC, Morel DR: Pharmacokinetics of pipecuronium in infants, children and adults. Anesthesiology 75:A777, 1991

82. Foldes FF, Nagashima H, Nguyen HD, Duncalf D, Goldiner PL: Neuromuscular and cardiovascular effects of pipecuronium. Can J Anaesth 37:549–555, 1990
83. Larijani GE, Bartkowski RR, Azad SS, Seltzer JL, Weinberger MJ, Beach CA, Goldberg ME: Clinical pharmacology of pipecuronium bromide. Anesth Analg 68:734–739, 1989
84. Stanley JC, Mirakhur RK, Bell PF, Sharpe TDE, Clarke RSJ: Neuromuscular effects of pipecuronium bromide. Eur J Anaesthesiol 8:151–156, 1991
85. Wierda JMKH, Richardson FJ, Agoston S: Dose-response relation and time course of action of pipecuronium bromide in humans anesthetized with nitrous oxide and isoflurane, halothane, or droperidol and fentanyl. Anesth Analg 68:208–213, 1989
86. Deam RK, Soni N: Effects of pipecuronium and pancuronium on the isolated rabbit heart. Br J Anaesth 62:287–289, 1989
87. Stanley JC, Carson IW, Gibson FM, McMurray TJ, Elliott P, Lyons SM, Mirakhur RK: Comparison of the haemodynamic effects of pipecuronium and pancuronium during fentanyl anaesthesia. Acta Anaesthesiol Scand 35:262–266, 1991
88. Tassonyi E, Neidhart P, Pittet JF, Morel DR, Gemperle M: Cardiovascular effects of pipecuronium and pancuronium in patients undergoing coronary artery bypass grafting. Anesthesiology 69:793–796, 1988
89. Wierda JMKH, Karuczek GF, Vandenbroom RHG, Pinto I, Kersten-Kleef UW, Meijer DKF, Agoston S: Pharmacokinetics and cardiovascular dynamics of pipecuronium bromide during coronary artery surgery. Can J Anaesth 37:183–191, 1990
90. Naguib M, Abdulatif M, Absood A: Comparative effects of pipecuronium and tubocurarine and plasma concentrations of histamine in humans. Br J Anaesth 67:320–322, 1991
91. Dubois R, Fleming NW, Lee E: Effects of succinylcholine on the pharmacodynamics of pipecuronium and pancuronium. Anesth Analg 72:364–368, 1991
92. Caldwell JE, Canfell PC, Castagnoli KP, Lynam DP, Fahey MR, Fisher DM, Miller RD: The influence of renal failure on the pharmacokinetics and duration of action of pipecuronium bromide in patients anesthetized with halothane and nitrous oxide. Anesthesiology 70:7–12, 1989
93. Pittet JF, Tassonyi E, Schopfer C, Morel DR, Leemann P, Mentha G, LeCoultre C, Steinig DA, Benakis A: Dose requirements and plasma concentrations of pipecuronium during bilateral renal exclusion and orthotopic liver transplantation in pigs. Br J Anaesth 65:779–785, 1990
94. Khuenl-Brady KS, Sharma M, Chung K, Miller RD, Agoston S, Caldwell JE: Pharmacokinetics and disposition of pipecuronium bromide in dogs with and without ligated renal pedicles. Anesthesiology 71:919–922, 1989
95. Wierda JMKH, Szenohradszky J, DeWit APM, et al: Pharmacokinetics, urinary and biliary excretion of pipecuronium bromide. Eur J Anaesthesiol 8:451, 1991
96. Ornstein E, Matteo RS, Schwartz AE, Jamdar SC, Diaz J: Pharmacokinetics and pharmacodynamics of pipecuronium bromide (Arduan) in elderly surgical patients. Anesth Analg 74:841–844, 1992
97. Pittet JF, Tassonyi E, Morel DR, Gemperle G, Rouge JC: Neuromuscular effect of pipecuronium bromide in infants and children during nitrous oxide–alfentanil anesthesia. Anesthesiology 72:432–435, 1990
98. Pittet JF, Tassonyi E, Morel DR, et al: Pipecuronium-induced neuromuscular blockade during nitrous oxide–fentanyl, isoflurane, and halothane anesthesia in adults and children. Anesthesiology 71:210–213, 1989
99. Sarner JB, Brandom BW, Dong ML, Pickle D, Cook DR, Weinberger MJ: Clinical pharmacology of pipecuronium in infants and children during halothane anesthesia. Anesth Analg 71:362–366, 1990
100. Nguyen HD, Goldiner PL, Rabinowitz A, Nagashima H, Foldes FF: The neuromuscular effects of pipecuronium under enflurane anesthesia. Anesth Analg 66:S128, 1987
101. Abdulatif M, Naguib M: Neostigmine and edrophonium for reversal of pipecuronium neuromuscular blockade. Can J Anaesth 38:159–163, 1991
102. Meistelman C, Plaud B, Lira E, Donati F: Effects of the concentration of isoflurane on the recovery of pipecuronium neuromuscular blockade following neostigmine administration. Anesthesiology 73:A886, 1990
103. Organon Inc.: Product insert—ARDUAN (pipecuronium bromide). West Orange, NJ, 1990

104. Basta SJ, Savarese JJ, Ali HH, Embree PB, Schwartz AF, Rudd GD, Wastila WB: Clinical pharmacology of doxacurium chloride (BW A938U): a new long-acting nondepolarizing muscle relaxant. Anesthesiology 69:478–486, 1988
105. Faulds D, Clissold SP: Doxacurium: a review of its pharmacology and clinical potential in anaesthesia. Drugs 42:673–689, 1991
106. Katz JA, Fragen RJ, Shanks CA, Dunn K, McNulty B, Rudd GD: Dose-response relationships of doxacurium chloride in humans during anesthesia with nitrous oxide and fentanyl, enflurane, isoflurane, or halothane. Anesthesiology 70:432–436, 1989
107. Lynam DP, Caldwell JE, Miller RD: Isoflurane, halothane and narcotic anesthetic dose-response for BW A938U. Anesthesiology 67:A362, 1987
108. Lennon RL, Hosking MP, Houck PC, Rose SH, Wedel DJ, Gibson BE, Ascher JA, Rudd GD: Doxacurium chloride for neuromuscular blockade before tracheal intubation and surgery during nitrous oxide-oxygen-narcotic-enflurane anesthesia. Anesth Analg 68:255–260, 1989
109. Maddineni VR, Cooper R, Stanley JC, Mirakhur RK, Clarke RSJ: Clinical evaluation of doxacurium chloride. Anaesthesia 47:554–557, 1992
110. Murray DJ, Mehta MP, Choi WW, Forbes RB, Sokoll MD, Gergis SD, Rudd GD, Abou-Donia MM: The neuromuscular blocking and cardiovascular effects of doxacurium chloride in patients receiving nitrous oxide narcotic anesthesia. Anesthesiology 69:472–477, 1988
111. Murray DJ, Sokoll MD, Choi WW, Mehta MP, Forbes RB, Gergis SD: The neuromuscular blocking effect of doxacurium chloride during isoflurane anaesthesia. Eur J Anaesthesiol 7:395–402, 1990
112. Mehta MP, Murray D, Forbes R, Choi W, Gergis S, Sokoll M, Abou-Donia M, Rudd G: The neuromuscular pharmacology of BW A938U in anesthetized patients. Anesthesiology 65:A280, 1986
113. Savarese JJ, Wastila WB, Rudd GD, Welch RE, Samara B: Pharmacodynamics and pharmacokinetics of doxacurium chloride (BW A938U): background and overview. J Cardiothorac Anaesthesiol 4:14–19, 1990
114. Scott RPF, Norman J: Doxacurium chloride: a preliminary clinical trial. Br J Anaesth 62:373–377, 1989
115. Cook DR, Freeman JA, Lai AA, Robertson KA, Kang Y, Stiller RL, Aggarwal S, Abou-Donia MM, Welch RM: Pharmacokinetics and pharmacodynamics of doxacurium in normal patients and in those with hepatic or renal failure. Anesth Analg 72:145–150, 1991
116. Savarese JJ, Wastila WB: Current research in relaxant development. Semin Anaesth 5:304–311, 1986
117. Cashman JN, Luke JJ, Jones RM: Neuromuscular block with doxacurium (BW A938U) in patients with normal or absent renal function. Br J Anaesth 64:186–192, 1990
118. Dresner DL, Basta SJL, Ali HH, Schwartz AF, Embree PB, Wargin WA, Lai A, Brady KA, Savarese JJ: Pharmacokinetics and pharmacodynamics of doxacurium in young and elderly patients during isoflurane anesthesia. Anesth Analg 71:498–502, 1990
119. Koscielniak-Nielsen ZJ, Law-Min JC, Donati F, Bevan DR, Clement P, Wise R: Dose-response relations of doxacurium and its reversal with neostigmine in young adults and healthy elderly patients. Anesth Analg 74:845–850, 1992
120. Emmott RS, Bracey BJ, Goldhill DR, Yate PM, Flynn PJ: Cardiovascular effects of doxacurium, pancuronium and vecuronium in anaesthetized patients presenting for coronary artery bypass surgery. Br J Anaesth 65:480–486, 1990
121. Forbes RB, Murray DJ: Review of the hemodynamic profile of doxacurium chloride in healthy patients. J Cardiothorac Anaesthesiol 4:24–27, 1990
122. Reich DL, Konstadt SN, Thys DM, Hillel Z, Raymond R, Kaplan JA: Effects of doxacurium chloride on biventricular cardiac function in patients with cardiac disease. Br J Anaesth 63:675–681, 1989
123. Reich DL, Thys DM, Guffin AV, Kaplan JA: The hemodynamic effects of doxacurium during abdominal aortic surgery. J Cardiothorac Anaesthesiol 4:28–30, 1990
124. Stoops CM, Curtis CA, Kovach DA, et al: Hemodynamic effects of doxacurium chloride in patients receiving oxygen sufentanil anesthesia for coronary artery bypass grafting or valve replacement. Anesthesiology 69:365–370, 1988

125. Reich DL: Transient systemic arterial hypotension and cutaneous flushing in response to doxacurium chloride. Anesthesiology 71:783–785, 1989
126. Ensalada LM, Clark SK, Goldberg ME, McNulty SE, Lessin J, Seltzer JL, Raymond RN, Wise NM, Rudd GD: An evaluation of the hemodynamic effects of doxacurium during aortic valve replacement surgery for aortic stenosis in patients receiving oxygen fentanyl anesthesia. Anesthesiology 69:A886, 1988
127. Gosgnach ML, Coriat P, Le Bret F, Ammeur MB, Godet G, Samama M, Viars P: Doxacurium (BW 938) versus pancuronium in patients undergoing abdominal aortic surgery: effects on hemodynamics and LV function. Anesthesiology 69:A837, 1988
128. Goudsouzian NG, Alifimoff JK, Liu LMP, Foster V, McNulty B, Savarese JJ: Neuromuscular and cardiovascular effects of doxacurium in children anesthetized with halothane. Br J Anaesth 62:263–268, 1989
129. Sarner JB, Brandom BW, Cook DR, Dong ML, Horn MC, Woelfel SK, Davis PJ, Rudd D, Foster VJ, McNulty BF: Clinical pharmacology of doxacurium chloride (BW A938U) in children. Anesth Analg 67:303–306, 1988
130. Nana A, Cardan E, Domokos M: Blood catecholamine changes after pancuronium. Acta Anaesthesiol Scand 17:83–87, 1973

13

DAVID G. SILVERMAN | RAJINDER K. MIRAKHUR

Intermediate-Acting Relaxants of the 1980s

The 1980s witnessed the introduction of atracurium and vecuronium, the first nondepolarizing relaxants (NDRs) of "intermediate duration." These drugs have expanded the use of NDRs for relatively short procedures, allowed the use of higher doses of relaxant to accelerate the onset of block, and have facilitated NDR titration by continuous infusion and intermittent bolus administration. The Dur_{25} (time until twitch response recovers to 25% of baseline height), RI_{25-75} (recovery index, the interval between time to 25% recovery and time to 75% recovery of twitch height), and the Dur_{95} after an ED_{95} dose of atracurium or vecuronium average approximately 25, 13, and 50 minutes; these times are approximately 40–60% of those for the long-acting agents (see Table 12-1).

◆ ATRACURIUM

Atracurium besylate (Tracrium) is a bisquaternary benzylisoquinolinium compound with an ED_{95} of 0.20–0.25 mg · kg^{-1} and an RI_{25-75} of 13–15 minutes; after 2 times its ED_{95}, pronounced twitch depression typically is attained in 2.3–4 minutes.[1-9] Atracurium's major advantage is its *relatively rapid metabolism*[1,2,9-15]: its $t_{1/2elim}$ is as brief as 21 minutes.[10,11] Clearance of atracurium occurs in the peripheral as well as central compartments and is relatively independent of organ elimination (and the factors that compromise organ elimination).[5,12] Less than 10% is excreted by the kidney.[16]

The *rapid metabolism* of atracurium is in contrast to the slower metabolism of long-acting agents and of vecuronium or rocuronium, which are highly dependent on redistribution. Atracurium manifests little accumulation[2,8,11,17-20]; its $t_{1/2elim}$[11] and RI_{25-75}[1] are virtually unchanged by large doses. Atracurium's *duration is also less affected* by inhalational anesthesia,[21] obesity,[22] phenytoin,[23] old age,[24] renal failure,[11,13,16,25-28] or liver failure.[15,22,28,29] However, changes have been noted: as examples, atracurium's clearance and $t_{1/2elim}$ may be compromised in the elderly[30,31] and occasionally by organ failure.[32] Its spontaneous degradation is accelerated by alkalosis[5,11] and by hyperthermia.[33]

In adults, the mean *infusion rate* during nitrous oxide–narcotic anesthesia to maintain twitch response at 5% of baseline is 6.0–8.0 µg · kg^{-1} · min^{-1} (0.36–0.48 mg · kg^{-1} · hr^{-1}).[34,35] After the infusion is stopped, the RI$_{25-75}$ usually is 10–12 minutes and the Dur$_{95}$ is 25–30 minutes. As for other NDRs, infusion requirements vary among patients, and the relaxant should be titrated to effect.

As for other NDRs (Chap. 10), the bolus[36,37] and infusion[38,39] dose requirements for atracurium are increased in the 2- to 10-year-old *pediatric population*, and recovery is faster in these children than in adults.[36–40] In children, the mean infusion rates to achieve 90–99% twitch depression were 8.3–8.8 µg · kg^{-1} · min^{-1} during halothane anesthesia[38,39] and 9.3 µg · kg^{-1} · min^{-1} during nitrous oxide–narcotic anesthesia.[38] Atracurium's µg · kg^{-1} · min^{-1} requirements remain relatively constant for infants weighing more than 5 kg.[36,39] Infants, especially smaller neonates[40] and those less than 3 months old,[41] require less atracurium to produce a given degree of block than do older children.[40–43] During infusion in infants less than 1 month old, 25% less was required.[39] In contrast to NDRs that are wholly dependent on organ elimination, the duration of action of atracurium is not markedly prolonged in neonates.[40,42] The RI$_{25-75}$ may be longer in neonates,[43] but it nevertheless has been concluded that "prompt recovery can be expected in all healthy pediatric patients following a standard intubating dose of atracurium 0.5 mg · kg^{-1}."[40]

Atracurium is essentially two molecules of *laudanosine* connected by an *acrylate bridge*. It is metabolized by a variety of means, including (1) *organ elimination*, particularly hepatic[12,44]; (2) *ester hydrolysis* to a quaternary acid and a quaternary alcohol by nonspecific esterases (which may be compromised by a carboxylesterase inhibitor)[45]; (3) spontaneous *Hofmann elimination* (approximately one third) to laudanosine and a quaternary monoacrylate[10,12,19,46,47]; and (4) an alternative route of non-enzyme-catalyzed degradation that may entail nucleophilic substitution.[48,49]

There is in vitro evidence to suggest that, in very high concentrations, *atracurium's metabolites as a result of Hofmann elimination* (e.g., *acrylates*) may disturb the *cellular membranes* of skin and hepatocytes.[50–54] However, this has not been substantiated in other studies.[55,56] The acrylate concentrations generated in routine clinical practice are below those implicated in laboratory studies,[46,55,57] especially in light of the relatively large amount of atracurium that undergoes more "routine" organ elimination and ester hydrolysis to nonacrylate metabolites. The acrylates typically are scavenged effectively by conjugation to glutathione.[58] The highest plasma concentration achieved after 0.6 mg · kg^{-1} was 10 µM[57]; in the laboratory, drug-induced leakage was not seen until concentrations above 30 µM were reached.[55] It has also been suggested that the acrylate metabolites may have the potential to induce allergic side effects,[51] but this has not been confirmed after atracurium. Other studies have documented atracurium's lack of toxicity in various animal models. In clinical doses, neither atracurium, d-tubocurarine, pancuronium, nor vecuronium caused developmental toxicity during organogenesis.[59] Administration on days 6–18 of pregnancy caused no adverse effects in pregnant rabbits or their fetuses.[60] After long-term administration of atracurium to rats, dogs, or monkeys,[60] no hematological, clinical chemistry, or histopathological changes were noted.

Laudanosine, atracurium's primary metabolite via Hofmann elimination, is a potential *cerebral stimulant*.[61–65] A tertiary isoquinoline alkaloid, laudanosine is capable of crossing the blood-brain barrier.[62] Laudanosine increases the anesthetic requirements for halothane in rabbits,[65] but the sensitivity of rabbits is not shared by all species. In patients receiving an atracurium infusion during thiopental–nitrous oxide–fentanyl anesthesia, the plasma level of thiopental at the time of awakening was 20% higher (this difference was judged to be "too modest to be of clinical significance").[66] Progressive changes noted in *response to laudanosine infusions* in dogs were an increased frequency and amplitude on the electroencephalogram (EEG; 2 µg · mL^{-1}), spikes on the EEG (10 µg · mL^{-1}), myoclonic jerks and facial twitches (14 µg · mL^{-1}), and clonic seizures (>17 µg · mL^{-1}).[61] To elicit epileptiform activity typically would require between 14 and 22 mg · kg^{-1} of atracurium.[62,67] An *atracurium dose* of 0.5 mg · kg^{-1} typically results in a laudanosine level below 0.20 µg · mL^{-1},[25] which is far lower than that implicated in laboratory studies. However, a slightly higher incidence of seizures has been noted in patients who received "high-dose" atracurium infusion (12–15 µg · kg^{-1} · min^{-1} for a total dose of 130–435 mg) and isoflurane for neurosurgical procedures[68]; perhaps laudanosine enters the CNS more readily if there is a lesion of the blood-brain barrier.

Under normal conditions, the $t_{1/2elim}$ of laudanosine is approximately 10 times longer than that of atracurium.[69] The potential for *elevated plasma levels of laudanosine* is increased by prolonged atracurium administration in the context of decreased renal clearance[13,70,71] or decreased hepatic metabolism.[29,72–74] Plasma clearance of laudanosine as well as atracurium is not necessarily compromised significantly by renal failure alone.[16,75] Atracurium infusions lasting up to 36 hours have been used safely in patients with renal failure.[76] The levels generated in different settings are summarized in Table 13-1.

Atracurium is *without significant direct autonomic (or antimuscarinic) effects;* it does not elicit the increase in heart rate and blood pressure that is seen after pancuronium.[5,80] As for other relaxants without autonomic effects, it may be associated with bradycardia,[81] probably due to the unopposed vagomimetic effects of induction agents.[80] Being a benzylisoquinolinium compound, atracurium may cause significant *histamine release* after rapid bolus administration of more than twice its ED$_{95}$ (i.e., >0.5 mg · kg^{-1}).[2,8,20,82–96]

TABLE 13-1
Laudanosine Levels During Atracurium Administration

Atracurium Dose and Clinical Setting	Laudanosine Level ($\mu g \cdot mL^{-1}$)
0.5 mg · kg^{-1} bolus[25]	<0.20
6–12-hr infusions of atracurium for 95% twitch depression	
In normal renal function[13]	1.0
In renal failure[13]	6.0
0.5 mg · kg^{-1} bolus, followed by 0.75 mg · kg^{-1} · hr^{-1} infusion intraoperatively:	
In normal renal function[71]	0.37
In renal failure[71]	0.77
0.5 mg · kg^{-1} · hr^{-1} during renal transplantation[77]	0.6–2.7
Long-term infusions in ICU patients[13,75,78,79]	1.9–5.1
Continuous infusion during liver transplantation[73]	<1.02
0.5 mg · kg^{-1} bolus in patients with renal failure[70]	<0.76

This dose-related effect limits the usefulness of atracurium for a rapid-sequence intubation where rapid bolus administration of ≥3 times the ED$_{95}$ of an NDR is planned. As for other benzylisoquinolinium compounds (Chap. 11), such anaphylactoid (not anaphylactic) responses usually are limited to cutaneous reactions but certainly may include decreased blood pressure or increased bronchomotor tone.[89,92,93,97–100] The latter may be more likely in the patient with asthma.[98,100]

Doses less than 0.5 mg · kg^{-1} generally produce few clinically significant cardiovascular effects. As detailed in Chapter 11, histamine-mediated effects may be prevented by pretreatment with H$_1$ and H$_2$ blockers.[94] Hypotension also may be avoided by (1) administering 0.1 mg · kg^{-1} doses at 30-second intervals, (2) dividing doses larger than 0.5 mg · kg^{-1} into smaller doses spaced 60 seconds apart, or (3) infusing such doses over 60–75 seconds.[20,90,94] The histamine-related effects are less in children and the elderly.[101,102]

Atracurium may also be indirectly responsible for *other cardiovascular changes. Histamine* is a known inducer of catecholamine release.[103,104] Such release may have been responsible for hypertension and dysrhythmias after a relatively large dose of atracurium (e.g., 0.6–0.7 mg · kg^{-1}) was administered to patients with a *pheochromocytoma*.[105] In addition, at relatively high concentrations, *laudanosine* may exert cardiovascular effects,[51–63] including decreased blood pressure and increased norepinephrine release.[106]

Atracurium gradually loses potency at room temperature (5% per month), and it rapidly loses potency in lactated Ringer's solution because of the solution's pH.

◆ VECURONIUM

Vecuronium bromide (Norcuron), like pancuronium, is an aminosteroid. However, it is more likely to have a monoquaternary configuration. The absence of a methyl group from the nitrogen at 17 results in its lack of vagolytic effects, its increased lipophilicity, and its propensity for hepatic metabolism.[107] Vecuronium's ED_{95} is 0.04–0.06 mg · kg^{-1}. Its time course is similar to that for atracurium: its RI_{25-75} averages 13–15 minutes after a single bolus, and onset of a dose twice the ED_{95} typically occurs between 2.7 and 3.8 minutes.[3,108–111] Increasing the dose accelerates vecuronium's onset (within limits) but also prolongs its duration (Chap. 7).[111–117] Vecuronium is stable in solution for only 3 months; it thus is provided as a freeze-dried preparation that dissolves rapidly.

Vecuronium's main advantage is that it *does not elicit histamine release or induce cardiovascular effects*,[118–120] even in doses 8 times its ED_{95}.[112–116,121,122] However, *bradyarrhythmias* have been noted after vecuronium administration.[111,123–129] They are most likely due to unmasking of the vagotonic effects of opioids and other agents administered at the time of induction; vecuronium itself probably does not significantly increase vagal tone.[80,130] The hemodynamic stability after its administration has made vecuronium advantageous in the context of increased intracranial pressure.[131]

In contrast to atracurium, vecuronium's relatively short duration is dependent almost exclusively on *redistribution,* and its clearance is almost wholly dependent on *organ (liver) elimination*.[132] Only drug in the central (i.e., blood) compartment is metabolized. Within 30 minutes of an intravenous (IV) injection, more than 50% of vecuronium may be found in the liver.[133] Its $t_{1/2elim}$ is greater than atracurium's, approaching that of long-lasting agents.[134,135] Because it depends largely on redistribution into its relatively large volume of distribution for its short effect,[18,136,137] vecuronium *may produce a prolonged effect* after a continuous infusion,[138] a large dose, or multiple doses (after its peripheral storage sites are saturated).[18,110,114,116,139] The RI_{25-75} increased from 14 minutes to 30 minutes when the bolus dose was increased from 0.1 to 0.25 mg · kg^{-1},[116] and it increased from 8 minutes to 38 minutes as the dose was increased from 0.07 to 0.28 mg · kg^{-1}.[110] In another study, repeated doses of vecuronium were associated with increasing degrees of fade.[17] Alternatively, no appreciable prolongation was noted after as many as six repeated doses of 0.015 mg · kg^{-1} on recovery to 25% of control or after repeated administration of 2- to 3-mg boluses.[109,111] Thus, the *cumulative effects are relatively small* compared to those of the long-acting agents.

Like atracurium, vecuronium is well-suited for continuous intraoperative infusions.[34,140,141] Again, *infusion rate* requirements vary considerably among patients; rates of 1–2 μg · kg · min^{-1} (0.06–0.12 mg · kg^{-1} · hr^{-1}) usually are necessary to maintain 90% block.[140] The infusion may need to be decreased as drug accumulates over time; as redistribution sites become saturated, times for recovery become prolonged.[34,138] The typical RI_{25-75} is 13–15 minutes and the 5–95% recovery interval is 30–35 minutes; these times may increase if drug has accumulated during a prolonged infusion. This is not a problem if the rate of infusion is titrated based on response to nerve stimulation.

As is the case for other NDRs (Chap. 10), *children* aged 2–10 years typically require more vecuronium[142–144] and experience faster onset[142,144] and recovery[134,142,145] than adults. Infants tend to need less vecuronium than older children,[142–144,146,147] but the differences are not always statistically significant.[142] In one study, children less than 1 year old required 0.06 mg · kg^{-1}, while those aged 1–15 years required 0.10 mg · kg^{-1}.[146] Infants also take significantly longer to recover.[142,147] Whereas the duration of a greater than 90% block after 0.15 mg · kg^{-1} was only 37 minutes in children aged 5–7 years, it was 111 minutes in infants less than 3 months old.[147] These data indicate that vecuronium bolus and infusion requirements in very young children are more age dependent than atracurium's dosing requirements. The elimination of vecuronium may be prolonged as a consequence of immature liver processes.[142,148]

In children undergoing nitrous oxide–narcotic anesthesia, the *vecuronium infusion rates* needed to maintain 90–95% adductor pollicis twitch depression after recovery to 10% of baseline from a bolus were 1.0 µg · kg^{-1} · min^{-1} in *neonates and infants*, 2.6 µg · kg^{-1} · min^{-1} in *children* 3–10 years old, and 1.5 µg · kg^{-1} · min^{-1} in adolescents.[144] These rates are consistent with the calculated amount of vecuronium eliminated at steady 50% block: 0.32, 0.65, and 0.48 µg · kg^{-1} · min^{-1} in infants, children, and adults, respectively.[148] The average infusion rates employed for *prolonged infusions in pediatric ICU patients* with adequate renal function were 1.8 µg · kg^{-1} · min^{-1} (0.11 mg · kg^{-1} · hr^{-1}) in *neonates* and 2.3 µg · kg^{-1} · min^{-1} (0.14 mg · kg^{-1} · hr^{-1}) in *infants and children*.[143] There was wide intersubject variability with respect to dosing and recovery.[143]

As for pancuronium, vecuronium is metabolized to a 3-hydroxy derivative with significant neuromuscular blocking properties.[149–152] The 3-OH derivative is 40–80% as potent as the parent compound; the 17-hydroxy and 3,17-dihydroxy derivatives are less than 5% as potent. This is consistent with the tendency for 3-OH congeners of the steroidal relaxants to be pharmacologically active.[152] The 3,17-desacetyl derivative is an unstable, short-lived intermediary product.[151] Clearance of the relatively potent *3-hydroxy derivative* is slightly slower than that of vecuronium, especially if the liver's capacity for storage and excretion is exceeded[153] or after prolonged infusion in patients with renal failure.[154,155] Of potential significance in light of reports of resistance to long-term vecuronium infusions in ICU patients,[156] the combined effect of vecuronium and its 3,17-desacetyl derivative (in low concentrations) was less than additive, indicating some antagonism.[149] This may be attributable to the competition among the competitors: the metabolite is a relatively weak, low-affinity antagonist whose rapid dissociation may increase the free fraction of receptors available to acetylcholine (ACh).[149]

Even though vecuronium is *dependent on hepatic elimination*,[134] vecuronium's kinetics and dynamics typically are not affected by mild to moderate liver disease, especially if ≤0.15 mg · kg^{-1} is administered.[157–159] However, its effects and those of its metabolites may be prolonged in *liver failure*,[132,158–160] especially when higher doses are used. In patients with *cholestasis*, 0.2 mg · kg^{-1} resulted in a $t_{1/2elim}$ of 98 ± 57 minutes vs. 58 ± 22 minutes in normal subjects.[160] The block induced by the 3-hydroxy derivative was prolonged by the exclusion of the liver in an animal model.[132] Of note, vecuronium metabolism appeared to be uniquely susceptible to prolongation by metronidazole in one animal study,[161] but this observation has not been confirmed.[143,162,163]

The *duration of a bolus dose* of vecuronium may be prolonged in the *elderly*,[164,165] as may the effect of an infusion,[166] presumably owing to reduced clearance and increased volume of distribution. However, the increase generally is not marked after a single dose.[102] The RI may increase by 200–300%,[164,166] but the results of different studies vary widely. After a 0.1 mg · kg^{-1} bolus in elderly patients anesthetized with a nitrous oxide–narcotic technique, clearance was 2.6 mL · kg · $^{-1}$min^{-1} (vs. 5.6 in young adults), the $t_{1/2elim}$ was 125 (vs. 78) minutes, and the RI_{25-75} was 49 (vs. 15) minutes.[164] Others have not reported such prolongation,[102,167] perhaps because the decrease in clearance was offset by a decrease in volume of distribution and because of wide intersubject variability.[167] The neostigmine dose required to reverse a vecuronium-induced block was increased in elderly patients,[168] perhaps as a result of the slower rate of spontaneous recovery in the elderly.[164,165]

Obesity also may be associated with delayed recovery after vecuronium: after 0.1 mg · kg^{-1}, the RI_{25-75} and Dur_{75} were 33 and 82 minutes in obese patients, significantly greater than the corresponding times of 13 and 50 minutes in controls.[22] Delayed recovery in obese patients may be attributable to delayed elimination as a result of altered hepatic function, decreased hepatic blood flow, or a relative overdose (because of dosing according to total body weight), which limits the impact of redistribution on clinical recovery.[22] There was relatively little difference in pharmacokinetic indices between obese and control subjects when vecuronium was administered according to ideal body weights.[169,170]

Although it had been reported that vecuronium's disposition is largely undisturbed by *renal failure*,[135,171,172] its duration may be prolonged in this setting,[173–176] especially if repeated doses or infusions are administered.[26,176–179] The $t_{1/2elim}$ is increased in pronounced renal failure,[154,173,176] but to a far lesser degree than for pancuronium. Infusion requirements are decreased by approximately 20% in patients with renal failure.[26] Desacetyl vecuronium (the

3-hydroxy metabolite) is more dependent on renal clearance than vecuronium (22% vs. 9%) and has been implicated in prolonged paralysis in ICU patients receiving prolonged infusions.[155] However, its normal clearance is only slightly longer than that of its parent compound, and questions remain as to its distribution and as to its potential to cause long-term neuromuscular dysfunction (Chap. 11).

Discussion Questions ◆

a. Is *atracurium's clinical duration* markedly affected by changes in relative amounts of extracellular fluid and lipid volumes in the *elderly*?
b. Can *atracurium* or *vecuronium* be administered in the same syringe as *thiopental*?
c. What *cardiovascular changes* may be encountered when *vecuronium* is used during a high-dose fentanyl induction?
d. What features of *vecuronium* make it well-suited for rapid tracheal intubation in the patient with *increased intracranial pressure*?
e. During train-of-four monitoring, is there much difference in the *height of T_1 at which T_4 returns during recovery* from atracurium, vecuronium, pancuronium, and *d*-tubocurarine?

Answers ◆

a. *Atracurium's duration* is not markedly prolonged by the increased lipid compartment and decreased organ function that are noted in the *elderly*. Its metabolism occurs in the peripheral as well as central compartments and is relatively independent of changes in organ function.
b. *Atracurium* and *vecuronium* should not be mixed with *thiopental*. They are acidic solutions and thiopental is an alkaline solution; they will precipitate. The *relaxant-thiopental precipitate* has been associated with marked histamine release and cardiopulmonary collapse (Chap. 11).
c. Although it apparently has no direct cardiovascular effects, *vecuronium* administration at induction of anesthesia may be associated with an increased incidence of *bradycardia* when narcotics are also administered. Most likely, this is due to the unopposed vagal effects of the narcotics. It is reversible with vagolytic therapy.
d. If one elects to avoid SCh prior to rapidly intubating the trachea of a patient with *increased intracranial pressure*, *vecuronium* may be a logical choice. It is devoid of significant histamine release and cardiovascular effects at 8 times its ED_{95}. This allows the use of a high dose (e.g., $3-4 \times ED_{95}$) to accelerate onset. Vecuronium does not compromise cerebral perfusion pressure in patients with brain tumors.[131] However, one must be aware of the potential for bradyarrhythmias and for dose-related prolongation of vecuronium-induced block. In addition, even

high-dose vecuronium does not ensure onset of total paralysis that is as rapid as that attained after SCh (Chap. 7). It is possible that this limitation will be largely overcome by rocuronium (Chap. 14).

e. The *height of T_1 at which T_4 becomes detectable* during recovery is similar after atracurium (22–33%), vecuronium (29–32%), pancuronium (31%), and *d*-tubocurarine (29%).[180] Slight differences may be noted during onset of block.[181–183] Despite the minor differences, the general relationships between T_1 and T_4 (see Table 4-1) tend to apply to all commonly used NDRs.

References ◆

1. Ali HH, Basta SJ, Sunder N, Gionfriddo M, Lineberry C: Clinical pharmacology of atracurium: a new intermediate acting non-depolarizing relaxant. Semin Anesth 1:57, 1982
2. Basta SJ, Ali HH, Savarese JJ, Sunder N, Gionfriddo M, Cloutier G, Lineberry C, Cato AE: Clinical pharmacology of atracurium besylate (BW 33A): a new non-depolarizing muscle relaxant. Anesth Analg 61:723–729, 1982
3. Gramstad L, Lilleaasen P, Minsaas BB: Onset time and duration of action of atracurium, Org NC45 and pancuronium. Acta Anaesthesiol Scand 25:484, 1981
4. Gibson FM, Mirakhur RK, Lavery GG, Clarke RSJ: Potency of atracurium: a comparison of single dose and cumulative dose techniques. Anesthesiology 62:657–659, 1985
5. Hughes R, Chapple DJ: The pharmacology of atracurium: a new competitive neuromuscular blocking agent. Br J Anaesth 53:31–44, 1981
6. Hunter JM, Jones RS, Utting JE: Use of atracurium during general surgery monitored by the train-of-four stimuli. Br J Anaesth 54:1243–1250, 1982
7. Katz RL, Stirt J, Murray AL, Lee C: Neuromuscular effects of atracurium in man. Anesth Analg 61:730–734, 1982
8. Mirakhur RK, Lavery GG, Clarke RS, Gibson FM, McAteer E: Atracurium in clinical anaesthesia: effect of dosage on onset, duration and conditions for tracheal intubation. Anaesthesia 40:801–805, 1985
9. Ward S, Wright D: Combined pharmacokinetic and pharmacodynamic study of a single bolus dose of atracurium. Br J Anaesth 55:35S, 1983
10. Stiller RL, Cook DR, Chakravorti S: *In vitro* degradation of atracurium in human plasma. Br J Anaesth 57:1085–1088, 1985
11. Ward S, Weatherley BC: Pharmacokinetics of atracurium and its metabolites. Br J Anaesth 58:6S-1010S, 1986
12. Fisher DM, Canfell PC, Fahey MR, Rosen JI, Rupp SM, Sheiner LB, Miller RD: Elimination of atracurium in humans: contribution of Hofmann elimination and ester hydrolysis versus organ-based elimination. Anesthesiology 65:6–12, 1986
13. Ward S, Boheimer N, Weatherley BC, Simmonds RJ, Dopson TA: Pharmacokinetics of atracurium and its metabolites in patients with normal renal function, and in patients in renal failure. Br J Anaesth 59:697–706, 1987
14. deBros FM, Lai A, Scott R, et al: Pharmacokinetics and pharmacodynamics of atracurium during isoflurane anesthesia in normal and anephric patients. Anesth Analg 65:743–746, 1986
15. Cook DR, Brandom BW, Stiller RL, Woelfel S, Lai A, Slater J: Pharmacokinetics of atracurium in normal and liver failure patients. Anesthesiology 61:A433, 1984
16. Shearer ES, O'Sullivan EP, Hunter JM: Clearance of atracurium and laudanosine in the urine and by continuous venovenous haemofiltration. Br J Anaesth 67:569–573, 1991
17. Ali HH, Savarese JJ, Basta SJ, Sunder N, Gionfriddo M: Evaluation of cumulative properties of three new non-depolarizing neuromuscular blocking drugs BW A444U, atracurium, and vecuronium. Br J Anaesth 55:107S–111S, 1983
18. Fisher DM, Rosen JI: A pharmacokinetic explanation for increasing recovery time fol-

lowing larger or repeated doses of nondepolarizing muscle relaxants. Anesthesiology 65:286–291, 1986
19. Payne JP, Hughes R: Evaluation of atracurium in anaesthetized man. Br J Anaesth 53:45–54, 1981
20. Scott RPF, Savarese JJ, Basta SJ, Embree P, Ali HH, Sunder N, Hoaglin DC: Clinical pharmacology of atracurium given in high dose. Br J Anaesth 58:834–838, 1986
21. Rupp SM, Fahey MR, Miller RD: Neuromuscular and cardiovascular effects of atracurium during nitrous oxide–fentanyl and nitrous oxide–isoflurane anaesthesia. Br J Anaesth 55:67S–70S, 1983
22. Weinstein JA, Matteo RS, Ornstein E, Schwartz AE, Goldstoff M, Thal G: Pharmacodynamics of vecuronium and atracurium in the obese surgical patient. Anesth Analg 67:1149–1153, 1988
23. Ornstein E, Matteo RS, Schwartz AE, Silverberg PA, Young WL, Diaz J: The effect of phenytoin on the magnitude and duration of neuromuscular block following atracurium or vecuronium. Anesthesiology 67:191–196, 1987
24. d'Hollander AA, Luyckx C, Barvais L, De Ville A: Clinical evaluation of atracurium besylate requirement for a stable muscle relaxation during surgery: lack of age-related effects. Anesthesiology 59:237–240, 1983
25. Fahey MR, Rupp SM, Fisher DM, Miller RD, Sharma M, Canfell C, Castagnoli K, Hennis PJ: The pharmacokinetics and pharmacodynamics of atracurium in patients with and without renal failure. Anesthesiology 61:699–702, 1984
26. Gramstad L: Atracurium, vecuronium and pancuronium in end-stage renal failure: dose-response properties and interactions with azathioprine. Br J Anaesth 59:995–1003, 1987
27. Hunter JM, Jones RS, Utting JE: Use of atracurium in patients with no renal function. Br J Anaesth 54:1251–1258, 1982
28. Ward S, Neill EAM: Pharmacokinetics of atracurium in acute hepatic failure (with acute renal failure). Br J Anaesth 55:1169–1172, 1983
29. Parker CJR, Hunter JM: Pharmacokinetics of atracurium and laudanosine in patients with hepatic cirrhosis. Br J Anaesth 62:177–183, 1989
30. Kent AP, Parker CJR, Hunter JM: Pharmacokinetics of atracurium and laudanosine in the elderly. Br J Anaesth 63:661–666, 1989
31. Parker CJR, Hunter JM, Snowdon SL: Effect of age, sex and anaesthetic technique on the pharmacokinetics of atracurium. Br J Anaesth 69:439–443, 1992
32. Gyasi HK, Naguib M: Atracurium and severe hepatic disease: a case report. Can Anaesth Soc J 32:161, 1985
33. Benzer A, Mitterschiffthaler G, Pomaroli A, Müller L: Atracurium in whole body hyperthermia (letter). Anaesthesia 45:991, 1990
34. Ali HH, Savarese JJ, Embree PB, Basta SJ, Stout RG, Bottros H, Weakly JN: Clinical pharmacology of mivacurium chloride (W B1090U) infusion: comparison with vecuronium and atracurium. Br J Anaesth 61:541–546, 1988
35. Caldwell JE, Heier T, Kitts JB, Lynam DP, Fahey MR, Miller RD: Comparison of the neuromuscular block induced by mivacurium, suxamethonium or atracurium during nitrous oxide–fentanyl anaesthesia. Br J Anaesth 63:393–399, 1989
36. Fisher DM, Canfell PC, Spellman MJ, Miller RD: Pharmacokinetics and pharmacodynamics of atracurium in infants and children. Anesthesiology 73:33–37, 1990
37. Brandom BW, Rudd GD, Cook DR: Clinical pharmacology of atracurium in pediatric patients. Br J Anaesth 55:117S–121S, 1983
38. Goudsouzian NG, Martyn J, Rudd GD, Liu LMP, Lineberry CG: Continuous infusion of atracurium in children. Anesthesiology 64:171–174, 1986
39. Kalli I, Meretoja OA: Infusion of atracurium in neonates, infants and children: a study of dose requirements. Br J Anaesth 60:651–654, 1988
40. Meakin G, Shaw EA, Baker RD, Morris P: Comparison of atracurium-induced neuromuscular blockade in neonates, infants and children. Br J Anaesth 60:171–175, 1988
41. Meistelman C, Debaene B, Saint-Maurice C, Nebout T, Bargy F, Loose JP: Potency of atracurium in infants during halothane anesthesia. Anesthesiology 65:A290, 1986
42. Brandom BW, Woelfel SK, Cook DR, Fehr BL, Rudd GD: Clinical pharmacology of atracurium in infants. Anesth Analg 63:309–312, 1984

43. Meretoja OA, Kalli I: Spontaneous recovery of neuromuscular function after atracurium in pediatric patients. Anesth Analg 65:1042–1046, 1986
44. Nagashima H, Khilkin A, Ono K, Fu S, Duncalf D, Foldes FF: Effect of portacaval shunt and/or renal vessel ligation on disposition of muscle relaxants. Anesthesiology 59:A264 1983
45. Nigrovic V, Auen M, Wajskol A: Enzymatic hydrolysis of atracurium *in vivo*. Anesthesiology 62:606–609, 1985
46. Chapple DJ, Clark JS: Pharmacological action of breakdown products of atracurium and related substances. Br J Anaesth 55:11S–15S, 1983
47. Stenlake JB, Waigh RD, Unwin J, Dewar GH, Coker GG: Atracurium: conception and inception. Br J Anaesth 55:3S, 1983
48. Nigrovic V, Smith S: Inactivation pathways of atracurium: evidence for an additional route. Anesth Analg 66:S129, 1987
49. Nigrovic V, Smith S: Involvement of nucleophiles in the inactivation of atracurium. Br J Anaesth 59:617–621, 1987
50. Nigrovic V: New insights into the toxicity of neuromuscular-blocking drugs and their metabolites. Curr Opin Anaesth 4:603–607, 1991
51. Nigrovic V, Koechel DA: Atracurium: additional information needed (letter). Anesthesiology 60:606–607, 1984
52. Nigrovic V, Pandya JB, Klaunig JE: Reactivity and toxicity of atracurium and its metabolites *in vitro*. Can J Anaesth 36:262–268, 1989
53. Nigrovic V, et al: Potentiation of atracurium toxicity in isolated rat hepatocytes by inhibition of its hydrolytic degradation pathway. Anesth Analg 66:512–516, 1987
54. Nigrovic V, Klaunig JE, Smith SL, Schultz NE, Wajskol A: Comparative toxicity of atracurium and metocurine in isolated rat hepatocytes. Anesth Analg 65:1107–1111, 1986
55. Morley TJ, Dickins M: A study to investigate cytotoxicity of the neuromuscular blocking agent atracurium using primary rat hepatocyte culture. Hum Exp Toxicol 9:345–346, 1990
56. Reckendorfer H, Burgmann H, Sperlich M, Tüchy GL, Feigl W, Spieckermann PG, Weindlmayr-Göttel M, Schwarz S: Hepatotoxicity testing of atracurium and laudanosine in the isolated, perfused rat liver. Br J Anaesth 69:288–291, 1992
57. Weatherby BC, Williams SG, Neill EAM: Pharmacokinetics, pharmacodynamics and dose response relationships of atracurium administered I.V. Br J Anaesth 55:395, 1983
58. Delbressine LPC, Seuter-Berlage T, Seuter ER: Identification of urinary mercapturic acid formed from acrylate, methacrylate and crotonate in the rat. Xenobiotica 11:241–247, 1981
59. Fujinaga M, Baden JM, Mazze RI: Developmental toxicity of nondepolarizing muscle relaxants in cultured rat embryos. Anesthesiology 76:999–1003, 1992
60. Skarpa M, Dayan AD, Follenfant M, James DA, Moore WB, Thomson PM, Lucke JN, Morgan M, Lovell R, Medd R: Toxicity testing of atracurium. Br J Anaesth 55:27S–29S, 1982
61. Chapple DJ, Miller AA, Ward JB, et al: Cardiovascular and neurological effects of laudanosine. Br J Anaesth 59:218–225, 1987
62. Hennis PJ, Fahey MR, Canfell PC, et al: Pharmacology of laudanosine in dogs. Anesthesiology 65:56–60, 1986
63. Ingram MD, Sclabassi RJ, Stiller RL, Cook DR, Bennett MH: Cardiovascular and electroencephalographic effects of laudanosine in "nephrectomized" cats. Anesth Analg 64:A232, 1985
64. Lanier WL, Milde JH, Michenfelder JD: The cerebral effects of pancuronium and atracurium in halothane-anesthetized dogs. Anesthesiology 63:589–597, 1985
65. Shi W, Fahey MR, Fisher DM, et al: Laudanosine (a metabolite of atracurium) increases the minimum alveolar concentration of halothane in rabbits. Anesthesiology 63:584–588, 1985
66. Beemer GH, Bjorksten AR, Dawson PJ, Crankshaw DP: Production of laudanosine following infusion of atracurium in man and its effects on awakening. Br J Anaesth 63:76–80, 1989
67. Mercier J, Mercier E: Action de quelques alcaloides secondaires de l'opium sur l'electrocorticogramme du chien. C R Soc Biol (Paris) 149:760–762, 1955

68. Beemer GH, Dawson PJ, Bjorksten AR, Edwards NE: Early postoperative seizures in neurosurgical patients administered atracurium and isoflurane. Anaesth Intensive Care 17:504–509, 1989
69. Agoston S, Vandenbrom RHG, Wierda JMKH: Clinical pharmacokinetics of neuromuscular blocking drugs. Clin Pharmacokinet 22:94–115, 1992
70. Fahey MR, Rupp SM, Canfell C, Fisher DM, Miller RD, Sharma M, Castagnoli K, Hennis PJ: Effect of renal failure on laudanosine excretion in man. Br J Anaesth 57:1049–1051, 1985
71. Schwarz S, Lackner FX, Hrska F, Weindlmayr-Goettel M, Tüchy G, Steinbereithner K: Metabolism of atracurium in patients with renal failure. Anesthesiology 73:A917, 1990
72. Pittet JF, Schopfer C, Morel DR, Mentha G, Benakis A, Tassonyi E: Plasma levels of laudanosine, but not of atracurium are increased during the anhepatic phase of orthotopic liver transplantation in pigs. Anesthesiology 69:A486, 1988
73. Lawhead RG, Matsumi M, Peters KR, Landers DF, Becker GL, Earl RA: Plasma laudanosine levels in patients given atracurium during liver transplantation. Anesth Analg 76:569–573, 1993
74. Vine P, Boheimer N, Ward S, Weatherley B, Buick A, Smith I: Laudanosine pharmacokinetics after bolus atracurium in patients with hepato-biliary dysfunction. Br J Anaesth 58:1327P, 1986
75. Parker CJR, Jones JE, Hunter JM: Disposition of infusions of atracurium and its metabolite, laudanosine, in patients in renal and respiratory failure in an ITU. Br J Anaesth 61:531–540, 1988
76. Griffiths RB, Hunter JM, Jones RS: Atracurium infusion in patients with renal failure on an I.T.U. Anaesthesia 41:375, 1986
77. Lepage JY, Athouel A, Vecherini MF, Malinovsky JM, Cozian A: Evaluation of proconvulsant effect of laudanosine in renal transplant recipient. Anesthesiology 75:A781, 1991
78. Hennis PJ, Fahey MR, Canfell PC, et al: Pharmacology of atracurium during isoflurane anesthesia in normal and anephric patients. Anesth Analg 65:743–746, 1986
79. Yate PM, Flynn PJ, Arnold RW, et al: Clinical experience and plasma laudanosine concentrations during atracurium infusion in the intensive therapy unit. Br J Anaesth 59:211–217, 1987
80. Lavery GG, Mirakhur RK, Clarke RSJ, Gibson FM: The effect of atracurium, vecuronium and pancuronium on heart rate and arterial pressure in normal individuals. Eur J Anaesthesiol 3:459–468, 1986
81. Carter ML: Bradycardia after the use of atracurium. Br Med J 287:247–248, 1983
82. Barnes PK, DeRenzy-Martin N, Thomas VJE, Watkins J: Plasma histamine levels following atracurium. Anaesthesia 41:821–824, 1986
83. Basta SJ, Savarese JJ, Ali HH, Moss J, Gionfriddo M: Histamine-releasing potencies of atracurium, dimethyl tubocurarine and tubocurarine. Br J Anaesth 55:105S–106S, 1983
84. Cork RC, Gallo JA, Puchi P: Histamine and hemodynamic response after atracurium vs. vecuronium. Anesth Analg 66:S32, 1987
85. Fox MA: Atracurium in normal doses may release histamine (letter). Anesthesiology 60:386, 1984
86. Goudsouzian NG, Young ET, Moss J, Liu MP: Histamine release during the administration of atracurium or vecuronium in children. Br J Anaesth 58:1229–1233, 1986
87. Lavery GG, Boyle MM, Mirakhur RK: Probable histamine liberation with atracurium: a case report. Br J Anaesth 57:811–813, 1985
88. Lavery GG, Clarke RSJ, Watkins J: Histaminoid response after intradermal and intravenous administration of atracurium, vecuronium and tubocurarine: a comparative study. Eur J Anaesthesiol 3:439–447, 1986
89. Mehr EH, Lindeman KS, Hirshman CA: Airway constriction following atracurium is due to histamine release. Anesthesiology 75:A974, 1991
90. Moyers JR, Carter JG, Fehr BL, Lineberry CC, Sokoll MD, Shimosato S: Circulatory effects of atracurium in patients with cardiovascular disease. Br J Anaesth 58:83S–88S, 1986
91. Pokar H, Brandt L: Haemodynamic effects of atracurium in patients after cardiac surgery. Br J Anaesth 55:139S, 1983

92. Siler JN, Mager JG Jr, Wyche MQ Jr: Atracurium: hypotension, tachycardia and bronchospasm. Anesthesiology 62:645–646, 1985
93. Smith DA, Wright DJ, Hammond JE: Influence of tubocurarine, pancuronium and atracurium on bronchomotor tone. Br J Anaesth 57:753–757, 1985
94. Scott RPF, Savarese JJ, Basta SJ, Sunder N, Ali HH, Gargarian M, Gionfriddo M, Batson AG: Atracurium: clinical strategies for preventing histamine release and attenuating the haemodynamic response. Br J Anaesth 57:550–553, 1985
95. Savarese JJ, Basta SJ, Ali HH, et al: Neuromuscular and cardiovascular effects of BW 33A (atracurium) in patients under halothane anesthesia. Anesthesiology 57:A262, 1982
96. Watkins J: Histamine release and atracurium. Br J Anaesth 58:19S–22S, 1986
97. Fisher M: Life threatening reaction to atracurium (letter). Br J Anaesth 60:598–599, 1988
98. Oh TE, Horton J: Adverse reactions to atracurium. Br J Anaesth 62:467–468, 1989
99. Rowlands DE: Life threatening reaction to atracurium. Br J Anaesth 60:599, 1988
100. Stirton-Hopkins C: Life threatening reaction to atracurium (letter). Br J Anaesth 60:597–598, 1988
101. Lavery GG, Mirakhur RK: Atracurium besylate in paediatric anaesthesia. Anaesthesia 39:1243–1246, 1984
102. Lowry KG, Mirakhur RK, Lavery GG, Clarke RSJ: Vecuronium and atracurium in the elderly: a clinical comparison with pancuronium. Acta Anaesthesiol Scand 29:405–408, 1985
103. Sheps SG, Maher FT: Histamine and glucagon tests in diagnosis of pheochromocytoma. JAMA 205:895–899, 1968
104. Vigorito C, Russo P, Picotti GB, et al: Cardiovascular effects of histamine infusion in man. J Cardiovasc Pharmacol 5:53–537, 1983
105. Amaranath L, Zanettin GG, Bravo EL, Barnes A, Estafanous FG: Atracurium and pheochromocytoma. Anesth Analg 67:1127–1130, 1988
106. Kinjo M, Nagashima H, Vizi ES: Effect of atracurium and laudanosine on the release of ^{3}H-noradrenaline. Br J Anaesth 62:683–690, 1989
107. Weindlmayr-Goettel M, Gilly H, Sipos E, Steinbereithner K: Lipid solubility of pancuronium and vecuronium determined by n-octanol/water partitioning. Br J Anaesth 70:579–580, 1993
108. Ali HH, Basta SJ, Savarese JJ, Gargarian M, Scott RFP, Sunder N, Gionfriddo M: Single twitch and train-of-four responses for atracurium and vecuronium. Anesth Analg 64:A187, 1985
109. Foldes F, Nagashima H, Boros M, Tassonyi E, Fitzal S, Agoston S: Muscular relaxation with atracurium, vecuronium and duador under balanced anaesthesia. Br J Anaesth 55:97S–103S, 1983
110. Fahey MR, Morris RB, Miller RD, Sohn YJ, Cronnelly R, Gencarelli P: Clinical pharmacology of ORG NC45 (Norcuron™): a new nondepolarizing muscle relaxant. Anesthesiology 55:6–11, 1981
111. Mirakhur RK, Ferres CJ, Clarke RSJ, Bali IM, Dundee JW: Clinical evaluation of ORG NC45. Br J Anaesth 55:119–124, 1983
112. Casson WR, Jones RM: Vecuronium induced neuromuscular blockade: the effect of increasing dose on speed of onset. Anaesthesia 41:354–357, 1986
113. Ginsberg B, Glass PS, Quill T, Shafron D, Ossey KD: Onset and duration of neuromuscular blockade following high-dose vecuronium administration. Anesthesiology 71:201–205, 1989
114. Rorvik K, Husby P, Gramstad L, Vamnes JS, Bitsch-Larsen L, Koller M-E: Comparison of large dose of vecuronium with pancuronium for prolonged neuromuscular blockade. Br J Anaesth 61:180–185, 1988
115. Tullock WC, Diana P, Cook DR, Wilks DH, Brandom BW, Stiller RL, Beach CA: Neuromuscular and cardiovascular effects of high-dose vecuronium. Anesth Analg 70:86–90, 1990
116. Feldman SA, Liban JB: Vecuronium--a variable dose technique. Anaesthesia 42:199–201, 1987
117. Silverman DG, Swift CA, Dubow HD, O'Connor TZ, Brull SJ: Variability of onset within and among relaxant regimens. J Clin Anesth 4:28–33, 1992

118. Marshall RJ, McGrath JC, Miller RD, Docherty JR, Lamar JC: Comparison of the cardiovascular actions of Org NC 45 with those produced by other non-depolarising neuromuscular blocking agents in experimental animals. Br J Anaesth 52:21S–29S, 1980
119. Saxena PR, Dhasmana KM, Prakash O: A comparison of systemic and regional hemodynamic effects of d-tubocurarine, pancuronium, and vecuronium. Anesthesiology 59:102–108, 1983
120. Salmenpera M, Peltola K, Takkunen O, Heinonen J: Cardiovascular effects of pancuronium and vecuronium during high-dose fentanyl anesthesia. Anesth Analg 62:1059–1064, 1983
121. Ferres CJ, Carson IW, Lyons SM, Orr IA, Patterson CC, Clarke RSJ: Haemodynamic effects of vecuronium, pancuronium and atracurium in patients with coronary artery disease. Br J Anaesth 59:305–311, 1987
122. Wierda JMKH, Maestrone E, Bencini AF, Boyer A, Rashkovsky OM, Lip H, Karliczek R, Ket JM, Agoston S: Haemodynamic effects of vecuronium. Br J Anaesth 52:194–198, 1989
123. Cozanitis DA, Pouttu J, Rosenberg PH: Bradycardia associated with the use of vecuronium: a comparative study with pancuronium with and without glycopyrronium. Anaesthesia 42:192–194, 1987
124. Dhamee MS, Olund T, Reynolds AC, Entress J, Kalbfleisch J: Cardiovascular effects of pancuronium, vecuronium and atracurium during induction of anaesthesia with sufentanil and lorazepam for myocardial revascularization. J Cardiothorac Anesth 4:336–339, 1990
125. Inoue K, El-Banayosy A, Stolarski L, Reichelt W: Vecuronium induced bradycardia following induction of anaesthesia with etomidate or thiopentone, with or without fentanyl. Br J Anaesth 60:10–17, 1988
126. Janik R, Dick W: Sufentanil: the effect on cardiocirculatory parameters and intubation conditions on administration of pancuronium or vecuronium. Anaesthesist 38:673–680, 1989
127. Milligan KR, Beers HT: Vecuronium-associated cardiac arrest. Anaesthesia 40:385, 1985
128. May JR: Vecuronium and bradycardia. Anaesthesia 40:710, 1985
129. Starr NJ, Sethna DH, Estafanous FG: Bradycardia and asystole following the rapid administration of sufentanil with vecuronium. Anesthesiology 64:521–523, 1986
130. Ridley S, Gaylard D, Lim M: Effect of vecuronium on dose response relationships for atropine-induced changes in heart rate. Anesthesiology 69:A478, 1988
131. Stirt JA, Maggio W, Haworth C, Minton MD, Bedford RF: Vecuronium: effect on intracranial pressure and hemodynamics in neurosurgical patients. Anesthesiology 67:570–573, 1987
132. Bencini AF, Houwertjes MC, Agoston S: Effects of hepatic uptake of vecuronium bromide and its putative metabolites on their neuromuscular blocking actions in the cat. Br J Anaesth 57:789–795, 1985
133. Bencini AF, Scaf AHJ, Sohn YJ, et al: Hepatobiliary disposition of vecuronium bromide in man. Br J Anaesth 58:988, 1986
134. Meistelman C, Agoston S, Kersten UW, Saint-Maurice C, Bencini AF, Loose J-P: Pharmacokinetics and pharmacodynamics of vecuronium and pancuronium in anesthetized children. Anesth Analg 65:1319–1323, 1986
135. Bencini AF, Scaf AHJ, Sohn YJ, Meistelman C, Lienhart A, Kersten UW, Schwarz S, Agoston S: Disposition and urinary excretion of vecuronium bromide in anesthetized patients with normal renal function or renal failure. Anesth Analg 65:245–251, 1986
136. Shanks CA: Pharmacokinetics of the nondepolarizing neuromuscular relaxants applied to calculation of bolus and infusion dosage regimens. Anesthesiology 64:72–86, 1986
137. Sohn YJ, Bencini AF, Scaf AHJ, et al: Comparative pharmacokinetics and dynamics of vecuronium and pancuronium in anesthetized patients. Anesth Analg 65:233–239, 1986
138. Noeldge G, Hinsken H, Buzello W: Comparison between the continuous infusion of vecuronium and the intermittent administration of pancuronium and vecuronium. Br J Anaesth 56:473–477, 1984
139. Sloan MH, Lerman J, Bissonnette B: Pharmacodynamics of high-dose vecuronium in children during balanced anesthesia. Anesthesiology 74:656–659, 1991

140. Mirakhur RK, Ferres CJ: Muscle relaxation with an infusion of vecuronium. Eur J Anaesthesiol 1:353–359, 1984
141. d'Hollander AA, Czerucki R, DeVille A, Cuvelier F: Stable muscle relaxation during abdominal surgery using combined intravenous bolus and demand infusion: clinical appraisal with ORG NC 45. Can Anaesth Soc J 29:136–141, 1982
142. Fisher DM, Miller RD: Neuromuscular effects of vecuronium (Org NC45) in infants and children during N_2O, halothane anesthesia. Anesthesiology 58:519–523, 1983
143. Fitzpatrick KTJ, Black GW, Crean PM, Mirakhur RK: Continuous vecuronium infusion for prolonged muscle relaxation in children. Can J Anaesth 38:169–174, 1991
144. Meretoja OA: Vecuronium infusion requirements in pediatric patients during fentanyl-N_2O-O_2 anesthesia. Anesth Analg 68:20–24, 1989
145. Woelfel SK, Dong ML, Brandom BW, et al: Vecuronium infusion requirements in children during halothane-narcotic-nitrous oxide, isoflurane-narcotic-nitrous oxide, and narcotic-nitrous oxide anesthesia. Anesth Analg 73:33, 1991
146. Schippers HC, Bell B, Erdmann W, Jackson Rees G: Dose response curve of vecuronium bromide in anesthetized neonates, infants and children. Anesthesiology 69:A761, 1988
147. Meretoja OA: Is vecuronium a long-acting neuromuscular blocking agent in neonates and infants? Br J Anaesth 62:184–187, 1989
148. Fisher DM, Castagnoli K, Miller RD: Vecuronium kinetics and dynamics in anesthetized infants and children. Clin Pharmacol Ther 37:402–406, 1985
149. Khuenl-Brady KS, Mair P, Koller J: Antagonism of vecuronium by one of its metabolites *in vitro*. Eur J Pharmacol 222:153–156, 1992
150. Durant NN, Marshall IG, Savage DS, et al: The neuromuscular autonomic blocking activities of pancuronium, Org NC 45 and other pancuronium analogues, in the cat. J Pharm Pharmacol 31:831, 1979
151. Marshall IG, Gibb AJ, Durant NN: Neuromuscular and vagal blocking actions of pancuronium bromide, its metabolites, and vecuronium bromide (ORG NC45) and its potential metabolism in the anaesthetized cat. Br J Anaesth 55:703–714, 1983
152. Ducharme J, Donati F: Pharmacokinetics and pharmacodynamics of steroidal muscle relaxants. Anesthesiol Clin North Am 11:283–307, 1993
153. Segredo V, Shin YS, Sharma ML, et al: Pharmacokinetics, neuromuscular effects, and biodisposition of 3-desacetylvecuronium (Org 7268) in cats. Anesthesiology 74:1052–1059, 1991
154. Smith CL, Hunter JM, Jones RS: Vecuronium infusions in patients with renal failure in an ITU. Anaesthesia 42:387–393, 1987
155. Segredo V, Matthay MA, Sharma ML, Gruenke LD, Caldwell JE, Miller RD: Prolonged neuromuscular blockade after long-term administration of vecuronium in two critically ill patients. Anesthesiology 72:566–570, 1990
156. Coursin DB, Klasek G, Goelzer SL: Increased requirements for continuously infused vecuronium in critically ill patients. Anesth Analg 69:518–521, 1989
157. Bell CF, Hunter JM, Jones RS, Utting JE: Use of atracurium and vecuronium in patients with oesophageal varices. Br J Anaesth 57:160–168, 1985
158. Hunter JM, Parker CJR, Bell CF, Jones RS, Utting JE: The use of different doses of vecuronium in patients with liver dysfunction. Br J Anaesth 57:758–764, 1985
159. Lebrault C, Berger JL, D'Hollander AA, Gomeli R, Henzel D, Duvaldestin P: Pharmacokinetics and pharmacodynamics of vecuronium (ORG NC45) in patients with cirrhosis. Anesthesiology 62:601–605, 1985
160. Lebrault C, Duvaldestin P, Henzel D, Chauvin M, Guesnon P: Pharmacokinetics and pharmacodynamics of vecuronium in patients with cholestasis. Br J Anaesth 58:983–987, 1986
161. McIndewar IC, Marshall RJ: Interactions between the neuromuscular blocking drug ORG NC45 and some anesthetic, analgesic and antimicrobial agents. Br J Anaesth 53:785–791, 1981
162. Anagnostou JM, Bell GC: Effects of metronidazole on neuromuscular transmission in rabbits. Anesth Analg 68:S10, 1989
163. d'Hollander A, Agoston S, Capouet V: Failure of metronidazole to alter a vecuronium neuromuscular blockade in humans. Anesthesiology 63:99–102, 1985
164. Lien CA, Matteo RS, Ornstein E, Schwartz AE, Diaz J: Distribution, elimination, and action of vecuronium in the elderly. Anesth Analg 73:39–42, 1991

165. McCarthy GJ, Elliott P, Mirakhur RK, Cooper R, Sharpe TDE, Clarke RSJ: Onset and duration of action of vecuronium in the elderly: comparison with adults. Acta Anaesthesiol Scand 36:383–386, 1992
166. d'Hollander AA, Massaux F, Nevelsteen M, Agoston S: Age-dependent dose-response relationship of ORG NC 45 in anaesthetized patients. Br J Anaesth 54:653–658, 1982
167. Rupp SM, Castagnoli KD, Fisher DM, Miller RD: Pancuronium and vecuronium pharmacokinetics and pharmacodynamics in younger and elderly patients. Anesthesiology 67:45–49, 1987
168. McCarthy GJ, Cooper R, Stanley JC, Mirakhur RK: Dose-response relationships for neostigmine antagonism of vecuronium-induced neuromuscular block in adults and the elderly. Br J Anaesth 69:281–283, 1992
169. Harrison MJ, Gunn K: Weight determined dosage of vecuronium bromide. Anaesthesia 44:692, 1989
170. Schwartz AE, Matteo RS, Ornstein E, et al: Pharmacokinetics and pharmacodynamics of vecuronium in the obese surgical patient. Anesth Analg 74:515, 1992
171. Fahey MR, Morris RB, Miller RD, Nguyen TL, Upton RA: Pharmacokinetics of Org NC45 (Norcuron) in patients with and without renal failure. Br J Anaesth 53:1049–1053, 1981
172. Hunter JM, Jones RS, Utting JE: Comparison of vecuronium, atracurium and tubocurarine in normal patients and in patients with no renal function. Br J Anaesth 56:941, 1984
173. Lynam DP, Cronnelly R, Castagnoli KP, Canfell C, Caldwell J, Arden J, Miller RD: The pharmacokinetics and pharmacodynamics of vecuronium in patients anesthetized with isoflurane with normal renal function or with renal failure. Anesthesiology 69:227–231, 1988
174. Meistelman C, Lienhart A, Leveque C, Bitker MO, Pigot B, Viars P: Pharmacology of vecuronium in patients with end-stage renal failure. Eur J Anaesthesiol 3:153–158, 1986
175. Peschaud JL, Kienlen J, Rey G, Marres F, Momas I, d'Athis F, du Cailar J: Pharmacodynamics of vecuronium in patients with and without renal failure. Anesthesiology 73:A916, 1990
176. Slater RM, Polard BJ, Doran BRH: Prolonged neuromuscular blockade with vecuronium in renal failure. Anaesthesia 43:250, 1988
177. Bevan DR, Donati F, Gyasi MB, Williams A: Cumulation of vecuronium in renal failure. Anesthesiology 61:A296, 1984
178. Goldberg ME, Marr AT, Starsnic MA, Ritter DE, Sosis M, Larijani GE: Does vecuronium accumulate in renal transplant patients? Anesth Analg 66:S68, 1987
179. Lepage JY, Malinge M, Cozian A, Pinaud M, Blanloeil Y, Souron R: Vecuronium and atracurium in patients with end-stage renal failure: a comparative study. Br J Anaesth 59:1004–1010, 1987
180. Mirakhur RK, Gibson FM, Clarke RSJ, Brady MM: Monitoring of neuromuscular block with atracurium, vecuronium, pancuronium and d-tubocurarine using train-of-four stimulation. Anesthesiology 65:A110, 1986
181. Fletcher JE, Sebel PS, Mick SA, Van Duys J, Ryan K: Comparison of the train-of-four fade profiles produced by vecuronium and atracurium. Br J Anaesth 68:207–208, 1992
182. Gibson FM, Mirakhur RK: Train-of-four fade during onset of neuromuscular block with nondepolarising neuromuscular blocking agents. Acta Anaesthesiol Scand 33:204–206, 1989
183. Raynes MM, Chisholm R, Woolner DF, Gibbs JM: A clinical comparison of atracurium and vecuronium in women undergoing laparoscopy. Anaesth Intensive Care 15:310–316, 1987

14

DAVID G. SILVERMAN / RAJINDER K. MIRAKHUR

Nondepolarizing Relaxants of the 1990s

The 1990s should benefit from the development of a nondepolarizing relaxant (NDR) of short duration (mivacurium) and one of more rapid onset (rocuronium). Their features are summarized in Table 12-1 and detailed below. Features shared with other agents are discussed in the relevant chapters.

◆ MIVACURIUM

Mivacurium chloride (Mivacron) is the first NDR with a brief duration of action. Mivacurium's ED_{95} is 0.06–0.08 mg · kg^{-1}. Consistent with most other NDRs, its onset time is 2.5–4.0 minutes after a dose of 2 times its ED_{95}; however, in contrast to other agents, the time to return of twitch height to 95% of baseline (Dur_{95}) is only 25–30 minutes after this dose of mivacurium.[1-13]

Mivacurium consists of three isomers, two of which (trans-trans and cis-trans) are far (>10-fold) more active than and more plentiful than the third (cis-cis) isomer.[3,14,15] This is rather fortunate, since the cis-cis isomer has a much longer half-time of elimination ($t_{1/2elim}$).[16]

Mivacurium's effective duration is approximately 33–50% that of atracurium or vecuronium and 200–300% that of succinylcholine (SCh). After a dose of 0.15 mg · kg^{-1} the *return of a detectable twitch* was evident within 10–15 minutes, the Dur_{95} was only 25 minutes, and T_4/T_1 was above 0.7 only 4 minutes later.[12] With block as deep as 99% twitch depression, *reversal after mivacurium takes place in less time* and with greater reliability than after other NDRs. The drug's rapid metabolism makes it practical to allow spontaneous recovery (without reversal) in many cases.[12,17]

Mivacurium is *metabolized by pseudocholinesterase* at a rate 70–88% of that for SCh.[12,18] It is metabolized to a monoester, a quaternary alcohol, and a dicarboxylic acid, each of which is inactive and does not readily cross the blood-brain barrier. Clearance averages 55–70 mL · kg^{-1} · min^{-1}.[3,19] This rate is at least 10-fold greater than the clearance rate of atracurium or vecuronium.[20,21] Mivacurium has been reported to have an in vivo $t_{1/2elim}$ of 16.9–18.4 minutes.[3,19] Clearance of the active isomers is much faster[14,16] than that of their less potent cis-cis counterpart, with a $t_{1/2elim}$ of only 2–3 minutes. In healthy individuals, the active isomers were "no longer present in the plasma" within 15 minutes of a 0.15 mg · kg^{-1} dose.[3]

Probably as a result of its rapid clearance, the *onset and depth of mivacurium-induced block may demonstrate high intersubject variability.*[22–24] The onset of mivacurium may be accelerated by pretreatment with a priming dose of mivacurium or of another NDR. Pancuronium may be particularly effective[24]; its inhibitory effect on pseudocholinesterase (Chap. 17) may temper the effect of rapid metabolism on mivacurium's onset. Onset may also be accelerated by increasing the intubating dose so long as one is cognizant of potential histamine release (see below).

The *recovery index* (RI_{25-75}) for mivacurium is relatively independent of dose (Fig. 14-1), and the overall *duration is less affected by a high dose or repeat dosing* than are the durations of most other NDRs.[1,5,12,25] Nevertheless, there is some prolongation of effect after high doses[1,23] or repeat doses.[25] Overall, it appears that increasing the dose 3-fold only increases the duration of action by approximately 50%.[1] The magnitude and duration of block appear to be less affected than other NDRs by *volatile agents*;[6] nevertheless, a decrease in ED_{95} and prolongation of block are noted with isoflurane[13] and especially enflurane.[4] These effects may be most marked during infusion.[26,27]

As noted above, the metabolism of mivacurium is primarily by pseudocholinesterase. As for SCh, pseudocholinesterase metabolism of mivacurium

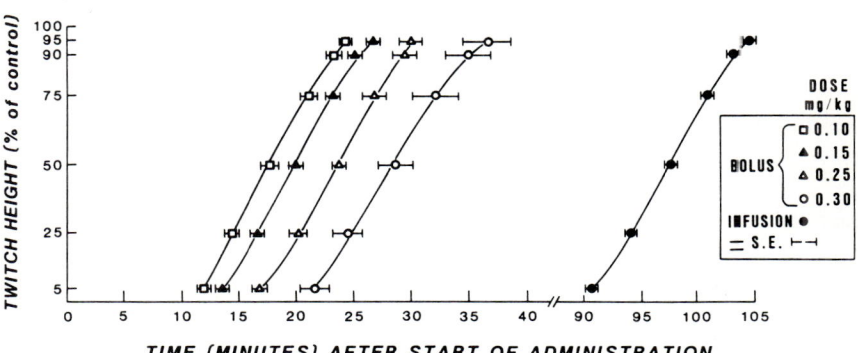

FIGURE 14-1 Comparative mean spontaneous recovery profiles (5–95% recovery) of response to single twitch stimulation after various bolus doses and after 38 infusions of mivacurium. Intervals from 25% to 75% and from 5% to 95% twitch recovery do not differ significantly among regimens. The data suggest that mivacurium evinces relatively little accumulation. (Reproduced with permission from Savarese JJ, et al: The clinical pharmacology of mivacurium chloride (BW1090U). Anesthesiology 68:723, 1988.[12])

begins before the relaxant reaches the neuromuscular junction (NMJ); as little as 0.03 mg · kg^{-1} of mivacurium (normally the ED$_{10}$ dose) may elicit 100% paralysis in patients who are homozygous for the *atypical pseudocholinesterase allele*[31] and thus are virtually incapable of rapid mivacurium hydrolysis. Mivacurium's t$_{½elim}$ increases as pseudocholinesterase activity decreases (but more so in rats than humans).[3,12,18,28,29] Even among "normal" patients, there may be a relationship between infusion requirements and pseudocholinesterase activity.[28,29] Significant prolongation of mivacurium is noted in the presence of *abnormal enzyme*.[4,30-35] (The multiple causes of abnormal enzyme activity are detailed in Chapter 17.) The block after 0.2 mg · kg^{-1} was prolonged up to 50% in patients who were heterozygous for the *atypical pseudocholinesterase* allele.[4,30] Block after 0.03 mg · kg^{-1} was markedly prolonged in four patients who were known to be homozygous for atypical pseudocholinesterase: it required 62 minutes (range, 26–128 minutes) for reappearance of the first response to train-of-four stimulation after what would normally have been the ED$_{10}$ dose.[31] Following administration of 0.12 mg · kg^{-1} to a 12 year-old who was later discovered to be homozygous for the atypical allele, response to the first stimulus of train-of-four stimulation was not noted for 3.5 hours.[32] As for SCh, the recovery from mivacurium can be accelerated by administration of purified human butyryl cholinesterase.[36]

Clearance may be reduced significantly in the context of *hepatic failure*.[3] Following 0.15 mg · kg^{-1}, clearance was less than 50% of normal in patients undergoing liver transplantation; t$_{½elim}$ increased to 34 minutes (vs. 18 minutes in controls), the Dur$_{25}$ averaged 57 minutes (vs. 19 minutes), RI$_{25-75}$ averaged 16 minutes (vs. 5.5 minutes), and the Dur$_{95}$ averaged 86 minutes (vs. 27 minutes).[3] This prolongation may be attributable to decreased pseudocholinesterase activity and increased volume of distribution. The consequences of *renal failure* tend to be less dramatic but are still apparent,[3,37] and occasionally appear to be marked.[38] In one series, t$_{½elim}$ increased to 34 minutes (vs. 18 in controls), the Dur$_{25}$ averaged 30 minutes (vs. 19 minutes), RI averaged 11.5 minutes (vs. 5.5 minutes), and Dur$_{95}$ averaged 51 minutes (vs. 27 minutes).[3] The effect of renal failure may be attributable, at least in part, to decreased pseudocholinesterase activity,[37] but this was not confirmed in a more recent report which concluded that the slightly longer duration of block in patients with renal failure "is not fully explained by the pharmacokinetics."[3] In a preliminary study in *elderly* patients, maximum block, time to maximum block, and times to 5%, 25%, and 95% recovery did not differ significantly from values in younger adults.[39]

As for other NDRs, recovery from mivacurium-induced block may be accelerated by anticholinesterase administration (i.e., *reversal*).[5,9,12,25,40-42] For example, neostigmine, 0.06 mg · kg^{-1}, accelerated the time between 25% to 95% recovery of twitch height after mivacurium from approximately 10 minutes to approximately 6 minutes.[12] Neostigmine-induced reversal of mivacurium-induced block takes approximately 33% and 67% of the time required for reversal after NDRs of long and intermediate duration, respectively. The effectiveness of neostigmine reversal is reassuring, for reversal agents inhibit pseudocholinesterase as well as acetylcholinesterase,[43–49] and thus theoretically may interfere with mivacurium's spontaneous recovery. This would be least likely with edrophonium, since it causes the least pseudocholinesterase inhibition (Chap. 17). In the context of markedly prolonged mivacurium-induced block due to pseudocholinesterase deficiency, reversal tends to be effective after 50–70% recovery of single twitch,[31] but earlier attempts at reversal may be unsuccessful.[32]

Mivacurium may be particularly beneficial when administered as a *continuous infusion*,[8,9,12,17,23,25,28,29,50] typically at rates between 6–8 µg · kg^{-1} · min^{-1} (0.36–0.48 mg · kg^{-1} · hr^{-1}) during balanced anesthesia and 4–5 µg · kg^{-1} · min^{-1} (0.24–0.30 mg · kg^{-1} · hr^{-1}) during enflurane anesthesia. These are approximately the same rates that are typically used for atracurium[25]; however, they constitute hourly rates that are 4–6 times the ED_{95} of mivacurium and only 1.5–2 times the ED_{95} of atracurium (because of mivacurium's very rapid metabolism) (Table 14-1). As for other NDRs, there is wide intersubject variability with respect to infusion requirements.

The *recovery time after an infusion* of mivacurium is half that after atracurium or vecuronium[28] and is not significantly different from that after a bolus dose (Fig. 14-1).[12,28] After infusions that maintained 95% twitch depression, spontaneous RI_{25-75} was approximately 6–7 minutes[12,17,23,27,28] and the time for T_4/T_1 to exceed 0.70 was approximately 17 minutes.[8,27] Recovery times may be slightly longer after a bolus dose plus infusion, which produced an RI_{25-75} of 9.6 minutes[50] and a time for recovery from 5% to 95% of baseline twitch height of 17 minutes[9] (vs. 14.5 minutes after a standard mivacurium infusion).[28] When the mivacurium-induced block was reversed with an anticholinesterase, the recovery time was similar to that after

TABLE 14-1
Infusion Rates and Recovery Times

Drug	Typical Infusion Rate (µg · kg^{-1} · min^{-1})	5% to 95% Recovery Time (min)	25% to 75% Recovery Time (min)
Succinylcholine*	20–60	8	5
Mivacurium	6–8	14	7
Atracurium	6–8	25	11
Vecuronium†	1–2	30	14
Rocuronium	10–11	30	14

Note: Rates and times are estimates for typical intraoperative infusions. Infusions should be titrated according to neuromuscular response, with attempts to taper as rapidly as possible in the ICU setting.
*Prolonged infusion of succinylcholine may lead to phase 2 block and delayed recovery.
†Prolonged infusion of vecuronium may lead to prolonged recovery due to accumulation of parent drug and metabolites.

SCh[8,9,25,41,50]: post infusion, recovery from T_1 at 8% of baseline to T_4/T_1 of 0.7 averaged 17 minutes if recovery was allowed to proceed spontaneously; 11 minutes after neostigmine, 0.04 mg · kg^{-1}; and 8 minutes after edrophonium, 0.75 mg · kg^{-1}.[8]

As is the case with other benzylisoquinolinium compounds, mivacurium may elicit *histamine release*. As with atracurium, cardiovascular effects are minimal with doses less than or equal to 2 times the ED_{95},[5,6,13,25,51,52] although facial flushing may be noted.[6,41] Rapid bolus administration of more than 2 times the ED_{95} elicits histamine release and may cause a transient (<5-minute) 12–59% decrease in mean blood pressure.[5,13,23,25,52,53] In one series, bolus injections of 0.15, 0.2, and 0.25 mg · kg^{-1} resulted in greater than 20% reductions in blood pressure in none of eight, four of seven, and three of eight patients[25]; all decreases in blood pressure occurred within 2 minutes, and spontaneous recovery commenced within 1 minute.[25] At doses of 0.20 and 0.25 mg · kg^{-1}, a slow bolus (over 60 seconds) occasionally caused transient hypotension in patients undergoing cardiac surgery.[54]

As discussed in Chapter 11, *histamine release may be reduced* by divided dosing or by injection over 60–75 seconds[5,52,54–56] and perhaps over as little as 30 seconds.[57] For example, the average peak histamine level after 0.25 mg · kg^{-1} increased to 132% of control after bolus administration over 10–15 seconds but did not change after injection over 60 seconds.[52] The tendency to release histamine is also less on repeated dosing.[52] Divided dosing with mivacurium has been shown to be effective.[57–61] A recent study indicated that 0.15 mg · kg^{-1} followed 30 seconds later by 0.10 mg · kg^{-1} provided good to excellent intubating conditions at 90 seconds after the initial dose of relaxant with an incidence similar to that after SCh; there was no significant difference in the hemodynamic profiles between the two groups.[57] However, it should be noted that divided dosing may expose more mivacurium to pseudocholinesterase, and thus the depth of block after divided dosing may be less than that achieved after rapid bolus administration of the same total dose.[58]

Consistent with other NDRs (Chap. 10), the use of *mivacurium in children* aged 2–10 years is characterized by a higher ED_{95} (0.09–0.12 mg · kg^{-1}), higher infusion requirements (13–16 µg · kg^{-1} · min^{-1} or 0.78–0.96 mg · kg · hr^{-1}), faster onset, faster recovery, and less pronounced evidence of histamine release.[26,62–64] In children recovering from an infusion that maintained 95% twitch height depression, the Dur_{95} was 19 minutes during halothane anesthesia and 12 minutes during nitrous oxide–narcotic anesthesia.[26] These times were accelerated to 6 minutes and 3.3 minutes after edrophonium-induced reversal.[26] In children recovering from a bolus dose, reversal with edrophonium, 0.3 mg · kg^{-1} (and atropine, 0.03 mg · kg^{-1}), when T_1 returned to 43% ± 2% of control resulted in 95% recovery in 3.3 ± 0.6 (SEM) minutes.[63] As is the case for other NDRs, *infants are more sensitive* than older children to the same µg · kg^{-1} dose and especially the same µg · m^{-2} dose.[65] The ED_{95} in infants was 0.075 mg · kg^{-1} or 1.4 mg · m^{-2}.[65]

◆ ROCURONIUM

Rocuronium (ORG 9426, Zemuron [United States and Canada], Esmeron), a desacetoxy derivative of vecuronium, is a new aminosteroid of relatively low potency. Its ED_{95} is 0.25–0.30 mg · kg^{-1}. Rocuronium shares the intermediate duration of action of atracurium and vecuronium; however, the *onset* of rocuronium-induced block is considerably faster.[66–97]

The most striking feature of rocuronium is the brief time it requires in order to cause detectable twitch depression (*"lag time"*).[68,75,92] Its accelerated onset then persists until maximum twitch depression is attained. In patients receiving thiopental, fentanyl, and 65% nitrous oxide in oxygen, the lag time after 0.5 mg · kg^{-1} of rocuronium was one-half that after 0.085 mg · kg^{-1} of vecuronium (36 and 71 seconds, respectively).[92] On stimulation with single twitch at 10-second intervals, 0.6 mg · kg^{-1} (approximately 2 × ED_{95}) had a lag time at the adductor pollicis of only 25.8 ± 6.2 (SD) seconds and achieved maximum twitch depression in 88.9 ± 36.9 seconds (and had a Dur_{25} of 30.5 ± 7.5 minutes).[68] In that study, the degrees of adductor pollicis twitch depression averaged 89% and 98% at 60 and 90 seconds, respectively.[68] At 90 seconds, 17 of 20 patients had excellent and 3 of 20 patients had good *intubating conditions*.[68] The onset of rocuronium was 10–15 seconds faster after 0.9 mg · kg^{-1},[70] but still slower than after SCh. Similar overall intubating conditions were reported in other studies.[75,78,85,92,93] In patients receiving propofol, alfentanil, and nitrous oxide in oxygen, rocuronium, 0.6 mg · kg^{-1}, and SCh, 1 mg · kg^{-1}, produced 95% twitch depression in 1.2 ± 0.5 minutes and 0.8 ± 0.1 minute, respectively (single twitch at 0.1 Hz).[85] Of the 20 patients who received rocuronium, 17 had excellent and 3 had good intubating conditions at 1 minute; of the 10 patients who received SCh, 8 had excellent, 1 had good, and 1 had poor conditions.[85] Another group reported onset times of 74 and 131 seconds, respectively, after SCh and 2 times the ED_{95} of rocuronium.[73]

The *shorter lag time* after rocuronium may be attributable to its *low potency*, which leads to the administration of a higher "molecular load." This, in turn, is faster at overcoming the delays posed by buffered diffusion (Chap. 7).[98] This effect may be augmented by rocuronium's relatively low plasma binding (and hence three times greater free plasma concentration compared to vecuronium).[99] Other features of rocuronium-induced block are similar to vecuronium-induced block. Rocuronium's propensity to elicit fade differs only slightly from that of vecuronium.[100,101] The relative prejunctional effects of these compounds are similar,[100,101] as is their potential to induce channel block.[77] In view of its potential use as an agent to facilitate rapid intubation of the trachea, it is important to note that there appears to be little interaction between rocuronium and anesthetic induction agents.[102]

It should be noted that rapid onset has not been attained in every rocuronium-treated subject,[66,68,75,82] and a regimen that ensures intersubject consistency needs to be established before an NDR such as rocuronium can be recommended without qualifications for rapid-sequence intubation.[103] Perhaps this will be accomplished with higher doses, priming techniques (but not necessarily[74]), or a combination of rocuronium and other relaxants. It should be borne in mind that "excellent" conditions are not always attained with SCh, and they are not necessarily required for intubation unless coughing or any movement is unacceptable.

As with other NDRs, onset time is shorter and sensitivity to NDR less at the larynx and diaphragm than at the adductor pollicis (Chap. 3).[104] While 0.5 mg · kg^{-1} typically caused greater than 95% depression of T_1 at the adductor pollicis, it typically caused less than 80% depression at the larynx.[104] However, after rocuronium, 0.5 mg · kg^{-1}, maximum block (77% ± 5%) was attained in 1.4 ± 0.1 minutes at the larynx, while maximum block (99% ± 1%) was attained in 2.4 ± 0.2 (SEM) minutes at the adductor pollicis. At each site, the onset was faster than after a comparable dose of vecuronium, after which maximum block was obtained in 3.3 minutes at the larynx and 5.7 minutes at the adductor pollicis.[105] The time for onset of rocuronium at the larynx was only slightly longer than the 0.9 minute reported for SCh.[106]

As for vecuronium, *redistribution* is primarily responsible for the decline in rocuronium's plasma concentration. Rocuronium's measured $t_{1/2elim}$ appears to be longer than that for vecuronium,[88] possibly because its low potency leads to the use of high doses that allow detectable levels to be present for a longer time. The $t_{1/2elim}$ averaged approximately 97 minutes in patients undergoing general anesthesia with isoflurane.[69] No putative metabolites have been detected. The 17-hydroxy metabolite is approximately 20 times less potent than the parent molecule and thus is unlikely to contribute to neuromuscular block.[77] This may prove to be an *advantage over vecuronium,* which has an active (3-OH) metabolite.

Rocuronium is less lipid soluble than vecuronium and has a smaller volume of distribution.[93] As with vecuronium, the *duration* of action of rocuronium increases with *increased doses:* the Dur_{25} increased from 30 minutes to 45 minutes as the dose was increased from 0.6 to 0.9 mg · kg^{-1},[70] RI_{25-75} increased from 7 minutes to 18 minutes, and the Dur_{25} increased from 14 minutes to 43 minutes as the dose was increased from 0.3 to 0.68 mg · kg^{-1}.[82] As with vecuronium, the effect of rocuronium is likely to be prolonged in hepatic failure,[80,96] obesity, and in the elderly.[107,108]

Rocuronium's action is prolonged by *hepatic failure* and by removal of the liver from the circulation.[80,96] In one study, $t_{1/2elim}$ increased to 173 minutes (vs. 79 minutes in controls), while clearance decreased from 3.4 to 3.0 mL · min^{-1} · kg^{-1} and the volume of distribution increased from 0.17 to 0.32 L · kg^{-1}.[80]

Although studies in the cat have suggested that rocuronium is predominantly excreted via the *liver* (predominantly unchanged),[96] up to 30% is excreted by the *kidneys* in man.[93] *Renal failure* is without marked statistically significant clinical effects,[69,88] nor was renal pedicle ligation in the cat.[96] In one study, clearance was reduced in patients with renal failure, but half-lives and recovery times were not significantly prolonged[69]; however, there was greater interindividual variation. In another study,[88] total plasma clearance and the volume of the central compartment did not differ between control and renal transplant patients. However, the volume of distribution was greater in the renal transplant patients (264 ± 19 mL · kg^{-1}) than in control patients (207 ± 14 mL · kg^{-1}). This resulted in a longer elimination half-life in renal transplant patients (97.2 ± 17.3 minutes) compared to controls (70.9 ± 4.7 minutes). The authors concluded that renal failure and renal transplantation alter the distribution but not the clearance of rocuronium. In cats, renal pedicle ligation slowed plasma clearance, but this effect was offset by increased hepatic clearance, resulting in relatively little prolongation of clinical effect.[96]

In a recent series of 100 patients, there was no difference in potency between *elderly and younger patients;* however, the onset was 20% slower, and the recovery index (RI_{25-75}) and the Dur_{25} were 25–40% longer in the elderly group.[109] These observations are consistent with the data reported for other NDRs (except atracurium) and probably reflect the decreases in hepatic and renal perfusion associated with aging.

The requisite rocuronium *infusion rate* to maintain 90–95% twitch depression is approximately 10–11 μg · kg^{-1} · min^{-1} (0.60–0.66 mg · kg · hr^{-1}) under balanced anesthesia and 8 μg · kg^{-1} · min^{-1} (0.48 mg · kg · hr^{-1}) under isoflurane anesthesia.[110] Postinfusion recovery is similar to that after vecuronium. In *children,* the rate to maintain 95% depression was 12.3 μg · kg^{-1} · min^{-1} (0.74 mg · kg · hr^{-1}) when halothane was used; the RI_{25-75} was 12.6 minutes and the time for T_4/T_1 to exceed 0.75 averaged 29 minutes.[111] Consistent with what is observed with other NDRs, rocuronium's rate of onset appears to be faster in children (1.5–7.5 years).[95,97,112]

In low doses, rocuronium has a *cardiovascular profile* similar to that of vecuronium.[72,77,87,92,93] Like vecuronium, it does not cause histamine release.[113,114] However, at doses approaching 3–5 times its ED_{95}, it may cause increased heart rate.[72,77,82] In animals, the vagolytic dose was 4.4–7.4 times the neuromuscular blocking dose.[72,77] Doses of 1.1 and 2.5 mg · kg^{-1} did not induce cardiovascular changes in two patients.[66] In patients undergoing coronary artery bypass surgery, 2 times the ED_{95} of rocuronium was associated with a 7% increase in heart rate, while an equivalent dose of vecuronium was associated with a 4–5% decrease.[115] Administration of 0.6 mg · kg^{-1} to children (aged 4–12 years) receiving halothane resulted in a transient increase in heart rate from 82 to 94 beats · min^{-1}.[97] No change in heart rate was noted on assessment 5 minutes after 0.8 mg · kg^{-1}.[95] As expected, this NDR does not trigger malignant hyperthermia.[116]

Discussion Questions ◆

a. Why might it be easier to maintain an *infusion* with *mivacurium* than with *SCh?*

b. Will *reversal with neostigmine* accelerate return of twitch height if administered at 25% recovery of twitch height after *mivacurium*? Is it necessary to use a reversal agent?

c. What special features about *mivacurium* make use of a *nerve stimulator* particularly desirable during its administration?

d. Why might it be argued that the discrepancy between the concentrations achieved at the *diaphragm* and *adductor pollicis* during onset of block is greater for *mivacurium* than for other NDRs (which are metabolized less rapidly)?

e. What features of *rocuronium* contribute to its relatively *fast onset*?

f. Compare high-dose (e.g., $4 \times ED_{95}$) vecuronium and high-dose *rocuronium* as NDRs for *rapid-sequence induction*.

g. Categorize each long-, intermediate-, and short-acting relaxant's dependence on *renal elimination* as: 100%, 80–100%, 60–90%, 40–60%, 10–20%, or less than 10%.

h. Why is the calculated ED_{95} of a short- or intermediate-duration NDR higher when a *traditional cumulative dosing technique* is used than when a single bolus is administered?

i. Why would increasing the *dose of rocuronium* from 0.3 to 0.9 mg · kg^{-1} improve *intubating conditions*?

Answers ◆

a. *Mivacurium's* brief duration and relatively little accumulation allow it to be titrated as effectively as SCh and permit nearly as rapid recovery. Recovery times after an infusion have been similar; however, after a bolus plus infusion of mivacurium, the recovery tends to take longer. In such cases, recovery may be accelerated to the rate of recovery after SCh by administering an anticholinesterase, provided the block is not too profound.[8,9,25]

   In some aspects, mivacurium is superior to *SCh* for continuous infusions. It avoids the undesirable systemic effects of SCh and will not produce the dual (phase 1 plus phase 2) block that may complicate maintenance of and recovery from an SCh infusion. In light of this, it may be more readily reversed by anticholinesterase administration in patients with pseudocholinesterase deficiency.[33]

b. After mivacurium, *neostigmine accelerated recovery* from 75% block by 4 minutes (40%) vs. the spontaneous recovery pattern.[12] "While this difference is statistically significant, in many cases such a minor acceleration of recovery may not be clinically important."[12] Additionally, it was noted that T_4/T_1 is greater than 0.7 within only 4 minutes of spontaneous recovery to Dur_{95},[12] and that once a T_4/T_1 ratio of 0.4 is attained during recovery, a T_4/T_1 of 0.7 or greater is attained in 5.2 ± 2.3 (SD) minutes (range, 2.1–10.4 minutes).[117] The latter may be particularly relevant since visual assessment of the response to ulnar nerve stimulation may miss fade when T_4/T_1 is greater than 0.4, but it can usually detect fade when T_4/T_1 is less than 0.4 (Chap. 5). Thus, if no fade is apparent, one may be able to withhold reversal agent and simply wait for spontaneous recovery. Obviously, the adequacy of recovery should be assessed clinically. Furthermore, the effectiveness of subsequent spontaneous recovery can only be relied on if a normal pattern of recovery is apparent (i.e., there is no evidence of a pseudocholinesterase deficiency).

c. Several features about *mivacurium* make use of the *nerve stimulator* particularly helpful during its administration. Most of these features are direct consequences of mivacurium's rapid clearance. This may lead to "surprisingly" rapid return of movement; it provides for prompt responses to titration (e.g., continuous infusion); and it may allow anesthesiologists to rely on spontaneous recovery rather than reversal. In addition, the rare patient with a significant pseudocholinesterase deficiency or abnormality will be particularly sensitive to this drug.

d. It may be that the discrepancy between onset of block at the *diaphragm* and at the *adductor pollicis* (Chap. 3) is greater for *mivacurium* than for any other NDR. Two factors must be taken into account: (1) the diaphragm and vocal cord muscles are less sensitive than the adductor pollicis to NDRs, and (2) the onset of block at the diaphragm (and vocal cords) is faster than onset at the adductor pollicis. After a bolus dose of vecuronium, these factors tend to "offset" one another, so that the diaphragm and adductor pollicis ultimately develop similar depths of block.[105] Because equilibration of muscle relaxant at the diaphragm occurs earlier in the distribution phase, the diaphragm is exposed to a higher plasma concentration of relaxant. The rapid metabolism of mivacurium may serve to accentuate the impact of faster onset at the diaphragm, since the concentration may have decreased more markedly by the time equilibration is achieved at the adductor pollicis. This may explain why good to excellent intubating conditions have been reported despite only partial mivacurium-induced paralysis of the adductor pollicis muscle.[9,50] Conversely, block of the adductor pollicis does not ensure excellent intubating conditions. Mivacurium-induced paralysis of laryngeal muscles actually may start to regress relatively long before it decreases at the adductor pollicis.

e. *Rocuronium's rapid onset* may be attributable to the large molecular load delivered to the NMJ. Such molecular loading leads to more rapid attainment of desired concentrations in the NMJ. The large number of rocuronium molecules at the NMJ is a consequence of rocuronium's *low potency* (i.e., more molecules are required for a given effective dose)[98] and *low protein binding* (i.e., more free drug).[99]

f. "High-dose" rocuronium may prove to be preferable to high-dose vecuronium for rapid attainment of paralysis. The onset of rocuronium is faster than onset of an equipotent dose of vecuronium. Neither drug elicits significant histamine release; however, rocuronium may cause some vagolysis in doses greater than 4 times its ED_{95}. It should be remembered that the duration of each agent increases in proportion to the dose that is administered. Overall duration may be decreased by replacing high-dose vecuronium (e.g., >4 × ED_{95}) with a moderate dose of rocuronium (e.g., 3 × ED_{95}).

g. *Dependence on renal elimination* (i.e., percent excreted in urine):
   - 95–100%: gallamine, decamethonium, doxacurium
   - 60–95%: metocurine, pancuronium, pipecuronium, alcuronium, fazadinium
   - 40–60%: d-tubocurarine
   - 10–20%: vecuronium, rocuronium
   - <10%: atracurium, mivacurium, SCh

   Remember, NDRs are highly ionized, water-soluble substances that are filtered by the renal glomerulus and are not reabsorbed in the proximal tubule.

h. The calculated ED_{95} of a short- or intermediate-duration NDR is higher when a *cumulative dosing technique* is used because the effects of an earlier dose wane before a subsequent dose has reached its peak effect. This may be particularly evident for mivacurium,[22] which may be partially metabolized even before it reaches the NMJ.

i. There are two major reasons why increasing the dose of rocuronium from 0.3 to 0.9 mg · kg^{-1} should improve intubating conditions:
   1. As detailed in Chapter 7, increasing the dose of relaxant increases its rate of onset. This is logical, since you are delivering more molecules of relaxant to the effector sites.
   2. As detailed in Chapter 3, increasing the dose of relaxant above the ED_{95} for the adductor pollicis increases the likelihood of achieving total paralysis of the diaphragm and vocal cords. The ED_{95} at these sites may be 1.5–2 times greater than that at the adductor pollicis. Thus, a dose of approximately 0.6 mg · kg^{-1} may be required to provide an average of 95% depression of laryngeal and diaphragmatic function in most patients. To ensure complete paralysis of these muscles in virtually all patients would require an even larger dose. If one wished to administer rocuronium to provide rapid-sequence intubating conditions with minimal risk of coughing or movement, then a dose ≥ 0.9 mg · kg^{-1} may be required. (It remains to be determined whether such a dose would provide intubating conditions rapidly enough in all settings.)

References ◆

1. Basta SJ: Clinical pharmacology of mivacurium chloride: a review. J Clin Anesth 4:153–163, 1992

2. Basta SJ, Savarese JJ, Ali HH, et al: The neuromuscular pharmacology of NW B1090U in anesthetized patients. Anesthesiology 63:A318, 1985
3. Cook DR, Freeman JA, Lai AA, Kang Y, Stiller RL, Aggarwal S, Harrelson JC, Welch RM, Samara B: Pharmacokinetics of mivacurium in normal patients and in those with hepatic or renal failure. Br J Anaesth 69:580–585, 1992
4. Caldwell JE, Kitts JB, Heier T, Fahey MR, Lynam DP, Miller RD: The dose-response relationship of mivacurium chloride in humans during nitrous oxide–fentanyl or nitrous oxide–enflurane anesthesia. Anesthesiology 70:31–35, 1989
5. Choi WW, Mehta MP, Murray DJ, Sokoll MD, Forbes RB, Gergis SD, Abou-Donia M, Kirchner J: Neuromuscular and cardiovascular effects of mivacurium chloride in surgical patients receiving nitrous oxide–narcotic or nitrous oxide–isoflurane anaesthesia. Can J Anaesth 36:641–650, 1989
6. From RP, Pearson S, Choi WW, Abou-Donia M, Sokoll MD: Neuromuscular and cardiovascular effects of mivacurium chloride (BW B1090U) during nitrous oxide-fentanyl-thiopentone and nitrous oxide-halothane anaesthesia. Br J Anaesth 64:193–198, 1990
7. Gergis SD, Abou-Doria M, Kirchner J: Neuromuscular and cardiovascular effects of mivacurium chloride in surgical patients receiving nitrous oxide narcotic or nitrous oxide isoflurane anesthesia. Can J Anaesth 36:641–650, 1989
8. Goldhill DR, Whitehead JP, Emmott RS, Griffith A, Bracey BJ, Flynn PJ: Neuromuscular and clinical effects of mivacurium chloride in healthy adult patients during nitrous oxide–enflurane anesthesia. Br J Anaesth 67:289–295, 1991
9. Goldberg ME, Larijani GE, Azad SS, Sosis M, Seltzer JL, Ascher J, Weakly JN: Comparison of tracheal intubating conditions and neuromuscular blocking profiles after intubating doses of mivacurium chloride or succinylcholine in surgical outpatients. Anesth Analg 69:93–99, 1989
10. Pearson KS, From RP, Choi WW, Abou-Donia M, Sokoll MD: Neuromuscular and cardiovascular effects of mivacurium chloride (BW B1090U) during nitrous oxide-narcotic, nitrous oxide–halothane and nitrous oxide–isoflurane anesthesia in surgical patients. Middle East J Anaesthesiol 10(5):469–478, 1990
11. Savarese JJ, Ali HH, Basta SJ, Embree PB, Schwartz A, Halleem-Bottros L, Weakly JN, Batson AG: Ninety and 120-second tracheal intubation with BW B109U: clinical conditions with and without priming after fentanyl-thiopental induction. Anesthesiology 65:A283, 1986
12. Savarese JJ, Ali HH, Basta SJ, Embree PB, Scott RPF, Sunder N, Weakly JN, Wastila WB, El-Sayad HA: The clinical neuromuscular pharmacology of mivacurium chloride (BW B1090U): a short-acting nondepolarizing ester neuromuscular blocking drug. Anesthesiology 68:723–732, 1988
13. Weber S, Brandom BW, Powers DM, Sarner JB, Woelfel SK, Cook DR, Foster VJ, McNulty BF, Weakly JN: Mivacurium chloride (BW B1090U)-induced neuromuscular blockade during nitrous oxide–isoflurane and nitrous oxide–narcotic anesthesia in adult surgical patients. Anesth Analg 67:495–499, 1988
14. Head-Rapson AG, Devlin JC, Lovell GG, Parker CJR, Hunter JM: The pharmacokinetics of the isomers of mivacurium chloride in the healthy adult. Br J Anaesth 70:487P, 1993
15. Wray DL, Belmont MR, Maehr RB, Welch R, Wastila W: The pharmacokinetics of two isomers of mivacurium in the cat. Anesthesiology 75:A305, 1991
16. Lien CA, Schmith VD, Wargin WA, Kudlak DD, Savarese JJ: Pharmacokinetics and pharmacodynamics of mivacurium stereoisomers during a two-step infusion. Anesthesiology 77:A910, 1992
17. Diefenbach C, Mellinghoff H, Lynch J, Buzello W: Mivacurium: dose-response relationship and administration by repeated injection or infusion. Anesth Analg 74:420–423, 1992
18. Cook DR, Stiller RL, Weakly NJ: In vitro metabolism of mivacurium chloride (BW 1090) and succinylcholine. Anesth Analg 68:452–456, 1989
19. deBros F, Basta SJ, Ali HH, Wargin W, Welch R: Pharmacokinetics and pharmacodynamics of BW B1090U in healthy surgical patients receiving N_2O/O_2 isoflurane anesthesia. Anesthesiology 67:A609, 1987
20. Fahey MR, Rupp SM, Fisher DM, Miller RD, Sharma M, Canfell C, Castagnoli K, Hennis PJ: The pharmacokinetics and pharmacodynamics of atracurium in patients with and without renal failure. Anesthesiology 61:699–702, 1984

21. Lynam DP, Cronnelly R, Castagnoli KP, Canfell C, Caldwell J, Arden J, Miller RD: The pharmacokinetics and pharmacodynamics of vecuronium in patients anesthetized with isoflurane with normal renal function or with renal failure. Anesthesiology 69:227–231, 1988
22. Silverman DG, Brull SJ: Depth of block after divided doses of mivacurium spaced 60 seconds apart. Anesth Analg 77:164–167, 1993
23. Brandom BW, Woelfel SK, Cook DR, Weber S, Powers DM, Weakly JN: Comparison of mivacurium and suxamethonium administered by bolus and infusion. Br J Anaesth 62:488–493, 1989
24. Brandom BW, Meretoja OA, Taivainen T, Wirtavuori K: Accelerated onset and delayed recovery of neuromuscular block induced by mivacurium preceded by pancuronium in children. Anesth Analg 76:998–1003, 1993
25. Caldwell JE, Heier T, Kitts JB, Lynam DP, Fahey MR, Miller RD: Comparison of the neuromuscular block induced by mivacurium, suxamethonium or atracurium during nitrous oxide–fentanyl anaesthesia. Br J Anaesth 63:393–399, 1989
26. Alifimoff JK, Goudsouzian NG: Continuous infusion of mivacurium in children. Br J Anaesth 63:520–524, 1989
27. Powers DM, Brandom BW, Cook DR, Byers R, Sarner JB, Simpson K, Weber S, Woelfel SK, Foster VJ: Mivacurium infusion during nitrous oxide–isoflurane anesthesia: a comparison with nitrous oxide–opioid anesthesia. J Clin Anesth 4:123–126, 1992
28. Ali HH, Savarese JJ, Embree PB, Basta SJ, Stout RG, Bottros H, Weakly JN: Clinical pharmacology of mivacurium chloride (W B1090U) infusion: comparison with vecuronium and atracurium. Br J Anaesth 61:541–546, 1988
29. Brandom BW, Sarner JB, Woelfel SK, Dong ML, Horn MC, Borland LM, Cook DR, Foster VJ, McNulty BF, Weakly JN: Mivacurium infusion requirements in pediatric surgical patients during nitrous oxide–halothane and during nitrous oxide–narcotic anesthesia. Anesth Analg 71:16–22, 1990
30. Ostergaard D, Jensen FS, Jensen E, Viby-Mogensen J: Mivacurium induced neuromuscular blockade (NMB) in patients heterozygous for the atypical gene for plasma cholinesterase. Anesthesiology 71:A782, 1989
31. Ostergaard D, Jensen E, Jensen FS, Viby-Mogensen J: The duration of action of mivacurium-induced neuromuscular block in patients homozygous for the atypical plasma cholinesterase gene. Anesthesiology 75:A774, 1991
32. Peterson RS, Bailey PL, Kalameghan R, Ashwood ER: Prolonged neuromuscular block after mivacurium. Anesth Analg 76:194–196, 1993
33. Goudsouzian NG, d'Hollander AA, Viby-Mogensen J: Prolonged neuromuscular block from mivacurium in two patients with cholinesterase deficiency. Anesth Analg 77:183–185, 1993
34. Bevan DR: Prolonged mivacurium-induced neuromuscular block. Anesth Analg 77:4–6, 1993
35. Maddineni VR, Mirakhur RK: Prolonged neuromuscular block following mivacurium. Anesthesiology 78:1181–1184, 1993
36. Bownes PB, Hartman GS, Chiscolm D, Savarese JJ: Antagonism of mivacurium blockade by purified human butyryl cholinesterase in cats. Anesthesiology 77:A909, 1992
37. Phillips BJ, Hunter JM: Use of mivacurium chloride by constant infusion in the anephric patient. Br J Anaesth 67:653P–654P, 1991
38. Mangar D, Kirchhoff GT, Rose PL, Castellano FC: Prolonged neuromuscular block after mivacurium in a patient with end-stage renal disease. Anesth Analg 76:866–867, 1993
39. Basta SJ, Dresner DL, Shaff LP, Lai AA, Welch R: Neuromuscular effects and pharmacokinetics of mivacurium in elderly patients under isoflurane anesthesia. Anesth Analg 68:S18, 1989
40. Curran MJ, Shaff L, Savarese JJ, Ali HH, Risner M: Comparison of spontaneous recovery and neostigmine-accelerated recovery from mivacurium neuromuscular blockade. Anesthesiology 69:A528, 1988
41. Poler SM, Watcha MF, White PF: Mivacurium as an alternative to succinylcholine during outpatient laparoscopy. J Clin Anesth 4:127–133, 1992
42. Belmont MR, Maehr RB, Wastila WB, Savarese JJ: Pharmacodynamics and pharmaco-

kinetics of benzylisoquinolinium (curare-like) neuromuscular blocking drugs. Anesthesiol Clin North Am 11:251–281, 1993
43. Mirakhur RK, Lavery TD, Briggs LP, Clarke RSJ: Effects of neostigmine and pyridostigmine on serum cholinesterase activity. Can Anaesth Soc J 29:55–58, 1982
44. Mirakhur RK: Edrophonium and plasma cholinesterase activity. Can Anaesth Soc J 33:588–590, 1986
45. Sunew KY, Hicks RG: Effects of neostigmine and pyridostigmine on duration of succinylcholine action and pseudocholinesterase activity. Anesthesiology 49:188–191, 1978
46. Cook DR, Chakravorti S, Brandom BW, Stiller RL: Effects of neostigmine, edrophonium and succinylcholine on the *in vitro* metabolism of mivacurium: clinical correlates. Anesthesiology 77:A948, 1992
47. Bishop MJ, Hornbein TF: Prolonged effect of succinylcholine after neostigmine and pyridostigmine administration in patients with renal failure. Anesthesiology 58:384–386, 1983
48. Baraka A, Wakid N, Mansour R, Haddad W: Effect of neostigmine and pyridostigmine on the plasma cholinesterase activity. Br J Anaesth 53:849–851, 1981
49. Sakuma N, Hasimoto Y, Iwatsuki N: Effects of neostigmine and edrophonium on human erythrocyte acetylcholinesterase activity. Br J Anaesth 68:316–317, 1992
50. Shanks CA, Fragen RJ, Pemberton D, Katz JA, Risner ME: Mivacurium-induced neuromuscular blockade following single bolus doses and with continuous infusion during either balanced or enflurane anesthesia. Anesthesiology 71:362–366, 1989
51. Savarese JJ, Rosow CE, Embree PB, Schwartz AF, Basta SJ: A quantal analysis of the dose-response of mivacurium for plasma histamine increase, facial erythema, and arterial pressure decrease. Anesthesiology 69:A527, 1988
52. Savarese JJ, Ali HH, Basta SJ, Scott RPF, Embree PB, Wastila WB, Abou-Donia MM, Gelb C: The cardiovascular effects of mivacurium chloride (BW B1090U) in patients receiving nitrous oxide-opiate-barbiturate anesthesia. Anesthesiology 70:386–394, 1989
53. Forbes RB, Choi WW, Mehta MP, et al: Cardiovascular effects of BW B1090U during nitrous oxide-oxygen-narcotic anesthesia. Anesthesiology 67:A360, 1987
54. Stoops CM, Curtis CA, Kovach DA, McCammon RL, Stoelting RK, Warren TM, Miller D, Bopp SK, Jugovic DJ, Abou-Donia MM: Hemodynamic effects of mivacurium chloride administered to patients during oxygen-sufentanil anesthesia for coronary artery bypass grafting or valve replacement. Anesth Analg 68:333–339, 1989
55. Cheng M, Lee C, Yang E, Cantley E: Comparison of fast and slow bolus injections of mivacurium chloride under narcotic–nitrous oxide anesthesia. Anesthesiology 69:A877, 1988
56. Powers D, Simpson K, Morici M, Benckart D, Maher T, Torpey DJ: The hemodynamic effects of mivacurium chloride in patients undergoing coronary artery bypass graft during fentanyl/valium anesthesia. Anesthesiology 69:A530, 1988
57. Ali HH, Brull SJ, Witkowski T, Kopman A, Silverman DG, Goudsouzian NG, Bartkowski R, Weakly N: Efficacy and safety of divided dose administration of mivacurium for rapid tracheal intubation. Anesthesiology 79:A934, 1993
58. Flashburg M, Molbegott L, Baker T: Speed and ease of endotracheal intubation at 75 seconds after prior priming at two, three and five minutes with mivacurium compared to succinylcholine at 75 seconds. Anesthesiology 79:A935, 1993
59. Flashburg M, Baker T: Speed and ease of endotracheal intubation at fixed times after mivacurium with priming. Anesthesiology 79:A936, 1993
60. Molbegott L, Baker T: Speed and ease of endotracheal intubation after mivacurium doses of various multiples of ED95 with and without priming compared to SCh. Anesthesiology 79:A933, 1993
61. Peterman R, Axelrod E, Brown M: Rapid sequence induction with mivacurium. Anesthesiology 79:A937, 1993
62. Brandom BW, Sarner JB, Dong ML, Woefel SK, Cook DR, Borland LM, Davis PJ, Foster VJ, McNulty BS: Mivacurium chloride (BW B1090U) infusion requirements in children during halothane or narcotic anesthesia. Anesth Analg 67:S20, 1988
63. Goudsouzian NG, Alifimoff JK, Eberly C, Smeets R, Griswold J, Miler V, McNulty BF,

Savarese JJ: Neuromuscular and cardiovascular effects of mivacurium in children. Anesthesiology 70:237–242, 1989
64. Sarner JB, Brandom BW, Woelfel SK, Dong M-L, Horn MC, Cook DR, McNulty BF, Foster VJ: Clinical pharmacology of mivacurium chloride (BW B1090U) in children during nitrous oxide–halothane and nitrous oxide–narcotic anesthesia. Anesth Analg 68:116–121, 1989
65. Woelfel SK, Brandom BW, McGowan FX Jr, Cook DR: Dose-response relationship of mivacurium chloride (Mivacron®) in infants during nitrous oxide–halothane anesthesia. 75:A775, 1991
66. Booij LHDJ, Knape HTA: The neuromuscular blocking effect of Org 9426: a new intermediately-acting steroidal non-depolarising muscle relaxant in man. Anaesthesia 46:341–343, 1991
67. Bartkowski R, Witkowski T, Azad SS, Marr A, Lessin J: A comparison of onset and recovery of neuromuscular block after ORG9426 and vecuronium. Anesthesiology 75:A1071, 1991
68. Cooper R, Mirakhur RK, Clarke RSJ, Boules Z: Comparison of intubating conditions after administration of ORG 9426 (rocuronium) and suxamethonium. Br J Anaesth 69:269–273, 1992
69. Cooper R, Maddineni VR, Mirakhur RK, Wierda JMKH, Brady M, Fitzpatrick KTJ: Time course of neuromuscular effect and pharmacokinetics of rocuronium bromide (ORG 9426) during isoflurane anesthesia in patients with and without renal failure. Br J Anaesth 71:222–226, 1993
70. Cooper RA, Mirakhur RK, Maddineni VR: Neuromuscular effects of rocuronium bromide (Org 9426) during fentanyl and halothane anaesthesia. Anaesthesia 48:103–105, 1993
71. Cantineau JP, Porte F, Homs JB, Liu N, Duvaldestin P: Neuromuscular blocking effect of ORG 9426 on human diaphragm. Anesthesiology 75:A785, 1991
72. Cason B, Baker DG, Hickey RF, Miller RD, Agoston SS: Cardiovascular and neuromuscular effects of three steroidal neuromuscular blocking drugs in dogs (ORG 9616, ORG 9426, ORG 9991). Anesth Analg 70:382–388, 1990
73. Dubois M, Shearrow T, Tran D, Kataria B, Rever L, Gadde P, Lea D: ORG 9426 used for endotracheal intubation: a comparison with succinylcholine. Anesthesiology 75:A1066, 1991
74. Foldes F, Nagashima H, Nguyen HD, Schiller WS, Mason MM, Ohta Y: The neuromuscular effects of ORG 9426 in patients receiving balanced anesthesia. Anesthesiology 75:191–196, 1991
75. Huizinga ACT, Vandenbrom RHG, Wierda JMKH, Hommes FDM, Hennis PJ: Intubating conditions and onset of neuromuscular block of rocuronium (Org 9426): a comparison with suxamethonium. Acta Anaesthesiol Scand 36:463–468, 1992
76. Lambalk LM, DeWit APM, Wierda JMKH, Hennis PJ, Agoston S: Dose-response relationship and time course of action of Org 9426: a new muscle relaxant of intermediate duration evaluated under various anaesthetic techniques. Anaesthesia 46:907–911, 1991
77. Muir AW, Houston J, Green KL, Marshall RJ, Bowman WC, Marshall IG: Effects of a new neuromuscular blocking agent (Org 9426) in anaesthetized cats and pigs and in isolated nerve-muscle preparations. Br J Anaesth 63:400–410, 1989
78. Mirakhur R, Cooper R, McCarthy G, Elliott P: Comparison of the intubating conditions and some neuromuscular effects following administration of ORG 9426 and succinylcholine. Anesth Analg 74:S210, 1992
79. Mayer M, Doenicke A, Hofmann A, Peter K: Onset and recovery of rocuronium (ORG 9426) and vecuronium under enflurane anaesthesia. Br J Anaesth 69:511–512, 1992
80. Magorian T, Wood P, Caldwell JE, Szenohradszky J, Segredo V, Sharma H, Gruenke LD, Miller RD: Pharmacokinetics, onset, and duration of action of rocuronium in humans: normal vs. hepatic dysfunction. Anesthesiology 75:A1069, 1991
81. Mayer M, Doenicke A, Angster R, Hoffmann A, Peter K: ORG 9426: the increase of dose shortens the onset time. Anesthesiology 75:A1070, 1991
82. Mellinghoff H, Diefenbach C, Buzello W: Neuromuscular and cardiovascular properties of ORG 9426. Anesthesiology 75:A807, 1991

83. Nagashima H, Nguyen HD, Kinsey A, Rosa M, Hollinger I, et al: The human dose response of Org 9426. Anesthesiology 71:A773, 1989
84. Powers D, Lefebvre D, Knos G, Cyran J, Brandom B: Intubation conditions after administration of ORG 9426 during nitrous oxide-fentanyl-midazolam anesthesia. Anesth Analg 74:S240, 1992
85. Puhringer FK, Khuenl-Brady KS, Koller J, Mitterschiffthaler G: Evaluation of the endotracheal intubating conditions of rocuronium (ORG 9426) and succinylcholine in outpatient surgery. Anesth Analg 75:37–40, 1992
86. Plaud B, Meistelman C, Donati F: Organon 9426 neuromuscular blockade at the adductor muscles of the larynx and adductor pollicis in man. Anesthesiology 75:A784, 1991
87. Quill TJ, Begin M, Glass PSA, Ginsberg B, Gorback MS: Clinical responses to ORG 9426 during isoflurane anesthesia. Anesth Analg 72:203–206, 1991
88. Szenohradszky J, Fisher DM, Segredo V, Caldwell JE, Bragg P, Sharma ML, Gruenke LD, Miller RD: Pharmacokinetics of rocuronium bromide (ORG 9426) in patients with normal renal function or patients undergoing cadaver renal transplantation. Anesthesiology 77:899–904, 1992
89. Tullock WC, Wilks DH, Brandom BW, Cook DR: ORG 9426: onset, intubating conditions and clinical duration. Anesthesiology 75:A789, 1991
90. Vandenbrom RHG, Wierda JMKH, Huizinga ACT, Hennis PJ: Intubation conditions and time-course of action of ORG 9426. Anesthesiology 75:A788, 1991
91. Witkowski T, Bartkowski R, Azad SS, Marr A, Lessin J: Onset of Org 9426: a comparison with atracurium and vecuronium. Anesth Analg 74:S351, 1992
92. Wierda JMKH, DeWit APM, Kuizenga K, Agoston S: Clinical observations on the neuromuscular blocking action of Org 9426, a new steroidal nondepolarizing agent. Br J Anaesth 64:521–523, 1990
93. Wierda JMHK, Kleef UW, Lambalk LM, et al: The pharmacodynamics and pharmacokinetics of ORG 9426: a new nondepolarizing neuromuscular blocking agent in patients anaesthetized with nitrous oxide, halothane and fentanyl. Can J Anaesth 38:430–435, 1991
94. Lapeyre G, Dubois M, Lea D, et al: Effects of three intubating doses of Org 9426 in humans. Anesthesiology 73:A906, 1990
95. O'Kelly B, Frossard J, Meistelman C, Ecoffey C: Neuromuscular blockade following Org 9426 in children during N_2O-halothane anesthesia. Anesthesiology 75:A787, 1991
96. Khuenl-Brady K, Castagnoli KP, Canfell PC, Caldwell JE, Agoston S, Miller RD: The neuromuscular blocking effects and pharmacokinetics of ORG 9426 and ORG 9616 in the cat. Anesthesiology 72:669–674, 1990
97. Vuksanaj D, Skjonsby B, Dunbar B: Pharmacokinetics and pharmacodynamics of intubating dose of ORG9426 (rocuronium) in children. Anesthesiology 79:A1127, 1993
98. Bowman WC, Rodger IW, Houston J, Marshall RJ, McIndewar I: Structure:action relationships among some desacetoxy analogues of pancuronium and vecuronium in the anesthetized cat. Anesthesiology 69:57–62, 1988
99. Chaudry I, Foldes FF, Ohta Y, Nagashima H: The protein binding of Org 9426 and its inhibitory effect on human cholinesterases. Anesthesiology 75:A786, 1991
100. Tian L, Mehta MP, Prior C, Marshall IG: Relative pre- and postjunctional effects of a new vecuronium analogue, Org 9426, at the rat neuromuscular junction. Br J Anaesth 69:284–287, 1992
101. Shiraishi H, Suzuki H, Suzuki T, Katsumata N, Ogawa S: Fading responses in the evoked EMG after rocuronium in cats. Can J Anaesth 39:1099–1104, 1992
102. Khuenl-Brady KS, Agoston S, Miller RD: Interaction of ORG 9426 and some of the clinically used intravenous anaesthetic agents in the cat. Acta Anaesthesiol Scand 36:260–263, 1992
103. Silverman DG, Swift CA, Dubow HD, O'Connor TZ, Brull SJ: Variability of onset times within and among relaxant regimens. J Clin Anesth 4:28–33, 1992
104. Meistelman C, Plaud B, Donati F: Rocuronium (ORG 9426) neuromuscular blockade at the adductor muscles of the larynx and adductor pollicis in humans Can J Anaesth 39:665–669, 1992
105. Donati F, Meistelman C, Plaud B: Vecuronium neuromuscular blockade at the adductor muscles of the larynx and adductor pollicis. Anesthesiology 74:833–837, 1991

106. Meistelman C, Plaud B, Donati F: Neuromuscular effects of succinylcholine on the vocal cords and adductor pollicis muscles. Anesth Analg 73:278–282, 1991
107. Fiset P, Balendran P, Bevan DR: Onset, duration, and recovery from Org 9426 in the elderly. Anesthesiology 73:A881, 1990
108. Matteo RS, Ornstein E, Schwartz AE, Stone JG, Ostapkovich N, Spencer HK, Dee CM: Pharmacokinetics and pharmacodynamics of ORG 9426 in elderly surgical patients. Anesthesiology 75:A1065, 1991
109. Bevan DR, Fiset P, Balendran P, Law-Min JC, Ratcliffe A, Donati F: Pharmacodynamic behaviour of rocuronium in the elderly. Can J Anaesth 40:127–132, 1993
110. Shanks CA, Fragen RJ, Ling D, Pemberton D, Dunn K, Howard K: Infusion requirements of ORG 9426 in patients receiving balanced, enflurane or isoflurane anesthesia. Anesthesiology 75:A1068, 1991
111. Brandom BW, Woelfel SK, Sarner JB, Cook DR: ORG-9426 infusion requirements in children during halothane anesthesia. Anesthesiology 75:A1072, 1991
112. Woelfel SK, Brandom BW, Cook DR, Sarner JB: Effects of bolus administration of ORG-9426 in children during nitrous oxide–halothane anesthesia. Anesthesiology 76:939–942, 1992
113. Davis GK, Szlam F, Lowdon JD, Levy JH: Evaluation of histamine release following Org 9426 administration using a new radioimmunoassay. Anesthesiology 75:A818, 1991
114. Mayer M, Doenicke A, Lorenz W, Nebauer AE, Rull T, Kapp B, Peter K: Histamine releasing potency of rocuronium. Anesthesiology 77:A906, 1992
115. McCoy EP, Maddineni VR, Elliott P, Mirakhur RK, Carson IW, Cooper RA: Haemodynamic effects of rocuronium during fentanyl anaesthesia: comparison with vecuronium. Can J Anaesth 40:703–708, 1993
116. Williams CH, Chandra P, Serda R, Martinez M: Malignant hyperthermia induction in susceptible swine following exposure to Organon 9426. Anesth Analg 74:S350, 1992
117. Brull SJ, Connelly NR, Garwood S, Garcia R, Silverman DG: Recovery of train-of-four after mivacurium. Anesthesiology 79:A925, 1993

15

DAVID G. SILVERMAN | RAJINDER D. MIRAKHUR

Reversal of Nondepolarizing Block

Anticholinesterases used for reversal of neuromuscular block are quaternary ammonium compounds that allow the concentration of acetylcholine (ACh) to increase in the neuromuscular junction (NMJ) and thereby compete more effectively for cholinergic receptors. They bind reversibly to acetylcholinesterase, which otherwise rapidly breaks down ACh to acetate and choline. Neostigmine, pyridostigmine, and edrophonium each bind to the anionic site of cholinesterase by electrostatic attachment. However, they differ in their binding to the esteratic site. Neostigmine and pyridostigmine attach by covalent linking of their *carbamyl group,* which can result in hydrolysis of the acetylcholinesterase molecule. Edrophonium attaches by reversible hydrogen binding at that site, recombining with acetylcholinesterase in a competitive manner.[1] It may also act by means other than acetylcholinesterase inhibition (discussed below). In addition to reversibly binding to acetylcholinesterase, these agents may also (1) bind at (or allow increased ACh activity at) presynaptic sites,[2-6] thereby increasing ACh release at the given motor nerve terminal and perhaps from branches throughout the given motor unit; (2) produce direct stimulation of the end-plate (nicotinic) receptor[7-9]; or (3) alter the configuration of receptor channels.

Following anticholinesterase administration, the *time to recovery* from nondepolarizing block is a composite of the *antagonism* by the anticholinesterase and *spontaneous recovery* from the given neuromuscular blocking agent. The onset of reversal is fastest for edrophonium and slowest for pyridostigmine (Table 15-1). Interestingly, none of the reversal regimens used clinically was able to fully reverse a ≥95% block caused by persistent bathing of a rat diaphragm preparation in a pancuronium solution.[10] In other words, there is a ceiling effect.[10-14]

◆ FACTORS AFFECTING REVERSAL

A multitude of factors influence the *time to effective recovery*. These factors include the following:

1. The degree of paralysis at the time of antagonism.[11,13,15–33] The deeper the block, the longer the time to adequate reversal. Except perhaps after mivacurium, it may be best to withhold reversal agents until the response to single twitch or train-of-four stimulation is at least 10% of control.
2. The pharmacokinetics and pharmacodynamics of the relaxant. Spontaneous recovery is more rapid (and reversal "easier") after atracurium, vecuronium, and rocuronium than after *d*-tubocurarine or pancuronium,[26,34–37] and it is especially rapid after mivacurium.[38]
3. Blood levels of the relaxant.[11,17,23,39,40] An NMJ to blood gradient for relaxant facilitates recovery[39] but is not necessarily required for partial antagonism.[39,41]
4. The means of relaxant administration. Reversal 2 minutes after discontinuing an infusion typically is slower than during recovery after a bolus.[26]
5. The specific antagonist.
6. The dose of antagonist.
7. Underlying neuromuscular dysfunction.
8. Drug interactions that may selectively affect the relaxant or reversal agent. For example, recovery and reversal are slowed and more likely to be associated with persistent fade in the presence of inhalational anesthesia (the effects of inhalational agents occur in the order enflurane > isoflurane > halothane) (Chap. 9).[42–46]
9. Organ dysfunction (Chap. 10).
10. Acid-base and electrolyte disturbances (Chap. 10), most notably respiratory acidosis.[47–49]
11. Patient age. Children (but not necessarily neonates) have faster spontaneous recovery, lower dose requirements for reversal, and a lesser incidence of residual weakness (Chap. 10),[29,50–52] and reversal in the pediatric patient may be successful at greater depths of block.[22,53] The elderly may have reduced relaxant clearance, delayed recovery, and less efficient reversal (Chap. 10),[54,55] factors not wholly offset by the reduced clearance rate of reversal agents.[56]

TABLE 15-1
Some Properties of Specific Anticholinesterases

Agent	(Brand Name)	Typical Dose ($mg \cdot kg^{-1}$)	Peak Effect (min)	Metabolism/ Elimination
Neostigmine	(Prostigmine)	0.04–0.07	7–10	Liver ≥ kidney
Pyridostigmine	(Mestinon)	0.14–0.25	10–15	Mostly kidney (75%)
Edrophonium	(Tensilon)	0.5–1.0	1–3	Mostly kidney (70%)

◆ ANTIMUSCARINIC AGENTS

The accumulation of ACh as a result of anticholinesterase administration is not specific to the NMJ. *Nicotinic effects* occur at preganglionic autonomic ganglia as well as at the NMJ. *Muscarinic effects* occur due to binding at the sinus node, smooth muscles, and glands; these effects include bradycardia, intestinal hypermotility, bronchospasm, and increased secretions. Muscarinic effects are antagonized by administration of *antimuscarinic agents* (atropine or glycopyrrolate).[41,57–62] A typical dose during reversal with 0.05 mg · kg^{-1} of neostigmine is either atropine, 0.015–0.02 mg · kg^{-1}, or glycopyrrolate, 0.008–0.01 mg · kg^{-1}.

The most *significant differences* between the two antimuscarinic agents in the context of reversal are the following: (1) Atropine has a faster onset (1 minute vs. 2–3 minutes).[60] (2) Atropine is more likely to induce initial tachycardia. (3) Glycopyrrolate is a more effective antisialagogue.[41,57,60–62] (4) Atropine, because it is a tertiary amine, crosses the blood-brain barrier and placenta and may cause delayed emergence or disorientation.[63–66] (Glycopyrrolate and the relaxants themselves are charged quaternary amines.) Of note, the transient increase in heart rate as a result of atropine (or glycopyrrolate) administration appears to be greater when reversing *d*-tubocurarine as opposed to pancuronium.[67] This difference may be attributable to pancuronium's vagolytic and sympathomimetic properties (Chap. 11).

◆ ANTICHOLINESTERASE AGENTS

Neostigmine is the most commonly employed reversal agent and the most reliable in the context of deep block.[17–19,26,31,68] However, even neostigmine is not reliable in the context of extremely profound block. Increasing the dose beyond 0.07–0.08 mg · kg^{-1} generally does not increase the effectiveness of reversal.[10,13,22] Neostigmine is metabolized by cholinesterases in the NMJ and liver; up to 50% is eliminated via the kidneys.[69] The onset of effect of a typical clinical dose occurs in about 3 minutes, with a peak effect within 10 minutes; a decline to 50% of peak effectiveness is seen within approximately 60 minutes.[70]

Neostigmine is used with either atropine or glycopyrrolate. Simultaneous administration of atropine with neostigmine typically causes transient tachycardia (within 1–2 minutes) and then some decrease in heart rate (10–20 minutes later).[60,67,71,72] Glycopyrrolate is more commonly employed because its slightly slower onset and longer duration (peak at 3–5 minutes) more closely resemble those of neostigmine (peak at 7–10 minutes).[59–61,73–75] It thus may be preferable in patients with cardiovascular disease.[62,76–78] A *mixture* of 0.010–0.015 mg · kg^{-1} glycopyrrolate and 0.05–0.07 mg · kg^{-1} neostigmine has been recommended.[59–61] However, if one is particularly concerned about even transient muscarinic effects (e.g., bradycardia), then prior administration of glycopyrrolate or the use of atropine may be preferable. A patient on atenolol[79] and two heart transplant recipients[80] developed transient heart block and sinus arrest after receiving glycopyrrolate and neostigmine simultaneously. An alternative may be to split a dose of atropine and give it before and after neostigmine.[81]

Pyridostigmine is 20% as potent as neostigmine and has a slower onset, 40% longer duration, and less severe muscarinic effects.[67,70,82-84] A typical clinical dose exerts its peak effect within 12 minutes and declines to 50% of peak effectiveness at approximately 80 minutes.[70] In view of its slow time course, pyridostigmine is best accompanied by glycopyrrolate.[57] Pyridostigmine is the agent most commonly employed in the daily (oral) therapy of patients with myasthenia gravis because of its long duration. Of the three commonly employed anticholinesterases, it is the most (75%[83]) dependent on renal clearance.

Edrophonium is the least potent of the three commonly employed anticholinesterase agents, with a dose requirement that is 12-20 (and even 35) times greater than that for neostigmine.[30,40,85-94] Edrophonium has the fastest onset, reaching peak effect in 1-2 minutes.[40,41,93-96] It may act predominantly by means other than acetylcholinesterase inhibition,[8,97-102] such as by increasing the release of ACh presynaptically[6] or by altering the configuration of receptor channels.

Edrophonium can provide a rapid, satisfactory, and sustained antagonism provided that *residual block is not intense* (all four responses to train-of-four stimulation are present) and that the *accumulated mass of relaxant is modest.*[88] Because of its faster onset, edrophonium may be advantageous for reversal of light and moderate depths of block caused by short-acting relaxants.[27,33,88,103-105] When given in equipotent doses, neostigmine and edrophonium have similar rates of distribution and elimination[14,41] and similar durations of antagonism. Except in the context of deep block, edrophonium reversal is associated with the least degree of fade,[96,106] perhaps attributable to the rapidity of its effects or to its propensity for presynaptic activity. The latter mechanism promotes release of ACh, which would offset the use-dependent rundown of ACh that may be responsible for fade (Chaps. 2 and 4).

In 1983, Miller and Cronnelly aptly noted that "Only when edrophonium has been used for thousands of patients will its proper position in regard to neostigmine and pyridostigmine be established."[91] It has since become evident that the *extent of antagonism by edrophonium* is highly dependent on its dose and on the depth of block.* When it is given in small doses (e.g., 0.2 mg · kg^{-1}) to reverse a moderate or deep block, edrophonium's onset, effectiveness, and duration are inadequate.[25] For *moderate depths of block,* these limitations may be overcome by increasing the dose to 0.8-1.0 mg · kg^{-1},[17,26,31,95] such that plasma levels remain sufficiently high to maintain effective concentrations in the NMJ.

*References 17-19, 22, 26, 27, 30, 31, 40, 68, 85, 87-90, 93, 96, 105, and 107-109.

At intense levels of block, the requisite dose of *edrophonium* is disproportionately large,[31,40,68,87] and the response is variable and often inadequate. For example, the *neostigmine:edrophonium potency ratio* for reversal of atracurium block was 17:1 at 90% twitch depression and 35:1 at 99% twitch depression.[87] As the depth of block increases, the ability to reverse train-of-four fade with edrophonium decreases markedly.[68,87] In light of these factors, *edrophonium is not an appropriate choice for reversal of deep block.** This is particularly evident after large doses of long-acting relaxant.[26,30,68,93,95,107,108,113]

The potential limitations of *edrophonium* in the presence of *deep block* are even more evident when monitoring *recovery of train-of-four:* (1) When reversal was attempted at 10% T_1 recovery from pancuronium-induced block, a dose of edrophonium that was 12 times that for neostigmine was required to achieve 80% recovery of T_1, while 25 times as much edrophonium was needed to achieve a T_4/T_1 ratio of 0.5.[68] (2) When T_1 was only 1% of baseline during atracurium-induced block, the calculated dose of edrophonium for return of T_4/T_1 to ≥0.70 at 10 minutes was 60 times greater than that calculated for neostigmine.[87] (3) When T_1 was 10% of control, edrophonium, 1.0 mg · kg^{-1}, provided a $T_4/T_1 \geq 0.7$ at 9 minutes after vecuronium and failed to achieve this ratio within 37 minutes in half of the patients who had received pancuronium.[108]

Reversal by *edrophonium* is highly sensitive to the presence of *inhalational anesthetics,* with increased dose requirements for recovery of twitch height and resolution of fade.[43] In addition, although the dose of edrophonium required for reversal did not differ significantly among infants, children, and adults,[114] the effects were highly variable in infants, and a relatively large dose of edrophonium[114] (but not necessarily of neostigmine[50]) may be required.

Edrophonium is typically administered with atropine because of their similarly rapid onset.[40,115–117] The dose of atropine required is lower than that used with neostigmine, since edrophonium elicits less severe muscarinic effects,[27,40,114] but this advantage may be lost at high doses. Typically doses of 0.005–0.01 mg · kg^{-1} are given, but higher doses may occasionally be required.[107,118,119] Edrophonium also may be given with *glycopyrrolate*[120]; 0.005 and 0.01 mg · kg^{-1} may be administered 30–60 seconds prior to edrophonium but may be associated with extreme changes in heart rate.[117,120,121]

◆ ANTICHOLINESTERASE OVERDOSE AND POISONING

Overdosage with anticholinesterases may cause *excessive muscarinic effects and altered neuromuscular function.* These effects may range from insignificant changes to the lethal effects of *organophosphate insecticides* (para-

---

*References 17–19, 23, 25–27, 30, 31, 68, 89, 95, 107, 108, and 110–113.

thion, naphthyl carbymates) and *"nerve gas"* (e.g., tabun, soman, sarin, and venom X).

Neuromuscular effects of an overdosage of anticholinesterases or of their administration in the absence of a muscle relaxant may first lead to an SCh-like block with prolonged depolarization of the end-plate. Loss of synchronization between the end-plate depolarization and the development of an action potential may lead to muscle fibrillation.[122] Especially with neostigmine and pyridostigmine, this may be followed by weakness, with depressed peak tetanic contraction and *tetanic fade,* especially in the context of inhalational anesthesia.[123,124] In the clinical setting, this is typically seen on repeat dosing.[21,125] The fade has been attributed to postsynaptic desensitization (as a result of a persistent excess of ACh) or to exhaustion of available ACh in the presynaptic nerve terminal.[3,123–129] Evidence for a *presynaptic effect* includes the finding that, in the presence of anticholinesterases, a single nerve impulse may elicit repetitive nerve action potentials; these lead to summated twitch responses that fade rapidly.[3,5,6,10,123,124,129,130] Even without "over-reversal," a typical dose of reversal agent may aggravate neuromuscular dysfunction: neostigmine reversal has resulted in increased weakness and caused a myotonic response in patients with underlying neuromuscular disorders.[131]

In contrast to the reversible agents that are used clinically, the *poisonous agents* essentially are noncompetitive and *not readily reversible.* Their common mechanism involves *phosphorylation of cholinesterase;* the phosphorus-enzyme bond abolishes cholinesterase activity. As above, the *nicotinic effects of nerve gas–induced ACh excess* include muscle fasciculations, repetitive firing, decreased peak tetanic tension, and tetanic fade, with weakness that may progress to paralysis. We may also see altered autonomic activity as a result of increased ACh at preganglionic terminals. The *muscarinic effects* of ACh excess include excessive secretions (bronchial, salivary, ocular, intestinal), bronchospasm, bradycardia, intestinal hypermotility, vomiting, miosis, and sweating. *Central nervous system* effects include disorientation, loss of consciousness, convulsions, and depression of ventilatory drive that may precipitate or contribute to respiratory arrest.[132]

Treatment of anticholinesterase toxicity includes administering *atropine* to counteract potentially lethal muscarinic effects, administering *oximes* such as *pralidoxime* (PAM) to bind the offending agent and thereby spare the portion of the victim's cholinesterase that has not yet been destroyed, and administering *benzodiazepines* to decrease seizures.[133–136]

Discussion Questions ◆

a. Why might it be wise to *wait until there is at least partial return* of a single twitch *before reversing* a nondepolarizing block after pancuronium?

b. Would your *selection of reversal agent* be different if T_1 was 10% of baseline as opposed to ≥25% of baseline during recovery from pancuronium? Why or why not?
c. Is the *rate of reversal* of pancuronium-induced block markedly different if the single twitch has returned to 10% vs. >25% of baseline?
d. *Establish guidelines for reversal* based on the number of responses to train-of-four stimulation and presence or absence of fade after an intermediate- or long-acting NDR.
e. Does the *time since relaxant administration* affect the reversibility of a given degree of block?
f. Discuss the *reasons for reversal* in the context of 100% recovery of twitch height and train-of-four response by visual and tactile assessment after a long-acting (e.g., pancuronium) and intermediate-acting (e.g., atracurium) block.
g. Discuss the *reasons why one might elect not to administer reversal* in the above context.
h. Is apparently adequate reversal of pancuronium by *clinical criteria or visual assessment of train-of-four responses* at the end of surgery a reliable predictor of normal neuromuscular function in the postanesthesia care unit (PACU)?
i. With which relaxants is *recurarization* most likely in the context of *renal failure?* Why is it uncommon?
j. Your patient is *slow to resume spontaneous ventilation* following a general anesthetic that included "typical" doses of thiopental, SCh, pancuronium, an inhalational agent, and neostigmine/atropine. What is your *differential diagnosis?*
k. Does *"priming" with a reversal agent* accelerate reversal?
l. What factors besides a residual effect from intraoperative neuromuscular block may account for a $T_4/T_1 < 0.70$ *in the PACU* in a patient who appeared adequately reversed and recovered in the operating suite?
m. Define *lower esophageal sphincter opening pressure* (or "barrier" pressure). How might reversal affect barrier pressure and the likelihood of regurgitation?
n. Why might we be concerned about reversal in the context of a *recent bowel anastomosis?*
o. Why are we concerned about *reversal* in the context of *asthma?*
p. Should you administer *atropine* before, during, or after injection of *edrophonium*, 1.0 mg · kg^{-1}, for reversal of neuromuscular block? Why?
q. Is *glycopyrrolate* a reasonable choice when administering *edrophonium?*
r. Are the requirements for an *antimuscarinic agent* the same in *adults* and *children?*
s. What are the roles of atropine, diazepam, and pralidoxime in the treatment of the *nerve gas victim?*

t. Why might prophylactic *pretreatment with low-dose pyridostigmine* be helpful for *soldiers* at risk of exposure to nerve gas?

u. Would an assay of *cholinesterase activity* be helpful in determining if a patient has been *poisoned with organophosphates?* Why or why not?

v. How should you adjust the dose of *neostigmine* if the patient has received *physostigmine?*

w. During *long-term exposure to anticholinesterases,* the increased availability of ACh in the NMJ gradually causes down-regulation of the postsynaptic receptors. How might this affect the response to SCh or an NDR?

x. Why might it be easier to regulate the effects of *SCh after edrophonium* than it would be after *neostigmine or pyridostigmine?*

Answers ◆

a. *Neuromuscular function after reversal is a composite* of (1) the degree of "spontaneous" recovery prior to reversal, (2) the extent of antagonism of block due to reversal, and (3) the amount of spontaneous recovery (i.e., as may result from clearance) concomitant with reversal. At *deep levels of block,* antagonism alone may be insufficient and "spontaneous" recovery may also be required for return of normal function. Spontaneous recovery will be slower for long-acting agents. Regardless of whether you administer the reversal agent when $T_1 = 0-1\%$ or wait until $T_1 = 10\%$, the total time to achieve adequate reversal plus recovery from the time when $T_1 = 0$ is the same.[13,22,29,31] Attempts at early reversal may actually make titration to desired effect more difficult. Furthermore, high doses or repeated doses of the reversal agents themselves may alter neuromuscular function.

b. The *depth of block* influences *selection of reversal agent.* Avoid *edrophonium* if T_1 is ≤10% of baseline, especially after a long-acting relaxant. If edrophonium, 0.5–1.0 mg · kg^{-1}, is given when T_1 is ≤10%, reversal is slow and may be inadequate, even at 30 minutes.[23,27,31] Some workers recommend using edrophonium only if three or more responses to train-of-four stimulation are present[17,18,26,27,30,31,89]; this corresponds to a T_1 of ≥20%. The limited effectiveness of edrophonium may also be seen when T_1 is less than 10% after shorter-acting NDRs.[17,18,30]

c. Recovery is much faster if T_1 has returned to >25% of its baseline height than if $T_1 = 10\%$. When $T_1 > 25\%$ (i.e., three and probably all four twitches of the train-of-four response are visible) during recovery from *pancuronium,* a T_4/T_1 ratio above 0.70 generally is attained in 5–7 minutes after *neostigmine,* 0.05 mg · kg^{-1}. When $T_1 = 10\%$ during recovery from pancuronium block, it typically takes more than 20 minutes to achieve a T_4/T_1 ratio above 0.70 after neostigmine, 0.05 mg · kg^{-1}.

d. *Guidelines for reversal:*

1. *Extremely deep block* (i.e., no twitches in response to single twitch or train-of-four stimulation): probably should withhold reversal until there is evidence of recovery.
2. *Relatively deep block* (one or two twitches in response to train-of-four stimulation, T_1 = 5–15%): neostigmine, 0.07 mg · kg^{-1}, is preferable to edrophonium, especially after a long-acting relaxant.
3. *Moderate block* (three twitches, $T_1 \geq 20\%$): neostigmine, 0.04–0.07 mg · kg^{-1}, or edrophonium, 1.0 mg · kg^{-1}.
4. *Light block* (all four twitches, fade, $T_1 \geq 25\%$): edrophonium, 0.5–1.0 mg · kg^{-1}, or neostigmine, 0.03–0.07 mg · kg^{-1}. Edrophonium may be preferable because it produces faster recovery with less severe muscarinic effects.
5. *"No" detectable block* (four twitches, no observed fade): low-dose edrophonium, 0.25–0.5 mg · kg^{-1}, or neostigmine, 0.03–0.05 mg · kg^{-1}, or possibly nothing if absence of fade can be reliably demonstrated.

e. *Recent dosing* with a bolus dose of a nondepolarizing agent and/or maintenance with a continuous infusion provide higher plasma concentrations of relaxant. These high plasma concentrations may limit removal of relaxant from the NMJ and compromise reversal.[11,17,25,30,40]

f. There are potential advantages to *reversal in the context of apparent "100%" recovery*. Reversal, which may be accomplished in this setting with a low dose of an anticholinesterase,[137] "ensures" adequate recovery. It may be indicated because of the *lack of sensitivity of routine clinical testing*. Absence of train-of-four (T_4/T_1) fade by *tactile or visual assessment* generally means that the T_4/T_1 ratio is above 0.40 but not necessarily above 0.70; moderate degrees of fade between 0.40 and 0.70 are not consistently detected (Chap. 5). The use of double-burst stimulation may improve accuracy, but not entirely (Chaps. 4 and 5). Additionally, T_4/T_1 actually may "decline" during transport from the OR to the PACU.[138] Furthermore, a T_4/T_1 ratio of 0.70 does not necessarily guarantee full neuromuscular transmission and ability to protect one's airway (Chap. 6). A T_4/T_1 ratio as high as 0.9 may be associated with heaviness of the eyelids, blurred vision, difficulty swallowing, and generalized discomfort.[139-141] Even when the T_4/T_1 ratio is normal and no weakness is apparent, as many as 70% of receptors may be occupied (Chap. 4).

g. *Reversal is not totally benign*. It may elicit excess *ACh-mediated effects* (bradycardia, muscle weakness, salivation, increased bowel activity, nausea and vomiting). It may cause sinus arrest in heart transplant recipients.[80] Patients who underwent reversal had a higher incidence of nausea and vomiting.[142]

Excessive administration of the reversal agents themselves may cause block or random hyperactivity, with spontaneous twitching and repetitive firing with fade on stimulation. However, it is highly unlikely that a single dose of neostigmine will cause significant weakness.[16,21,24,143,144]

Reversal may not always be necessary. Even without reversal, adequate recovery after an NDR of intermediate or short duration should be achieved relatively rapidly even if T_4/T_1 has been overestimated by visual or tactile assessment. Although visual assessment may fail to identify fade even at a T_4/T_1 ratio of 0.4, adequate recovery after intermediate- and short-acting relaxants should be quite rapid. After *atracurium* and moderate doses of *vecuronium*, it is likely that the mechanographic T_4/T_1 will be above 0.75 within 10 minutes after a ratio of ≥0.40; after these agents, T_4/T_1 typically progresses from as low as 0.25 to ≥0.75 in less than 20 minutes.[145] During recovery after mivacurium, T_4/T_1 was greater than 0.70 at 5.2 ± 2.3 minutes (range, 2.1–10.4 minutes in 34 trials[146]) after a T_4/T_1 ratio of 0.4 was recorded.

h. A relatively large number of patients may exhibit train-of-four fade and/or signs and symptoms of *residual weakness in the PACU* despite apparently adequate reversal at the end of surgery.[34,36,75,138,147–149] Clearly, judging the adequacy of reversal by a single parameter (e.g., visual assessment of train-of-four fade) is subject to inaccuracy (Chap. 5).

Residual weakness is far more common (up to 42%) after *long-acting relaxants*[34,75,147] and perhaps after high doses of vecuronium.[147] Fortunately, this generally does not result in significant morbidity. Residual weakness is far less likely after atracurium, routine doses of vecuronium, and especially mivacurium. It also appears to be less likely in children than adults.[52]

It should be noted that factors such as *peripheral cooling* or excess reversal may also contribute to a decline in T_4/T_1 in the PACU.[148,150–153] Peripheral cooling may have a disproportionate (and perhaps misleading) effect on neuromuscular monitoring in the particular limb used even if neuromuscular function is adequate (Chap. 10).

i. The effects of all NDRs, with the possible exception of atracurium, are prolonged in patients with *renal failure*. This is most notable for long-acting relaxants. *Gallamine, doxacurium,* and to a slightly lesser extent *pancuronium and pipecuronium* are predominantly renally excreted and might best be avoided in patients with *renal failure*. Otherwise, altered pharmacokinetics as a result of renal failure should not result in disproportionately greater prolongation of the effects of relaxants as opposed to antagonists. The clearance of antagonists is likewise reduced by renal failure. Hence, so long as at least partial spontaneous recovery is evident prior to reversal, the *duration of a reversal agent* typically outlasts that remaining for the relaxant and its metabolites.[41,154,155] This is especially true for *pyridostigmine;* its duration is prolonged to the greatest extent (>3×) because it is 75% renally excreted (vs. 50% for neostigmine and 70% for edrophonium).[14,70,82,156] Renal failure resulted in an increase from a normal elimination half-life for pyridostigmine of 112 minutes to 379 minutes and a decrease in clearance from 9 to 2 mL · kg^{-1} · min^{-1}.[82] Neostigmine was prolonged to a slightly lesser degree; its elimination half-life more than doubled.[69]

j. The following might result in a prolonged period of *postoperative respiratory depression:*
  1. A relative excess of active relaxant (e.g., if it was administered late in the procedure or in too high a maintenance dose, or if it accumulated during a prolonged surgical procedure).
  2. Altered metabolism of relaxant (organ dysfunction, atypical pseudocholinesterase).
  3. Inadequate reversal or reversal prior to adequate spontaneous recovery (i.e., reversal in the presence of very deep block).
  4. Interactions with anesthetic agents or with other drugs such as aminoglycoside antibiotics.
  5. Underlying neuromuscular and muscular disease (e.g., myasthenia gravis, myasthenic syndrome).
  6. Hypothermia with decreased nerve conduction, muscle contractility, muscle blood flow, and metabolism.
  7. pH, P_{CO_2}, and electrolyte abnormalities.
  8. Depressed CNS function from anesthetic agents, opiates, or atropine or from a preexisting or acute CNS disorder.
  9. Respiratory reflexes (e.g., depressed Hering-Breuer reflex due to controlled ventilation, reflex laryngeal apnea).

     Central depression may be distinguished from peripheral paralysis by assessing the ventilatory pattern (Table 15-2).

k. *Priming* with a small dose of *reversal agent* prior to administration of the "full" dose has been reported to be useful,[157,158] but this has not been substantiated by other investigators.[13,159,160] Its proponents argue that it accelerates reversal without compromising neuromuscular block prior to administration of the full reversal dose. The technique has not gained widespread acceptance.

TABLE 15-2
Respiratory Patterns in the Presence of CNS Depression and Paralysis

	Rate	Depth	Tvg	Tremors
CNS Depression	slow	normal–deep	no	no
Peripheral Paralysis	rapid, jerky	shallow	yes	yes

l. Following apparently adequate recovery and reversal in the OR, $T_4/T_1 <$ 0.70 *in the PACU* may be due to inaccurate assessment in the OR (i.e., a mistaken impression that there was adequate reversal), inaccurate assessment in the PACU, excessive reversal agent, administration of other agents with blocking properties, and peripheral cooling. Even though administration of reversal agents improves neuromuscular function, there may be enough relaxant still around, and drugs such as aminoglycoside antibiotics and calcium entry blockers may exacerbate residual block. If there are no accompanying clinical signs of weakness, then a phenomenon that is limited to the site of peripheral testing must be considered. It has recently been shown that a cool extremity is associated with decreased responses to train-of-four stimulation (Chap. 10).[148,151,153]

m. *Barrier pressure* is the pressure differential between the lower esophageal sphincter and the stomach. *Atropine* alone has been shown to decrease *barrier pressure* for 1 hour and thus allow for possible regurgitation (if there is an incompetent sphincter). Simultaneous administration of neostigmine and atropine is associated with a significant decrease at 1 and 2 minutes, with a return toward normal by 3 minutes.[161] Administration of a prokinetic drug such as metoclopramide does not prevent the relaxation of the lower esophageal sphincter. Of note, patients who underwent reversal with neostigmine may have higher rates of nausea and vomiting than nonreversed controls.[142]

n. *Anticholinesterases* may increase *bowel activity* even if they are accompanied by an antimuscarinic agent.[162-165] It has been suggested that this (as well as neostigmine-induced reduction of mesenteric blood flow) may compromise the integrity of bowel anastomoses.[162,163,166] This theoretical concern generally is not a problem if one avoids unopposed muscarinic stimulation. However, neostigmine's effects on colonic motility are not fully prevented by atropine or glycopyrrolate,[167,168] and they may be particularly harmful in the presence of the sympathetic block that accompanies spinal or epidural anesthesia.[169] The effects may be attenuated by halothane.[165]

o. *Anticholinesterases* can result in increased *bronchomotor tone* and airway secretions. These effects are opposed by antimuscarinic agents.

p. It theoretically is best to give *atropine,* 0.007–0.01 mg · kg^{-1}, approximately 30 seconds before *edrophonium* because of the sudden effect that a high dose of edrophonium can have on the *heart rate.* This was found to be the case in infants and children, in whom administration of 0.01 mg · kg^{-1} of atropine prior to edrophonium, 1.0 mg · kg^{-1}, was found to be preferable to the simultaneous administration of these drugs.[114] However, these agents both have a rapid onset, and many anesthesiologists give them simultaneously to adult patients.[40,115,117] A mixture of atropine, 0.01 mg · kg^{-1}, and edrophonium, 0.5 mg · kg^{-1}, has relatively minor effects on heart rate.[40,117] Higher doses of edrophonium may require larger doses of atropine,[107] but this has been disputed.[121]

q. *Glycopyrrolate,* which has a slower onset than atropine, is less suitable for simultaneous administration with *edrophonium:* 0.005 mg · kg^{-1} did not provide consistently adequate protection against edrophonium-induced decreases in heart rate,[115,117] and 0.01 mg · kg^{-1} was associated with excessive tachycardia.[117] Glycopyrrolate, 0.005 mg · kg^{-1} administered 1 minute before edrophonium provided better cardiovascular stability (than simultaneous administration) in children[121] and adults.[120] However, transient tachycardia may result, especially in adults who receive a higher dose of the antimuscarinic agent (e.g., 0.01 mg · kg^{-1}).[117,120]

r. *Muscarinic responses differ in adults and children.* For example, glycopyrrolate, 0.05 mg · kg^{-1}, is more effective at opposing edrophonium-induced bradycardia in adults[120] than in children.[121] The difference is attributable to a greater degree of vagal tone in children and adolescents. Overall, we tend to use higher doses of antimuscarinic agents in children and may elect to administer them prior to the anticholinesterases.

s. *Atropine* is the mainstay of therapy following *poisoning* with *nerve gas or organophosphorus insecticides.* It reverses the muscarinic effects of ACh excess. Autoinjectors with 2 mg of atropine citrate are carried on battlefields. Rapid initial atropinization with 2–4 mg and titration of additional atropine to *secretions* and *respiratory exchange* appear to be the "best indicators for casualty care."[133] Cumulative doses of atropine amounting to 10–20 mg may be required during the first 2–3 hours[133]; a dose of 453 mg was used in one case.[134] Titrating to *heart rate* alone may be misleading because of the magnitude of confounding variables. The *size of the pupil* may be helpful; however, direct exposure of the conjunctiva to nerve gas will override the ocular effects of therapeutically effective doses of atropine.

Acute *treatment of CNS effects* seems best accomplished with *atropine* and *anticonvulsants* such as diazepam and midazolam.[133] Atropine, a tertiary amine, crosses the *blood-brain barrier.* Although this feature may be undesirable when one administers atropine along with a quaternary amine for reversal of a relaxant postoperatively, it may be a vital feature for treating the nerve gas victim. Benzodiazepines have abolished soman-induced seizure activity. In doses of 2.2 mg · kg^{-1} given intramuscularly 10 minutes prior to soman injection, diazepam prevented the development of neuropathologic lesions in experimental studies.[135]

Oximes such as *pralidoxime* actually *bind to the offending agent* and free up the victim's cholinesterase.[170] Such agents have been effective in the treatment of cholinergic crisis following anticholinesterase overdose in patients with myasthenia gravis. Autoinjectors with 600 mg of pralidoxime (2 *PAM* chloride) are carried on battlefields.[133] In the emergency room setting, 1-gm boluses have been used to treat poisoning due to organophosphate insecticides. If two such doses are not effective, intravenous infusion at a rate of 0.5 gm/hr has been helpful.[136] No untoward side effects were noted with doses as high as 28 gm.[134] Unfortunately, oxime therapy is not effective if the anticholinesterase has had enough time to irreversibly destroy the victim's cholinesterase. For an agent like GD (soman), this may be 50% complete in 2 minutes; for GB (sarin) it is 5 hours; and for commercial pesticides and VX it may require days.[133]

t. In view of the potential for rapid destruction of the victim's cholinesterase by *nerve gas,* it has been recommended that soldiers be *pretreated with pyridostigmine* in doses approximately 1/10th to 1/20th that taken by patients with myasthenia gravis. The goal of such pretreatment is to "protect" some of the cholinesterase in a potential victim from irreversible destruction by an agent such as soman.[171,172] Experience has shown that pyridostigmine bromide tablets, 30 mg taken every 8 hours, greatly reduce the lethality of exposure to GD (soman).[133] This dose typically provides sufficient *reversible carbamylation* of cholinesterase while not compromising normal cholinergic functions. Free cholinesterase becomes available when the pyridostigmine-acetylcholinesterase complex separates. Studies in an isolated limb model suggest that such pretreatment should not affect the intraoperative use of NDRs.[173] However, it has been proposed that a decrease in ACh metabolism may result in less choline being available for resynthesis of ACh.[172]

u. An assay of *cholinesterase activity* would identify inactivation and destruction of cholinesterase by *organophosphate poisoning or nerve gas,* since these actions reduce cholinesterase activity.

v. The *dose of neostigmine* should not be changed because of *physostigmine* administration. Physostigmine, an anticholinesterase with a tertiary amine structure, is used to treat central anticholinergic syndrome that may be induced by atropine that has crossed the blood-brain barrier. In the doses used for this purpose (1–2 mg/70 kg), physostigmine lacks significant ability to reverse nondepolarizing block.[174] However, at least on theoretical grounds, it may oppose an NDR-induced block by (1) slight inhibition of acetylcholinesterase and (2) inhibition of phosphodiesterase (thereby allowing release of more ACh).[175,176]

w. The effects of *long-term exposure to anticholinesterases* (e.g., in battlefield exposure) on neuromuscular block may manifest as follows: (1) First, during exposure to the anticholinesterases, the patient demonstrates decreased response to NDRs, increased sensitivity to SCh and decreased metabolism of SCh. (2) Subsequent down-regulation of ACh receptors will be associated with an increased sensitivity to NDRs and, if the anticholinesterase is no longer present, a decreased responsiveness to SCh. (3) Eventually one sees diffuse abnormalities resembling a polyneuropathy.

x. The relative lack of *pseudocholinesterase inhibition* by *edrophonium*[102] might have an advantage if SCh had to be administered only a short time after a previous NDR-induced block had been reversed. Both *neostigmine* and *pyridostigmine* cause profound pseudocholinesterase inhibition.[99,101,102,177–179] At 5 minutes after neostigmine, 0.05 mg · kg^{-1}, and pyridostigmine, 0.25 mg · kg^{-1}, serum cholinesterase activity was depressed 70% and 63%, respectively.[178] Greater than 33% depression persisted for 15 minutes after neostigmine and 60 minutes after pyridostigmine.[178] Following neostigmine, 5 mg, or pyridostigmine, 25 mg, the effect of SCh was prolonged from a control of 11.1 minutes to 13.1 and 23.9 minutes, respectively.[179]

References ◆

1. Wilson IB: The interaction of tensilon and neostigmine with acetylcholinesterase. Arch Int Pharmacodyn Ther 54:204, 1955
2. Baker T, Stanec A: Drug actions at mammalian motor nerve endings: the suppression of neostigmine-induced fasciculations by vecuronium and isoflurane. Anesthesiology 67:942–947, 1987
3. Blaber LC, Bowman WC: Studies on the repetitive discharge evoked in ulnar nerve and skeletal muscle after injection of anticholinesterase drugs. Br J Pharmacol 20:326–344, 1963
4. Raines A, Henderson TR, Dretchen KL: Effects of calcium channel blocking agents on neostigmine-induced fasciculations. Eur J Pharmacol 173:11–17, 1989
5. Riker WF, Okamoto MO: Pharmacology of motor nerve terminals. Annu Rev Pharmacol 9:173–208, 1969
6. Blaber LC: The mechanism of the facilitatory action of edrophonium in cat skeletal muscle. Br J Pharmacol 46:498–507, 1972
7. Fiekers JF: Interactions of edrophonium, physostigmine and methanesulfonyl fluoride with the snake end-plate acetylcholine receptor-channel complex. J Pharmacol Exp Ther 234:539–549, 1985
8. Wachtel RE: Comparison of anticholinesterases and their effects on acetylcholine-activated ion channels. Anesthesiology 72:496–503, 1990
9. Riker WF, Wescoe WC: The direct action of prostigmine on skeletal muscle: its relationship to the choline esters. J Pharmacol Exp Ther 88:58, 1946
10. Bartkowski RR: Incomplete reversal of pancuronium neuromuscular blockade by neostigmine, pyridostigmine, and edrophonium. Anesth Analg 66:594–598, 1987
11. Baraka A: Irreversible tubocurarine neuromuscular block in the human. Br J Anaesth 39:891–894, 1967
12. Bevan DR, Donati F, Kopman AF: Reversal of neuromuscular blockade. Anesthesiology 77:785–805, 1992
13. Magorian TT, Lynam DP, Caldwell JE, Miller RD: Can early administration of neostigmine, in single or repeated doses, alter the course of neuromuscular recovery from a vecuronium-induced neuromuscular blockade? Anesthesiology 73:410–414, 1990
14. Morris RB, Cronnelly R, Miller RD, et al: Pharmacokinetics of edrophonium and neostigmine when antagonizing d-tubocurarine neuromuscular block in man. Anesthesiology 54:399–402, 1981
15. Baraka A: Irreversible curarization. Anaesth Intensive Care 5:244–246, 1977
16. Beemer GH, Bjorksten AR, Dawson PJ, Dawson RJ, Robertson BA: Determinants of reversal time of competitive neuromuscular block by anticholinesterases. Br J Anaesth 66:469–475, 1991
17. Caldwell JE, Robertson EN, Baird WLM: Antagonism of profound neuromuscular blockade induced by vecuronium or atracurium: comparison of neostigmine with edrophonium. Br J Anaesth 58:1285–1289, 1986
18. Caldwell JE, Robertson EN, Baird WLM: Antagonism of vecuronium and atracurium: comparison of neostigmine and edrophonium administered at 5% twitch height recovery. Br J Anaesth 59:478–481, 1987

19. Donati F, Lahoud J, McCready D, Bevan DR: Neostigmine, pyridostigmine and edrophonium as antagonists of deep pancuronium blockade. Can J Anaesth 34:589–593, 1987
20. Engbaek J, Ostergaard D, Skovgaard LT, Viby-Mogensen J: Reversal of intense neuromuscular blockade following infusion of atracurium. Anesthesiology 72:803–806, 1990
21. Goldhill DR, Wainwright AP, Stuart CS, Flynn PJ: Neostigmine after spontaneous recovery from neuromuscular blockade: effect on depth of blockade monitored with train-of-four and tetanic stimuli. Anaesthesia 44:293–299, 1989
22. Gwinnutt CL, Walker RWM, Meakin G: Antagonism of intense atracurium-induced neuromuscular block in children. Br J Anaesth 67:13–16, 1991
23. Hennart D, d'Hollander A, Plasman C, et al: Importance of the level of paralysis recovery for a rapid antagonism of atracurium neuromuscular blockade with moderate doses of edrophonium. Anesthesiology 64:384–387, 1986
24. Jones JE, Hunter JM, Utting JE: Use of neostigmine in the antagonism of residual neuromuscular blockade produced by vecuronium. Br J Anaesth 59:1454–1458, 1987
25. Katz RL: Neuromuscular effects of d-tubocurarine, edrophonium and neostigmine in man. Anesthesiology 28:327–336, 1967
26. Kopman AF: Recovery times following edrophonium and neostigmine reversal of pancuronium, atracurium and vecuronium steady-state infusions. Anesthesiology 65:572–578, 1986
27. Kopman AF: Edrophonium antagonism of pancuronium induced neuromuscular blockade in man: a reappraisal. Anesthesiology 51:139–42, 1979
28. Katz RL: Clinical neuromuscular pharmacology of pancuronium. Anesthesiology 34:550–556, 1971
29. Meistelman C, Debaene B, d'Hollander A, Saint-Maurice C: Importance of the level of paralysis recovery for a rapid antagonism of vecuronium with neostigmine in children during halothane anesthesia. Anesthesiology 69:97, 1988
30. Mirakhur RK, Gibson FM, Lavery GG: Antagonism of vecuronium-induced neuromuscular blockade with edrophonium or neostigmine. Br J Anaesth 59:473–477, 1987
31. Rupp SM, McChristian JW, Miller RD, Taboada JA, Cronnelly R: Neostigmine and edrophonium antagonism of varying intensity neuromuscular blockade induced by atracurium, pancuronium or vecuronium. Anesthesiology 64:711–717, 1986
32. Beemer GH, Rozental P: Postoperative neuromuscular function. Anaesth Intensive Care 14:41–45, 1986
33. Cashman JN, Jones RM, Adams AP: Atracurium recovery: prediction of safe reversal times with edrophonium. Anaesthesia 44:805–807, 1989
34. Bevan DR, Smith CE, Donati F: Postoperative neuromuscular blockade: a comparison between atracurium, vecuronium, and pancuronium. Anesthesiology 69:272–276, 1988
35. Gencarelli PJ, Miller RD: Antagonism of ORG NC45 (vecuronium) and pancuronium neuromuscular blockade by neostigmine. Br J Anaesth 54:53–56, 1982
36. Hutton P, Burchett KR, Madden AP: Comparison of recovery after neuromuscular blockade by atracurium or pancuronium. Br J Anaesth 60:36–42, 1988
37. Fisher DM, Rosen JI: A pharmacokinetic explanation for increasing recovery time following larger or repeated doses of nondepolarizing muscle relaxants. Anesthesiology 65:286–291, 1986
38. Savarese JJ, Ali HH, Basta SJ, Embree PB, Scott RPF, Sunder N, Weakly JN, Wastila WB, El-Sayad HA: The clinical neuromuscular pharmacology of mivacurium chloride (BW B1090U): a short-acting nondepolarizing ester neuromuscular blocking drug. Anesthesiology 68:723–732, 1988
39. Agoston S, Feldman SA, Miller RD: Plasma concentrations of pancuronium and neuromuscular blockade after injection into the isolated arm, bolus injection, and continuous infusion. Anesthesiology 51:119–122, 1979
40. Cronnelly R, Morris RB, Miller RD: Edrophonium: duration of action and atropine requirement in humans during halothane anesthesia. Anesthesiology 57:261–266, 1982
41. Cronnelly R, Morris RB: Antagonism of neuromuscular blockade. Br J Anaesth 54:183–194, 1982
42. Dernovoi B, Agoston S, Barvais L, Baurain M, Lefebvre R, d'Hollander A: Neostigmine

antagonism of vecuronium paralysis during fentanyl, halothane, isoflurane, and enflurane anesthesia. Anesthesiology 66:698–701, 1987
43. Gill SS, Bevan DR, Donati F: Edrophonium antagonism of atracurium during enflurane anaesthesia. Br J Anaesth 64:300–305, 1990
44. Gencarelli PJ, Miller RD, Eger II EI, Newfield P: Decreasing enflurane concentrations and d-tubocurarine neuromuscular blockade. Anesthesiology 56:192–194, 1982
45. Delisle S, Bevan DR: Impaired antagonism of pancuronium during enflurane anaesthesia in man. Br J Anaesth 54:441–445, 1982
46. Gyermek L: Halogenated vapor anesthetics adversely influence edrophonium reversal. Int J Clin Pharmacol Ther Toxicol 26:75, 1988
47. Miller RD, Van Nyhuis LS, Eger EI II, Vitez TS, Way WL: The effect of acid-base balance on neostigmine antagonism of d-tubocurarine-induced neuromuscular blockade. Anesthesiology 42:377–383, 1975
48. Miller RD, Roderick LL: The influence of acid-base changes on neostigmine antagonism of pancuronium neuromuscular blockade. Br J Anaesth 50:317–324, 1978
49. Tammisto T, Wirtavouri K, Salmenpera M: Effect of hypo- or hypercarbia on the neostigmine antagonism of pancuronium-induced neuromuscular blockade in man. Br J Anaesth 53:116P, 1981
50. Fisher DM, Cronnelly R, Miller RD, Sharma M: The neuromuscular pharmacology of neostigmine in infants and children. Anesthesiology 59:220–225, 1983
51. Meakin G, Sweet PT, Bevan JC, Bevan DR: Neostigmine and edrophonium as antagonists of pancuronium in infants and children. Anesthesiology 59:316, 1983
52. Baxter MRN, Bevan JC, Samuel J, Donati F, Bevan DR: Postoperative neuromuscular function in pediatric day-care patients. Anesth Analg 72:504–508, 1991
53. Goudsouzian NG, d'Hollander AA, Viby-Mogensen J: Prolonged neuromuscular block from mivacurium in two patients with cholinesterase deficiency. Anesth Analg 77:183–185, 1993
54. Marsh RHK, Chjmielewski AT, Goat VA: Recovery from pancuronium: a comparison between old and young patients. Anaesthesia 35:1193–1196, 1980
55. McCarthy GJ, Cooper R, Stanley JC, Mirakhur RK: Dose-response relationships for neostigmine antagonism of vecuronium-induced neuromuscular block in adults and the elderly. Br J Anaesth 69:281–283, 1992
56. Young WL, Matteo RS, Ornstein E: Duration of action of neostigmine and pyridostigmine in the elderly. Anesth Analg 67:775–778, 1988
57. Mirakhur RK, Briggs P, Clarke RSJ, Dundee JW, Johnston HML: Comparison of atropine and glycopyrrolate in a mixture with pyridostigmine for the antagonism of neuromuscular block. Br J Anaesth 53:1315–1320, 1981
58. Mirakhur RK, Clarke RSJ, Dundee JW, McDonald JR: Anticholinergic drugs in anaesthesia: a survey of their present position. Anaesthesia 33:133–138, 1978
59. Mirakhur RK, Dundee JW, Jones CJ, Coppel DL, Clarke RSJ: Reversal of neuromuscular blockade: dose determination studies with atropine and glycopyrrolate given before or in a mixture with neostigmine. Anesth Analg 60:557–562, 1981
60. Mirakhur RK, Jones CJ, Dundee JW: Heart rate changes following reversal of neuromuscular block with glycopyrrolate or atropine given before or with neostigmine. Indian J Anaesth 29:83–87, 1981
61. Mirakhur RK, Dundee JW, Clarke RSJ: Glycopyrrolate-neostigmine mixture for antagonism of neuromuscular block: comparison with atropine-neostigmine mixture. Br J Anaesth 49:825–829, 1977
62. Mirakhur RK, Dundee JW: Glycopyrrolate: pharmacology and clinical use. Anaesthesia 38:1195–1204, 1983
63. Proakis AG, Harris GB: Comparative penetration of glycopyrrolate and atropine across the blood-brain and placental barriers in anesthetized dogs. Anesthesiology 48:339–344, 1978
64. Simpson KH, Smith RJ, Davies RJ, Davies LF: Comparison of the effects of atropine and glycopyrrolate on cognitive function following general anesthesia. Br J Anaesth 59:966, 1987
65. Tune L, Holland A, Folstein M, Damlouji N, Gardner T, Coyle J: Association of postoperative delirium with raised serum levels of anticholinergic drugs. Lancet 2:651–653, 1981

66. Sheref SE: Pattern of CNS recovery following reversal of neuromuscular blockade: comparison of atropine and glycopyrrolate. Br J Anaesth 57:188, 1985
67. Fogdall RP, Miller RD: Antagonism of d-tubocurarine- and pancuronium-induced neuromuscular blockades by pyridostigmine in man. Anesthesiology 39:504–509, 1973
68. Donati F, McCarroll SM, Antzaca C, McCreedy D, Bevan DR: Dose-response curves for edrophonium, neostigmine, and pyridostigmine after pancuronium and d-tubocurarine. Anesthesiology 66:471–476, 1987
69. Cronnelly R, Stanski DR, Miller RD, et al: Renal function and the pharmacokinetics of neostigmine in anesthetized patients. Anesthesiology 51:222–226, 1979
70. Miller RD, Van Nyhuis LS, Eger II EI, Vitez TS, Way WL: Comparative times to peak effect and durations of action of neostigmine and pyridostigmine. Anesthesiology 41:27–33, 1974
71. Samra SK, Pandit UA, Pandit SK, Kothary SP: Modification by halogenated anaesthetics of chronotropic response during reversal of neuromuscular blockade. Can Anaesth Soc J 30:48–52, 1983
72. Baraka A: Safe reversal: II. Atropine-neostigmine mixture. An electrocardiographic study. Br J Anaesth 40:30–34, 1968
73. Goldhill DR, Embree PB, Ali HH, Savarese JJ: Reversal of pancuronium: neuromuscular and cardiovascular effects of a mixture of neostigmine and glycopyrronium. Anaesthesia 43:443, 1988
74. Ramamurthy S, Shaker MH, Winnie AP: Glycopyrrolate as a substitute for atropine in neostigmine reversal of muscle relaxant drugs. Can Anaesth Soc J 19:399–411, 1972
75. Ostheimer GW: A comparison of glycopyrrolate and atropine during reversal of nondepolarizing neuromuscular block with neostigmine. Anesth Analg 56:182–186, 1977
76. Bali IM, Mirakhur RK: Comparison of glycopyrrolate, atropine and hyoscine in a mixture of neostigmine for reversal of neuromuscular block following closed mitral valvotomy. Acta Anaesthesiol Scand 24:321–325, 1980
77. Cozanitis DA, Dundee JW, Merrett JD, Jones CJ, Mirakhur RK: Evaluation of glycopyrrolate and atropine as adjuncts to reversal of nondepolarising neuromuscular blocking agents in a "true-to-life" situation. Br J Anaesth 523:85–89, 1980
78. Mostafa SM, Vucevic M: Comparison of atropine and glycopyrronium in patients with pre-existing cardiac disease. Anaesthesia 39:1207–1213, 1984
79. Lonsdale M, Stuart J: Complete heart block following glycopyrronium/neostigmine mixture (letter). Anaesthesia 44:448–449, 1989
80. Beebe DS, Shumway SJ, Maddock R: Sinus arrest after intravenous neostigmine in two heart transplant patients. Anesth Analg 78:779–782, 1994
81. Wettereslev J, Jarnvig I, Jorgensen LN, Olsen NV: Split-dose atropine versus glycopyrrolate with neostigmine for reversal of gallamine-induced neuromuscular blockade. Acta Anaesthesiol Scand 35:398–401, 1991
82. Katz RL: Pyridostigmin (Mestinon) as an antagonist of d-tubocurarine. Anesthesiology 28:528–534, 1967
83. Cronnelly R, Stanski DR, Miller RD, Sheiner LB: Pyridostigmine kinetics with and without renal function. Clin Pharmacol Ther 28:78–81, 1980
84. Williams NE, Calvey TN, Chan K: Plasma concentration of pyridostigmine during the antagonism of neuromuscular block. Br J Anaesth 55:27–31, 1983
85. Astley BA, Hughes R, Payne JP: Antagonism of atracurium-induced neuromuscular blockade by neostigmine or edrophonium. Br J Anaesth 58:1290–1295, 1986
86. Calvey TN, Williams NE, Muir KT: Plasma concentration of edrophonium in man. Clin Plasma Ther 19:813, 1976
87. Donati F, Smith CE, Bevan DR: Dose-response relationships for edrophonium and neostigmine as antagonists of moderate and profound atracurium blockade. Anesth Analg 68:13–17, 1989
88. Kopman AF: The current status of edrophonium: have we come "full circle"? Can J Anaesth 38:145–150, 1991
89. Lavery GG, Mirakhur RK, Gibson FM: A comparison of edrophonium and neostigmine for the antagonism of atracurium-induced neuromuscular block. Anesth Analg 64:867, 1985
90. Mirakhur RK: Antagonism of pancuronium and tubocurarine blocks by edrophonium or neostigmine: a comparative study. Eur J Anaesthesiol 4:411, 1987

91. Miller RD, Cronnelly R: A new look at an old drug. Anesthesiology 59:84–85, 1983
92. Smith CE, Donati F, Bevan DR: Dose-response relationship for edrophonium and neostigmine as antagonists of atracurium and vecuronium neuromuscular blockade. Anesthesiology 71:37–43, 1989
93. Ferguson A, Egerszegi P, Bevan DR: Neostigmine, pyridostigmine, and edrophonium as antagonists of pancuronium. Anesthesiology 53:390–394, 1980
94. Breen PJ, Doherty WG, Donati F, Bevan DR: The potencies of edrophonium and neostigmine as antagonists of pancuronium. Anaesthesia 40:844–847, 1985
95. Jones RM, Pearce AC, Williams JP: Recovery characteristics following antagonism of atracurium with neostigmine or edrophonium. Br J Anaesth 56:453–457, 1984
96. Bevan DR: Reversal of pancuronium with edrophonium. Anaesthesia 34:614–619, 1979
97. MacFarlane DW, Pelikan EW, Unna KR: Evaluation of curarising drugs in man: I. Antagonism to curarising effects of d-tubocurarine by neostigmine, m-hydroxyphenyltrimethylammonium and m-hydroxyphenylethyldimethylammonium. J Pharmacol Exp Ther 100:382–392, 1950
98. Randall LO, Lehmann G: Pharmacological properties of some neostigmine analogs. J Pharmacol Exp Ther 99:16–32, 1950
99. Sakuma N, Hasimoto Y, Iwatsuki N: Effects of neostigmine and edrophonium on human erythrocyte acetylcholinesterase activity. Br J Anaesth 68:316–317, 1992
100. Harper NJN, Bradshaw EG, Healy TEJ: Antagonism of alcuronium with edrophonium or neostigmine. Br J Anaesth 56:1089, 1984
101. Mirakhur RK, Lavery TD, Briggs LP, Clarke RSJ: Effects of neostigmine and pyridostigmine on serum cholinesterase activity. Can Anaesth Soc J 29:55–58, 1982
102. Mirakhur RK: Edrophonium and plasma cholinesterase activity. Can Anaesth Soc J 33:588–590, 1986
103. Baird WLM, Bowman WC, Kerr WJ: Some actions of ORG NC45 and of edrophonium in the anaesthetized cat and in man. Br J Anaesth 54:375–385, 1982
104. Casson WR, Jones RM, Skelly AM, Robinson PD, Adams AP: Reversal of profound atracurium induced paralysis: anticholinesterases compared using train of four stimulation. Anesthesiology 63:A360, 1985
105. Yang E, Lee C, Tran B: Optimum dose of edrophonium for reversal of atracurium neuromuscular block. Anesth Analg 63:A283, 1984
106. Donati F, Ferguson A, Bevan DR: Twitch depression and train-of-four ratio after antagonism of pancuronium with edrophonium, neostigmine, or pyridostigmine. Anesth Analg 62:314–316, 1983
107. Engbaek J, Ording H, Ostergaard D, Viby-Mogensen J: Edrophonium and neostigmine for reversal of the neuromuscular blocking effect of vecuronium. Acta Anaesthesiol Scand 29:544–546, 1985
108. Power SJ, Jones RM: Reversal of profound paralysis: use of large doses of edrophonium to antagonize vecuronium and pancuronium neuromuscular blockade. Acta Anaesthesiol Scand 33:478–481, 1989
109. Shorten GD, Ali HH, Goudsouzian NG: Neostigmine and edrophonium antagonism of moderate neuromuscular block induced by pancuronium or tubocurarine. Br J Anaesth 70:160–162, 1993
110. Lahoud J, Donati F, Bevan DR, et al: Neostigmine, edrophonium and pyrdostigmine as antagonists of deep pancuronium block. Can Anaesth Soc J 33:S88–S89, 1986
111. Rupp SM, McChristian JW, Miller RD: Neostigmine antagonizes a profound neuromuscular blockade more rapidly than edrophonium. Anesthesiology 61:A297, 1984
112. Sanfilippo M, Vilardi V, Fierro G, Rosa G, Pelaia P, Gasparetto A: Neostigmine and edrophonium as antagonists of atracurium and pancuronium. Acta Anaesthesiol Scand 32:437–440, 1988
113. Abdulatif M, Naguib M: Neostigmine and edrophonium reversal of the neuromuscular blocking effect of pipecuronium. Can J Anaesth 38:159–163, 1991
114. Fisher DM, Cronnelly R, Sharma M, Miller RD: Clinical pharmacology of edrophonium in infants and children. Anesthesiology 61:428–433, 1984
115. Azar I, Pham AN, Karambelkar DJ, Lear E: The heart rate following edrophonium-atropine and edrophonium-glycopyrrolate mixtures. Anesthesiology 59:139–141, 1983

116. Mehta MP, Choi WW, Kumar V, Gergis SD, Sokoll MD: Safety and efficacy of OH 101—mixture of edrophonium and atropine. A reversal agent. Anesth Analg 65:S96, 1986
117. Mirakhur RK: Antagonism of the muscarinic effects of edrophonium with atropine or glycopyrrolate: a comparative study. Br J Anaesth 57:1216–1220, 1985
118. Urquhart ML, Ramsey FM, Royster RL, Morell RC, Gerr P: Heart rate and rhythm following an edrophonium/atropine mixture for antagonism of neuromuscular blockade during fentanyl/N_2O/O_2 anesthesia. Anesthesiology 67:561–565, 1987
119. Naguib M, Gomaa M, Absood GH: Atropine-edrophonium mixture: a dose-response study. Anesth Analg 67:650, 1988
120. Dodd P, Day SJ, Goldhill DR, Macleod DM, Withington PS, Yate PM: Glycopyrronium requirements for antagonism of the muscarinic side effects of edrophonium. Br J Anaesth 62:77–81, 1989
121. Goldhill DR, Pyne A, Jones CJ: Antagonism of neuromuscular blockade: the cardiovascular effects in children of the combination of edrophonium and glycopyrronium. Anaesthesia 43:930–934, 1988
122. Mirakhur RK, McCarthy GJ: Basic pharmacology of reversal agents. Anesthesiol Clin North Am 11:237–250, 1993
123. Eriksson LI, Wyon N, Lennmarken C: Repetitive administration of neostigmine may cause increased neuromuscular block. Anesth Analg 74:S89, 1992
124. Payne JP, Hughes R, Azawi S: Neuromuscular blockade by neostigmine in anaesthetized man. Br J Anaesth 52:69–76, 1980
125. Astley BA, Katz RL, Payne JP: Electrical and mechanical responses after neuromuscular blockade with vecuronium, and subsequent antagonism with neostigmine or edrophonium. Br J Anaesth 59:983–988, 1987
126. Albuquerque EX, Akaike A, Shaw KP, Rickett DL: The interaction of anticholinesterase agents with the acetylcholine receptor-ionic channel complex. Fundam Appl Toxicol 4:S27–S33, 1984
127. Chang CC, Chen SM, Hong SJ: Reversal of the neostigmine induced tetanic fade and endplate potential rundown with respect to autoregulation of transmitter release. Br J Pharmacol 95:1255–1261, 1988
128. Chang CC, Hong SJ, Ko JL: Mechanisms of the inhibition by neostigmine of tetanic contraction in the mouse diaphragm. Br J Pharmacol 87:757–762, 1986
129. Riker WF, Standaert FG: The action of facilitatory drugs and acetylcholine on neuromuscular transmission. Ann NY Acad Sci 135:163–176, 1966
130. Miyamoto MD: The actions of cholinergic drugs on motor nerve terminals. Pharmacol Rev 29:221–247, 1978
131. Buzello W, Krieg N, Schlickewei A: Hazards of neostigmine in patients with neuromuscular disorders. Br J Anaesth 54:529–534, 1982
132. De Candole CA, Douglas WW, Evans CL, Holmes R, Spencer KEV, Torrance RW, Wilson KM: The failure of respiration in death by anticholinesterase poisoning. Br J Pharmacol 8:466–474, 1953
133. Dunn MA, Sidell FR: Progress in medical defense against nerve agents. JAMA 262:649–652, 1989
134. Milthers E, Clemmesen C, Nimb M: Poisoning with phosphostigmines: treated with atropine, pralidoxime methiodide and diacetyl monoxime. Dan Med Bull 10:122–129, 1963
135. Martin LJ, Doebler JA, Shih TM, Anthony A: Protective effect of diazepam pretreatment on soman-induced brain lesion formation. Brain Res 325:287–289, 1985
136. Namba T, Nolte C, Jackrel J, Grob D: Poisoning due to organophosphate insecticides: acute and chronic manifestations. Am J Med 50:475–492, 1971
137. Jones JE, Parker CJ, Hunter JM: Antagonism of blockade produced by atracurium or vecuronium with low doses of neostigmine. Br J Anaesth 61:560, 1988
138. Mitterschiffthaler G, Khunl-Brady KS, Koller J, Mair P, Wieser C, Wierda M: Residual neuromuscular blockade: a comparison of vecuronium (Vc), atracurium (Ac), alcuronium (Alc), pancuronium (Pc), and pipecuronium (Pip). Acta Anaesthesiol Scand 33(suppl 91):140, 1989
139. Engbaek J, Howardy-Hansen P, Ording H, Viby-Mogensen J: Precurarization with vecuronium and pancuronium in awake, healthy volunteers: the influence on neuromuscular transmission and pulmonary function. Acta Anaesthesiol Scand 29:117–120, 1985

140. Howardy-Hansen P, Jorgensen BC, Ording H, Viby-Mogensen J: Pretreatment with nondepolarizing muscle relaxants: the influence on neuromuscular transmission and pulmonary function. Acta Anaesthesiol Scand 24:419–422, 1980
141. Howardy-Hansen P, Moller J, Hansen B: Pretreatment with atracurium: the influence on neuromuscular transmission and pulmonary function. Acta Anaesthesiol Scand 31:642–644, 1987
142. King MJ, Milazkiewicz R, Carli F, Deacock AR: Influence of neostigmine on postoperative vomiting. Br J Anaesth 61:403–406, 1988
143. Fox MA, Keens SJ, Utting JE: Neostigmine in the antagonism of the action of atracurium. Br J Anaesth 59:468, 1987
144. Johnson RA, Harper NJN: Antagonism of moderate degrees of vecuronium-induced neuromuscular block by small doses of neostigmine. Br J Anaesth 62:483, 1989
145. Erkola O, Karhunen U, Sandelin-Hellqvist: Spontaneous recovery of residual neuromuscular blockade after atracurium or vecuronium during isoflurane anaesthesia. Acta Anaesthesiol Scand 33:290–294, 1989
146. Brull SJ, Connelly NR, Garwood S, Garcia R, Silverman DG: Recovery of train-of-four after mivacurium. Anesthesiology 79:A925, 1993
147. Brull SJ, Ehrenwerth J, Connelly NR, Silverman DG: Assessment of residual curarization using low-current stimulation. Can J Anaesth 38:164–168, 1991
148. Pedersen T, Viby-Mogensen J, Bang U, Olsen NV, Jensen E, Engbaek J: Does perioperative tactile evaluation of the train-of-four response influence the frequency of postoperative residual neuromuscular blockade? Anesthesiology 73:835–839, 1990
149. Viby-Mogensen J, Jorgensen BC, Ording H: Residual curarization in the recovery room. Anesthesiology 50:539–541, 1979
150. Ali HH, Shorten GS: Nerve stimulation and residual neuromuscular block (letter). Anesthesiology 74:956–957, 1991
151. Eriksson LI, Jensen E, Viby-Mogensen J, Lennmarken C: Train-of-four (TOF) response following prolonged neuromuscular monitoring: influence of peripheral temperature. Anesthesiology 71:A827, 1989
152. Engbaek J, Skovgaard LT, Friis B, Kann T: The effect of temperature on the evoked EMG response. Anesthesiology 70:A810, 1989
153. Eriksson LI, Jensen E, Viby-Mogensen J, Lennmarken C: Influence of peripheral hypothermia on the train-of-four response in the absence of neuromuscular blockade (abstract). Acta Anaesthesiol Scand 33:157, 1989
154. Bevan DR, Archer D, Donati F, Ferguson A, Higgs BD: Antagonism of pancuronium in renal failure: no recurarization. Br J Anaesth 54:63–68, 1982
155. Miller RD, Cullen DJ: Renal failure and postoperative respiratory failure: recurarization? Br J Anaesth 48:253–256, 1976
156. Morris RB, Cronnelly R, Miller RD, et al: Pharmacokinetics of edrophonium in anephric and renal transplant patients. Br J Anaesth 53:1311–1314, 1981
157. Abdulatif M, Naguib M: Accelerated reversal of atracurium blockade with divided doses of neostigmine. Can Anaesth Soc J 33:723–728, 1986
158. Naguib M, Abdulatif M, Absood GH: Accelerated reversal of atracurium blockade with priming doses of edrophonium. Anesthesiology 66:397–400, 1987
159. Donati F, Smith CE, Bevan DR: "Priming" with neostigmine: failure to accelerate reversal of single twitch and train-of-four responses. Can J Anaesth 36:30–34, 1989
160. Szalados JE, Donati F, Bevan DR: Edrophonium priming for antagonism of atracurium neuromuscular blockade. Can J Anaesth 37:197–201, 1990
161. Turner DAB, Smith G: Evaluation of the combined effects of atropine and neostigmine on the lower oesophageal sphincter. Br J Anaesth 57:956–959, 1985
162. Aitkenhead AR: Anaesthesia and bowel surgery. Br J Anaesth 56:95, 1984
163. Ball CMA, Lewis CB: Effect of neostigmine of integrity of ileorectal anastomoses. Br Med J 2:587–588, 1968
164. Hannington-Kiff JG: Timing of atropine and neostigmine in the reversal of muscle relaxants. Br Med J 1:418–20, 1969
165. Wilkins JL, Hardcastle JD, Mann CV, et al: Effects of neostigmine and atropine on motor activity of ileum, colon and rectum of anaesthetized subjects. Br Med J 1:793–794, 1970

166. Hunter AR: Colorectal surgery for cancer: the anaesthetist's contribution? (editorial). Br J Anaesth 58:825–826, 1986
167. Ball CMA: Neostigmine and anastomosis dehiscence. Proc R Soc Med 63:752, 1970
168. Child CS: Prevention of neostigmine-induced colonic activity. Anaesthesia 39:1083, 1984
169. Carlstedt A, Nordgren S, Fasth S, Appelgren L, Hulten L: Epidural anesthesia and postoperative colorectal motility: a possible hazard to a colorectal anastomosis. Int J Colon Dis 4:144–149, 1989
170. Childs AF, Davies DR, Green AL, Rutland JP: The reactivation by oximes and hydroxamic acids of cholinesterase inhibited by organo-phosphorus compounds. Br J Pharmacol 10:462–465, 1955
171. Dirnhuber P, French MC, Green M, Leadbeater L, Stratton JA: The protection of primates against soman poisoning by pretreatment with pyridostigmine. J Pharm Pharmacol 31:295–299, 1979
172. Carter ML, Karalliedde L: Effect of pretreatment with oral pyridostigmine. Br J Anaesth 68:113, 1992
173. Turner GA, Williams JD, Baker DJ: Effect of pretreatment with oral pyridostigmine on subsequent activity of alcuronium in non-anaesthetized subjects. Br J Anaesth 66:365–369, 1991
174. Baraka A: Antagonisms of neuromuscular block by physostigmine in man. Br J Anaesth 50:1075–1077, 1978
175. Standaert FG, Dretchen KL: Cyclic nucleotides in neuromuscular transmission. Anesth Analg 60:91–99, 1981
176. Curley WH, Dretchen KL, Standaert FG: Inhibition by physostigmine of neural phosphodiesterase. Fed Proc 39:410, 1980
177. Bishop MJ, Hornbein TF: Prolonged effect of succinylcholine after neostigmine and pyridostigmine administration in patients with renal failure. Anesthesiology 58:384–386, 1983
178. Baraka A, Wakid N, Mansour R, Haddad W: Effect of neostigmine and pyridostigmine on the plasma cholinesterase activity. Br J Anaesth 53:849–851, 1981
179. Sunew KY, Hicks RG: Effects of neostigmine and pyridostigmine on duration of succinylcholine action and pseudocholinesterase activity. Anesthesiology 49:188–191, 1978

16

DAVID G. SILVERMAN | FRANÇOIS DONATI

Neuromuscular Effects of Depolarizing Relaxants

◆ MECHANISMS OF ACTION

The depolarizing agents, succinylcholine (SCh) and decamethonium, generally have a more flexible structure that allows more free bond rotation than their nondepolarizing (competitive, stabilizing) counterparts.[1] They cause prolonged end-plate *depolarization* by remaining in the neuromuscular junction (NMJ) and *binding repeatedly* to the alpha subunits of cholinoceptors.

Like acetylcholine (ACh), these agents depolarize the end-plate and generate a muscle action potential (MAP). However, in contrast to ACh, these agents are not metabolized by acetylcholinesterase in the NMJ and thus may cause persistent end-plate depolarization. Until SCh or decamethonium leaves the junction and the end-plate returns toward its resting state, the end-plate is "incapable" of generating subsequent MAPs. This flaccid paralysis (termed *phase 1 depolarizing block*) apparently is characterized by a spatial voltage gradient[2,3] with inactivation of "dual-gated" sodium channels in the perijunctional area (i.e., at the rim of the end-plate)[4,5] (Chaps. 1 and 2).

As discussed in Chapter 2, the initial effects of a depolarizing relaxant at cholinoceptors may be followed by *channel block* and *desensitization*.[6-12] The precise mechanisms are not totally understood but appear to entail (1) direct occlusion of receptor channels, (2) distortion of the receptor subunits, and/or (3) direct interruption (poisoning) of the muscle cell's cytoplasmic mechanisms.[13,14] These mechanisms oppose subsequent depolarization and may promote development of a block with features of a *nondepolarizing block* (termed *phase 2* or dual block[4,15-17]). Alternatively, the end-plate may be altered as a consequence of activation of the Na-K pump[12] by the prolonged ion flux through open channels.

Depolarizing agents tend to exert their effect relatively quickly. Succinylcholine or suxamethonium (British) has a shorter duration of action than decamethonium and has virtually replaced it in clinical settings. Succinylcholine is rapidly metabolized by pseudocholinesterase in the plasma, whereas decamethonium is dependent on organ elimination. If not for its rapid time course, SCh would probably be a drug mainly of historical interest.[11] As detailed in Chapter 18, depolarizing block has the potential to elicit many undesirable effects. The advent of vecuronium and atracurium in the early 1980s (Chap. 13) led Durant and Katz to speculate that their 1982 review "[might] well be a requiem for suxamethonium."[11] However, SCh's rapid onset paralyzed the competition. Presently it is being attacked on both flanks: mivacurium provides nondepolarizing block of short duration; rocuronium provides nondepolarizing block of rapid onset (Chap. 14). It remains to be seen which, if any, of the challengers will be successful.

◆ SUCCINYLCHOLINE (SUXAMETHONIUM)

Succinylcholine chloride (Anectine, Quelicin) is essentially two molecules of ACh, each with a monoquaternary nitrogen, that are connected via methyl groups by an ester bond (see Fig. 2-1). The ester bond is hydrolyzed by pseudocholinesterase in the plasma but not by acetylcholinesterase in the NMJ (Chap. 17). When first tested in 1906, SCh was considered to be ineffective (because it was administered to curarized cats).[18] Its properties became apparent several years later, and it was introduced into clinical practice in the early 1950s.[19,20]

The *onset of SCh-induced block* typically is heralded by *fasciculations*. These rippling, uncoordinated contractions progress from the eyes to the shoulders, the abdomen, the hands, and then the feet. Fasciculations are most likely the consequence of *presynaptic binding,* which causes either (1) simultaneous "one-time" depolarization of multiple end-plates (since this occurs simultaneously throughout a given motor unit, it most likely originates as a result of SCh activity at the nerve itself—i.e., at presynaptic cholinoceptors),[15,21–25] or (2) brief, "tetanic" contractions as a consequence of a series of nerve action potentials that is initiated when SCh binds to presynaptic cholinoceptors[26] (this would account for the increased strength of the initial contractions). Either of these presynaptic mechanisms would account for the effectiveness of pretreatment with a small (defasciculating) dose of a nondepolarizing relaxant (NDR), especially those agents that tend to elicit fade,[24,27] and with agents with a presynaptic effect such as diphenylhydantoin (Dilantin).[24,28]

The *onset of SCh-induced block* also is typified by transiently *increased muscle twitch tension*. This may be detected at the adductor pollicis muscle, especially after small doses[29] and in infants,[30] but it is far more prominent at the *masseter muscle*.[31–37] The increase in jaw tension averages 0.5 kg but may be much higher.[31] It appears to be dose-related at low doses[32] but not at high doses (a probable ceiling effect).[30,31] Depending on the means of assessment, the duration of this effect has been reported to range from less than 150 seconds[31] to more than 10 minutes.[37] Clinically significant rigidity is seen in only 0.01–1% of patients; it is influenced by the use of halothane, the route of SCh injection (IV > IM), and even geography.[38–42]

The relation of *masseter spasm* to malignant hyperthermia and its implications with respect to testing and management are controversial[31,35-38,41,43-46]; they are discussed in Chapter 19. Pretreatment with a *large (paralyzing) dose* of an NDR abolishes the increase in masseter tone, but a *small (defasciculating) dose* of an NDR does not significantly decrease it.[47]

Consistent with other relaxants, SCh has a log-linear dose-response curve. The ED_{95} of SCh has been reported to be within the range of 0.15–0.50 mg · kg^{-1},[48-56] with wide intersubject variability.[49,50,56] It tends to be slightly lower in the presence of nitrous oxide and volatile anesthetic agents.[29,51,53,54] The dose-response curve for SCh (or decamethonium) is shifted to the right after a defasciculating dose of an NDR, which increases the ED_{50} by as much as a factor of 2 and/or decreases the duration of subsequent SCh-induced block.[24,29,57-74] A dose of 1–1.5 mg · kg^{-1} is usually administered to facilitate tracheal intubation in adults. This dosage typically provides excellent intubating conditions, with *paralysis within 60–90 seconds* and *complete recovery (in normals) in 10–15 minutes*.[29,55,56,75]

Succinylcholine exhibits rapid first-order elimination kinetics (see Fig. 8-1).[48,76,77] In patients with adequate pseudocholinesterase activity, the *metabolism of SCh is very rapid*, with a t$_{1/2elim}$ of 2–4 minutes.[48] As much as 60–80% of a dose of SCh may be metabolized within 2 minutes of injection, such that only a small percentage of the parent drug is available at the time of maximum block (Chap. 17).[77] The *intramuscular route* is characterized by a 2- to 3-minute latency period and a duration that is 10–20 minutes longer than the IV route.[75,78-80] Following an IM dose of 4 mg · kg^{-1}, maximum effect is noted in 3–4 minutes and recovery typically occurs within 20–25 minutes.

As for NDRs, the onset of SCh is faster at the *diaphragm* and *larynx* than at the adductor pollicis.[81-83] Onset at the masseter is also faster.[34,47] The *diaphragm appears to be less sensitive* than the thumb to SCh,[83,84] as is the case for NDRs. In contrast, the *laryngeal adductor muscles are highly sensitive to SCh;* i.e., they do not demonstrate the sparing that characterizes their response to NDRs.[81,83-85] Hence, SCh-induced block is both rapid and intense at the laryngeal muscles.[81] The difference between the diaphragm and the larynx has been attributed to their different fiber types[81]: in contrast to NDRs, SCh more effectively blocks the fast-contracting fibers[86-89] that are found in the laryngeal adductors.[90,91] It has been suggested that the difference may be due to the larger number of ACh receptors in fast-twitch as opposed to slow-twitch fibers,[92,93] but several factors may interact in clinical settings (Chap. 1, question i; Chap. 3).

Several studies have addressed these relationships, and the following observations have been recorded:

1. After 1 mg · kg^{-1}, thumb adduction was abolished in 1.1 minutes, reappeared in 4.6 minutes, returned to 50% in 8.3 minutes, and recovered fully in 12.2 minutes,[94] while diaphragm movements returned within 5.6 minutes and spontaneous ventilation returned in 7.3 minutes.[94]

2. After 1 mg · kg^{-1} in the presence of halothane, apnea averaged 5.8 minutes, while the times for adductor pollicis twitch height to return to 25% and 95% of baseline (Dur$_{25}$ and Dur$_{95}$) averaged 5.6 minutes and 9.3 minutes, respectively.[95]
3. Following 0.8 mg · kg^{-1}, maximum twitch height depression was attained by 50 seconds at the diaphragm and by 80 seconds at the adductor pollicis; the time for complete recovery of twitch height was 9 minutes at the diaphragm and 11 minutes at the adductor pollicis.[82]
4. When grip strength was 50% of control due to SCh-induced block, maximum inspiratory and expiratory pressures and voluntary ventilation were approximately 80% of control.[84]

Children, most notably infants, require higher doses of SCh on a mg · kg^{-1} basis.[96–99] SCh distributes throughout the extracellular fluid; thus, its *steady-state volume of distribution* (V_{ss}) is increased in infants and children.[97,99,100] In one study, the ED$_{90}$ values for neonates, infants, and children were 0.52, 0.61, and 0.35 mg · kg^{-1}, respectively.[99] The *rate of recovery* appears to be fastest in children and slowest in adults.[48,56,97,101] The Dur$_{90}$ after 1.0 mg · kg^{-1} was approximately 4–5 minutes in children[97] and 12–15 minutes in adults.[75] However, this may be due to the greater effectiveness of the same mg · kg^{-1} dose in adults as a consequence of their smaller V_{ss}.

Prior to the availability of relatively short-acting NDRs, SCh was often administered as a *continuous infusion.* However, it has recently been shown that infusion or intermittent bolus administration of a short-acting NDR may be a suitable alternative (Chap. 14). *Infusion requirements* for SCh vary markedly among patients[56,102,103]: in one series, SCh requirements ranged from 1.7 to 15.2 mg · kg^{-1} · hr^{-1}.[56] To maintain 90–95% twitch height depression, SCh may be infused initially at 2.4–6.0 mg · kg^{-1} · hr^{-1} (40–100 µg · kg^{-1} · min^{-1}). The rate should be titrated with the aid of a nerve stimulator. After cessation of an infusion in normal individuals, the time for recovery from 5% to 95% of baseline twitch height averaged 6.5 ± 2.8 minutes during N$_2$O-narcotic anesthesia.[102] The potential for prolonged block is discussed below.

◆ DECAMETHONIUM

Decamethonium bromide (Syncurine) is a depolarizing relaxant that was studied extensively in the past but is no longer routinely administered, primarily because it has a slower onset and longer duration than SCh.[4,104–108] The typical dose is 0.05–0.07 mg · kg^{-1}. Like SCh, it is not metabolized in the NMJ. It is dependent on *renal excretion,* and thus its action may be unduly prolonged in renal failure. Decamethonium has been called a partial agonist[1]; it does not always elicit opening of the receptor channel,[109] and it tends to interfere with ion translocation by blocking the channel directly.[110]

It has a relatively high tendency to slide through the receptor channel to inactivate cytoplasmic processes and *readily causes phase 2 block*. These negative features outweigh its tendency to produce less ganglionic block.[1]

◆ PHASE 1 AND PHASE 2 BLOCK

The *typical depolarizing block* (*phase 1 block*) is characterized by depression of twitch height *without fade;* i.e., the depression of the evoked response does not become more pronounced during rapid stimulation. This is in contrast to the competitive block caused by NDRs, which is characterized by fade in response to tetanic or train-of-four stimulation even before there is evidence of single twitch depression (Chaps. 2 and 4). Additionally, phase 1 block does not cause posttetanic facilitation, and it is enhanced (rather than diminished) by anticholinesterase therapy.[16,111–113]

During persistent exposure to a depolarizing agent, phase 1 block may evolve into varying degrees of *phase 2 block*.[12,16,114,115] The latter has features of competitive nondepolarizing block (fade, posttetanic facilitation, probably reversible with an anticholinesterase).[5,15,56,103,116–118] The development of significant phase 2 block is most likely in the context of decreased pseudocholinesterase activity. It occurs more commonly after large doses[15,119] or with prolonged infusions (e.g., >3 mg · kg^{-1} · hr^{-1} of SCh for more than 2 hours[53,56,103,112,120]), especially in children.[121] Phase 2 block may also be noted with lower doses, especially in the context of inhalational anesthesia.[15,53,106,112,122–125] Initially, phase 2 block often is associated with an increased dose requirement (*tachyphylaxis*), possibly due to competition; it then may cause decreased requirements (*bradyphylaxis*) as the more persistent competitive block predominates.[5,15,53,119,126–128]

Because *phase 1 block decreases as circulating SCh is cleared* whereas *phase 2 block tends to persist*,[129] it has been recommended that one allow 10 minutes to elapse after discontinuing an SCh infusion before determining whether one should "reverse" phase 2 block.[129] This period is approximately three times the half-life of SCh in normal patients.[48,129] At this time, phase 1 block should be gone, and the administration of an *anticholinesterase to selectively reverse phase 2 block* is more likely to be effective.[13,53,112,113,118,129–131] Successful reversal is most likely when there is posttetanic facilitation and fade (e.g., $T_4/T_1 < 0.5$). If plasma levels of SCh persist (as in patients with abnormal cholinesterase activity), anticholinesterase therapy is usually ineffective and actually may exacerbate phase 1 block. When neostigmine was administered to a patient with atypical pseudocholinesterase who had twitch depression and a T_4/T_1 of 0.25 at 3 hours after administration of SCh, the T_4/T_1 ratio improved to 0.9, but T_1 remained at 25% of control. This apparent persistence of phase 1 block responded to administration of 45 mg of *exogenous cholinesterase*.[132] Such treatment may be provided by blood or plasma (which typically retain cholinesterase activity)[133] or cholinesterase derived from plasma (e.g., cholase)[134-136]; however, blood products may carry the risk of infection. Alternatively, one may simply allow the effects of SCh to resolve gradually and spontaneously over the ensuing few hours.

The onset of *phase 2 block* is influenced by *volatile anesthetics*. In a recent assessment of *SCh infusion*,[53] all patients initially developed phase 1 (depolarizing) block. Infusion rates to maintain 95% twitch depression averaged 54 and 58 µg · kg^{-1} · min^{-1} in groups anesthetized with enflurane and fentanyl, respectively. With time, tachyphylaxis (with doubling of infusion requirements) and *phase 2 block* occurred: the T_4/T_1 ratio decreased to 0.5, 0.25, and 0 after 31, 46, and 59 minutes in the enflurane group (at cumulative SCh doses of 2.2, 3.2, and 4.2 mg · kg^{-1}, respectively). Corresponding figures for the fentanyl group were 52, 73, and 86 minutes (at doses of 3.4, 5.0, and 5.9 mg · kg^{-1}). Ten minutes after the infusion was stopped, T_4/T_1 remained below 0.5 in most enflurane patients who had received more than 6 mg · kg^{-1} SCh and in most fentanyl patients who had received 13 mg · kg^{-1}. The block in each of the patients who did not recover spontaneously during this observation period was successfully antagonized with subsequent administration of atropine and neostigmine.[53]

Discussion Questions ◆

a. Is a *muscle action potential* generated for the duration of a depolarizing block? Why or why not?
b. Does dosing on a mg · m^{-2} (as opposed to mg · kg^{-1}) basis minimize or accentuate the apparent difference between *adult and infant requirements* for SCh?
c. Describe the effect of depolarizing block on the response to *tetanic stimulation*.
d. Why might the development of *phase 2 block* during SCh infusion initially be associated with *tachyphylaxis*?
e. Why is a *decline in plasma concentration* of SCh more closely paralleled by a decrease in *phase 1* rather than *phase 2 block*?
f. Why might it be detrimental to administer an *anticholinesterase* for reversal of phase 2 block while *plasma concentrations of SCh* remain elevated?
g. Compare the relative *time courses of fasciculations* and depression of adductor pollicis twitch height after SCh.
h. How does *defasciculation with a small dose of nondepolarizing agent* (to decrease the unwanted SCh-induced effects discussed in Chap. 18) affect the required dose of SCh and its duration?
i. What is the effect of *SCh administration on existing nondepolarizing block*?
j. What is the effect of *SCh on subsequent nondepolarizing block*?

k. What evidence suggests a *presynaptic effect of SCh,* in addition to its postsynaptic effects?

Answers ◆

a. The *end-plate depolarization* that results from SCh initially generates a *muscle action potential* (MAP), but SCh then "prevents" triggering of subsequent MAPs. The depolarizing current may be visualized as opening the upper gate of "dual-gated" Na^+ channels that border the end-plate and separate it from the remainder of the muscle cell (Chap. 1). Opening of the gate allows propagation of the MAP. This is followed by prompt closure of the lower "inactivation" gate, with subsequent inability of the end-plate to propagate another MAP. The inactivation gate remains closed until the end-plate potential dissipates and the gates return to their resting states (i.e., the resting gradients are re-established).

b. On a mg · kg^{-1} basis, *infants and children have higher SCh dose requirements* than adults, and undergo SCh-induced block of briefer duration (as much as 50% shorter).[97–99] Administering SCh on a mg · m^{-2} basis "corrects" for differences with respect to relative *extracellular fluid* and thereby reduces the age-related differences in dose requirement and time course.[99,100] A linear relationship exists between log-dose on a mg · m^{-2} basis and the maximum intensity of block in infants, children, and adults.[97] The mean ED_{90} is approximately 10 mg · m^{-2}.[99] However, in certain neonates, there may be some resistance to SCh as a result of end-plate immaturity[98]; i.e., there may be fewer receptor sites, thereby reducing the likelihood of SCh-induced depolarizing block and, conversely, increasing the likelihood of nondepolarizing block.

c. *Depolarizing (phase 1) block* causes decreased magnitude of the evoked responses to both *single twitch and tetanic stimulation,* without fade or posttetanic facilitation. In contrast to nondepolarizing block, depolarizing block tends to maintain *presynaptic ACh mobilization* and actually may augment it, owing to SCh activity at presynaptic cholinoceptors.[23] Unblocked and many partially "blocked" motor units respond with repetitive firing and increased muscle contraction (the normal summated response to tetanic stimulation).

d. As the features of *phase 2 block* evolve, *tachyphylaxis* (higher requirements) may develop. In other words, the development of phase 2 block is associated with a lesser degree of twitch depression from a given rate of SCh infusion.[5] The competitive feature of phase 2 block may oppose the ability of SCh to sustain phase 1 block, as it decreases the number of receptors that are available for SCh binding.[137] Eventually tachyphylaxis will give way to bradyphylaxis (lower requirements) as the more persistent phase 2 block predominates.

e. *Phase 1 block* depends on SCh at the end-plate receptor, which is in equilibrium with that in the NMJ and plasma. The relatively low affinity of depolarizing agents for receptors results in rapid washout (and hence rapid recovery from phase 1 block) once the plasma concentration decreases. Several potential mechanisms have been proposed for the persistence of phase 2 block: large amounts of SCh with low activity "hanging around" at the end-plate receptors; SCh-induced block of presynaptic cholinoceptors; and persistent SCh-induced channel block or desensitization. Recovery from nondepolarizing agents (and apparently from SCh during phase 2 block) lags behind decreases in plasma concentration. Channel block, in particular, may persist despite low plasma levels of SCh.

f. The *administration of an anticholinesterase to reverse phase 2 block* elicits unpredictable effects and may exacerbate the phase 1 component in patients who are receiving SCh concurrently or who have atypical pseudocholinesterase.[111,113,129–131] In these settings, plasma concentrations of SCh remain elevated and phase 1 block, which typically dissipates on clearance of SCh, may persist. Anticholinesterase administration would be detrimental because (1) it would further compromise clearance of SCh by also inhibiting pseudocholinesterase,[118,138,139] and (2) it would allow a buildup of ACh in the NMJ, which would reinforce the SCh-induced depolarizing block.

g. With single twitch nerve stimulation at 1.0 Hz, *100% twitch depression* occurred only 6 ± 16 seconds after the *end of fasciculations*. However, at a stimulating frequency of 0.1 Hz, twitch ablation occurred 52 ± 32 seconds later.[140] (The effect of stimulating rate on the apparent rate of onset is discussed in Chapter 4.)

h. Following a *defasciculating dose of NDR,* a dose of SCh that is approximately 50% above normal may be indicated to ensure timely onset of paralysis at the airway musculature; a dose of ≥1.5 mg · kg^{-1} has been recommended.[24,29,57–70,72,73] The rationale appears to be one of normalizing the time course[17,58,60,64,74] and degree of SCh-induced block. Likewise, a higher dose of decamethonium may be required.[71] If a *larger dose* is not used, pretreatment with an NDR may delay the onset, compromise the effectiveness, or shorten the duration of SCh-induced block. The increased dose may delay return of twitch height or resumption of spontaneous ventilation, but such a delay generally is not clinically significant. However, it should be noted that studies in which doses above the ED$_{100}$ for SCh were employed may have masked changes in the effect of SCh that would be noted at lower doses or during a slow infusion. Additionally, it should be noted that, because of its unique anticholinesterase activity, a defasciculating dose of *pancuronium* tends to increase the duration of SCh-induced block (Chap. 17).[59,67,68,72,141]

i. The *effect of SCh on existing block by an NDR* depends on the depth of block, the dose of SCh, and the means of assessment. *A small (subparalyzing) dose of SCh* (e.g., 0.1 mg · kg^{-1}) typically decreases the depth of an existing nondepolarizing block, probably by "competing" with the NDR at postsynaptic cholinoceptors or by causing the release of additional ACh by binding presynaptically.[142-146] Depending on the degree of NDR-induced block, SCh may also produce a depolarizing block.[143,147,148] A *large dose of SCh* typically first decreases the nondepolarizing block and then causes a relatively persistent depolarizing block.[143-145,149,150]

The *confusing nature of the interactions* was evidenced by the finding that administration of SCh, 0.2 mg · kg^{-1}, in the context of 50% recovery from tubocurarine block enhanced the twitch response but depressed tetanic contraction.[151] In another study, a dose of 25 mg of SCh at a stage of recovery between 8% and 50% resulted in a marked increase in twitch height which then leveled off at 5–20 minutes at a point higher than would have been expected if SCh had not been given.[152] A 75-mg dose caused the same pattern initially but then a depression of twitch height.[152]

The effects of SCh after pancuronium are even more confusing. As noted above (question h), in addition to its effects as an NDR, pancuronium interferes with pseudocholinesterase and may lead to a prolonged effect of SCh (Chap. 17).

j. Even after apparent recovery from SCh or decamethonium, the effectiveness of *subsequent NDR* often is increased (Chap. 9).[142,153-161] This may be manifested as faster onset, decreased dose requirements, increased effectiveness of a given plasma concentration, or a longer duration of action. The mechanism has not been clearly elucidated, and augmentation of nondepolarizing block has not always been noted.[150,162-164] One theory proposes that the presynaptic actions of SCh lead to depletion of ACh or of the Ca^{2+} that facilitates ACh release, leading to less effective competition by ACh for receptor sites. The augmentation is most marked in the context of SCh-induced phase 2 block.[122] Regardless of the degree of augmentation, the clinical nature of the nondepolarizing block is not altered, and the relationship of the T_4/T_1 ratio to the decline in twitch height is not distorted.[159]

k. *Presynaptic effects of SCh* are suggested by (1) repetitive neural responses to a single stimulus, (2) posttetanic neural repetitive activity, and (3) simultaneous contraction (fasciculations) of the muscles supplied by the branches of a motor unit and their inhibition by drugs with presynaptic activity, such as tubocurarine and diphenylhydantoin.[24,165]

References ◆

1. Taylor P: Neuromuscular blocking agents. In Goodman LS, Gilman A (eds): Goodman and Gilman's The Pharmacological Basis of Therapeutics, 6th ed. New York, Macmillan, 1980, pp 221–234

2. Waud DR: The nature of "depolarization block." Anesthesiology 29:1014–1024, 1968
3. Waud DR, Waud BE: Depolarization block and phase II block at the neuromuscular junction. Anesthesiology 43:10–20, 1975
4. Betz WJ, Caldwell JH, Kinnamon SC: Increased sodium conductance in the synaptic region of rat skeletal muscle fibres. J Physiol (Lond) 352:189–202, 1984
5. Katz AM, Messineo FC, Herbette L: Ion channels in membranes. Circulation 65:I2–I10, 1982
6. Gage PW, Hammill OP: Effects of anesthetics on ion channels in synapses. Int Rev Physiol (Neurophysiol) 25:1–46, 1981
7. Katz B, Thesleff S: A study of the "desensitization" produced by acetylcholine at the motor end-plate. J Physiol 138:63–80, 1957
8. Peper K, Bradley RJ, Dreyer F: The acetylcholine receptor at the neuromuscular junction. Physiol Rev 62:1271–1340, 1982
9. Sine SM, Steinbach JH: Agonists block currents through acetylcholine receptor channels. Biophys J 46:277–284, 1984
10. Standaert FG: Donuts and holes: molecules and muscle relaxants. Semin Anesth 3:251–261, 1984
11. Durant NN, Katz RL: Suxamethonium. Br J Anaesth 54:195–208, 1982
12. Gissen AJ, Nastuk WL: Succinylcholine and decamethonium: comparison of depolarization and desensitization. Anesthesiology 33:611, 1970
13. Neubig RR, Boyd ND, Cohen JB: Conformations of *Torpedo* acetylcholine receptor associated with ion transport and desensitization. Biochemistry 21:3460–3467, 1982
14. Sakmann B, Patlak J, Neher E: Single acetylcholine-activated channels show burst-kinetics in presence of desensitizing concentrations of agonist. Nature 286:71–73, 1980
15. Lee C: Dose relationships of phase II, tachyphylaxis and train-of-four fade in suxamethonium-induced dual neuromuscular block in man. Br J Anaesth 47:841–845, 1975
16. Churchill-Davidson HC, Christie TH, Wise RP: Dual neuromuscular block in man. Anesthesiology 21:144–149, 1960
17. Salpeter MM, Cooper DL, Levitt-Gilmour T: Degradation rates of acetylcholine receptors can be modified in the postjunctional plasma membrane of the vertebrate neuromuscular junction. J Cell Biol 103:1399, 1986
18. Hunt R, Taveau R de M: On the physiological action of certain cholin derivatives and new methods for detecting cholin. Br Med J 2:18, 1906
19. Brucke H, Ginzel KH, Klupp H, Pfaffenschlager F, Werner G: Bis-cholinester von Dicarbonsaüren als Muskelrelaxantien in der Narkose. Wien Klin Wochenschr 63:464, 1951
20. Foldes FF, McNall PG, Borrego-Hinjosa JM: Succinylcholine: a new approach to muscular relaxation in anesthesiology. N Engl J Med 247:596, 1952
21. Creese R, Head SD, Jenkinson DF: The role of the sodium pump during prolonged endplate currents in guinea-pig diaphragm. J Physiol 384:377–403, 1987
22. Bowman WC: Prejunctional and postjunctional cholinoceptors at the neuromuscular junction. Anesth Analg 59:935–943, 1980
23. Blaber LC: The effect of facilitatory concentrations of decamethonium on the storage and release of transmitter at the neuromuscular junction of the cat. J Pharmacol Exp Ther 175:664–672, 1970
24. Hartman GS, Fiamengo SA, Riker WF: Succinylcholine: mechanism of fasciculations and their prevention by *d*-tubocurarine or diphenylhydantoin. Anesthesiology 65:405–413, 1986
25. Kitamura S, Yoshiya I, Tashiro C, Negishi T: SCh causes fasciculation by prejunctional mechanism. Anesthesiology 55:A22, 1981
26. Standaert FG: Release of transmitter at the neuromuscular junction. Br J Anaesth 54:131–145, 1982
27. Erkola O: Train-of-four fade of non-depolarizing muscle relaxants: an insight into the mechanism of precurarization. Ann Fr Anesth Reanim 7:299–304, 1988
28. Raines A, Standaert FG: Pre and postjunctional effects of diphenylhydantoin at the cat soleus neuromuscular junction. J Pharmacol Exp Ther 153:361–366, 1966
29. Szalados JE, Donati F, Bevan DR: Effect of *d*-tubocurarine pretreatment on

succinylcholine twitch augmentation and neuromuscular blockade. Anesth Analg 71:55–59, 1990
30. Meakin G, Walker RWM, Dearlove OR: Myotonic and neuromuscular blocking effects of increased doses of suxamethonium in infants and children. Br J Anaesth 65:816–818, 1990
31. Leary NP, Ellis FR: Masseteric muscle spasm as a normal response to suxamethonium. Br J Anaesth 64:488–492, 1990
32. Plumley MH, Bevan JC, Saddler JM, Donati F, Bevan DR: Dose-related effects of succinylcholine on the adductor pollicis and masseter muscles in children. Can J Anaesth 37:15–20, 1990
33. Saddler JM, Bevan JC, Plumley MH, Polomeno RC, Donati F, Bevan DR: Jaw muscle tension after succinylcholine in children undergoing strabismus surgery. Can J Anaesth 37:21–25, 1990
34. Smith CE, Donati F, Bevan DR: Effects of succinylcholine at the masseter and adductor pollicis muscles in adults. Anesth Analg 69:158–162, 1989
35. Van Der Spek AFL, Fang WB, Ashton-Miller JA, et al: Increased masticatory muscle stiffness during limb flaccidity associated with succinylcholine administration. Anesthesiology 69:11–16, 1988
36. Van Der Spek AFL, Fang WB, Ashton-Miller JA, Stohler CS, Carlson DS, Schork MA: The effects of succinylcholine on mouth opening. Anesthesiology 67:459–465, 1987
37. Van Der Spek AFL, Reynolds PI, Fang WB, Ashton-Miller JA, Stohler CS, Schork MA: Changes in resistance to mouth opening induced by depolarizing and nondepolarizing neuromuscular relaxants. Br J Anaesth 64:21–27, 1990
38. Berry FA, Lynch C III: Succinylcholine and trismus (letter). Anesthesiology 70:161–162, 1989
39. Christian AF, Ellis FR, Halsall PJ: Is there a relationship between masseteric muscle spasm and malignant hyperpyrexia? Br J Anaesth 62:540–544, 1989
40. Ording H: Incidence of malignant hyperthermia in Denmark. Anesth Analg 64:700–704, 1985
41. Rosenberg H: Succinylcholine and trismus. Anesthesiology 70:162–163, 1989
42. Schwartz L, Rockoff MA, Koka BV: Masseter spasm with anesthesia: incidence and implications. Anesthesiology 61:772–775, 1984
43. Gronert GA: Management of patients in whom trismus occurs following succinylcholine (letter). Anesthesiology 68:653–654, 1988
44. Rosenberg H: Trismus is not trivial (editorial). Anesthesiology 67:453–455, 1987
45. Rosenberg H: Management of patients in whom trismus occurs following succinylcholine (letter). Anesthesiology 68:654–655, 1988
46. Saddler FM: Jaw stiffness—an ill understood condition (editorial). Br J Anaesth 67:515–516, 1991
47. Smith CE, Saddler JM, Bevan JC, Donati F, Bevan DR: Pre-treatment with non-depolarizing neuromuscular blocking agents and suxamethonium-induced increases in resting jaw tension in children. Br J Anaesth 64:577–581, 1990
48. Cook DR, Wingard LB Jr, Taylor FH: Pharmacokinetics of succinylcholine in infants, children and adults. Clin Pharmacol Ther 20:493–498, 1976
49. Chestnut RJ, Healy TEJ, Harper NJN, Faragher EB: Suxamethonium: the relation between dose and response. Anaesthesia 44:14–18, 1989
50. Katz RL, Norman J, Seed RF, Conrad L: A comparison of the effects of suxamethonium and tubocurarine in patients in London and New York. Br J Anaesth 41:1041–1047, 1969
51. Miller RD, Way WL, Dolan WM, Stevens WC, Eger EI II: Comparative neuromuscular effects of pancuronium, gallamine, and succinylcholine during forane and halothane anesthesia in man. Anesthesiology 35:509–514, 1971
52. Smith C, Donati F, Bevan DR: Dose response curves for succinylcholine: single versus cumulative techniques. Anesthesiology 69:338–342, 1988
53. Donati F, Bevan DR: Effect of enflurane and fentanyl on the clinical characteristics of long-term succinylcholine infusion. Can Anaesth Soc J 29:59–64, 1982
54. Szalados JE, Donati F, Bevan DR: Nitrous oxide potentiates succinylcholine neuromuscular blockade in humans. Anesth Analg 72:18–21, 1991

55. Caldwell JE: Comparison of the neuromuscular block induced by mivacurium, suxamethonium or atracurium during nitrous oxide–fentanyl anaesthesia. Br J Anaesth 63:393–399, 1989
56. Katz RL, Ryan JF: The neuromuscular effects of suxamethonium in man. Br J Anaesth 41:381–390, 1969
57. Blitt CD, Carlson GL, Rolling GD, et al: A comparative evaluation of pretreatment with nondepolarizing blockers prior to the administration of succinylcholine. Anesthesiology 55:687–689, 1981
58. Cullen DJ: The effect of pretreatment with nondepolarizing muscle relaxants on the neuromuscular blocking action of succinylcholine. Anesthesiology 35:572–578, 1971
59. Ferguson A, Bevan DR: Mixed neuromuscular block: the effect of precurarization. Anaesthesia 36:661–666, 1981
60. Freund FG, Rubin AP: The need for additional succinylcholine after d-tubocurarine. Anesthesiology 36:185–187, 1972
61. Manchikanti L, Grow JB, Colliver JA, Canella MG, Hadley CH: Atracurium pretreatment for succinylcholine-induced fasciculations and postoperative myalgia. Anesth Analg 64:1010–1014, 1985
62. Miller RD: The advantages of giving d-tubocurarine before succinylcholine. Anesthesiology 37:568, 1972
63. Masey SA, Glazebrook CW, Goat VA: Suxamethonium: a new look at pretreatment. Br J Anaesth 55:729–733, 1983
64. Miller RD, Way WL: The interaction between succinylcholine and subparalyzing doses of d-tubocurarine and gallamine in man. Anesthesiology 35:567–570, 1971
65. O'Sullivan EP, Williams NE, Calvey TN: Differential aspects of neuromuscular blocking agents on suxamethonium-induced fasciculations and myalgia. Br J Anaesth 60:367–371, 1988
66. Pauca AL, Reynolds RC, Strobel GE: Inhibition of suxamethonium relaxation by tubocurarine and gallamine pretreatment during induction of anaesthesia in man. Br J Anaesth 47:1067–1073, 1975
67. Nishizawa M: Influence of small doses of vecuronium and pancuronium on succinylcholine-induced neuromuscular blockade. Masui 39:1188–1197, 1990
68. Ivankovich AD, Sidell N, Cairoli VJ, Dietz AA, Albrecht RF: Dual action of pancuronium on succinylcholine block. Can Anaesth Soc J 24:228–241, 1977
69. Lindgren L, Klemola UM, Saarnivaara L: Optimal time interval between pretreatment with alcuronium and suxamethonium during anesthetic induction. Acta Anaesthesiol Scand 32:244–247, 1988
70. Cook WP, Schultetus RR, Caton D: A comparison of d-tubocurarine pretreatment and no pretreatment in obstetric patients. Anesth Analg 66:756–760, 1987
71. Campkin NTA, Hood JR, Feldman SA: Resistance to decamethonium neuromuscular block after prior administration of vecuronium. Anesth Analg 77:78–80, 1993
72. Erkola O, Salmenpera A, Kuoppamaki R: Five nondepolarizing muscle relaxants in precurarization. Acta Anaesthesiol Scand 27:427–432, 1983
73. Chestnutt WN, Lowry KG, Dundee JW, Pandit SK, Mirakhur RK: Failure of two benzodiazepines to prevent suxamethonium-induced muscle pain. Anaesthesia 40:263–269, 1985
74. Eisenkraft JB, Herlich A, Book WJ, Mann SM, Hubbard M: Precurarization does not alter dose-response to succinylcholine. Anesthesiology 69:A493, 1988
75. Walts LF, Dillon JB: Clinical studies on succinylcholine chloride. Anesthesiology 38:372–376, 1967
76. Levy G: Kinetics of pharmacologic activity of succinylcholine in man. J Pharmacol Sci 56:1687–1688, 1967
77. Dal Santo G: Kinetics of distribution of radioactive labeled muscle relaxants: III. Investigations with ^{14}C-succinyldicholine and ^{14}C-succinylmonocholine during controlled conditions. Anesthesiology 29:435–443, 1969
78. Beldavs J: Intramuscular succinylcholine for endotracheal intubation in infants and children. Can Anaesth Soc J 6:141–147, 1959
79. Liu LMP, De Cook TH, Goudsouzian NG, et al: Dose response to intramuscular succinylcholine in children. Anesthesiology 55:599–601, 1981

80. Sutherland GA, Bevan JC, Bevan DR: Neuromuscular blockade in infants following intramuscular succinylcholine in two or five per cent concentration. Can Anaesth Soc J 30:342–346, 1983
81. Meistelman C, Plaud B, Donati F: Neuromuscular effects of succinylcholine on the vocal cords and adductor pollicis muscles. Anesth Analg 73:278–282, 1991
82. Pansard JL, Chauvin M, Lebrault C, Gauneau P, Duvaldestin P: Effect of an intubating dose of succinylcholine and atracurium on the diaphragm and the adductor pollicis in humans. Anesthesiology 67:326–330, 1987
83. Smith CE, Donati F, Bevan DR: Potency of suxamethonium at the diaphragm and at the adductor pollicis. Anesth Analg 67:625–630, 1988
84. Williams JP, Bourke DL: Effects of succinylcholine on respiratory and nor-respiratory muscle strength in humans. Anesthesiology 63:299–303, 1985
85. Foldes FF, Monte AP, Brunn HM Jr, Wolfson B: Studies with muscle relaxants in unanesthetized subjects. Anesthesiology 22:230–236, 1961
86. Choi WW, Gergis SD, Sokoll MD: Effects of succinylcholine chloride on the response of fast and slow muscle in the cat. Acta Anaesthesiol Scand 28:516–520, 1984
87. Muir AW, Marshall RJ: Comparative neuromuscular blocking effects of vecuronium, pancuronium, ORG 6368 and suxamethonium in the anaesthetized domestic pig. Br J Anaesth 59:622–629, 1987
88. Muir AW, Houston J, Green KL, Marshall RJ, Bowman WC, Marshall IG: Effects of a new neuromuscular blocking agent (Org 9426) in anaesthetized cats and pigs and in isolated nerve-muscle preparations. Br J Anaesth 63:400–410, 1989
89. Secher NH, Robe N, Secher O: Effect of tubocurarine on human soleus and gastrocnemius muscles. Acta Anaesthesiol Scand 26:231–234, 1982
90. Johnson MA, Polgar W, Weightman D, Appleton D: Data on the distribution of fibre types in thirty-six human muscles: an autopsy study. J Neurol Sci 18:111–129, 1973
91. Sanders I, Aviv J, Kraus WM, Racenstein MM, Biller HF: Transcutaneous electrical stimulation of the recurrent laryngeal nerve in monkeys. Ann Otol Rhinol Laryngol 96:38–42, 1987
92. Meistelman C, Plaud B, Donati F: Rocuronium (ORG 9426) neuromuscular blockade at the adductor muscles of the larynx and adductor pollicis in humans. Can J Anaesth 39:665–669, 1992
93. Sterz R, Pagala M, Peper K: Postjunctional characteristics of the endplates in mammalian fast and slow muscles. Pflugers Arch 398:48–54, 1983
94. Healy TEJ, Birmingham AT, Chatterjee SC: A comparison of the effect of induction of anaesthesia by thiopentone or Althesin on the duration of action of suxamethonium. Postgrad Med J (June suppl) 90–92, 1972
95. Viby-Mogensen J: Correlation of succinylcholine duration of action with plasma cholinesterase activity in subjects with genotypically normal enzyme. Anesthesiology 53:517–520, 1980.
96. Nightingale DA, Gloss AG, Bachman L: Neuromuscular blocking effects of succinylcholine in infants and children. Anesthesiology 27:736, 1983
97. Cook DR, Fischer CG: Neuromuscular blocking effects of succinylcholine in infants and children. Anesthesiology 42:662–665, 1975
98. Goudsouzian NG, Liu LMP: The neuromuscular response of infants to a continuous infusion of succinylcholine. Anesthesiology 60:97–101, 1984
99. Meakin G, McKiernan EP, Morris P, Baker D: Dose-response curves for suxamethonium in neonates, infants and children. Br J Anaesth 62:655–658, 1989
100. Walts LF, Dillon JB: The response of newborns to succinylcholine and d-tubocurarine. Anesthesiology 31:35–38, 1969
101. Cunliffe M, Lerman J, McLeod ME, Burrows FA: Neuromuscular blockade for rapid intubation in children: pancuronium is slower than succinylcholine. Anesthesiology 63:A474, 1985
102. Goldberg ME, Larijani GE, Azad SS, Sosis M, Seltzer JL, Ascher J, Weakly JN: Comparison of tracheal intubating conditions and neuromuscular blocking profiles after intubating doses of mivacurium chloride or succinylcholine in surgical outpatients. Anesth Analg 69:93–99, 1989
103. Ramsey FM, Lebowitz PW, Savarese JJ, Ali HH: Clinical characteristics of long-term

succinylcholine neuromuscular blockade during balanced anesthesia. Anesth Analg 59:110–116, 1980
104. Burns BD, Paton WDM: Depolarization of the motor end plate by decamethonium and acetyl-choline. J Physiol (Lond) 115:41–73, 1951
105. Thesleff S: The mode of neuromuscular block caused by acetylcholine, nicotine, decamethonium and succinylcholine. Acta Physiol Scand 34:218–231, 1955
106. de Jong RH, Freund FG: Characteristics of the neuromuscular block with succinylcholine and decamethonium in man. Anesthesiology 28:583–591, 1967
107. Alderson AM, MacLagan J: The action of decamethonium and tubocurarine on the respiratory and limb muscles of the cat. J Physiol (Lond) 173:38–56, 1964
108. Paton WDM, Zaimis EJ: The action of d-tubocurarine and of decamethonium on respiratory and other muscles in the cat. J Physiol 112:311–331, 1951
109. Katz B, Miledi R: The characteristics of "end plate noise" produced by different depolarizing drugs. J Physiol (Lond) 231:549–574, 1973
110. Adams PR, Sakmann B: Decamethonium both blocks and opens end plate channels. Proc Natl Acad Sci USA 75:2994–2998, 1978
111. Gissen AJ, Katz RL, Karis JH, Papper EM: Neuromuscular block in man during prolonged arterial infusion with succinylcholine. Anesthesiology 27:242–249, 1966
112. Katz RL, Wolfe CE, Papper EM: The non-depolarizing neuromuscular blocking action of suxamethonium in man. Anesthesiology 24:784–789, 1963
113. Lee C: Train-of-four fade and edrophonium antagonism of neuromuscular block by succinylcholine in man. Anesth Analg 55:663–667, 1976
114. Jenden DJ: The effect of drugs upon neuromuscular transmission in the isolated guinea pig diaphragm. J Pharmacol Exp Ther 114:398, 1955
115. Zaimis E: Motor end plate differences as a determining factor in the mode of action of neuromuscular blocking substances. J Physiol 122:238–251, 1953
116. Churchill-Davidson HC, Katz PL: Dual, phase II, or desensitization block? Anesthesiology 33:536–538, 1966
117. Katz RL: Electromyographic and mechanical effects of suxamethonium and tubocurarine on twitch, tetanic and post-tetanic responses. Br J Anaesth 45:849–859, 1973
118. Savarese JJ, Ali HH, Murphy JD, Padget C, Lee C-M, Ponitz J: Train-of-four nerve stimulation in the management of prolonged neuromuscular blockade following succinylcholine. Anesthesiology 42:106–111, 1975
119. Churchill-Davidson HC, Christie TH, Wise RP: Dual neuromuscular block in man. Anesthesiology 21:144–149, 1960
120. Futter ME, Donati F, Bevan DR: Prolonged suxamethonium infusion during nitrous oxide anaesthesia supplemented with halothane or fentanyl. Br J Anaesth 55:947–953, 1983
121. Bevan JC, Donati F, Bevan DR: Prolonged infusion of suxamethonium in infants and children. Br J Anaesth 58:839–843, 1986
122. Foldes FF, Wnuck A, Hamer-Hodges RJ, et al: The mode of action of depolarizing relaxants. Anesth Analg 36:23–37, 1957
123. Fogdall RP, Miller RD: Neuromuscular effects of enflurane alone and in combination with d-tubocurarine, pancuronium and succinylcholine in man. Anesthesiology 42:173–178, 1975
124. Hilgenberg JC, Stoelting RK: Characteristics of succinylcholine-produced phase II neuromuscular block during enflurane, halothane, and fentanyl anesthesia. Anesth Analg 60:192, 1981
125. Zaimis E: The neuromuscular junction: area of uncertainty. In Zaimis E (ed): Neuromuscular Junction. Berlin, Springer-Verlag, 1976, pp 1–18
126. Donati F, Bevan DR: Long-term succinylcholine infusion during isoflurane anesthesia. Anesthesiology 58:6–10, 1983
127. Lee C, Barnes A, Katz RL: Magnitude, dose-requirement and mode of development of tachyphylaxis to suxamethonium in man. Br J Anaesth 50:189–194, 1978
128. Sugai N, Hughes R, Payne JP: The skeletal muscle response to repeated administration of suxamethonium and its interaction with edrophonium in anaesthetized man. Br J Clin Pharmacol 2:487, 1975
129. Donati F, Bevan DR: Antagonism of phase II succinylcholine block by neostigmine. Anesth Analg 64:773–776, 1985

130. Baraka A: Suxamethonium-neostigmine interaction in patients with normal or atypical cholinesterase. Br J Anaesth 49:479–484, 1977
131. Viby-Mogensen J: Succinylcholine neuromuscular blockade in subjects homozygous for atypical plasma cholinesterase. Anesthesiology 55:429–434, 1981
132. James MFM, Howe HC: Prolonged paralysis following suxamethonium and the use of neostigmine. Br J Anaesth 65:430–432, 1990
133. Epstein HM, Jarzemsky D, Zuckerman L, Vagher P: Plasma cholinesterase activity in bank blood. Anesth Analg 59:211–214, 1980
134. Goedde HW, Atland K, Schloot W: Therapy of prolonged apnea after suxamethonium with purified pseudocholinesterase: new data on kinetics of the hydrolysis of succinyldicholine and succinylmonocholine and further data on N-acetyltransferase polymorphism. Ann NY Acad Sci 151:742, 1968
135. Scholler KL, Goedde HW, Benkmann HG: The use of serum cholinesterase in succinylcholine apnoea. Can Anaesth Soc J 24:396–400, 1977
136. Benzer A, Luz G, Oswald E, et al: Succinylcholine-induced prolonged apnea in a 3-week old newborn: treatment with human plasma cholinesterase. Anesth Analg 74:137–138, 1992
137. Lee C: Self-antagonism: a possible mechanism of tachyphylaxis in suxamethonium-induced neuromuscular block in man. Br J Anaesth 48:1097–1102, 1976
138. Bevan DR, Donati F: Succinylcholine apnoea: attempted reversal with anticholinesterases. Can Anaesth Soc J 30:536–539, 1983
139. Viby-Mogensen J: Cholinesterase and succinylcholine. Dan Med Bull 30:129–150, 1983
140. Connelly NR, Silverman DG, Brull SJ: Temporal correlation of succinylcholine-induced fasciculations to loss of twitch response at different stimulating frequencies. J Clin Anesth 4:190–193, 1992
141. Stovner J, Oftedal N, Holmboe J: The inhibition of cholinesterases by pancuronium. Br J Anaesth 47:949–954, 1975
142. Katz RL: Modification of the action of pancuronium by succinylcholine and halothane. Anesthesiology 35:602–606, 1971
143. Scott RPF, Norman J: Effect of suxamethonium given during recovery from atracurium. Br J Anaesth 61:292–296, 1988
144. Young RB: Suxamethonium for peritoneal closure. Anaesthesia 34:716, 1979
145. Feldman SA: Rational use of muscle relaxants and anticholinesterase in clinical practice. In Feldman SA (ed): Muscle Relaxants. Philadelphia, WB Saunders, 1979, p 219
146. Huang KC, Simpson PM: Succinylcholine enhances the recovery from atracurium induced paralysis. Anesthesiology 75:A783, 1991
147. Black AMS: Effect of suxamethonium given during recovery from atracurium (correspondence). Br J Anaesth 62:348–349, 1989
148. Rouse JM, Bevan DR: Mixed neuromuscular block. Anaesthesia 34:608–617, 1979
149. Buzello W, Krieg N, Kuhls E, Schlickewei A: Modification of pancuronium-induced nondepolarizing neuromuscular block by succinylcholine in anesthetized humans. Anesthesiology 59:573–576, 1983
150. Walts LF, Dillon JB: Clinical studies of the interaction between d-tubocurarine and succinylcholine. Anesthesiology 31:39–44, 1969
151. Sugai N, Payne JP: The interaction of tubocurarine and suxamethonium at different stages of recovery from tubocurarine-induced neuromuscular blockade in anaesthetized man. Br J Anaesth 47:1061–1066, 1975
152. Gray TC: The mechanism of reversal of nondepolarizing relaxants. International Congress Series No. 168. Amsterdam, Excerpta Medica, 1968, pp 431–436
153. Donati F, Gill SS, Bevan DR, Ducharme J, Theoret Y, Varin F: Pharmacokinetics and pharmacodynamics of atracurium with and without previous suxamethonium administration. Br J Anaesth 66:557–561, 1991
154. d'Hollander AA, Agoston S, DeVille A, et al: Clinical and pharmacological actions of a bolus injection of suxamethonium: two phenomena of distinct duration. Br J Anaesth 55:131–134 1983
155. Krieg N, Hendrickx HHL, Crul JF: Influence of suxamethonium on the potency of ORG NC 45 in anaesthetized patients. Br J Anaesth 53:259–262, 1981
156. Ono K, Manabe N, Ohta Y, Morita K, Kosaka F: Influence of suxamethonium on the

action of subsequently administered vecuronium or pancuronium. Br J Anaesth 62:324–326, 1989
157. Olkkola KT, Schwilden H: Quantitation of the interaction between atracurium and succinylcholine using closed-loop feedback control of infusion of atracurium. Anesthesiology 73:614–618, 1990
158. Swen J, Koot HWJ, Bencini A, Ket JM, Hermans J, Agoston S: The interaction between suxamethonium and the succeeding non-depolarizing neuromuscular blocking agents. Eur J Anaesthesiol 7:203–209, 1990
159. Yang J, Brull SJ, Turner J, Connelly NR, O'Connor TZ, Silverman DG: Effect of succinylcholine on the rate and nature of recovery from nondepolarizing blockade. Anesth Analg 72:S330, 1991
160. Dubois MY, Fleming NW, Lea DE: Effects of succinylcholine on the pharmacodynamics of pipecuronium and pancuronium. Anesth Analg 72:364, 1991
161. Feldman S, Fauvel N: Potentiation and antagonism of vecuronium by decamethonium. Anesth Analg 76:631–634, 1993
162. Walts LF, Rusin DW: The influence of succinylcholine on the duration of pancuronium neuromuscular blockade. Anesth Analg 56:22, 1977
163. Ali H, Savarese J, Basta S, Sunder N, Gionfriddo M, Lineberry C, Batson AG: Does succinylcholine modify the response to atracurium? Anesth Analg 64:A188, 1985
164. Brown TC, Meretoja OA, Clare D, et al: Does suxamethonium influence the subsequent dose requirements of alcuronium and its reversibility in children? Anaesth Intens Care 18:479, 1990
165. Standaert FG, Adams JE: The actions of succinylcholine on the mammalian motor nerve terminal. J Pharmacol Exp Ther 149:113–123, 1965

17

DAVID G. SILVERMAN | FRANÇOIS DONATI

Factors Affecting Pseudocholinesterase and the Pharmacokinetics and Pharmacodynamics of Succinylcholine

◆ METABOLISM OF SUCCINYLCHOLINE

The *short clinical duration of succinylcholine* (SCh) is due to rapid metabolism as well as redistribution. It is metabolized primarily by *pseudocholinesterase* (also commonly referred to as plasma cholinesterase or butyryl cholinesterase), an extracellular enzyme in the plasma. In contrast to acetylcholine (ACh), SCh is *not metabolized by acetylcholinesterase* in the neuromuscular junction (NMJ).

The *two stages of SCh metabolism* that are catalyzed by *pseudocholinesterase* are (1) hydrolysis of SCh to choline and succinylmonocholine, which has weak relaxant properties, and (2) subsequent slower metabolism of succinylmonocholine to succinic acid and a second molecule of choline.[1-5] In typical clinical doses, the rate of elimination is directly proportional to SCh concentration in the plasma (first-order elimination kinetics),[6-8] with an elimination half-life ($t_{1/2elim}$) between 2–5 minutes and a rate constant (K_{el}) of approximately 0.14 min^{-1} ($t_{1/2}$ = 0.693/K_{el}).[6,8] *Redistribution* also plays an important role in the termination of SCh-induced block.[7,9] *Alkaline hydrolysis* (5% per hour) and organ elimination (e.g., *renal excretion*) typically contribute relatively little to SCh elimination.[10] Assuming a dose of 60 mg, a weight of 60 kg, and a plasma volume of 3.5 L, the rate of disappearance of SCh from the plasma has been estimated as 27 mg (7.7 mg · L^{-1}) during the first minute and 10 mg (2.9 mg · L^{-1} · min^{-1}) during each of the following 2 minutes.[6]

◆ PSEUDOCHOLINESTERASE ACTIVITY AND GENETICS

A patient's level of *pseudocholinesterase activity* may be determined by measuring the ability of pseudocholinesterase to hydrolyze a substrate such as benzoylcholine or butyrylthiocholine. There is a wide margin of safety, with a *wide range of adequate values*.[11,12] Below the normal range for a given laboratory, the duration of[11,13] and sensitivity to[14,15] SCh are inversely related to pseudocholinesterase activity. In a laboratory whose normal range of *pseudocholinesterase activity* was 650–1,700 units · L^{-1}, *recovery to 100% twitch height* after 1 mg · kg^{-1} of SCh occurred at 22, 13, 11, 10, and 9 minutes in the context of pseudocholinesterase activities of 200, 400, 600, 1,000, and 1,600 units · L^{-1}, respectively.[11] Pseudocholinesterase levels as low as 10% of control typically do not cause the clinical duration of SCh to exceed 22 minutes so long as the enzyme is qualitatively normal.[11,13,16] The remainder of this chapter will discuss genetic variations of pseudocholinesterase production (Table 17-1) and the effects of drug interactions and physiological states on pseudocholinesterase activity (Table 17-2).

Abnormal forms of pseudocholinesterase may be associated with marked prolongation of SCh-induced block. *Liver production* of pseudocholinesterase appears to be controlled by a single cholinesterase gene at the E_1 locus on chromosome 3 (chromosome site 3q26), with the potential for a variety of nucleotide variations.[17–29] The most notable are *usual* (u), *atypical* (dibucaine-resistant) (a), *fluoride-resistant* (f), and *silent* (s). Approximately one in 25 patients is heterozygous for an atypical allele ($E_1^u E_1^a$); approximately one in 2,500 is homozygous for the atypical autosomal recessive allele ($E_1^a E_1^a$).[30–32] The incidence of homozygous $E_1^f E_1^f$ or $E_1^s E_1^s$ is less than 1:100,000,[31] but such variants may be increased in the Punjabi and Andhra Pradesh populations of India,[27,33] Alaskan Inuit populations,[34–37] and in Afrikaner South African populations.[38] The amino acid variations have been nicely summarized in a recent review[25]: E_1^a is due to replacement of asparagine with glycine at amino acid 70 at the E_1 locus, E_1^f entails replacement of threonine with methionine at amino acid 243 or glycine with valine at amino acid 390, and E_1^s can be due to an amino acid frame shift at one of three or more sites.

Abnormal pseudocholinesterase production may be identified and its effects quantified in vitro. Testing has been complicated by the finding that the atypical variant is virtually incapable of metabolizing SCh in clinical concentrations but is still partially capable of hydrolyzing test substrates (e.g., ACh, benzoylcholine) in vitro.[4,5,25,39] Therefore, we have relied primarily on tests that quantify enzyme inhibition by dibucaine (Nupercaine), fluoride, or chloride. The *dibucaine number* (DN) measures the amount of enzyme that is inhibited by dibucaine[40]: normal enzyme has a high percentage of its ability to hydrolyze benzoylcholine inhibited by this local anesthetic, with DN =

80, whereas pseudocholinesterase from $E_1^a E_1^a$ individuals is highly resistant to dibucaine, with $DN = 10–25$. Heterozygotes ($E_1^a E_1^u$) typically have a DN between 40 and 60. The *fluoride number* (FN)[41] measures the amount of enzyme inhibited by sodium fluoride (instead of dibucaine). A normal FN is 60, whereas heterozygotes for the f allele have an FN between 15 and 25. This allele also is commonly associated with a decreased DN.[32] The f gene abnormality tends to be associated with less prolongation of the response to SCh than is the gene for the dibucaine-resistant ("atypical") variant. The *"silent"* nucleotide variant(s) is (are) associated with the production of a molecule that is incapable of hydrolyzing the choline ester bond; a patient who is homozygous for $E_1^s E_1^s$ (one in 100,000) has virtually no pseudocholinesterase activity.[32,34,42–44] A heterozygote $E_1^u E_1^s$ has approximately a 50% decrease in pseudocholinesterase activity but a normal DN and FN (since the enzyme produced by the E_1^u allele functions normally). It should be noted that not all genotypes based solely on the DN and FN are 100% accurate; therefore other inhibiting compounds (e.g., urea, or Ro2) may also be used to identify abnormal pseudocholinesterase production.[12,25,45]

The duration of SCh is prolonged only slightly in most *heterozygotes* (with one normal E_1^u allele), but it may be increased and prolonged for several hours in patients *homozygous* for abnormal genotypes or their combinations.[12,15,46–50] In such cases, complete twitch ablation persists for at least 2 hours, and subsequent recovery is complicated by phase 2 block with fade. It should be noted that $E_1^a E_1^f$ heterozygous patients are more sensitive than heterozygotes with one normal allele but are less sensitive than $E_1^a E_1^a$ homozygous patients.[49]

In addition to genetically determined production of abnormal enzyme, there may also be *genetically determined production of insufficient enzyme.*

TABLE 17-1
Pseudocholinesterase Activities in Cholinesterase Gene Variants

Genotype	Pseudocholinesterase Activity (% of Normal)	Dibucaine Number	Fluoride Number
$E_1^u E_1^u$	100	80	60
$E_1^u E_1^a$	50–75	40–70	40–50
$E_1^a E_1^a$	10–25	10–25	15–30
$E_1^u E_1^f$	60–75	70–80	40–50
$E_1^f E_1^f$	25–50	50–60	15–30
$E_1^u E_1^s$	50–60	80	60
$E_1^s E_1^s$	0–5	—	—
$E_1^a E_1^f$	25–50	40–50	20–30
$E_1^a E_1^s$	10–25	10–30	15–35
$E_1^s E_1^f$	25–35	50–70	20–40

The K,[29] J,[21] and H[28] variants have 33%, 66%, and 90% reduction in activity. Approximately one in 65 individuals has the K variant,[19] one in 150,000 has the J variant,[21,51] and only four families have been identified with the H variant.[28]

Alternatively, there are variants with *greater than normal activity* as a result of increased enzyme production[52–54] or increased activity per active site.[55]

Table 17-2 summarizes the effects of agents and conditions, which alter pseudocholinesterase activity and affect depolarizing block with SCh.

TABLE 17-2
Factors Affecting Activities of Pseudocholinesterase and Succinylcholine

Agent or Condition	Effect	Mechanism, Comments, References
I. MEDICATIONS AND POISONS		
ANTIBIOTICS	i	Less pronounced effect on depolarizing than nondepolarizing agents (see Chap. 9).[56]
ANTICHOLINESTERASES	I	Bind to varying degrees with pseudoChE in plasma as well as acetylChE in NMJ (Chap. 15). The inhibition of pseudoChE increases and prolongs the effects of SCh.
■ Echothiophate eye drops (Phospholine)	I	Irreversibly inhibits pseudoChE activity.[12,16,57] It takes the liver several weeks to restore normal enzyme levels.
■ Edrophonium, neostigmine, and pyridostigmine	I	Reversible inhibition of pseudoChE[58–63] (as well as desired inhibition of acetylChE); edrophonium has least effect on pseudoChE.[64] Neostigmine, 0.05 mg · kg^{-1}, and pyridostigmine, 0.25 mg · kg^{-1}, caused a 70% decrease at 5 min and a decrease that persisted for 60–120 min.[58] This may prolong the effect of SCh, which can then last for >30 min.
■ Organophosphate pesticides	I	Bind irreversibly to pseudoChE,[12,65] as do many agents for chemical warfare (Chap. 15).
■ Physostigmine	i	Prolongation was reported in a patient heterozygous for atypical ChE.[66]
ANTINEOPLASTICS	I	Agents such as cyclophosphamide and thiophosphoramide irreversibly inhibit pseudoChE.[12,65,67–69] However, prolongation may be prevented by appropriate SCh titration.[70] In addition, these drugs contain ammonium groups and thus may be capable of interacting with cholinoceptors.

(Continued)

I = increased effect of block, D = decreased effect of block, i = theoretical or minimal increase, d = theoretical or minimal decrease, ChE = cholinesterase (pseudoChE = pseudocholinesterase, acetylChE = acetylcholinesterase).

TABLE 17-2
(Continued)

Agent or Condition	Effect	Mechanism, Comments, References
BAMBUTEROL	I	Its bioconversion to terbutaline causes decreased pseudoChE activity with a peak effect reached in as little as 2 hours.[71-73] When administered 10–16 hr before surgery, 30 mg prolonged SCh-induced paralysis by >100%,[72] while 10 and 20 mg caused 30% and 50% prolongation, respectively.[73] At 2 hr after bambuterol administration, its depression of pseudoChE is maximal, and 30 mg is associated with 300% prolongation.[71] The prolongation may be associated with phase 2 block,[71,72] which may be reversed with edrophonium.[71,72]
CARDIOVASCULAR DRUGS		
■ Beta blockers	i	May slightly increase the potency of SCh and reduce fasciculations,[74,75] perhaps by an action similar to that of local anesthetics.[75] Beta blockers may also augment release of ACh as a consequence of an alpha-mediated increased release of catecholamines.[75] $Beta_2$-blockers may compromise the renal elimination of K^+ that results from SCh-mediated K^+ release[76,77]; however, this does not appear to be a consequence of even acute loading with the beta antagonist esmolol.[78]
—Esmolol	i/I	Varied results in vivo, ranging from no effect to 50% prolongation[79-81]; e.g., the time to 50% recovery of twitch height after 1 mg · kg^{-1} of SCh was 8.3 min (vs. 5.6 min).[79] *Potential mechanisms* include the following: (1) An esmolol-induced *decrease in cardiac output* can slow redistribution of SCh (a vital feature of rapid recovery from SCh). (2) The *membrane-stabilizing effects* of beta blockers may promote an increased effect of relaxants.[75,79] (3) *Competition for pseudoChE:* prolongation of SCh metabolism was suggested in vitro.[81] Because esmolol is metabolized by an esterase, it theoretically may compete for pseudoChE.[81,82] However, in contrast to rats and guinea pigs, the esterase responsible for esmolol metabolism in humans resides primarily in the cytosol of *red blood cells* and not in the plasma.[82] The potential decrease in pseudoChE activity is most likely of too little magnitude to significantly affect SCh duration.[79,81] (There was no change in the ability of pseudoChE to hydrolyze benzoylcholine in plasma obtained from subjects who received up to 1,400 μg · kg^{-1} of esmolol over 4 min.[81])
■ Ca^{2+} channel blockers	i	May occlude postsynaptic receptor channel and decrease muscle contraction.[83-85]

(Continued)

I = increased effect of block, D = decreased effect of block, i = theoretical or minimal increase, d = theoretical or minimal decrease, ChE = cholinesterase (pseudoChE = pseudocholinesterase, acetyChE = acetylcholinesterase).

TABLE 17-2

(Continued)

Agent or Condition	Effect	Mechanism, Comments, References
▪ Quinidine	I	Increases depth and duration of depolarizing and nondepolarizing block.[86]
▪ Trimethaphan	I	Decreases available pseudoChE; ganglionic block.[87,88]
GLUCOCORTICOIDS	i	May decrease enzyme synthesis in the liver[89]; alter neuromuscular function (Chap. 9).
INHALATIONAL ANESTHETICS		
▪ Nitrous oxide	I	Slight potentiation apparent within 6 min[90]; 0.3 mg · kg^{-1} of SCh caused 74% twitch depression with thiopental-N_2O vs. 50% depression after thiopental alone.[90]
▪ Volatile	I	Relatively little influence on depth of block[91,92] or onset time,[93] in comparison to effects on nondepolarizers. Presumably depresses pre- and postsynaptically. ED_{95} of SCh decreased more with isoflurane than halothane,[94] possibly due to the former's increasing blood flow. May lead to earlier onset of tachyphylaxis and dual block[91] and an increased likelihood of tetanic fade.[95]
INTRAVENOUS ANALGESICS AND SEDATIVES		
▪ Diazepam	—	May decrease fasciculations, K^+ change (in normal subjects), and muscle pains (Chap. 18), but 0.05 mg · kg^{-1} did not alter the magnitude or duration of block.[96]
▪ Ketamine	i	Slight increase, possibly due to altered ACh release[97] and a slight (probably insignificant) decrease in pseudoChE.
▪ Thiopental	—	Minimal effect.[98]
▪ Propanidid	I	Increased duration by 3–4 min due to pseudoChE inhibition[99] as well as probable postsynaptic action.[100] Such prolongation is not seen after thiopental or althesin.[98]
LOCAL ANESTHETICS	i	May block nerve action potential and ACh release and may cause channel block.[101,102] Can prolong block.[103]
▪ Esters	i	Are metabolized by, and thus compete for, available pseudoChE.[104–106]
NEUROL/PSYCHIATRIC MEDICATIONS		
▪ Chlorpromazine	i	Decreases pseudoChE activity.[107]
▪ Lithium	i/d	Competes with Na^+ and may cause decreased ACh release,[108] but data are not clear-cut.
▪ Monoamine oxidase inhibitors	i	Decrease pseudoChE activity.[32,109]
▪ Diphenylhydantoin (phenytoin), acute	i	Decreases SCh-induced fasciculations, presumably by suppressing prejunctional firing[110]; subsequent block by SCh was of increased magnitude and faster onset.[110]

(Continued)

I = increased effect of block, D = decreased effect of block, i = theoretical or minimal increase, d = theoretical or minimal decrease, ChE = cholinesterase (pseudoChE = pseudocholinesterase, acetylChE = acetylcholinesterase).

TABLE 17-2
(Continued)

Agent or Condition	Effect	Mechanism, Comments, References
■ Diphenylhydantoin, chronic	i	Proliferation of normal end-plate receptors theoretically may increase sensitivity to SCh but not predispose to SCh-induced hyperkalemia (Chaps. 9 and 22).
NONDEPOLARIZING RELAXANTS	D	Oppose SCh-induced block.
■ Defasciculating dose	D	Pretreatment with even a small dose of NDR necessitates use of a higher dose of SCh or decamethonium to reliably attain the typically rapid onset of depolarizing block (e.g., ≥1.5 mg · kg^{-1} of SCh) (Chap. 16). Subsequent recovery from the depolarizing agents may be characterized by fade.[111,112]
■ Intermediate dose	D	When 100 mg of SCh was injected after establishment of 25–50% block with vecuronium, complete block was delayed until 120–180 sec (vs. 60–90 sec in subjects without prior vecuronium), the time to 75% recovery of twitch height was shortened to 2–3 min (vs. 3–5 min), and the block was associated with a T_4/T_1 ratio < 0.3.[113] The effects of SCh administration on the NDR-induced block are discussed in Chapter 16.
■ Long-term	i	May lead to proliferation of cholinoceptors and increased sensitivity to depolarizing relaxants (after discontinuation of nondepolarizing agent) (Chap. 22).[114]
■ Pancuronium	D/i	Inhibits pseudoChE in clinical doses[115–119] and thus may prolong block.[117,120–123] In vitro, clinical concentrations of pancuronium cause 50% inhibition of benzoylcholine metabolism.[124] However, the decrease in ACh degradation typically is <15% after a defasciculating dose in humans.[118] It may not be appropriate to estimate the effect on in vivo clearance from effects on other substrates in vitro.[125] Pretreatment with pancuronium followed by an increased dose of SCh is more likely to cause phase 2 block in a heterozygous patient.[126] Negligible effect was noted when SCh, 0.3 mg · kg^{-1}, was given 20–60 min after pancuronium, 0.02–0.04 mg · kg^{-1}, in normal patients.[116]
■ Hexafluorenium	D/I	This competitive NDR strongly inhibits pseudoChE, thereby prolonging SCh-induced block.[127]
PERIOPERATIVE MEDICATIONS		
■ Metoclopramide	I	Inhibits pseudoChE activity[128–130]; 20 mg PO increased the duration of SCh from 8 min to 12.4 min.[129]

(Continued)

I = increased effect of block, D = decreased effect of block, i = theoretical or minimal increase, d = theoretical or minimal decrease, ChE = cholinesterase (pseudoChE = pseudocholinesterase, acetylChE = acetylcholinesterase).

TABLE 17-2
(Continued)

Agent or Condition	Effect	Mechanism, Comments, References
■ H$_2$ receptor antagonists	i	Onset normal; duration normal when one or two doses administered alone,[130,131] but duration was prolonged 200–250% by two oral doses of cimetidine + metoclopramide.[132] *Clinical doses of cimetidine and ranitidine* alone have minimal effect on subsequent pseudoChE activity.[133] IV ranitidine affects acetylChE, but pseudoChE is relatively undisturbed (Chap. 9).[134–136] However, *high doses* of ranitidine (2.5–20 mg · kg^{-1}) or cimetidine IV produced *immediate potentiation* of SCh-induced block followed by transient reversal and then a more *persistent potentiation*.[136,137] The increased block probably resulted from ACh accumulation; the transient reversal may have been due to development of a partial phase 2 (dual) block.[136] In very high doses (e.g., ranitidine, 60 mg · kg^{-1}), these agents may produce neuromuscular block by themselves,[138] perhaps as a consequence of their antiChE effects in the NMJ (which can reverse nondepolarizing block). These effects are not typically elicited in clinical settings, where serum ranitidine concentrations (4 µg · mL^{-1} after IV and 0.2 µg · mL^{-1} after oral dosing)[136] are far less than the concentrations used in rat models (8–67 µg · mL^{-1}).[136] "However, caution will need to be exercised in patients who are otherwise at risk of displaying prolonged paralysis" (e.g., low pseudoChE activity, concurrent medications).[136] It has also been noted that when cimetidine or ranitidine is given in close proximity to a relaxant, the drugs might interact "to produce unpredictable muscle relaxant activity."[134]
PHOSPHODIESTERASE INHIBITORS	i	Allow increased cAMP and thus increased ACh. This has relatively little impact on SCh-induced block in the clinical setting.
TOXINS		
■ *Clostridium botulinum* and *C. tetani*	I	Cause decreased ACh release and denervation-like syndrome[139–141] with supersensitivity to depolarizing agents.[142,143]
II. PATIENT STATUS		
CRITICAL ILLNESS NEUROPATHY	I	There is high incidence of neural damage (with primary axonal degradation) in ICU patients with sepsis and multiple organ failure.[144–152] This may predispose to SCh-induced hyperkalemia (Chap. 22).

(Continued)

I = increased effect of block, D = decreased effect of block, i = theoretical or minimal increase, d = theoretical or minimal decrease, ChE = cholinesterase (pseudoChE = pseudocholinesterase, acetylChE = acetylcholinesterase).

TABLE 17-2

(Continued)

Agent or Condition	Effect	Mechanism, Comments, References
CHRONIC DISEASE STATES	i	May be associated with decreased pseudoChE activity.[12]
DISUSE ATROPHY	I	Long-term disuse gives rise to receptor proliferation that may extend extrajunctionally and predispose to SCh-induced hyperkalemia (Chap. 22).
HYPERTHYROIDISM	d	Increased pseudoChE activity.[32]
HYPOPROTEINEMIA	i	Less bound, hence more free drug available.
INJURIES		
▪ Burns	I	Progressive *decrease in pseudoChE* for 5–6 days may persist for weeks (possible factors include dilution, transcapillary loss, decreased liver synthesis, circulating inhibitors).[151] Injury may lead to *hypersensitivity* and severe SCh-induced *hyperkalemia* (Chap. 22).[153]
▪ Denervation	I	Denervation hypersensitivity may predispose to SCh-induced *hyperkalemia* (Chap. 22).
LIVER FAILURE	i	Decreased pseudoChE activity.[16,45,154] Altered fluid and protein status (Chap. 10). In severe liver disease with 80% reduction of pseudoChE activity, the duration of apnea after an intubating dose of SCh increased to approximately 9 min.[16,45]
MALIGNANT HYPERTHERMIA	I	SCh definitely contraindicated. SCh-induced contractures may precipitate a malignant hyperthermia crisis (Chaps. 19 and 20). May be increased incidence of abnormal alleles for pseudoChE, especially E_1^f.[32]
MYASTHENIA GRAVIS	D/i	Depolarizers are less affected than NDRs[155] (Chap. 21). Some resistance to decamethonium[156,157] and SCh,[155,157–159] which is noted especially after low doses (e.g., 0.5 mg · kg^{-1} of SCh)[159]; onset of 1.0 mg · kg^{-1} may be slightly prolonged.[159] There is an increased incidence of SCh-induced phase 2 block.[155,157–162] In contrast to the decreased sensitivity to SCh that characterizes myasthenia gravis, an increased effect of SCh may occur if there is a residual effect of the anti-ChE therapy used to treat the disorder or if there is a reduction in pseudoChE levels to <20% of normal as a result of plasma exchange.[163–165]

(Continued)

I = increased effect of block, D = decreased effect of block, i = theoretical or minimal increase, d = theoretical or minimal decrease, ChE = cholinesterase (pseudoChE = pseudocholinesterase, acetylChE = acetylcholinesterase).

TABLE 17-2
(Continued)

Agent or Condition	Effect	Mechanism, Comments, References
OBESITY	—	Increased volume of distribution and increased total pseudoChE in proportion to increased weight.[166] Therefore, should dose according to total body weight.
OBSTETRICS		
▪ Pregnancy	i	Decreased pseudoChE activity to approximately 60–80% of normal.[16,167–172] However, the duration of SCh is relatively normal[170] or only slightly prolonged,[173] since remaining pseudoChE is adequate and an increased volume of distribution accelerates termination of SCh effect. Little, if any, correlation between pseudoChE concentration during pregnancy and SCh duration of action.[167] Maximum decrease may be reached during first trimester.[168] Faster onset,[173] probably due to increased cardiac output and administration of a relatively large dose. Pregnancy is associated with a relatively low incidence of SCh-induced fasciculations and myalgias.[174]
▪ Eclampsia	I	Decreases pseudoChE beyond that of normal pregnancy (typically by an additional 20%).[175] Effects of SCh are exaggerated by magnesium therapy.[175,176]
▪ Oral contraceptives	I	Decreased pseudoChE activity.[32,177]
▪ Post partum	I	PseudoChE activity is decreased for several days post partum,[167–172] to values lower than at delivery. This decrease may be associated with an increased time to 25% recovery (e.g., from 501 ± 21 sec to 685 ± 22 sec).[170]
OLD AGE	i	PseudoChE activity may be decreased by 25% in the elderly. The clinical effect of this is small.
PEDIATRICS		
▪ Children aged 1–12 yr	D	Increased volume of distribution and relatively high pseudoChE activity, hence greater SCh requirements, especially on a mg · kg^{-1} basis (Chap. 16).[178–181] Increased tendency toward phase 2 block with doses > 4 mg · kg^{-1}.
▪ Neonate	D	As for older children, increased requirements, especially on a mg · kg^{-1} basis.[178–186] Neonate and adult requirements tend to be similar on a mg · m^{-2} basis[181]; the increased volume of distribution[178,181] offsets the effects of decreased pseudoChE (50–60% of adult values).[187,188] The decrease in pseudoChE may lead to slight prolongation of effect, but this generally is offset by the increased volume of distribution and relatively high cardiac output. The al-

(Continued)

I = increased effect of block, D = decreased effect of block, i = theoretical or minimal increase, d = theoretical or minimal decrease, ChE = cholinesterase (pseudoChE = pseudocholinesterase, acetylChE = acetylcholinesterase).

TABLE 17-2
(Continued)

Agent or Condition	Effect	Mechanism, Comments, References
■ Neonate *(cont.)*	D	tered sensitivity in neonates (especially premature neonates) may also have a local neuroanatomic basis (i.e., it may result from the persistence of immature neuromuscular junctions). As noted in Chapters 2 and 16, block by a depolarizing relaxant "depends on a sharp demarcation between the chemically sensitive receptor channels of the end-plate and the chemically insensitive sodium channels in the perijunctional area of the muscle membrane. In contrast to the adult, in whom the boundary is sharp, infants whose junctions are not yet sensitive may have diffuse boundaries in which persistent fetal receptors are in the perijunctional margin. In this case, it would be harder to establish a blockade of neuromuscular transmission with a depolarizing agent."[189]
PSYCHIATRIC DISORDERS	I/D	There may be an increased incidence of the E_1^f allele and prolonged SCh-induced apnea in patients undergoing electroconvulsive shock therapy.[190] PseudoChE levels are reported to be normal in *affective disorders*[191] and are also reported normal *schizophrenia*,[186] but another report noted an increase in $E_1^a E_1^f$.[192] May be decreased in *Huntington's chorea* due to increase in $E_1^u E_1^f$.[190–192] Although one case of Huntington's chorea suggested a significant decrease of pseudoChE activity, this has not been substantiated.[193] Bipolar disorder (manic-depression) may be associated with increased pseudoChE activity.[32,194]
RENAL TRANSPLANT	i	May have decreased pseudoChE but also have increased volume of distribution.
SEPSIS	i	Leads to muscle weakness, catabolism, multiple organ failure, and electrolyte abnormalities.[151,195–197] This may predispose to SCh-induced hyperkalemia.
III. ACID-BASE/LYTES		
DECREASED K^+	d	May hyperpolarize and thereby oppose depolarization (but depends on rate and degree of change).[198]
INCREASED Ca^{2+}	d	Patients with hyperparathyroidism required 1.4 × more SCh.[199]

(Continued)

I = increased effect of block, D = decreased effect of block, i = theoretical or minimal increase, d = theoretical or minimal decrease, ChE = cholinesterase (pseudoChE = pseudocholinesterase, acetylChE = acetylcholinesterase).

TABLE 17-2
(Continued)

Agent or Condition	Effect	Mechanism, Comments, References
INCREASED Mg^{2+}	I	Multiple effects that, overall, lead to weakness: decreased ACh release, decreased end-plate sensitivity, decreased muscle contraction,[200] decreased K^+ release.[201,202] It may prolong block[176] (but not always[202]), decrease fasciculations,[203,204] and even blunt the typical 0.5 mEq · L^{-1} SCh-induced increase of K^+.[202] Overall effect is potentiation of depolarizing as well as nondepolarizing block.[204]

I = increased effect of block, D = decreased effect of block, i = theoretical or minimal increase, d = theoretical or minimal decrease, ChE = cholinesterase (pseudoChE = pseudocholinesterase, acetylChE = acetylcholinesterase).

Discussion Questions ◆

a. Is *SCh metabolized* in the *NMJ*? Why is this feature of SCh important?
b. Can a patient with *malnutrition* have low *pseudocholinesterase activity* yet still have a normal *dibucaine number*? Why or why not?
c. How often do we encounter patients who are $E_1^a E_1^a$ in *clinical practice*?
d. What does a *dibucaine number* of 80 tell you about the ability of a given patient's pseudocholinesterase to metabolize benzoylcholine?
e. List three genotypes with a *dibucaine number* that often is less than 30.
f. Does a marked decrease in *pseudocholinesterase activity* alter the ED_{95} of *SCh*? Why or why not?
g. In a patient who is *homozygous* for E_1^a, might you expect *apnea after 10 mg* of SCh? Why or why not?

Answers ◆

a. Succinylcholine is metabolized by *pseudocholinesterase* in the plasma but not by *acetylcholinesterase* in the NMJ. Breakdown of SCh in the NMJ is negligible. Thus, it continues to act in the NMJ until it diffuses back to the plasma along its concentration gradient.
b. Although the total amount of enzyme is decreased in states of decreased *pseudocholinesterase production,* the enzyme that is present is normal. It thus is inhibited by dibucaine and has a normal dibucaine number.
c. Although the incidence of $E_1^a E_1^a$ is 1:2,500, we may encounter patients who are *homozygous for atypical pseudocholinesterase* less commonly in clinical practice because (1) we avoid SCh in blood relatives of patients with known abnormalities (or such individuals are tested prior to surgery),[45] (2) many patients undergo surgery without exposure to SCh,

and (3) delayed recovery may be "masked" during a long surgical procedure. Alternatively, it should be remembered that other variants besides the $E_1^a E_1^a$ genotype may lead to ineffective or inadequate pseudocholinesterase.

d. A *DN = 80* indicates the presence of normal enzyme. The value means that a high percentage of enzyme activity, as measured by its *ability to hydrolyze* a substrate such as benzoylcholine, is *inhibited by dibucaine*. Atypical pseudocholinesterase exhibits far less inhibition. It should be remembered that the DN determines the quality of the enzyme that is present; it does not determine the amount of enzyme.

e. A *DN < 30* typically is noted with *genotypes* such as atyp/atyp ($E_1^a E_1^a$), atyp/silent ($E_1^a E_1^s$), or atyp/fluoride ($E_1^a E_1^f$).

f. In addition to prolonging the duration of SCh, a significant *pseudocholinesterase deficiency* also *increases the effectiveness* of a given dose. The decreased ED_{95} is due to the fact that pseudocholinesterase typically begins to metabolize SCh immediately on its injection (before it reaches the NMJ). The lack of metabolism has been associated with cases of violent fasciculations after a small dose of SCh[205,206] and with prolonged jaw rigidity and myalgias after SCh[207]; however, these findings are not limited to patients with pseudocholinesterase deficiencies.[206,208]

g. A dose of *10 mg of SCh* (0.15 mg · kg^{-1}) is well below the ED_{95} reported in most series (usually in the range of 0.3–0.5 mg · kg^{-1}) and probably would not cause apnea in a normal individual. A large percentage of the SCh would be metabolized prior to reaching the NMJ. In contrast, the dose of SCh probably would cause apnea in the patient who is homozygous for *atypical pseudocholinesterase*.

References ◆

1. Glick D: Some additional observations on the specificity of cholinesterase. J Biol Chem 137:357, 1941
2. Whittaker VP, Wijesundra S: The hydrolysis of succinyldicholine by cholinesterase. Biochem J 52:475, 1952
3. Foldes FF, McNall PG, Birch JH: The neuromuscular activity of succinylmonocholine iodide in man. Br Med J 1:967, 1954
4. Goedde HW, Heid KR, Altland K: Hydrolysis of succinyldicholine and succinylmonocholine in human serum. Mol Pharmacol 4:274–287, 1968
5. Kalow W: The distribution, destruction and elimination of muscle relaxants. Anesthesiology 20:505–518, 1959
6. Cook DR, Wingard LB Jr, Taylor FH: Pharmacokinetics of succinylcholine in infants, children, and adults. Clin Pharmacol Ther 20:493–498, 1976
7. Kvisselgard N, Moya F: Estimation of succinylcholine blood levels. Acta Anaesthesiol Scand 5:1–11, 1961
8. Levy G: Kinetics of pharmacologic activity of succinylcholine in man. J Pharmacol Sci 56:1687–1688, 1967
9. Dal Santo G: Kinetics of distribution of radioactive labeled muscle relaxants: III. Investigations with ^{14}C-succinyldicholine and ^{14}C-succinylmonocholine during controlled conditions. Anesthesiology 29:435–443, 1969

10. Holst-Larsen H: The hydrolysis of suxamethonium in human blood. Br J Anaesth 48:887–892, 1976
11. Viby-Mogensen J: Correlation of succinylcholine duration of action with plasma cholinesterase activity in subjects with the genotypically normal enzyme. Anesthesiology 53:517–520, 1980
12. Viby-Mogensen J: Cholinesterase and succinylcholine. Dan Med Bull 30:129–150, 1983
13. Ritter DM, Rettke SR, Ilstrup DM, Burritt MF: Effect of plasma cholinesterase activity on the duration of action of succinylcholine in patients with genotypically normal enzyme. Anesth Analg 67:1123–1126, 1988
14. Foldes F, Rhodes DH Jr: The role of plasma cholinesterase in anesthesiology. Anesth Analg 32:305–318, 1953
15. Smith CE, Lewis G, Donati F, Bevan DR: Dose-response relationship for succinylcholine in a patient with genetically determined low plasma cholinesterase activity. Anesthesiology 70:156–158, 1989
16. Pantuck EJ, Pantuck CB: Cholinesterases and anticholinesterases. In Katz RL (ed): Muscle Relaxants. Amsterdam, Excerpta Medica, 1975, p 143
17. Arpagaus M, Kott M, Vatsis KP, et al: Structure of the gene for human butyrylcholinesterase: evidence for a single copy. Biochemistry 29:124–131, 1990
18. Allderdice PW, Gardner HAR, Galutira D, et al: The cloned butyrylcholinesterase (BCHE) gene maps to a single chromosome site, 3q26. Genomics 11:452–454, 1991
19. Bartels CF, Jensen FS, Lockridge O, et al: DNA mutation associated with the human butyrylcholinesterase K-variant and its linkage to the atypical variant mutation and other polymorphic sites. Am J Hum Genet 50:1086–1103, 1992
20. Gaughan G, Park H, Priddle J, et al: Refinement of the localization of human butyrylcholinesterase to chromosome 3q26.1-q26.2 using a PCR-derived probe. Genomics 11:455–458, 1991
21. Garry PJ, Dietz AA, Lubrano T, et al: New allele at cholinesterase locus 1. J Med Genet 13:38–42, 1976
22. Lockridge O, Bartels CF, Vaughan TA, et al: Complete amino acid sequence of human serum cholinesterase. J Biol Chem 262:549–557, 1987
23. La Du BN, Primo-Parmo S, van der Spek AFL: Identification of DNA mutations responsible for serum butyrylcholinesterase variants will permit a better differentiation of aberrant drug responses. Anesthesiology 75:A372, 1991
24. McTiernan C, Adkins S, Chatonnet A, et al: Brain cDNA clone for human cholinesterase. Proc Natl Acad Sci USA 84:6682–6686, 1987
25. Pantuck EJ: Plasma cholinesterase: gene and variations. Anesth Analg 77:380–386, 1993
26. Prody CA, Zevin-Sonkin D, Gnatt A, et al: Isolation and characterization of full-length cDNA clones coding for cholinesterase from fetal human tissues. Proc Natl Acad Sci USA 84:3555–3559, 1987
27. Rao PR, Gopalam KB: High incidence of the silent allele at cholinesterase locus 1 in Vysyas of Andhra Pradesh (S. India). Hum Genet 52:139–141, 1979
28. Whittaker M, Britten JJ: E_{1b}, a new allele at cholinesterase locus 1. Hum Hered 37:54–58, 1987
29. Rubinstein HM, Dietz AA, Lubrano T: E_{1k}, another quantitative variant at cholinesterase locus 1. J Med Genet 15:27–29, 1978
30. Hanel HK, Viby-Mogensen J, Schaffalitzky de Muckadell OB: Serum cholinesterase variants in the Danish population. Acta Anaesthesiol Scand 22:505, 1978
31. Lehmann H, Lidell J: Human cholinesterase [pseudocholinesterase]: Genetic variants and their recognition. Br J Anaesth 41:243, 1969
32. Whittaker M: Plasma cholinesterase variants and the anaesthetist. Anaesthesia 35:174–197, 1980
33. Singh S, Amma MKP, Sareen KN, Goedde HW: A study of the pseudocholinesterase polymorphism among a Punjabi population. Hum Hered 21:388–393, 1971
34. Gutsche BB, Scott EM, Wright RC: Hereditary deficiency pseudocholinesterase in Eskimos. Nature 215:322–323, 1967
35. Scott EM, Wright RC: A third type of serum cholinesterase deficiency in Eskimos. Am J Hum Genet 28:253–256, 1976

36. Scott EM, Weaver DD, Wright RC: Discrimination of phenotypes in human serum cholinesterase deficiency. Am J Human Genet 22:363–369, 1970
37. Scott EM, Wright RC: Hereditary deficiency of pseudocholinesterase in Eskimos. Nature 215:322–333, 1967
38. Pannall PR, Potgieter GM, Raaubenheimer MM: Plasma cholinesterase variants—an unexpectedly high incidence of the silent allele. S Afr Med J 50:304–306, 1976
39. Davies RO, Marton AV, Kalow W: The action of normal and atypical cholinesterase of human serum upon a series of esters of choline. Can J Biochem Physiol 38:545–551, 1960
40. Kalow W, Genest K: A method for the detection of atypical forms of human serum cholinesterase: determination of dibucaine numbers. Can J Biochem Physiol 35:339–346, 1957
41. Harris H, Whittaker M: Differential inhibition of human serum cholinesterase with fluoride: recognition of two new phenotypes. Nature 191:496–498, 1961
42. Liddell J, Lehmann H, Silk E: A "silent" pseudocholinesterase gene. Nature 193:561–562, 1962
43. Hart SM, Mitchell JV: Suxamethonium in the absence of pseudocholinesterase. Br J Anaesth 34:207–209, 1962
44. Rubinstein HM, Dietz AA, Hodges LK, et al: Silent cholinesterase gene: variations in the properties of serum enzyme in apparent homozygotes. J Clin Invest 49:479–486, 1970
45. Viby-Mogensen J, Hanel HK: A Danish cholinesterase research unit. Acta Anaesthesiol Scand 21:405–412, 1977
46. Baraka A: Suxamethonium-neostigmine interaction in patients with normal or atypical cholinesterase. Br J Anaesth 49:479–484, 1977
47. James MFM, Howe HC: Prolonged paralysis following suxamethonium and the use of neostigmine. Br J Anaesth 65:430–432, 1990
48. Oshita S, Sari A, Fuju S, et al: Prolonged neuromuscular blockade following succinylcholine in a patient homozygous for the silent gene. Anesthesiology 59:71–73, 1983
49. Viby-Mogensen J: Succinylcholine neuromuscular blockade in subjects heterozygous for abnormal plasma cholinesterase. Anesthesiology 55:231–235, 1981
50. Viby-Mogensen J: Succinylcholine neuromuscular blockade in subjects homozygous for atypical plasma cholinesterase. Anesthesiology 55:429–434, 1981
51. Evans RT, Wardell J: On the identification and frequency of the J and K cholinesterase phenotypes in a Caucasian population. J Med Genet 21:99–102, 1984
52. Delbruck A, Henkel E: A rare genetically determined variant of pseudocholinesterase in two German families with high plasma cholinesterase activity. Eur J Biochem 99:65–69, 1979
53. Neitlich HW: Increased plasma cholinesterase activity and succinylcholine resistance: a genetic variant. J Clin Invest 45:380–387, 1966
54. Yoshida A, Motulsky AG: A pseudocholinesterase variant (E Cynthiana) associated with elevated plasma enzyme activity. Am J Hum Genet 21:486–497, 1969
55. Krause A, Lane AB, Jenkins T: A new high activity plasma cholinesterase variant. J Med Genet 25:677–681, 1988
56. Burkett L, Bilkhazi GM, Thamas KC, et al: Mutual potentiation of the neuromuscular effects of antibiotics and relaxants. Anesth Analg 58:107–115, 1979
57. Pantuck EJ: Ecothiopate iodide eye drops and prolonged response to suxamethonium. Br J Anaesth 38:406–407, 1966
58. Baraka A, Wakid N, Mansour R, Haddad W: Effect of neostigmine and pyridostigmine on the plasma cholinesterase activity. Br J Anaesth 53:849–851, 1981
59. Barrow MEH, Johnson JK: A study of the anticholinesterase and anticurare effects of some cholinesterase inhibitors. Br J Anaesth 38:420–431, 1966
60. Bentz EW, Stoelting RK: Prolonged response to succinylcholine following pancuronium reversal with pyridostigmine. Anesthesiology 44:258, 1976
61. Sunew KY, Hicks RG: Effects of neostigmine and pyridostigmine on duration of succinylcholine action and pseudocholinesterase activity. Anesthesiology 49:188–191, 1978
62. Katz RL, Ryan JF: The neuromuscular effects of suxamethonium in man. Br J Anaesth 41:381–390, 1969
63. Gissen AJ, Katz RL, Karis JH, Papper EM: Neuromuscular block in man during prolonged arterial infusion with succinylcholine. Anesthesiology 27:242–249, 1966

64. Sakuma N, Hasimoto Y, Iwatsuki N: Effects of neostigmine and edrophonium on human erythrocyte acetylcholinesterase activity. Br J Anaesth 68:316–317, 1992
65. Milthers E, Clemmesen C, Nimb M: Poisoning with phosphostigmines: treatment with atropine, pralidoxime methiodide and diacetyl monoxime. Dan Med Bull 10:122–129, 1963
66. Kopman AF, Strachovsky G, Lichtenstein L: Prolonged response to succinylcholine following physostigmine. Anesthesiology 49:142–143, 1978
67. Walker IR, Zapf PW, Mackay IR: Cyclophosphamide, cholinesterase and anesthesia. Aust NZ J Med 2:247, 1972
68. Wang RIH, Ross CA: Prolonged apnea following succinylcholine in cancer patients receiving AB-132. Anesthesiology 24:363, 1963
69. Zsigmond EK, Robins G: The effect of a series of anti-cancer drugs on plasma cholinesterase activity. Can Anaesth Soc J 19:75–82, 1972
70. Dillman JB: Safe use of succinylcholine during repeated anesthetics in a patient treated with cyclophosphamide. Anesth Analg 66:351–353, 1987
71. Bang U, Viby-Mogensen J, Wiren JE, et al: The effect of bambuterol (carbamylated terbutaline) on plasma cholinesterase activity and suxamethonium-induced neuromuscular blockade in genotypically normal patients. Acta Anaesthesiol Scand 34:596, 1990
72. Fisher DM, Caldwell JE, Sharma M, Wiren JE: The influence of bambuterol (carbamylated terbutaline) on the duration of action of succinylcholine-induced paralysis in humans. Anesthesiology 69:757–759, 1988
73. Staun P, Lennmarken C, Eriksson LI, et al: The influence of 10 mg and 20 mg of bambuterol on the duration of succinylcholine induced neuromuscular blockade. Acta Anaesthesiol Scand 34:498, 1990
74. Usubiaga JE: Neuromuscular effects of beta-adrenergic blockers and their interaction with skeletal muscle relaxants. Anesthesiology 29:484–492, 1968
75. Wislicki L, Rosenblum I: Effects of propranolol on the action of neuromuscular blocking drugs. Br J Anaesth 39:939–942, 1967
76. Brown MJ, Brown DC, Murphy MB: Hypokalemia from $beta_2$-receptor stimulation by circulating epinephrine. N Engl J Med 309:1414–1419, 1983
77. Goldhill DR, Martyn JAJ, Kim EM, Hoaglin DC: Effect in dogs of selective beta-blockade on potassium release after succinylcholine. Anesth Analg 65:S60, 1986
78. Halevy JD, Ornstein E, Matteo RS: Esmolol is not associated with an exaggerated succinylcholine mediated hyperkalemic response. Anesthesiology 69:A424, 1988
79. Murthy VS, Patel KD, Elangovan RG, Hwang TF, Solochek SM, Steck JD, Laddu AR: Cardiovascular and neuromuscular effects of esmolol during induction of anesthesia. J Clin Pharmacol 26:351–357, 1986
80. McCammon RL, Hilgenberg JC, Sandage BW Jr, Stoelting RK: The effect of esmolol on the onset and duration of succinylcholine-induced neuromuscular blockade. Anesthesiology 63:A317, 1985
81. Barabas E, Zsigmond EK, Kirkpatrick AF: The inhibitory effect of esmolol on human plasmacholinesterase. Can Anaesth Soc J 33:332–335, 1986
82. Sum CY, Stampfil HF: Biochemical characterization of esmolol esterase in blood. Fed Proc 43:561, 1984
83. Bikhazi GB, Leung I, Foldes FF: Ca-channel blockers increase potency of neuromuscular blocking agents *in vivo*. Anesthesiology 59:A269, 1983
84. Kraynack BJ, Lawson NW, Gintantas J, et al: Effects of verapamil on indirect muscle twitch responses. Anesth Analg 62:827–830, 1983
85. Salvatore A, Del Pozo E, Carlos R, Baeyens JM: Differential effects of calcium channel blocking agents on pancuronium- and suxamethonium-induced neuromuscular blockade. Br J Anaesth 60:495–499, 1988
86. Miller RD, Way WL, Katzung BG: The potentiation of neuromuscular blocking agents by quinidine. Anesthesiology 28:1036–1041, 1967
87. Poulton TJ, James FM, Lockridge O: Prolonged apnea following trimethaphan and succinylcholine. Anesthesiology 50:54–56, 1979
88. Tewfik GI: Trimethaphan: its effect on the pseudocholinesterase level of man. Anaesthesia 12:326–329, 1957
89. Foldes FF, Arai T, Gentsch HH, Zarday Z: The influence of glucocorticoids on plasma cholinesterase. Proc Soc Exp Biol Med 146:918–920, 1974

90. Szalados JE, Donati F, Bevan DR: Nitrous oxide potentiates succinylcholine neuromuscular blockade in humans. Anesth Analg 72:18–21, 1991
91. Donati F, Bevan DR: Effect of enflurane and fentanyl on the clinical characteristics of long-term succinylcholine infusion. Can Anaesth Soc J 29:59–64, 1982
92. Hilgenberg JC, Stoelting RK: Characteristics of succinylcholine-produced phase II neuromuscular block during enflurane, halothane, and fentanyl anesthesia. Anesth Analg 60:192, 1981
93. Connelly NR, Silverman DG, Brull SJ: Temporal correlation of succinylcholine-induced fasciculations to loss of twitch response at different stimulating frequencies. J Clin Anesth 4:190–193, 1992
94. Miller RD, Way WL, Dolan WM, Stevens WC, Eger EI II: Comparative neuromuscular effects of pancuronium, gallamine, and succinylcholine during forane and halothane anesthesia in man. Anesthesiology 35:509–514, 1971
95. Caldwell JE, Laster MJ, Magorian T, Heier T, Yasuda N, Lynam DP, Eger EI II, Weiskopf RB: The neuromuscular effects of desflurane, alone and combined with pancuronium or succinylcholine in humans. Anesthesiology 74:412–418, 1991
96. Eisenberg M, Balsley S, Katz RL: Effects of diazepam on succinylcholine-induced myalgia, potassium increase, creatinine phosphokinase elevation, and relaxation. Anesth Analg 58:314–317, 1979
97. Amaki Y, Nagashima H, Radnay PA, Foldes FF: Ketamine interaction with neuromuscular blocking agents in the phrenic nerve-hemidiaphragm preparation of the rat. Anesth Analg 57:238–243, 1978
98. Healy TEJ, Birmingham AT, Chatterjee SC: A comparison of the effect of induction of anaesthesia by thiopentone or Althesin on the duration of action of suxamethonium. Postgrad Med J (June suppl):90–92, 1972
99. Doenicke A, Krumey I, Kugler J, Klempa J: Experimental studies of the breakdown of Epontol: determination of propanidid in human serum. Br J Anaesth 40:415–428, 1968
100. Ellis FR: The neuromuscular interaction of propanidid with suxamethonium and tubocurarine. Br J Anaesth 40:818–824, 1968
101. Matsuo S, Rao DBS, Chaudry I, et al: Interaction of muscle relaxants and local anesthetics at the neuromuscular junction. Anesth Analg 57:580–587, 1978
102. Morita K, Matsuo S, Nagashima H, et al: In vivo muscle relaxant-local anesthetic interaction. Anesthesiology 51:S282, 1979
103. Naguib M, Farag H, Magbagbeola JA: Failure of lidocaine to modify suxamethonium-induced biochemical changes. Middle East J Anaesthesiol 9:375–382, 1988
104. Foldes FF, McNall PG, Davis DL, Ellis CH, Wnuck AL: Substrate competition between procaine and succinylcholine diiodide for plasma cholinesterase. Science 117:383–386, 1953
105. Usubiaga JF, Wikinski JA, Morales RL: Interaction of intravenously administered procaine, lidocaine and succinylcholine in anesthetized subjects. Anesth Analg 46:39–45, 1967
106. Zsigmond E, Eldertton TE: Abnormal reaction to procaine and succinylcholine in a patient with inherited atypical plasma cholinesterase. Can Anaesth Soc J 15:498–500, 1968
107. Erdös EG, Foldes FF, Bart N, Shanor SP: In vitro effects of chlorpromazine on human cholinesterases. Fed Proc 15:420, 1956
108. Hill GE, Wong KC, Hodges MR: Potentiation of succinylcholine neuromuscular blockade by lithium carbonate. Anesthesiology 44:439–442, 1976
109. Bodley PO, Halwax K, Potts L: Low serum pseudocholinesterase levels complicating treatment with phenelzine. Br Med J 3:510, 1969
110. Hartman GS, Fiamengo SA, Riker WF: Succinylcholine: mechanism of fasciculations and their prevention by d-tubocurarine or diphenylhydantoin. Anesthesiology 65:405–413, 1986
111. Campkin NTA, Hood JR, Feldman SA: Resistance to decamethonium neuromuscular block after prior administration of vecuronium. Anesth Analg 77:78–80, 1993
112. Sugai N, Hughes R, Payne JP: The effect of suxamethonium alone and its interaction with gallamine on the indirectly elicited tetanic and single twitch contractions of skeletal muscle in man during anaesthesia. Br J Clin Pharmacol 2:391–402, 1975

113. Baraka A: Rapid onset of suxamethonium block. Br J Anaesth 66:733, 1991
114. Berg DK, Hall ZW: Increased extrajunctional acetylcholine sensitivity produced by chronic post-synaptic neuromuscular blockade. J Physiol 244:659–676, 1975
115. Bowman WC: Non-relaxant properties of neuromuscular blocking drugs. Br J Anaesth 54:147–160, 1982
116. Katz RL: Modification of the action of pancuronium by succinylcholine and halothane. Anesthesiology 35:602–606, 1971
117. Ivankovich AD, Sidell N, Cairoli VJ, Dietz AA, Albrecht RF: Dual action of pancuronium on succinylcholine block. Can Anaesth Soc J 24:228–241, 1977
118. Stovner J, Oftedal N, Holmboe J: The inhibition of cholinesterases by pancuronium. Br J Anaesth 47:949–954, 1975
119. Mirakhur RK, Ferres CJ, Lavery TD: Plasma cholinesterase levels following pancuronium and vecuronium. Acta Anaesthesiol Scand 27:451–453, 1983
120. Ferguson A, Bevan DR: Mixed neuromuscular block: the effect of precurarization. Anaesthesia 36:661–666, 1981
121. Bennett EJ, Montgomery SJ, Dalal FY, Raj PP: Pancuronium and the fasciculations of succinylcholine. Anesth Analg 52:892–896, 1973
122. Erkola O, Salmenpera A, Kuoppamaki R: Five nondepolarizing muscle relaxants in precurarization. Acta Anaesthesiol Scand 27:427–432, 1983
123. Nishizawa M: Influence of small doses of vecuronium and pancuronium on succinylcholine-induced neuromuscular blockade. Masui 39:1188–1197, 1990
124. Whittaker M, Britten JJ: Inhibition of the plasma cholinesterase variants by pancuronium bromide and some of its analogues. Clin Chim Acta 108:89–94, 1980
125. Brandom BW, Meretoja OA, Taivainen T, Wirtavuori K: Accelerated onset and delayed recovery of neuromuscular block induced by mivacurium preceded by pancuronium in children. Anesth Analg 76:998–1003, 1993
126. Ostergaard D, Viby-Mogensen J, Hanel HK, Skovgaard LT: Pretreatment with pancuronium before suxamethonium administration in patients heterozygous for the usual and the atypical plasma cholinesterase gene. Acta Anaesthesiol Scand 35:502–507, 1991
127. Torda TAG, Foldes FF, Bailey MB, Klonymus DH, Kuwubara S: The interactions of neuromuscular blocking agents in man: the role of hexafluorenium. Anesthesiology 28:1010–1019, 1967
128. Kao YJ, Turner DR: Prolongation of succinylcholine block by metoclopramide. Anesthesiology 70:905–908, 1989
129. Kao YJ, Tellez J, Turner DR: Dose-dependent effect of metoclopramide on cholinesterases and suxamethonium metabolism. Br J Anaesth 65:220–224, 1990
130. Turner DR, Kao YJ, Bivona C: Neuromuscular block with suxamethonium following treatment with histamine type-2 antagonists or metoclopramide. Br J Anaesth 63:348–356, 1989
131. Woodworth GE, Sears DH, Grove TM, Ruff RH, Kosek PS, Katz RL: The effect of cimetidine and ranitidine on the duration of action of succinylcholine. Anesth Analg 68:295–297, 1989
132. Kambam JR, Dymond R, Krestow M: Effect of cimetidine on duration of action of succinylcholine. Anesth Analg 66:191–192, 1987
133. Kambam JR, Franks JJ: Cimetidine does not affect plasma cholinesterase activity. Anesth Analg 67:69–70, 1988
134. Gwee MCE, Cheah LS: Actions of cimetidine and ranitidine at some cholinergic sites: implications in toxicology and anesthesia. Life Sci 39:383–388, 1986
135. Hansen WE, Bertl S: Inhibition of cholinesterases by ranitidine. Lancet 1:235, 1983
136. Mishra Y, Ramzan I: Interaction between succinylcholine and ranitidine in rats. Can J Anaesth 40:32–37, 1993
137. Mishra Y, Ramsan I: Interaction between succinylcholine and cimetidine in rats. Can J Anaesth 39:370–374, 1992
138. Garg DC, Weidler DJ, Eshelman FN: Ranitidine bioavailability and kinetics in normal male subjects. Clin Pharmacol Ther 33:445–452, 1983
139. Gundersen CB: The effects of botulinum toxin on the synthesis, storage and release of acetylcholine. Prog Neurobiol 14:99, 1980

140. Martyn JAJ, White DA, Gronert GA, Jaffe RS, Ward JM: Up-and-down regulation of skeletal muscle acetylcholine receptors: effects on neuromuscular blockers. Anesthesiology 76:822–843, 1992
141. Simpson LL: Molecular pharmacology of botulinum toxin and tetanus toxin. Annu Rev Pharmacol Toxicol 26:427–453, 1986
142. Roth F, Wuthrich H: The clinical importance of hyperkalemia following suxamethonium administration. Br J Anaesth 41:311–316, 1969
143. Thesleff S: Supersensitivity of skeletal muscle produced by botulinum toxin. J Physiol 151:598–607, 1960
144. Bolton CF, Gilbert JJ, Hahn AF, Sibbald WJ: Polyneuropathy in critically ill patients. J Neurol Neurosurg Psychiatry 47:1223–1231, 1984
145. Coakley JH, Nagendran K, Honavar M, Hinds CJ: Preliminary observations on the neuromuscular abnormalities in patients with organ failure and sepsis. Intensive Care Med 19:323–328, 1993
146. Coronel B, Meracatello A, Couturiere J-C, et al: Polyneuropathy: potential cause of difficult weaning. Crit Care Med 18:486–489, 1990
147. Helliwall TR, Coakley JH, Wagenmakers AJM, et al: Necrotizing myopathy in critically ill patients. J Pathol 163:307–314, 1991
148. Hinds CJ, Nagendran K, Honauar M, Coakley JH: Muscle relaxants in intensive care patients (letter). Crit Care Med 21:1403–1404, 1993
149. Witt NJ, Bolton CF, Sibbald WJ: The incidence and early features of the polyneuropathy of critical illness. Neurology 35:74, 1985
150. Wokke JHJ, Jennekens FGI, van den Dord CJM, et al: Histological investigations of muscle atrophy and end plates in two critically ill patients with generalized weakness. J Neurol Sci 88:95–106, 1988
151. Witt NJ, Zochodne DW, Bolton CF, Grand'Maison F, Wells G, Young B. Sibbald WJ: Peripheral nerve function in sepsis and multiple organ failure. Chest 99:176–184, 1991
152. Zochodne DW, Bolton CF, Wells GA, Gilbert J, Hahn A, Brown J, et al: Critical illness polyneuropathy, a complication of sepsis and multiple organ failure. Brain 110:819–842, 1987
153. Viby-Mogensen J, Hanel HK, Hansen E, Sorensen B, Graae J: Serum cholinesterase activity in burned patients: I. Biochemical findings. Acta Anaesthesiol Scand 19:159–168, 1975
154. Ritter DM, Rettke SR, Ilstrup DM, Burritt MF: Effect of plasma cholinesterase activity on the duration of action of succinylcholine in patients with genotypically normal enzyme. Anesth Analg 67:1123–1126, 1988
155. Foldes F, McNall PG: Myasthenia gravis: a guide for anesthesiologists. Anesthesiology 23:837–872, 1962
156. Churchill-Davidson HC, Richardson AT: Neuromuscular transmission in myasthenia gravis. J Physiol 122:252–263, 1953
157. Johnson BR, Kim YI, Sanders DB: Neuromuscular blocking properties of suxamethonium and decamethonium in normal and myasthenic rat muscle. J Neurol Sci 59:431–440, 1983
158. Eisenkraft JB, Book WJ, Mann SM, Papatestas AE, Hubbard M: Resistance to succinylcholine in myasthenia gravis: a dose-response study. Anesthesiology 69:760–763, 1988
159. Wainwright AP, Brodrick PM: Suxamethonium in myasthenia gravis. Anaesthesia 42:950–957, 1987
160. Ginsberg H, Varejes L: The use of a relaxant in myasthenia gravis. Anaesthesia 10:177–178, 1955
161. Graham WJH, Grant AP: Dequanlinium in myasthenia gravis. Br Med J 1:153, 1959
162. Stanski DR, Lee RG, MacCannell KL, Karr GW: Atypical cholinesterase in a patient with myasthenia gravis. Anesthesiology 46:278–301, 1977
163. Lumley J: Prolongation of suxamethonium following plasma exchange. Br J Anaesth 52:1149–1150, 1980
164. Patterson JL, Walsh ES, Hall GM: Progressive depletion of plasma cholinesterase during daily plasma exchange. Br Med J 2:580, 1979
165. Wood GJ, Hall GM: Plasmapheresis and plasma cholinesterase. Br J Anaesth 50:945–949, 1978

166. Bentley JB, Borel JD, Vaughan RW, et al: Weight, pseudocholinesterase activity, and succinylcholine requirement. Anesthesiology 57:48–49, 1982
167. Blitt CD, Petty WC, Alberternst EE, Wright BJ: Correlation of plasma cholinesterase activity and duration of action of suxamethonium during pregnancy. Anesth Analg 56:78–83, 1977
168. Evans RT, Wroe JM: Plasma cholinesterase changes during pregnancy: their interpretation as a cause of suxamethonium-induced apnoea. Anaesthesia 35:651–654, 1980
169. Hazel B, Monier D: Human serum cholinesterase: variations during pregnancy and postpartum. Can Anaesth Soc J 18:272, 1971
170. Leighton BL, Cheek TG, Gross JB, Apfelbaum JL, Shantz BB, Gutsche BB, Rosenberg H: Succinylcholine pharmacodynamics in peripartum patients. Anesthesiology 64:202–205, 1986
171. Shnider SM: Serum cholinesterase activity during pregnancy, labor and the puerperium. Anesthesiology 26:335, 1965
172. Robson N, Robertson I, Whittaker M: Plasma cholinesterase changes during the puerperium. Anaesthesia 41:243–249, 1986
173. Carnie JC, Street MK, Kumar B: Emergency intubation of the trachea facilitated by suxamethonium. Br J Anaesth 58:498–501, 1986
174. Cook WP, Schultetus RR, Caton D: A comparison of d-tubocurarine pretreatment and no pretreatment in obstetric patients. Anesth Analg 66:756–760, 1987
175. Kambam JR, Perry SM, Entman S, Smith BE: Effect of magnesium on plasma cholinesterase activity. Am J Obstet Gynecol 159:309–311, 1988
176. Morris R, Giesecke AH: Potentiation of muscle relaxants by magnesium sulfate therapy in toxemia of pregnancy. South Med J 61:25, 1968
177. Robertson GS: Serum protein and cholinesterase changes in association with contraceptive pills. Lancet 1:232, 1967
178. Cook DR, Fischer CG: Neuromuscular blocking effects of succinylcholine in infants and children. Anesthesiology 42:662–665, 1975
179. Goudsouzian NG, Liu LMP: The neuromuscular response of infants to a continuous infusion of succinylcholine. Anesthesiology 60:97–101, 1984
180. Meakin G, McKiernan EP, Morris P, Baker D: Dose-response curves for suxamethonium in neonates, infants and children. Br J Anaesth 62:655–658, 1989
181. Walts LF, Dillon JB: The response of newborns to succinylcholine and d-tubocurarine. Anesthesiology 31:35–38, 1969
182. Churchill-Davidson HC, Wise RP: The response of the newborn infant to muscle relaxants. Can Anaesth Soc J 11:1, 1964
183. Stead AL: The response of the newborn infant to muscle relaxants. Br J Anaesth 27:124–130, 1955
184. Telford J, Keats AS: Succinylcholine in cardiovascular surgery of infants and children. Anesthesiology 18:841–848, 1957
185. Nightingale DA, Glass AG, Bachman L: Neuromuscular blockade by succinylcholine in children. Anesthesiology 27:736–741, 1966
186. DeCook TH, Goudsouzian NG: Tachyphylaxis and phase II block development during infusion of succinylcholine in children. Anesth Analg 59:639–643, 1980
187. Escobichon DJ, Stephens DG: Perinatal development of human esterases. Clin Pharmacol Ther 14:41, 1973
188. Zsgimond EK, Downs JR: Plasma cholinesterase activity in newborn and infants. Can Anaesth Soc J 18:278–285, 1971
189. Goudsouzian NG, Standaert FG: The infant and myoneural junction. Anesth Analg 65:1208–1217, 1986
190. Berry M, Whittaker M: Incidence of suxamethonium apnoea in patients undergoing E.C.T. Br J Anaesth 47:1195–1197, 1975
191. Propert DN: Pseudocholinesterase activity and phenotypes in mentally ill patients. Br J Psychiatry 134:477, 1979
192. Whittaker M, Berry M: The plasma cholinesterase variants in mentally ill patients. Br J Psychiatry 130:397–404, 1977
193. Costarino A, Gross JB: Patients with Huntington's chorea may respond normally to succinylcholine (letter). Anesthesiology 63:570, 1985

194. Plum CM: Study of cholinesterase activity in nervous and mental disorders. Clin Chem 6:332–340, 1960
195. Kohlschutter B, Baur H, Roth F: Suxamethonium-induced hyperkalemia in patients with severe intra-abdominal infections. Br J Anaesth 48:557–561, 1976
196. Khan TZ, Khan RM: Changes in serum potassium following succinylcholine in patients with infections. Anesth Analg 62:327–331, 1983
197. Roelofs RI, Cerra F, Beilka N, et al: Prolonged respiratory insufficiency due to acute motor neuropathy: a new syndrome? Neurology 33(suppl 2):240, 1983
198. Feldman SA: Effect of changes in electrolytes, hydration and pH upon the reactions to muscle relaxants. Br J Anaesth 35:546–551, 1963
199. Roland E, Villiers S, Lequeau F, Roupie E, Sarfati E, Eurin B: Succinylcholine dose-response in hyperparathyroidism. Anesthesiology 75:A808, 1991
200. Engbaek L: The pharmacological actions of magnesium ions with particular reference to the neuromuscular and cardiovascular systems. Pharmacol Rev 4:396–410, 1954
201. Aldrete JA, Zahler A, Aikawa JK: Prevention of succinylcholine induced hyperkalaemia by magnesium sulphate. Can Anaesth Soc J 17:477–484, 1970
202. James MFM, Cork RC, Ennett JE: Succinylcholine pretreatment with magnesium sulfate. Anesth Analg 65:373–376, 1986
203. DeVore JS, Asrami R: Magnesium sulfate prevents succinylcholine induced fasciculations in toxemic patients. Anesthesiology 52:76–77, 1980
204. Ghoneim MM, Long JP: The interaction between magnesium and other neuromuscular blocking agents. Anesthesiology 32:23–27, 1970
205. Glasser SA: Violent fasciculations after small dose succinylcholine infusion as a first sign of atypical pseudocholinesterase. Anesth Analg 63:869–870, 1984
206. Glasser SA: In response: Violent fasciculations may not signal pseudocholinesterase deficiency. Anesth Analg 64:557–558, 1985
207. Melvoll R, Stovner J, Whittaker M: Suxamethonium-induced jaw stiffness and myalgia associated with atypical cholinesterase: case report. Can Anaesth Soc J 27:283–285, 1980
208. Sosis M: Violent fasciculations may not signal pseudocholinesterase deficiency (letter). Anesth Analg 64:557, 1985

18

DAVID G. SILVERMAN | FRANÇOIS DONATI

Undesirable Effects of Succinylcholine

As discussed in Chapter 16, the benefits of succinylcholine (SCh) must be weighed against the potential side effects.[1-4] The potential risks should not and cannot be ignored. In November 1993, the Burroughs Wellcome Company sent a memo to anesthesia practitioners "to alert you to important changes being made to the product label for ANECTINE® brand succinylcholine."[5] Most notable was the statement that "Except when used for emergency tracheal intubation or instances where immediate securing of the airway is necessary, succinylcholine is contraindicated in children and adolescent patients."[5] The letter noted that "there have been several reports of cardiac arrest following administration of succinylcholine to apparently healthy children and adolescent patients who were subsequently found to have undiagnosed myopathies."[5] These effects are discussed below and for specific myopathies in Chapter 23. The letter (and the new package insert) also emphasized the risk of SCh-induced hyperkalemia "following major burns, multiple trauma, extensive denervation of skeletal muscle, or upper motor neuron injury."[5] The systemic effects of SCh are detailed below; their relation to specific injuries and disorders is detailed in Chapters 19, 20, 22, and 23.

◆ CARDIOVASCULAR EFFECTS

SCh exerts *cardiovascular effects* by increasing autonomic activity at preganglionic nicotinic ganglia and at cardiac muscarinic receptors and by increasing circulating catecholamines.[6-20] It has a biphasic action on the isolated mammalian heart, causing bradycardia in low doses and tachycardia in high doses or after longer exposure.[8,9] Selected perfusion of the sinoatrial node with SCh caused an increase in heart rate, but perfusion with succinylmonocholine caused a decrease in heart rate.[19] SCh typically causes increased heart rate and blood pressure in adults[18]; this increase may be associated with ventricular tachyarrhythmias in the presence of sympathomimetic agents or those that block the reuptake of catecholamines. Nevertheless, we are most concerned about a marked *bradycardia* as a consequence of increased muscarinic activity at the *sinus node*.[14,16,18] A prolonged QT interval was commonly noted after thiopental plus SCh in adults as well as children.[17] Bradycardia tends to be more common in anxious adults and even more prominent in *children*,[6,7,12,13] especially those receiving digitalis. Bradycardia has also been reported in the context of anesthetic techniques associated with a large degree of vagal tone (e.g., high-dose opioids). Although bradycardia and asystole have been described after a single dose of SCh,[20] the risk is greatest with *repeated SCh administration*,[10,18,21] even after a small self-taming dose.[22] Choline, a metabolite of SCh, may sensitize the myocardium to subsequent doses,[16] especially after the concentrations of SCh after the initial injection have declined. Other potential causes of severe bradyarrhythmias include hyperkalemia and underlying cardiac conduction abnormalities (as may be seen with many muscle disorders). *Intramuscular injection of SCh* may be less likely to cause bradycardia: 4 mg · kg^{-1} IM (with or without atropine) was not associated with severe bradycardia.[23] However, IM SCh has been implicated in occasional episodes of pulmonary edema and hemorrhage.[24]

SCh-induced *bradycardia may be prevented* by antimuscarinic therapy.[25,26] In adults and children, 0.01–0.02 mg · kg^{-1} of atropine or 0.005–0.01 mg · kg^{-1} of glycopyrrolate typically provides adequate protection.[12,25–28] Infants may require a vagolytic dose (0.03 mg · kg^{-1}) of atropine.[29] SCh-induced arrhythmias may also be alleviated by pretreatment with a small "defasciculating" dose of nondepolarizing relaxant (NDR).[25,26,30–33] Pretreatment with 0.3 mg · kg^{-1} of gallamine, a relaxant with marked vagolytic properties, was more effective than pretreatment with 0.006 mg · kg^{-1} of atropine in preventing a decrease in heart rate after a second dose of SCh.[25] *SCh-induced norepinephrine release also may be decreased* by pretreatment with a defasciculating dose of NDR.[31,32] Tubocurarine was more effective than alcuronium or pancuronium in preventing QT prolongations or ventricular premature contractions.[17]

SCh may elicit histamine release, and it has been implicated in cases of anaphylactoid reactions and anaphylaxis.[34–39] It may exacerbate *bronchospasm* and cause increased airway secretions. Especially if allowed to *precipitate with thiopental* in the same syringe or IV tubing, SCh may elicit acute changes in pulmonary vascular resistance and pulmonary capillary integrity that result in pulmonary edema and hemorrhage.[24,40–42] *Do not inject these agents simultaneously*. One study indicated that apparent type 1 hypersensitivity (allergic) reactions to SCh accounted for 34% of such reactions to neuromuscular blocking agents, even though the drug accounted for only 19% of total relaxant use.[35]

SCh-induced hyperkalemia and its severe cardiovascular consequences have been noted in a multitude of conditions (Chaps. 22 and 23).[43–46] SCh normally results in a 0.5–1.0 mEq · L^{-1} increase in plasma K$^+$ by increasing potassium efflux from cells[47-49]; the increase in children typically is less marked.[50,51] The degree of increase may be related to the degree of postoperative myalgias,[52] but this relationship is uncertain. In normal subjects, the *increase in K^+ may be blunted,* but not necessarily eliminated, with a variety of agents and techniques. We most commonly administer a defasciculating dose of an NDR,[53-56] but this does not always effectively blunt K^+ release.[33,57,58] Other possible forms of pretreatment include aspirin,[56] calcium gluconate,[52] diazepam[59] (but not consistently[53,60]), lidocaine[61] (but not consistently[62]), stretching,[63] magnesium,[64] and a self-taming dose (e.g., 10 mg) of SCh.[65] The SCh-induced increase in K^+ was not reduced by phenytoin[57] or verapamil.[66] Although beta blockers may stabilize membranes and thereby decrease K^+ release,[67,68] $beta_2$ (but not $beta_1$[69]) antagonists may impede $beta_2$-mediated K^+ elimination via the kidney.[70-74]

Severe hyperkalemia causes peaked T waves, loss of P waves, widened QRS, asystole, or ventricular tachycardia. We are particularly concerned about the potential for SCh-induced hyperkalemia in the context of conditions that predispose to the proliferation of highly sensitive extrajunctional receptors or incompetent muscle membranes (Chaps. 22 and 23). In such settings, the precipitous increase in K^+ may be considerable, and it is not reliably prevented by pretreatment with a defasciculating dose of an NDR or any of the other proposed means of prophylaxis.[33,74-78] It may be prevented by pretreatment with a large (e.g., ED_{100}) dose of an NDR; this suggests that the K^+ increase is mediated via an SCh effect at the postsynaptic nicotinic receptors (which are blocked by the high dose of NDR). However, such pretreatment is not useful in practice, since the SCh would not be necessary after paralysis is provided by the NDR. We are also concerned about the increase in K^+ after SCh in the context of preexisting hyperkalemia, as may be noted in the patient with renal failure who has not undergone recent dialysis.[79-80] Otherwise, the patient with renal failure is not at increased risk of developing SCh-induced hyperkalemia.

◆ EFFECT ON INTRACRANIAL PRESSURE

SCh commonly causes an increase in *intracranial blood flow,*[81-88] which may be particularly significant in patients with intracranial masses (and hence limited compliance).[81,84,85] The increase may be attributable to an SCh-induced increase in *motor activity* (including *afferent input from muscle spindle receptors*)[83,89-91]; the increase in *cerebral activity* required to process such information results in increased *cerebral blood flow.* In dogs, SCh caused a 500% increase in motor spindle activity, EEG arousal, a 180% increase in cerebral blood flow (which was only partially attributable to hypercapnia), and a 400% increase in intracranial pressure.[83] The SCh-induced increase in intracranial pressure may be prevented by pretreatment with a paralyzing dose of an NDR[83,85,88]; this tactic also prevents the electrophysiological changes induced by SCh[89,92] and has been shown to oppose SCh-induced activation of muscle spindles.[90] *The SCh-induced increase in intracranial pressure may be blunted,* but not always prevented, by a defasciculating dose of an NDR, by hyperventilation, by thiopental, and by deep general anesthesia.[83,87,88,92-95]

◆ EFFECT ON INTRAOCULAR PRESSURE

SCh also causes an increase in *intraocular pressure* (IOP). The rise in IOP peaks at 7.5–15.0 mmHg above baseline, at 2–3 minutes after injection.

Extraocular muscles (EOM) are designed to maintain steady contraction (Chap. 2). It traditionally has been taught that intense, persistent contractions as well as increases in intravascular pressure are primarily responsible for the SCh-induced rise in IOP.[96-123] However, the increases in IOP may occur despite prior detachment of the EOMs and in the absence of a change in blood pressure.[124] This suggests that the increased IOP may be largely due to increased resistance to outflow from the anterior chamber (due to SCh's cycloplegic effects on the ciliary muscle.)[124]

A marked increase in IOP may be particularly undesirable in the context of open globe injury or in the presence of severe narrow angle glaucoma. The effects of SCh have led to statements in the ophthalmologic literature such as "SCh is unsafe for intubation for the administration of general anesthesia in cases involving penetration or ocular injuries."[122] This position is controversial, for there are potential risks associated with the use of nondepolarizing as well as depolarizing agents (questions g and h), and many patients with penetrating eye injuries incur permanent damage whether or not SCh is used.[125] Reports from major eye centers suggest that SCh may be used safely—that is, without extrusion of eye contents.[126-128] One should assess the risks and benefits in the individual case.

Pretreatments that have been recommended include a defasciculating dose of an NDR[99,111,126,127,129-131] in the hope that the NDRs—which do not themselves cause ocular muscle contraction[98,132,133]—will lessen the impact of a subsequent dose of SCh. When SCh was given without a prior defasciculating dose, it caused an increase in IOP of 8.5 mm Hg in healthy humans and 11.3 mm Hg in cats; after pretreatment with gallamine, 20 mg, or *d*-tubocurarine, 3 mg, the SCh-induced increase was within a range of 1–2 mm Hg in healthy subjects and cats as well as in four subjects with glaucoma.[131] However, it appears that defasciculation alone is not always effective.* Other recommended pretreatments include:

1. diazepam[53,59,103,105,110,113,122] (but this does not prevent the rise in IOP consistently[59,113,122]);

---

*References 99, 101, 106, 109, 112, 113, 115, 122, and 134.

2. lidocaine[107,113] (but this does not always blunt the rise in IOP and systemic arterial pressure,[107,113,114,135] especially in doses below 1.5 mg · kg^{-1} [107]);
3. a self-taming (e.g., 10 mg) dose of SCh[121] (this small dose is designed to lessen the initial impact of a subsequent intubating dose, but it is not always effective[122,136] and may, itself, induce undesirable effects);
4. antihypertensive medications such as propranolol,[100] sublingual nifedipine,[108] and intranasal nitroglycerin[118];
5. pretreatment with acetazolamide (Diamox) in order to reduce the amount of aqueous fluid[137]; and
6. deep anesthesia (without ketamine).

◆ OTHER SYSTEMIC EFFECTS

Succinylcholine's *muscarinic activity* may affect *gastrointestinal, respiratory, and genitourinary* function. By stimulating muscarinic receptors in the GI tract, it causes increased GI secretions and possibly increased motility with intestinal (or bladder) "spasm." Its autonomic effects are comparable on both sides of the esophagogastric junction, and sphincter pressure actually may increase more than intragastric pressure.[138] This may lead one to assume that pretreatment with a defasciculating dose would not reduce the risk of gastroesophageal reflux; however, SCh-induced contractions of abdominal wall muscles (fasciculations) can increase *intragastric pressure* to as high as 40 cm H_2O in adults.[139–141] The abdominal fasciculations may be attenuated by a defasciculating dose of an NDR.[140] In contrast to adults, strong abdominal fasciculations are rarely encountered in small children, as they have weak abdominal musculature and less frequent fasciculations; a 4 cm H_2O increase has been noted.[142]

Although the SCh-induced changes in intragastric pressure may be undesirable, the risk of aspiration is unclear.[130,143] If one elects to pretreat with a defasciculating dose (as we do in many cases), he or she should do so with caution. Defasciculation may cause weakness of the airway musculature and thereby predispose to aspiration prior to induction.[144–147] In addition, it should be noted that avoiding SCh is not necessarily the best solution; coughing during intubation by a patient who is not adequately relaxed produces marked increases in intragastric pressure.[148,149]

A charged molecule, SCh does not cross the *placenta* as readily as more lipid-soluble drugs.[150,151] It can cross the primate placenta to some degree,[152] but is typically metabolized rapidly by the mother and fetus (which typically has low but adequate levels of pseudocholinesterase). It should be remembered that even a small amount of SCh may elicit symptoms in newborns with underlying neuromuscular disorders or in the presence of maternal and fetal deficiencies of normal pseudocholinesterase.[153,154]

◆ PERIOPERATIVE MUSCLE CHANGES

SCh-induced muscle changes, which may extend into the postoperative period, include myalgias, elevated serum creatine kinase (CK) levels, and myoglobinemia; they are discussed below. *Masseter rigidity* and *malignant hyperthermia* are among the most devastating effects of SCh; they are discussed in Chapters 19 and 20. *Rhabdomyolysis* is a potential consequence of SCh administration, especially in the presence of the myopathies discussed in Chapter 23.

SCh-induced myalgias occur in 20–75% of patients. The wide variability in reported incidence may be attributable to differences in premedication, age, sex, surgical procedure, anesthetic, time of ambulation, and the nature of assessment. Symptoms range from diffuse soreness to severe pain. They generally begin 12–24 hours postoperatively and last 24–48 hours, but can persist for several days. They commonly occur in young adults who undergo early ambulation. SCh-induced pain probably is due to *asynchronous depolarization* and contraction of muscle fibers,[48,155] with subsequent shearing among neighboring fibers.[155,156] The interfiber asynchrony that results from binding of SCh to pre- and postsynaptic sites within the NMJ is in contrast to the synchronous contraction of muscle fibers after normal neural discharge. Other potential causes of SCh-induced myalgias include residual changes in the muscle spindles and sarcolemma,[157] muscle electrolyte imbalance,[158] lactate production,[159] and pain secondary to positioning.

The likelihood of post-SCh *myalgias* may be increased following SCh-induced *fasciculations*. However, there are conflicting reports as to whether there is[63,160,161] or is not[33,58,162–166] a significant correlation between fasciculations and postoperative pain. Myalgias may be noted postoperatively in the absence of SCh, especially following abdominal insufflation for laparoscopy (but often to a lesser degree than that associated with SCh).[167–173] In one study of patients undergoing laparoscopy with SCh, vecuronium, or atracurium, 92%, 77%, and 89% of patients respectively reported myalgias.[171] The incidence of myalgias was not influenced by whether propofol or thiopental was used for induction.[174] In another study in awake volunteers, myalgias were noted after paralysis with vecuronium in the absence of surgery.[175]

The *incidence and severity of post-SCh myalgias* may be reduced by a "defasciculating dose" of an NDR (approximately 10% of the nondepolarizing agent's ED_{95}, typically given more than 3 minutes before the intubating dose of SCh) or other forms of pretreatment (Table 18-1). A recent report based on a meta-analysis of 45 published investigations noted that atracurium, *d*-tubocurarine, gallamine, pancuronium, diazepam, and lidocaine all significantly decreased the frequency of myalgias by about 30%; a self-taming dose of SCh was not found to be efficacious.[176] In some studies,

TABLE 18-1
Successful ("Yes") and Unsuccessful/Unreliable ("No") Means of Pretreatment Prior to Succinylcholine

	Fasciculations (References)		Post-SCh Myalgias (References)		Creatine Kinase, Myoglobin (References)	
	Yes	No	Yes	No	Yes	No
Tubocurarine (priming dose)	31, 32, 53, 54, 57, 105, 170, 178, 180, 184–187, 201–209	210, 211	160, 180, 194, 201, 203, 207, 211–215	57, 178, 208	54, 184–187, 194, 197, 199, 216	33, 57
Gallamine (prime)	58, 182, 202, 217	210, 211	58, 156, 211, 212		192	
Pancuronium (prime)	31, 177, 181, 205, 211, 217, 218	58, 202, 210	58, 211, 212, 218	177		
Alcuronium (prime)	32, 180, 181, 205, 219		180, 193		192, 193	
Vecuronium (prime)	31, 170, 180, 181	210	180			
Atracurium (prime)	178, 180, 209, 220		56, 172, 178, 208, 220	180, 221	56	
SCh (small self-taming dose)	185, 186, 218, 222, 223	58	164, 218	58, 162	187, 195	
Fentanyl/alfentanil	205, 233					
Benzodiazepines	59, 165, 188	53, 60, 105, 166, 170, 201, 206	59, 165, 188, 234	166, 193, 201, 207	59	166, 188, 193, 224
Phenytoin	57, 204			57		57
Barbiturates	225			225		
Lidocaine	209		61, 207, 226	193	224	193
Dantrolene	184, 227	228	227, 229		184, 228	
MgSO$_4$	230, 231	64		232		
Calcium			52	194		194
Chlorpromazine			194		194	
Salicylates (aspirin)			56, 215	194	56	
Vitamin E			194			194
Preop. stretching			63			

Note: The references have been categorized as to whether they indicate that the regimen prescribed constituted a "successful" (highly reliable) or "unsuccessful" (ineffective, relatively unreliable) means of preventing or blunting a given response.

pretreatment with one NDR decreased myalgias while pretreatment with another decreased fasciculations[58,177,178]; this may imply different causes (e.g., presynaptic vs. postsynaptic). Others have concluded that a large number of NDRs have similar effectiveness and hence are interchangeable.[179] In light of suggestions that SCh-induced fasciculations are due to binding of the drug to presynaptic receptor sites (Chap. 16), defasciculation with a nondepolarizing agent that has a strong prejunctional effect theoretically is preferable.[140,180-183]

In *children* over 12 months of age, SCh often causes an increase in *serum CK and/or myoglobin levels*,[184-199] especially in the presence of halothane. This increase may be more pronounced after masseter rigidity. It appears to be less pronounced in young infants than older children[186]; interestingly, infants less than 12 months old tend to respond to SCh with gross muscle movements rather than fine fasciculations (which may lead to shearing).[186,200] Others have noted no correlation between serum myoglobin levels and the incidence of fasciculations.[185,196] The increase in CK levels is most prominent within the first 6 hours of SCh administration.[195] Myoglobinuria is relatively rare in adults, especially in the absence of halothane; however, otherwise normal patients may occasionally experience a marked increase in myoglobin levels after SCh and a minor surgical procedure.[192,193,201] It appears that some people may be "reactors."[166] In normal subjects, the *release of CK or myoglobin may be reduced*, but not necessarily eliminated, by a defasciculating dose of an NDR, sedatives, local anesthetics, and dantrolene.

Severe *rhabdomyolysis* and hyperkalemia may occur in the context of malignant hyperthermia, other myopathies (even an occult myopathy), massive tissue injury, and a myriad of neurological disorders (see Chaps. 19, 20, 22, 23). In addition to severe electrolyte abnormalities, this may lead to acute rhabdomyolytic renal failure.

The means that have been recommended to reduce the incidence or severity of SCh-induced *fasciculations, myalgias, and release of CK and myoglobin* are listed in Table 18-1.

Discussion Questions ◆

a. Why and when should one be concerned about potential *hyperkalemia* from SCh in the patient with *renal failure?*
b. Why might one theoretically be more concerned about *SCh-induced hyperkalemia* in patients receiving *beta-blocking agents?*
c. How reliably is the SCh-induced increase in *intracranial pressure* blunted by a *defasciculating dose* of an NDR?
d. Why or why not might an NDR be a better choice than SCh for rapid *tracheal intubation* in the patient with *increased intracranial pressure?*
e. What is the time course of the change in *IOP* following a bolus dose of SCh?

f. How might the effect of SCh on *IOP* be blunted? Do any of these techniques provide guaranteed safety?
g. Might a *nondepolarizing agent* be a better choice in the patient with increased *IOP*? Why or why not?
h. In what underlying conditions is the likelihood of SCh-induced *gastric reflux* increased?
i. What are the potential *problems associated with defasciculation* prior to rapid-sequence induction?
j. List the means that have been recommended to reduce the incidence or severity of SCh-induced *fasciculations, myalgias, and release of CK and myoglobin*.

Answers ◆

a. SCh should be avoided if the patient with *renal failure* already has marked hyperkalemia, as the "normal" K^+ release (e.g., 0.5–1.0 mEq · L^{-1}) associated with SCh may not be tolerated.[79,80] Otherwise, if the preoperative K^+ is normal, SCh may be a suitable choice,[130] since renal failure per se does not predispose to increased K^+ release.

b. It appears that *beta$_2$ receptors modulate serum K^+ levels*.[70] Administration of salbutamol, a beta$_2$ agonist, reduced the rise in K^+ after SCh,[71] probably by promoting K^+ elimination and/or reuptake into cells. Alternatively, beta$_2$ blockers may increase K^+ levels after SCh.[68,72,73] Pretreatment with 0.25 mg · kg^{-1} of propranolol resulted in increased levels of K^+ after SCh for many minutes,[73] while no effect was noted with the selective beta$_1$ antagonist esmolol.[69] Thus, esmolol is "safe" at induction (Chap. 17). Beta blockers may actually decrease K^+ release (and reduce fasciculations) by membrane stabilization in man.[67,68] In contrast to beta$_2$ blockers, the Ca^{2+} channel blocker verapamil does not increase serum K^+ after SCh[66]; however, the latter may exaggerate the clinical effects of otherwise high levels of K^+.

c. There is evidence to suggest that the SCh-induced *increase in intracranial pressure* may be blunted by a *defasciculating dose* of an NDR, but the benefits are uncertain. A defasciculating dose of metocurine was reported to be effective in humans.[88] However, a defasciculating dose of pancuronium or tubocurarine has not prevented an increase in intracranial pressure. Even though a typical defasciculating dose of pancuronium virtually abolished visible SCh-induced fasciculations in dogs, it did not eliminate the SCh-induced increase in *muscle afferent activity,* the EEG "arousal," or the increase in cerebral blood flow.[93]

d. *Nondepolarizing agents* are not associated with an increase in *intracranial pressure* and may actually decrease cerebral activity (Chap. 11). Alternatively, they may not be as effective as SCh for managing the patient with a difficult airway or full stomach. Struggling or coughing during

intubation (due to inadequate block) may cause more severe changes in intracranial pressure than those associated with SCh.
e. The SCh-induced increase in *IOP* typically is detected soon after the onset of fasciculations and lasts for the duration of SCh-induced block. It is noted after 1 minute, peaks in 2–3 minutes, and typically *persists for 5–7 minutes* in adults as well as children.[102,119] In cats, the increase in tension persisted for 10–20 minutes at the eye, vs. 1 minute at the tibialis muscle.[120]
f. No means of *pretreatment* is consistently effective for preventing the increases in IOP associated with SCh. Means that blunt fasciculations may *blunt the increase in IOP*. There are reports that a defasciculating dose of gallamine or tubocurarine is helpful, but there is no guarantee that *defasciculation* with an NDR will be effective. The use of IV lidocaine, acetazolamide (Diamox), deep anesthesia (with sedatives, neuroleptics, narcotics, and inhalational anesthetics), and avoidance of hypercarbia and venous compression are also recommended, but likewise are not always successful. It has recently been shown that nifedipine, 10 mg sublingually, or nitroglycerin, 2 mg/3 mL intranasally, or IV beta-blocking agents may be helpful; their effectiveness may be attributable to the correlation between hemodynamic and IOP changes after intubation.

Although we lack a practical means to guarantee stable IOP, the experiences at major eye centers indicate that SCh can be used successfully (commonly after a defasciculating dose) in a large number of open eye surgeries, without reports of loss of global contents. In a 10-year experience with penetrating eye injuries, the team at Wills Eye Hospital in Philadelphia noted no expulsion of global contents; they feel that SCh may be employed safely.[126,127]
g. There is uncertainty as to which is the *best relaxant regimen* for avoidance of increased *IOP*. Many feel that, if *a nondepolarizing agent* can be used effectively for intubation, then it is preferable.[98,99,109,115,122] NDRs do not increase IOP.[98,132,133] However, it is difficult to ensure deep block with nondepolarizing agents during a rapid-sequence induction. Unless the patient is deeply anesthetized, tracheal intubation may precipitate coughing and bucking, with increased IOP[97,117,128,132] and increased *intragastric* pressures[142,149] (which may translate into increased venous pressure). Obviously, one must take into account the patient's cardiovascular status and airway morphology as well as the risk for pulmonary aspiration of gastric contents. It is particularly important to assess the airway for potential difficulty during induction and intubation before administering a high dose of an NDR. Furthermore, since only a small percentage of patients with penetrating eye injuries recover useful sight in the injured eye,[125] the risks, benefits, and priorities for a given case should be assessed according to the given injury and the individual patient's preanesthetic status.
h. The *risk of regurgitation* that is associated with SCh is unclear.[130,143] Normally an *intragastric pressure* above 30 cm H$_2$O is required to over-

come the esophagogastric junction. However, a lesser pressure may induce reflux if the esophagogastric junction is distorted (e.g., by hiatal hernia or displacement of the stomach during pregnancy).[140] Reflux may also be more likely in the context of compromised gastric emptying; a dilated stomach would be more prone to a pressure increase as a result of abdominal muscle fasciculations. Overall, since fasciculations may play a critical role in the SCh-induced increase in gastric pressure,[140,149] defasciculation may be helpful.

i. *Defasciculation* may lead to muscular weakness and passive regurgitation and pulmonary aspiration of gastric contents, since cricoid pressure typically is not applied until induction of general anesthesia.[144–146] A defasciculating dose prior to SCh[147] or a priming dose prior to a larger dose of an NDR (Chap. 7) can decrease pulmonary function in a dose-related manner. It may also lead to patient anxiety. In addition, it may increase the SCh requirement or delay the onset of SCh-induced paralysis (Chap. 16).

j. The following have been suggested to *prevent fasciculations, myalgias, and/or increases in CK or myoglobin levels*. They typically exhibit inconsistent efficacy (Table 18-1):

   1. A defasciculating dose of NDR given 3–5 minutes before SCh, especially an NDR with a relatively large degree of presynaptic activity (e.g., gallamine or *d*-tubocurarine). Although not always effective, this approach generally is considered to be the most reliable.
   2. Administration of a "self-taming" (e.g., 10 mg) dose of SCh. In susceptible patients, this may cause weakness on its own.
   3. Barbiturates, benzodiazepines, opioids, diphenylhydantoin, chlorpromazine, local anesthetics, and other stabilizing agents.
   4. Dantrolene.
   5. Magnesium.
   6. Calcium.
   7. Miscellaneous drugs, including aspirin and vitamin E.
   8. Preoperative exercises, stretching.

References ◆

1. Cook DR: Succinylcholine: an argument to abandon its elective use in pediatric anesthesia. Anesthesiol Rep 1:84–88, 1988
2. Delphin E, Jackson D, Rothstein P: Use of succinylcholine during elective pediatric anesthesia should be reevaluated. Anesth Analg 66:1190–1192, 1987
3. Lee C: Succinylcholine: its past, present and future. Semin Anesth 3:293–302, 1984
4. Durant NN, Katz RL: Suxamethonium. Br J Anaesth 54:195–208, 1982
5. Kent RS: Dear Anesthesia Practitioner (letter). Burroughs Wellcome Co., November 1993
6. Craythorne NWB, Turndorf H, Dripps RD: Changes in pulse rate and rhythm associated with the use of succinylcholine in anesthetized children. Anesthesiology 18:698–702, 1957

7. Digby-Leigh M, McLoyd D, Belton MK, et al: Bradycardia following intravenous administration of succinylcholine in anesthetized children. Anesthesiology 58:519–523, 1957
8. Galindo AH, Davis TB: Succinylcholine and cardiac excitability. Anesthesiology 23:32–40, 1962
9. Goat VA, Feldman SA: The dual action of suxamethonium on the isolated rabbit heart. Anaesthesia 27:149, 1972
10. Lupprian KG, Churchill-Davidson HC: Effect of suxamethonium on cardiac rhythm. Br Med J 2:1774, 1960
11. Leiman BC, Katz J, Butler BD: Mechanisms of succinylcholine-induced arrhythmias in hypoxic or hypoxic:hypercarbic dogs. Anesth Analg 66:1292–1297, 1987
12. Lerman J, Chinyanga HM: The heart rate response to succinylcholine in children: a comparison of atropine and glycopyrrolate. Can Anaesth Soc J 30:377–381, 1983
13. Leigh MD, McCoy DD, Belton K, et al: Bradycardia following intravenous administration of succinylcholine chloride in infants and children. Anesthesiology 18:698–702, 1957
14. Nigrovic V: Succinylcholine, cholinoceptors and catecholamines: proposed mechanism of early adverse haemodynamic reactions. Can Anaesth Soc J 31:382–394, 1984
15. Ohmura A, Wong KC, Shaw L: Cardiac effects of succinyldicholine and succinylmonocholine. Can Anaesth Soc J 23:567–573, 1976
16. Schoenstadt DA, Witcher CE: Observations on the mechanism of succinyldicholine-induced cardiac arrhythmias. Anesthesiology 24:358–362, 1963
17. Saarnivaara L, Lindgren L: Prolongation of QT interval during induction of anaesthesia. Acta Anaesthesiol Scand 27:126–130, 1983
18. Williams CH, Deutsch S, Linde HW, Bullough JW, Dripps RD: Effects of intravenously administered succinyldicholine on cardiac rate, rhythm, and arterial blood pressure in anesthetized man. Anesthesiology 22:947–954, 1961
19. Yasuda I, Hirano T, Amaha K, Fudeta H, Obara S: Chronotropic effects of succinylcholine and succinylmonocholine on the sinoatrial node. Anesthesiology 57:289–292, 1982
20. Sorenson M, Engbaek J, Viby-Mogenson J, Guldager H, Molke Jensen F: Bradycardia and cardiac asystole following a single injection of suxamethonium. Acta Anaesthesiol Scand 28:232, 1984
21. Graf K, Ström G, Wahlin A: Circulatory effects of succinylcholine in man. Acta Anaesthesiol Scand Suppl 14:1, 1963
22. Magee DA, Sweet PT, Holland AJ: Cardiac effects of self-taming of succinylcholine and repeated succinylcholine administration. Can Anaesth Soc J 29:577–580, 1982
23. Hannallah RS, Oh TH, McGill WA, Epstein BS: Changes in heart rate and rhythm after intramuscular succinylcholine with or without atropine in anesthetized children. Anesth Analg 65:1329–1332, 1986
24. Cook DR, Westman H, Rosenfeld L, et al: Pulmonary edema in infants: possible association with intramuscular succinylcholine. Anesth Analg 60:220–223, 1981
25. Stoelting RK: Comparison of gallamine and atropine as pretreatment before anesthetic induction and succinylcholine administration. Anesth Analg 56:493–495, 1977
26. Viby-Mogensen J, Wisberg K, Sorensen O: Cardiac effects of atropine and gallamine in patients receiving suxamethonium. Br J Anaesth 52:1137–1142, 1980
27. Green DW, Bristow AB, Fischer M: Glycopyrrolate and atropine in the prevention of bradycardia and dysrhythmias following repeated doses of suxamethonium in children. Br J Anaesth 55:1163P, 1983
28. Sorensen O, Eriksen S, Hommelgaard P, Viby-Mogensen J: Thiopental-nitrous oxide-halothane anesthesia and repeated succinylcholine: comparison of preoperative glycopyrrolate and atropine administration. Anesth Analg 59:686, 1980
29. Cook DR, Fischer CG: Neuromuscular blocking effects of succinylcholine in infants and children. Anesthesiology 42:662–665, 1975
30. Magee DA, Sweet PT, Holland AJ: Effect of atropine on bradydysrhythmias induced by succinylcholine following pretreatment with d-tubocurarine. Can Anaesth Soc J 29:573–576, 1982
31. Oshita S, Denda S, Fujiwara Y, Takeshita H, Kosaka F: Pretreatment with d-tubocurarine, vecuronium, and pancuronium attenuates succinylcholine-induced increases in plasma norepinephrine concentrations in humans. Anesth Analg 72:84–88, 1991

32. Kautto UM: Effects of precurarization on the blood pressure and heart rate changes induced by suxamethonium facilitated laryngoscopy and intubation. Acta Anaesthesiol Scand 25:391–396, 1981
33. Stoelting RK, Peterson C: Adverse effects of increased succinylcholine dose following d-tubocurarine pretreatment. Anesth Analg 54:282–288, 1975
34. Assem ES, Frost PG, Levis RD: Anaphylactic-like reaction to suxamethonium. Anaesthesia 36:405–410, 1981
35. Fisher MM, Munro I: Life-threatening anaphylactoid reactions to muscle relaxants. Anesth Analg 62:559–564, 1983
36. Harle DG, Baldo BA, Fisher MM: Detection of IgE antibodies to suxamethonium after anaphylactoid reactions during anaesthesia. Lancet 1:930–932, 1984
37. Royston D, Wilkes RG: True anaphylaxis to suxamethonium chloride. Br J Anaesth 50:611, 1978
38. Vervloet D, Nizankowska E, Arnaud A, Senft M, Alazia M, Charpin J: Adverse reactions to suxamethonium and other muscle relaxants under general anaesthesia. J Allergy Clin Immunol 71:552, 1983
39. Youngman PR, Taylor KM, Wilson JD: Anaphylactoid reactions to neuromuscular blocking agents: a commonly undiagnosed condition? Lancet 2:597, 1983
40. Moneret-Vautrin DA, Widmer S, Gueant JL, Kamel L, Laxenaire MC, Mouton C, Gerard H: Simultaneous anaphylaxis to thiopentone and a neuromuscular blocker: a study of two cases. Br J Anaesth 64:743–745, 1990
41. Watkins J, Clarke RSJ: Report of a symposium: adverse responses to intravenous agents. Br J Anaesth 50:1159, 1978
42. Wright PJ, Shortland JR, Stevens JD, Parsons MA, Watkins J: Fatal haemopathological consequences of general anaesthesia. Br J Anaesth 62:104–107, 1990
43. Birch AA Jr, Mitchell GD, Playford GA, Lang CA: Changes in serum potassium response to succinylcholine following trauma. JAMA 210:490–493, 1969
44. Fung DL, White DA, Jones BJ, Gronert GA: The onset of disuse-related potassium efflux to succinylcholine. Anesthesiology 75:650–653, 1991
45. Gronert GA, Theye RA: Pathophysiology of hyperkalemia induced by succinylcholine. Anesthesiology 43:89–99, 1975
46. Yentis SM: Suxamethonium and hyperkalaemia. Anaesth Intensive Care 18:91–101, 1990
47. Klupp H, Kraupp O: The liberation of potassium from muscles under the influence of muscle relaxants. Arch Int Pharmacodyn Ther 98:340–354, 1954
48. Paton WDM: The effects of muscle relaxants other than muscle relaxation. Anesthesiology 20:453, 1959
49. Weintraub HD, Heisterkamp DV, Cooperman LH: Changes in plasma potassium concentration after depolarizing blockers in anaesthetized man. Br J Anaesth 41:1048–1052, 1969
50. Dierdorf SF, McNiece WL, Rao CC, Wolfe TM, Means LJ: Failure of succinylcholine to alter plasma potassium in children with myelomeningocoele. Anesthesiology 64:272–273, 1986
51. Henning RD, Bush GH: Plasma potassium after halothane-suxamethonium induction in children. Anaesthesia 37:802–805, 1982
52. Shrivastava OP, Chatterji S, Kachhawa S, Daga SR: Calcium gluconate pretreatment for prevention of succinylcholine-induced myalgia. Anesth Analg 62:59–62, 1983
53. Erkola O, Salmenpera M, Tammisto T: Does diazepam pretreatment prevent succinylcholine-induced fasciculations? A double-blind comparison of diazepam and tubocurarine pretreatments. Anesth Analg 59:932–934, 1980
54. Evers W, Racz GB, Levy AA: Changes in plasma potassium and calcium levels and in the electrocardiogram after a single dose of succinylcholine preceded by d-tubocurarine. Can Anaesth Soc J 23:383–394, 1976
55. Konchigeri HN, Tay CH: Influence of pancuronium on potassium efflux produced by succinylcholine. Anesth Analg 55:474–477, 1976
56. Naguib M, Farag H, Magbagbeola JA: Effect of pretreatment with lysine acetyl salicylate on suxamethonium-induced myalgia. Br J Anaesth 59:606–610, 1987
57. Kuo WS, Ho ST, Hu OY, Li CH, Hwing CS: The study of pretreatment with diphenylhydantoin or d-tubocurarine on succinylcholine-induced adverse effects. Ma Tsui Hsueh Tsa Chi 23:323–328, 1990

58. O'Sullivan EP, Williams NE, Calvey TN: Differential aspects of neuromuscular blocking agents on suxamethonium-induced fasciculations and myalgia. Br J Anaesth 60:367–371, 1988
59. Fahmy NR, Malek NS, Lappas DG: Diazepam prevents some adverse effects of succinylcholine. Clin Pharmacol Ther 26:395–398, 1979
60. Raffe MR, Crimi AJ, Ruff J: Effect of diazepam pretreatment on succinylcholine-induced muscle fasciculation in the dog. Am J Vet Res 43:510–512, 1982
61. Chatterji S, Thind SS, Daga SR: Lignocaine pretreatment for suxamethonium: a clinicobiochemical study. Anaesthesia 38:867–870, 1983
62. Naguib M, Farag H, Magbagbeola JA: Failure of lidocaine to modify suxamethonium-induced biochemical changes. Middle East J Anaesthesiol 9:375–382, 1988
63. Magee DA, Robinson RJ: Effect of stretch exercises on suxamethonium induced fasciculations and myalgia. Br J Anaesth 59:596–601, 1987
64. James MF, Cork RC, Dennett JE: Succinylcholine pretreatment with magnesium sulfate. Anesth Analg 65:373–376, 1986
65. Magee DA, Gallagher EG: "Self-taming" of suxamethonium and serum potassium concentration. Br J Anaesth 56:977–980, 1984
66. Roth JL, Nugent M, Gronert GA: Verapamil does not alter succinylcholine-induced increases in serum potassium during halothane anesthesia in normal dogs. Anesth Analg 64:1202–1204, 1985
67. Maryniak JK, Henderson AM, Woodall NM, Lim M, Simpson JC: Beta-adrenoreceptor blockade and suxamethonium-induced rise in plasma potassium. Anaesthesia 42:71–74, 1987
68. Usubiaga JE: Neuromuscular effects of beta-adrenergic blockers and their interaction with skeletal muscle relaxants. Anesthesiology 29:484–492, 1968
69. Halevy JD, Ornstein E, Matteo RS: Esmolol is not associated with an exaggerated succinylcholine mediated hyperkalemic response. Anesthesiology 69:A424, 1988
70. Brown MJ, Brown DC, Murphy MB: Hypokalemia from $beta_2$-receptor stimulation by circulating epinephrine. N Engl J Med 309:1414–1419, 1983
71. Inaba H, Ohwada T, Sato J, Mizuguchi T, Hirasawa H: Effects of salbutamol and hyperventilation on the rise in serum potassium after succinylcholine administration. Acta Anaesthesiol Scand 31:524–528, 1987
72. Goldhill DR, Martyn JAJ, Kim EM, Hoaglin DC: Effect in dogs of selective beta-blockade on potassium release after succinylcholine. Anesth Analg 65:S60, 1986
73. McCammon RL, Stoelting RK: Exaggerated increase in serum potassium following succinylcholine in dogs with beta blockade. Anesthesiology 61:723–725, 1984
74. Iwasaki H, Namika A, Omote K, et al: Response differences of paretic and healthy extremities to pancuronium and neostigmine in hemiplegic patients. Anesth Analg 64:864–866, 1985
75. Koller ME, Breivik H, Greider P, Jones DJ, Smith RB: Synergistic effect of acidosis and succinylcholine-induced hyperkalemia in spinal cord transected rats. Acta Anaesthesiol Scand 28:87–90, 1984
76. Moorthy SS, Hilgenberg JC: Resistance to nondepolarizing muscle relaxants in paretic upper extremities of patients with residual hemiplegia. Anesth Analg 59:624–627, 1980
77. Smith RB, Grenvik A: Cardiac arrest following succinylcholine in patients with central nervous system injuries. Anesthesiology 33:558–560, 1970
78. Smith RB: Hyperkalaemia following succinylcholine administration in neurological disorders: a review. Can Anaesth Soc J 18:199–201, 1971
79. Koide M, Waud BE: Serum potassium concentrations after succinylcholine in patients with renal failure. Anesthesiology 36:142–145, 1972
80. Miller RD, Way WL, Hamilton WK, et al: Succinylcholine-induced hyperkalemia in patients with renal failure? Anesthesiology 36:138–141, 1972
81. Bormann BE, Smith RB, Bunegin L, et al: Does succinylcholine raise intracranial pressure? Anesthesiology 53:S262, 1980
82. Cottrell JE, Hartung J, Giffin JP, et al: Intracranial and hemodynamic changes after succinylcholine administration in cats. Anesth Analg 62:1006–1009, 1983
83. Lanier WL, Milde JH, Michenfelder JD: Cerebral stimulation following succinylcholine in dogs. Anesthesiology 64:551–559, 1986

84. Marsh ML, Dunlop BJ, Shapiro HM, Gagnon RL, Rockoff MA: Succinylcholine-intracranial pressure effects in neurosurgical patients. Anesth Analg 59:A550, 1980
85. Minton MD, Grosslight K, Stirt JA, Bedford RF: Increases in intracranial pressure from succinylcholine: prevention by prior nondepolarizing blockade. Anesthesiology 65:165–169, 1986
86. Stullken EH Jr, Sokoll MD: Anesthesia and subarachnoid intracranial pressure. Anesth Analg 54:494–498, 1975
87. Shapiro HM, Wyte S, Harris A, Galindo A: Acute intraoperative intracranial hypertension in neurosurgical patients: mechanical and pharmacological factors. Anesthesiology 57:242–244, 1982
88. Stirt JA, Grosslight KR, Bedford RF, Vollmer D: "Defasciculation" with metocurine prevents succinylcholine-induced increases in intracranial pressure. Anesthesiology 67:50–53, 1987
89. Brinling JC, Smith CE: A characterization of the stimulation of mammalian muscle spindles by succinylcholine. J Pharmacol Exp Ther 129:56–60, 1960
90. Granit R, Skoglund S, Thesleff S: Activation of muscle spindles by succinylcholine and decamethonium: the effects of curare. Acta Physiol Scand 28:134–151, 1953
91. Motokizawa F, Fujimori B: Arousal effect of afferent discharges from muscle spindles upon electroencephalograms in cats. Jpn J Physiol 14:344–353, 1964
92. Mori K, Iwabuchi K, Fujita M: The effects of depolarizing muscle relaxants on the electroencephalogram and the circulation during halothane anesthesia in man. Br J Anaesth 45:605–610, 1973
93. Lanier WL, Iaizzo PA, Milde JH: Cerebral function and muscle afferent activity following intravenous succinylcholine in dogs anesthetized with halothane: the effects of pretreatment with a defasciculating dose of pancuronium. Anesthesiology 71:87–95, 1989
94. Thiagarajah S, Sophie S, Lear E, Azar I, Frost EA: Effect of suxamethonium on the ICP of cats with and without thiopentone pretreatment. Br J Anaesth 60:157–160, 1988
95. McLeskey CH, Cullen BF, Kennedy RD, Galindo A: Control of cerebral infusion pressure during induction of anesthesia in high-risk neurosurgical patients. Anesth Analg 53:985–992, 1974
96. Eakins KE, Katz RL: The action of succinylcholine on the tension of extraocular muscle. Br J Pharmacol 26:205, 1966
97. Wynands JE, Crowell DE: Intraocular tension in association with succinylcholine and endotracheal intubation: a preliminary report. Can Anaesth Soc J 7:39–43, 1960
98. Badrinath SK, Vazeery A, McCarthy RJ, Ivankovich AD: The effect of different methods of inducing anesthesia on intraocular pressure. Anesthesiology 65:431–435, 1986
99. Cunningham AJ, Barry P: Intraocular pressure—physiology and implications for anaesthetic management. Can Anaesth Soc J 33:195–208, 1986
100. Cook JH, Feneck RO, Smith MB: Effect of pretreatment with propranolol on intra-ocular pressure changes during induction of anaesthesia. Eur J Anaesthesiol 3:449–457, 1986
101. Cook JH: The effect of suxamethonium on intraocular pressure. Anaesthesia 36:359–365, 1981
102. Craythorne NWB, Rottenstein HS, Dripps RD: The effect of succinylcholine on intraocular pressure in adults, infants, and children during general anesthesia. Anesthesiology 21:59–66, 1960
103. Cunningham AJ, Albert O, Cameron J, Watson AG: The effect of intravenous diazepam on rise of intraocular pressure following succinylcholine. Can Anaesth Soc J 28:591–596, 1981
104. Dillon JB, Sabawala P, Taylor DB, et al: Depolarizing neuromuscular blocking agents and intraocular pressure *in vivo*. Anesthesiology 18:439–442, 1957
105. Fjeldborg P, Hecht PS, Busted N, Nissen AB: The effect of diazepam pretreatment on the succinylcholine-induced rise in intraocular pressure. Acta Anaesthesiol Scand 29:415–417, 1985
106. Feneck RO, Cook JH: Failure of diazepam to prevent the suxamethonium-induced rise in intraocular pressure. Anaesthesia 38:120–127, 1983

107. Grover VK, Lata K, Sharma S, Kaushik S, Gupta A: Efficacy of lignocaine in the suppression of the intraocular pressure response to suxamethonium and tracheal intubation. Anaesthesia 44:22–25, 1989
108. Indu B, Batra YK, Puri GD, Singh H: Nifedipine attenuates the intraocular pressure response to intubation following succinylcholine. Can J Anaesth 36:269–272, 1989
109. Jantzen JPAH: Hackett GH, Earnshaw G: Succinylcholine and open eye injury (letter). Anesthesiology 64:524–525, 1986
110. Kruger AE, Roelofse JA: Precautions against intraocular pressure changes during endotracheal intubation—a comparison of pretreatment with intravenous lignocaine and diazepam. S Afr Med J 63:887–888, 1983
111. Konchigeri HN, Lee YE, Venugopal K: Effect of pancuronium on intraocular pressure changes induced by succinylcholine. Can Anaesth Soc J 26:479–481, 1979
112. Lavery GG, McGalliard JN, Mirakhur RK, Shepherd WF: The effects of atracurium on intraocular pressure during steady state anaesthesia and rapid sequence induction: a comparison with succinylcholine. Can Anaesth Soc J 33:437–442, 1986
113. Mahajan RP, Grover VK, Munjal VP, Singh H: Double-blind comparison of lidocaine, tubocurarine and diazepam pretreatment in modifying intraocular pressure increases. Can J Anaesth 34:41–45, 1987
114. Murphy DF, Eustace P, Unwin A, Magner JB: Intravenous lignocaine pretreatment to prevent intraocular pressure rise following suxamethonium and tracheal intubation. Br J Ophthalmol 70:596–598, 1986
115. Meyers EF, Krupin T, Johnson M, et al: Failure of nondepolarizing neuromuscular blockers inhibit succinylcholine-induced intraocular pressure: a controlled study. Anesthesiology 48:149–151, 1978
116. Murphy DF: Anesthesia and intraocular pressure. Anesth Analg 64:520–530, 1985
117. McDiarmid IR, Halloway KB: Factors affecting intraocular pressure. Proc R Soc Med 69:601–602, 1976
118. Mahajan RP, Grover VK, Sharma SL, Singh H: Intranasal nitroglycerin and intraocular pressure during general anesthesia. Anesth Analg 67:631–636, 1988
119. Pandey K, Gadola RP, Dumar S: Time course of intraocular hypertension produced by suxamethonium. Br J Anaesth 44:191–196, 1972
120. Pryn SJ, Van Der Spek AFL: Comparative pharmacology of succinylcholine on jaw, eye and tibialis muscle. Anesthesiology 73:A859, 1990
121. Verma RS: "Self-taming" of succinylcholine-induced fasciculations and intraocular pressures. Anesthesiology 50:245–247, 1979
122. Varghese C, Chopra SK, Daniel R, Kaur B: Intraocular pressure profile during general anesthesia. Ophthalmic Surg 21:856–859, 1990
123. Warner LO, Bremer DL, Davidson PJ, Rogers GL, Beach TP: Effects of lidocaine, succinylcholine, and tracheal intubation on intraocular pressure in children anesthetized with halothane–nitrous oxide. Anesth Analg 69:687–690, 1989
124. Kelly RE, Dinner M, Turner LS, Barrett H, Abramson DH, Daines P: Succinylcholine increases intraocular pressure in the human eye with extraocular muscles detached. Anesthesiology 79:948–952, 1993
125. Bourke DL: Open eye injuries (letter). Anesthesiology 63:727, 1985
126. Libonati MM, Leahy JJ, Ellison N: The use of succinylcholine in open eye surgery. Anesthesiology 62:637–640, 1985
127. Libonati MM, Leahy JJ, Ellison N: Succinylcholine and open eye injury (letter). Anesthesiology 64:525, 1986
128. Donlon JV Jr: Succinylcholine and open eye injury: II. (letter). Anesthesiology 64:525–526, 1986
129. Katz RL, Eakins KE: The action of neuromuscular blocking agents on extraocular muscle and intraocular pressure. Proc R Soc Med 61:1217–1220, 1969
130. Miller RD, Savarese JJ: Pharmacology of muscle relaxants and their antagonists. In Miller RD (ed): Anesthesia, 3rd ed. New York, Churchill Livingstone, 1990, pp 389–435
131. Miller RD, Way WL, Hickey RF: Inhibition of succinylcholine-induced increased intraocular pressure by nondepolarizing muscle relaxants. Anesthesiology 29:123, 1968

132. Schneider MJ, Stirt JA, Finholt DA: Atracurium, vecuronium and intraocular pressure in humans. Anesth Analg 65:877–882, 1986
133. Maharaj RJ, Humphrey D, Kaplan N, Kadwa H, Blignaut P, Brock-Utne JG, Welsh N: Effects of atracurium on intraocular pressure. Br J Anaesth 56:459–463, 1984
134. Giala MM, Balamoutsos NG, Tsakona EA, Vasiliadov S, Macris SG: Failure of gallamine to inhibit succinylcholine-induced increase in intraocular pressure. Anesthesiology 51:578, 1979
135. Polek WV, Baughman VL, Laurito CE, Riegler FX, VadeBorcouer TR: Adequate serum lidocaine levels fail to control the hemodynamic response to intubation. Anesth Analg 68:S225, 1989
136. Meyers EF, Singer P, Otto A: A controlled study of the effect of succinylcholine self-taming on intraocular pressure. Anesthesiology 53:72, 1980
137. Carballo AS: Succinylcholine and acetazolamide (Diamox) in anaesthesia for ocular surgery. Can Anaesth Soc J 12:486, 1965
138. Smith G, Dalling R, Williams TIR: Gastro-oesophageal pressure gradient changes produced by induction of anaesthesia and suxamethonium. Br J Anaesth 50:1137–1143, 1978
139. Andersen N: Changes in intragastric pressure following the administration of suxamethonium. Br J Anaesth 34:363–367, 1962
140. Miller RD, Way WL: Inhibition of succinylcholine-induced increased intragastric pressure by nondepolarizing relaxants and lidocaine. Anesthesiology 34:185–188, 1971
141. Roe RB: The effect of suxamethonium on intragastric pressure. Anaesthesia 17:179–181, 1962
142. Salem MR, Wong AY, Lin YH: The effect of suxamethonium on the intragastric pressure in infants and children. Br J Anaesth 44:166–170, 1972
143. Gibbs CP, Modell JH: Management of aspiration pneumonitis. In Miller RD (ed): Anesthesia, 3rd ed. New York, Churchill Livingstone, 1990, pp 1293–1320
144. Bruce DL, Downs JB, Kulkarni PS, et al: Precurarization inhibits maximal ventilatory effort. Anesthesiology 61:618–621, 1984
145. Massey SA, Glazebrook CW, Goat VA: Suxamethonium: a new look at pretreatment. Br J Anaesth 55:729–733, 1983
146. Rao TLK, Jacobs HK: Pulmonary function following "pretreatment" dose of pancuronium in volunteers. Anesth Analg 59:659–661, 1980
147. Motsch J, Fuchs W, Hoch P, Kaas V, Hutschenreuter K: Side effects and changes in pulmonary function after fixed dose precurarization with alcuronium, pancuronium or vecuronium. Br J Anaesth 59:1528–1532, 1987
148. Lacour D: Prevention of rise in intra-gastric pressure due to suxamethonium fasciculations by prior dose of d-tubocurarine. Acta Anaesthesiol Scand 14:5, 1970
149. Spence AA, Moir DD, Finlay WEI: Observations on intragastric pressure. Anaesthesia 22:249, 1967
150. Moya F, Kvisselgaard N: The placental transfer of succinylcholine. Anesthesiology 22:1, 1961
151. Parer JT: Uteroplacental circulation and respiratory gas exchange. In Shnider SM, Levinson G (eds): Anesthesia for Obstetrics. Baltimore, Williams & Wilkins Co, 1987, p 17
152. Drabkova J, Crul JF, vander Kleihn E: Placental transfer of ^{14}C labelled succinylcholine in near-term Macaca mulatta monkeys. Br J Anaesth 45:1087–1095, 1973
153. Cherala SR, Eddie DN, Sechzer PH: Placental transfer of succinylcholine causing transient respiratory depression in the newborn. Anaesth Intensive Care 17:202–204, 1989
154. Hinkle AJ, Dorsch JA: Maternal masseter muscle rigidity and neonatal fasciculations after induction for emergency cesarean section. Anesthesiology 79:175–177, 1993
155. Roth F, Wuthrich H: The clinical importance of hyperkalemia following suxamethonium administration. Br J Anaesth 41:311–316, 1969
156. Waters DJ, Mapleson WW: Suxamethonium pains: hypothesis and observation. Anaesthesia 26:127, 1971
157. Rack PMH, Westbury DR: The effects of suxamethonium and acetylcholine on the behaviour of cat muscle spindles during dynamic stretching, and during fusimotor stimulation. J Physiol (Lond) 186:698, 1966
158. Churchill-Davidson HC: Suxamethonium pains and early electrolyte changes. Anaesthesia 33:454, 1978

159. Konig W: Uber Beschwerden nach Anwendung von Succinylcholin. Anaesthesist 5:50, 1956
160. Churchill-Davidson HC: Suxamethonium (succinylcholine) chloride and muscle pains. Br Med J 1:74, 1954
161. Collier C: Suxamethonium pains and fasciculations. Proc R Soc Med 68:105, 1975
162. Brodsky JB, Brock-Utne JG: Does "self-taming" with succinylcholine prevent postoperative myalgia? Anesthesiology 50:265–267, 1979
163. Hegarty P: Postoperative muscle pain. Br J Anaesth 11:209, 1956
164. Strom J, Jansen EC: Pain-reducing effect of self-taming suxamethonium. Acta Anaesthesiol Scand 28:40–43, 1984
165. Verma RS: Diazepam and suxamethonium muscle pain (a dose-response study). Anaesthesia 37:688–690, 1982
166. Fisher QA, Fisher E, Matjasko MJ: Midazolam pretreatment does not ameliorate myoglobinemia or the clinical side effects of succinylcholine. J Clin Anesth 5:414–418, 1993
167. Brodsky JB, Ehrenwerth J: Postoperative muscle pains and suxamethorium. Br J Anaesth 52:215–217, 1980
168. Collins RM, Docherty PW, Plantevin OM: Postoperative morbidity following gynaecological outpatient laparoscopy: a reappraisal of the science. Anaesthesia 39:819–822, 1984
169. Dodson ME: Laparoscopy and suxamethonium muscle pain (letter). Br J Anaesth 50:84, 1978
170. Mingus ML, Herlich A, Eisenkraft JB: Attenuation of suxamethonium myalgias: effect of midazolam and vecuronium. Anaesthesia 45:834–837, 1990
171. Sosis M, Goldberg M, Marr AT, Cubler AJ, Larijani G: Succinylcholine does not contribute to postoperative pain after outpatient laparoscopy. Anesth Analg 66:S163, 1987
172. Trepanier CA, Brousseau C, Lacerte L: Myalgia in outpatient surgery: comparison of atracurium and succinylcholine. Can J Anaesth 35:255–259, 1989
173. Zahl K, Apfelbaum JL: Muscle pain occurs after outpatient laparoscopy despite substitution of vecuronium for succinylcholine. Anesthesiology 70:408–411, 1989
174. Smith I, Ding Y, White PF: Muscle pain after outpatient laparoscopy–influence of propofol versus thiopental and enflurane. Anesth Analg 76:1181–1184, 1993
175. Topulos GP, Lansing RW, Banzett RB: The experience of complete neuromuscular blockade in awake humans. J Clin Anesth 5:369–374, 1993
176. Pace NL: Prevention of succinylcholine myalgias: a meta-analysis. Anesth Analg 70:477–483, 1990
177. Brodsky JB, Brock-Utne JG, Samuels SI: Pancuronium pretreatment and postsuccinylcholine myalgia. Anesthesiology 51:259, 1979
178. Sosis M, Broad T, Larijani GE, Marr AT: Comparison of atracurium and d-tubocurarine for prevention of succinylcholine myalgia. Anesth Analg 657–659, 1987
179. Blitt CD, Carlson GL, Rolling GD, Hameroff SR, Otto CW: A comparative evaluation of pretreatment with nondepolarizing blockers prior to the administration of succinylcholine. Anesthesiology 55:687–689, 1981
180. Erkola O: Effects of precurarisation on suxamethonium-induced postoperative myalgia during the first trimester of pregnancy. Acta Anaesthesiol Scand 34:63–67, 1990
181. Erkola O: Complications of neuromuscular blockers: interaction with concurrent medications and other neuromuscular blockers. Anesthesiol Clin North Am 11:427–444, 1993
182. Erkola O, Salmenpera A, Kuoppamaki R: Five nondepolarizing muscle relaxants in precurarization. Acta Anaesthesiol Scand 27:427–432, 1983
183. Erkola O: Train-of-four fade of non-depolarizing muscle relaxants: an insight into the mechanism of precurarization. Ann Fr Anesth Reanim 7:299–304, 1988
184. Asari H, Inoue K, Maruta H, Hirose Y: The inhibitory effect of intravenous d-tubocurarine and oral dantrolene on halothane-succinylcholine-induced myoglobinemia in children. Anesthesiology 61:332–333, 1984
185. Blanc VR, Vaillancourt G, Brisson G: Succinylcholine, fasciculations and myoglobinaemia. Can Anaesth Soc J 33:178–184, 1986

186. Cozanitis DA, Erkola O, Klemola UM, Makela V: Precurarisation in infants and children less than three years of age. Can J Anaesth 34:17–20, 1987
187. Charak DS, Dhar CL: Suxamethonium-induced changes in serum creatine phosphokinase. Br J Anaesth 53:955–957, 1981
188. Eisenberg M, Balsley S, Katz RL: Effects of diazepam on succinylcholine-induced myalgia, potassium increase, creatine phosphokinase elevation, and relaxation. Anesth Analg 58:314–317, 1979
189. Harrington JF, Ford DJ, Striker TW: Myoglobinemia and myoglobinuria after succinylcholine in children. Anesthesiology 59:A439, 1983
190. Innes RKR, Stromme JH: Rise in creatinine phosphokinase associated with agents used in anaesthesia. Br J Anaesth 45:185–189, 1973
191. Inagaki M, Kohyama A, Sakata S, Tonogai R, Yamada Y: Serum myoglobin levels following administration of succinylcholine during nitrous oxide-oxygen-halothane anesthesia. Jpn J Anesth 29:1476–1482, 1981
192. Laurence AS: Biochemical changes following suxamethonium. Serum myoglobin, potassium and creatinine kinase changes before commencement of surgery. Anaesthesia 40:854–859, 1985
193. Laurence AS: Myalgia and biochemical changes following intermittent suxamethonium administration: effects of alcuronium, lignocaine, midazolam and suxamethonium pretreatments on serum myoglobin, creatine kinase and myalgia. Anaesthesia 42:503–510, 1987
194. McLoughlin C, Elliott P, McCarthy G, Mirakhur RK: Muscle pains and biochemical changes following suxamethonium administration after six pretreatment regimens. Anaesthesia 47:202–206, 1992
195. Plotz J, Braun J: Failure of "self-taming" doses of succinylcholine to inhibit increases in postoperative serum creatine kinase activity in children. Anesthesiology 56:207–209, 1982
196. Ryan JF, Kagen LJ, Hyman AI: Myoglobinemia after a single dose of succinylcholine. N Engl J Med 285:824–827, 1971
197. Sekino N, Hiroki K, Namatame R, Tano M, Fukatsu O, Nishimura M, Fujihara T, Ogata K: Effect of induction methods of pediatric anesthesia on serum myoglobin. Masui 39:284–292, 1990
198. Tammisto T, Airaksinen M: Increase of creatine kinase activity in serum as sign of muscular injury caused by intermittently administered suxamethonium during halothane anaesthesia. Br J Anaesth 38:510–515, 1966
199. Tammisto T, Leikkonen P, Airaksinen M: The inhibitory effect of d-tubocurarine on the increase of serum creatine kinase activity produced by intermittent suxamethonium administration during halothane anaesthesia. Acta Anaesthesiol Scand 11:333–340, 1967
200. Cook DR, Fischer CG: Characteristics of succinylcholine neuromuscular blockade in neonates. Anesth Analg 57:63–66, 1978
201. Chestnutt WN, Lowry KG, Dundee JW, Pandit SK, Mirakhur RK: Failure of two benzodiazepines to prevent suxamethonium-induced muscle pain. Anaesthesia 40:263–269, 1985
202. Cullen DJ: The effect of pretreatment with nondepolarizing muscle relaxants on the neuromuscular blocking action of succinylcholine. Anesthesiology 35:572–578, 1971
203. Horrow JC, Lambert DH: The search for an optimal interval between pretreatment dose of d-tubocurarine and succinylcholine. Can Anaesth Soc J 31:528–533, 1984
204. Hartman GS, Fiamengo SA, Riker WF: Succinylcholine: mechanism of fasciculations and their prevention by d-tubocurarine or diphenylhydantoin. Anesthesiology 65:405–413, 1986
205. Lindgren L, Saarnivaara L: Effect of competitive myoneural blockade and fentanyl on muscle fasciculations caused by suxamethonium in children. Br J Anaesth 55:747–751, 1983
206. Manchikanti L: Diazepam does not prevent succinylcholine-induced fasciculations and myalgia: a comparative evaluation of the effect of diazepam and d-tubocurarine pretreatments. Acta Anaesthesiol Scand 28:523–528, 1984

207. Melnick B, Chalasani J, Uy NT, Phitayakorn P, Mallett SV, Rudy TE: Decreasing post-succinylcholine myalgia in outpatients. Can J Anaesth 34:238–241, 1987
208. Marr AT, Sosis M: Effectiveness of atracurium in preventing succinylcholine myalgia. J Am Assoc Nurse Anesth 57:128–130, 1989
209. Pinchak AC, Sung JC, Hagen JF, Hall F: Waiting time alters inhibition of succinylcholine fasciculations by atracurium. Anesth Analg 64:A265, 1985
210. Ferres CJ, Mirakhur RK, Craig HJ, Browne ES, Clarke RS: Pretreatment with vecuronium as a prophylactic against post-suxamethonium muscle pains: comparison with other non-depolarizing neuromuscular blocking drugs. Br J Anaesth 55:735–741, 1983
211. Konchigeri HN, Jadhav KB, Akkineni S, Patel KP: Comparative effects of nondepolarizing muscle relaxants on succinylcholine-induced fasciculations and postoperative pain. South Med J 70:1083–1085, 1977
212. Bennetts FE, Khalil KI: Reduction of post-suxamethonium pain by pretreatment with four non-depolarizing agents. Br J Anaesth 53:531–536, 1981
213. Lamoreaux LF, Urbach KF: Incidence and prevention of muscle pain following the administration of succinylcholine. Anesthesiology 21:394–396, 1960
214. Morris DDB, Dunn GH: Suxamethonium chloride administration and postoperative muscle pain. Br Med J 1:383, 1957
215. McLoughlin C, Nesbitt GA, Howe JP: Suxamethonium induced myalgia and the effect of pre-operative administration of oral aspirin: a comparison with a standard treatment and an untreated group. Anaesthesia 43:565–567, 1988
216. Miller RD: Advantages of giving d-tubocurarine before succinylcholine (letter). Anesthesiology 37:568–569, 1972
217. Jansen EC, Hansen PH: Objective measurement of SCh-induced fasciculations and the effect of pretreatment with pancuronium or gallamine. Anesthesiology 51:159–160, 1979
218. Wald-Oboussier G, Lohmann C, Viell B, Doehn M: "Self-taming": an alternative to the prevention of succinylcholine-induced pain. Anaesthesist 36:426–430, 1987
219. Lindgren L, Klemola UM, Saarnivaara L: Optimal time interval between pretreatment with alcuronium and suxamethonium during anesthetic induction. Acta Anaesthesiol Scand 32:244–247, 1988
220. Manchikanti L, Grow JB, Colliver JA, Canella MG, Hadley CH: Atracurium pretreatment for succinylcholine-induced fasciculations and postoperative myalgia. Anesth Analg 64:1010–1014, 1985
221. Budd A, Scott RF, Blogg CE, Goat VA: Adverse effects of suxamethonium: failure of prevention by atracurium or fazadinium. Anaesthesia 40:642–646, 1985
222. Baraka A: Succinylcholine pretreatment unsatisfactory (letter). Anesthesiology 48:298, 1978
223. Baraka A: Self-taming of succinylcholine-induced fasciculations. Anesthesiology 46:292, 1977
224. Umino M, Miura M, Kondo T, Ohi K, Yoshino A, Kubota Y: Effect of thiamylal and diazepam on release of myoglobin and creatine phosphokinase by succinylcholine during halothane anesthesia. Bull Tokyo Med Dent Univ 32:91–96, 1985
225. Manani G, Valenti S, Segatto A, Angel A, Meroni M, Giron GP: The influence of thiopentone and alfathesin on succinylcholine-induced fasciculations and myalgias. Can Anaesth Soc J 28:253–258, 1981
226. Haldia KN, Chatterji S, Kackar GN: Intravenous lignocaine for prevention of muscle pains after succinylcholine. Anesth Analg 52:849, 1974
227. Collier D: Dantrolene and suxamethonium: the effect of preoperative dantrolene on the action of suxamethonium. Anaesthesia 34:152–158, 1979
228. Laurence AS: Oral dantrolene prevents rise of myoglobin due to suxamethonium. Anaesthesia 40:907–910, 1985
229. Laurence AS, McKean JF: Dantrolene and suxamethonium: myalgia, biochemical changes and serum dantrolene levels following oral dantrolene pre-treatment in laparoscopy patients. Eur J Anaesthesiol 7:493–500, 1990
230. DeVore JS, Asrami R: Magnesium sulfate prevents succinylcholine induced fasciculations in toxemic patients. Anesthesiology 52:76–77, 1980

231. Ghoneim MM, Long JP: The interaction between magnesium and other neuromuscular blocking agents. Anesthesiology 32:23–27, 1970
232. Chestnutt WN, Dundee JW: Failure of magnesium sulphate to prevent suxamethonium induced muscle pains. Anaesthesia 40:488–490, 1985
233. Lindgren L, Saarnivaara L: Increase in intragastric pressure during suxamethonium-induced muscle fasciculations in children: inhibition by alfentanil. Br J Anaesth 60:176, 1988
234. Davies AO: Oral diazepam premedication reduces the incidence of postsuccinylcholine muscle pains. Can Anaesth Soc J 30:603, 1983

19

DAVID G. SILVERMAN | HENRY ROSENBERG

Malignant Hyperthermia: Etiology, Risks, and Assessment of Susceptibility

First formally described by Denborough and Lovell in 1960,[1] *malignant hyperthermia* (MH) is an inherited myopathy characterized by an inability of the *sarcoplasmic reticulum* (and possibly mitochondria and sarcolemma) to modulate cytoplasmic calcium levels,[2-8] especially in the presence of triggering agents. The *increased myoplasmic Ca^{2+}* results in excess muscle contraction (contractures), glycolysis, and heat production. There is eventual uncoupling of oxidative phosphorylation, with decreased adenosine triphosphate (ATP) levels causing membrane instability and rhabdomyolysis. A vicious cycle develops as hypermetabolism, acidosis, and hyperthermia lead to further loss of control.[9-13] In addition to this classic form, which is characterized by ineffective Ca^{2+} modulation, MH may be the common end point following exposure to *triggering agents* in a number of neuromuscular disorders associated with excessive levels of myoplasmic Ca^{2+}, contractures, and excess metabolism.

◆ TRIGGERING AGENTS

It is possible for a patient to undergo multiple anesthetic experiences without an MH episode and then to develop MH during a subsequent anesthetic.[14,15] The *anesthetic agents* most commonly incriminated are *halothane* and *succinylcholine* (SCh),[16-20] but all potent volatile agents may precipitate an MH crisis and MH-like symptoms.[21,22] The inciting agents precipitate a *destructive increase in metabolism*, apparently disturbing muscle structure and calcium homeostasis to a degree that cannot be tolerated by MH-susceptible muscle.[10,11,13,23-25] The release itself is not specific to MH-susceptible individuals[26,27]; however, the degree of Ca^{2+} release or its consequences are abnormal in MH-susceptible muscle. For example, halothane-induced release of Ca^{2+} from the sarcoplasmic reticulum is greater in MH-susceptible muscle,[25] an effect that may be mediated by unsaturated fatty acids[28] as a consequence of altered lipase activity.[23,28–31] It is offset by dantrolene (Chap. 20).[6,13,25,32–34]

Anesthetics generally *considered to be safe* include barbiturates, nitrous oxide, narcotics, ester-type local anesthetics, amide-type local anesthetics,[35–37] and nondepolarizing relaxants (NDRs) and anticholinesterases.[38] Nevertheless, a recent review of published cases of MH noted that some episodes of apparent MH have occurred in the absence of volatile agents or depolarizing relaxants.[15] (However, MH-like signs may be secondary to other conditions—e.g., sepsis, pheochromocytoma.) MH-like signs and symptoms also have been documented in an awake, unmedicated individual.[39]

Barbiturates actually may delay the onset of MH.[40] *Droperidol* seems to be safe, and decreases contractures during in vitro testing.[41,42] *Ketamine* does not trigger MH; however, it may delay the early diagnosis of MH by causing tachycardia. Phenothiazines might best be avoided: they may induce the neuroleptic malignant syndrome (Chap. 20), they increase intracellular Ca^{2+}, and they may cause MH-susceptible muscle to develop contractures in vitro[43] (but this has been disputed).[41] Elevated levels of serum Ca^{2+} and large doses of digoxin do not initiate an MH response.[44]

As detailed in Chapter 20, dantrolene can prevent and abort MH episodes. *Nondepolarizing relaxants* may mitigate the effects of SCh and even of volatile agents.[40] Tubocurarine had previously been implicated as a triggering agent,[45] but this now is considered highly unlikely.[46] It is best to choose a relaxant that does not promote tachycardia. Other drugs, though not implicated in triggering MH themselves or in altering triggering by other agents, may modify the course of an MH reaction. Although administration of an alpha-adrenoceptor antagonist did not alter the initial response to SCh in MH-susceptible pigs, it limited the severity of the MH response.[47]

◆ SUCCINYLCHOLINE AND JAW MUSCLE RIGIDITY

The onset of action of SCh may be marked by a transient increase in muscle tension that is far more prominent in the *muscles of mastication* than in the adductor pollicis (Chap. 16).[48–57] Masseter muscles have fibers that typically respond with *slow tonic contractures;* thus, jaw contractions are more prominent than contractions of peripheral muscles.[58] The prominent contractions may also be due in part to the heterogeneity of fiber types in the masseter muscle, which permits integration of refined movements and maximal closing forces.[58,59] Clinically detectable masseter spasm is observed in patients at the high end of the spectrum of masseter responsiveness,[60] whether the responsiveness is normal or of pathologic origin.

Halothane decreases the mechanical threshold of muscle[61] and thus may exacerbate SCh-induced masseter contractions. There is a 0.01–1% incidence of masseter stiffness in all children in whom anesthesia is induced with the *combination of halothane and SCh*,[20,62-64] especially in those undergoing strabismus surgery or other surgery related to a muscle imbalance or abnormality.[62] Although most common with halothane and SCh, masseter stiffness may also follow induction with other agents.

Extreme jaw contraction, or *trismus,* is characterized by spasm (rigidity) such that for several minutes the mouth can barely be opened. Trismus may occur even after abolition of the nerve stimulator-induced twitch response in the periphery[54] or at the masseter itself.[50] Masseter rigidity may be accompanied by creatine kinase (CK) elevation, myoglobinuria, and myalgias. The likelihood and severity of these sequelae are decreased by dantrolene. Trismus *may herald the onset of MH*,[16,18,64-76] which typically becomes evident 10–20 minutes after resolution of the spasm but sometimes immediately after or up to several hours later.[65] When individuals who have shown evidence of masseter rigidity undergo a subsequent workup, the incidence of MH susceptibility (based on in vitro testing of muscle biopsies) is approximately 50% in children and 25% in adults.[18,65,68,77] Additionally, masseter muscle rigidity *may precede hyperkalemia-precipitated cardiac arrest* in patients with an undiagnosed myopathy (usually the apparently normal child with as yet undiagnosed Duchenne's dystrophy; see Chap. 23).

◆ TESTS FOR MALIGNANT HYPERTHERMIA

The *caffeine and halothane contracture test* (CHCT) detects MH susceptibility by measuring the contracture threshold of muscle strips exposed to halothane and/or caffeine.[78-81] MH-susceptible muscles, as well as muscles affected by some other disorders (Chap. 23), exhibit a low threshold,[82,83] most consistently to halothane.[78]

Criteria are not universally agreed on, and testing is not 100% reliable. A positive result on in vitro testing does not necessarily indicate that the patient will develop MH on subsequent exposures. A variety of neuromuscular diseases are associated with abnormal halothane contracture tests as well as varying degrees of MH susceptibility. The test currently used in the United States has an *80–85% specificity*.[83] Until recently, the CHCT was considered to be *virtually 100% sensitive;* i.e., patients who tested negative had not developed an MH crisis on subsequent exposure to triggering agents.[84,85] However, it was recently reported that four patients who tested negative on CHCT had clinical episodes that were highly suggestive of MH. Of potential note, the testing was conducted and evaluated according to European criteria rather than North American criteria (question h). The false-negative CHCT results have led to the suggestion that if the perioperative *clinical and biochemical findings* suggest MH, a diagnosis of MH is warranted, even if the CHCT result is negative.[86] Although it may be argued on theoretical grounds that dantrolene may alter test sensitivity, there is no good evidence to support this conjecture.

Other tests of muscle status may also help in the assessment of MH susceptibility. *Routine CK levels* are clearly positive (i.e., >1,000–2,000 IU) in many MH-susceptible patients, but levels are variable and may be normal.[87–92] Muscle lactate levels may be high[13]; *phosphocreatine levels* are low,[13] and inorganic phosphate/phosphocreatine, phosphodiester/phosphocreatine, or *inorganic phosphate/ATP ratios* are increased (as may be detected by nuclear magnetic resonance spectroscopy).[31,93–95] However, alterations of these indices also may be seen with myotonic dystrophy, muscle injury, and denervating disorders.[93,96–99] Combinations of the different parameters may be most sensitive.[94] During effort, susceptible muscle may evidence marked intracellular acidosis.[99] Although initial studies suggested that MH-susceptible patients responded abnormally to tourniquet-induced ischemia,[100,101] this has not been substantiated.[102,103]

◆ PREVALENCE AND RISK FACTORS

The overall *prevalence of MH susceptibility* has been estimated as 1:15,000 anesthetic episodes in children and 1:50,000 anesthetic episodes in adults.[104] MH susceptibility is genetically transmitted,[30,105–107] and the prevalence varies in different populations. In a recent review of 503 cases worldwide, ages ranged from newborn (reacting to anesthesia for cesarean section) to 73 years, with 52% of cases occurring in children under 15 years.[15]

A number of disorders are associated with varying degrees of risk for MH.[81,90,108–110] A *relatively high degree of risk* is associated with King's syndrome or *King Denborough syndrome* (musculoskeletal abnormalities including myopathy, hypotonia, low-set ears, slanted eyes, pectus deformity, malar hypoplasia, and short stature; cryptorchidism; and retardation),[90,111,112] *Evan's myopathy,* and *central core disease* (weakness, cores with decreased mitochondria in Type I fibers).[113,114] A *lower risk* is associated with proximal muscle weakness (e.g., limb girdle), nonspecific and subclinical myopathies,[90,115,116] Duchenne's muscular dystrophy,[92,117,118] and the neuroleptic malignant syndrome.[119,120] Approximately 50% of biopsy specimens from patients with *Duchenne's or Becker's dystrophy* develop halothane-induced contractures (Chap. 23).[81,109] An *uncertain link* has been postulated for muscle imbalance such as strabismus,[62] ptosis, squint, and kyphoscoliosis; osteogenesis imperfecta[121]; pectus excavatum; hyperkalemic periodic paralysis[92]; and myotonia.[122] A history of apparent heat stroke has been implicated, since stress-induced MH may resemble heat stroke, but a cause-and-effect relationship is unlikely.[123] Although sudden infant death syndrome was reported to be associated at times with overheating and was more likely in families with a myopathy,[124] its relationship to MH has not been confirmed and is controversial.

Discussion Questions ◆

a. Is *increased jaw tension* a common consequence of *SCh* administration? How frequently do we encounter masseter spasm?
b. What is the differential diagnosis of *SCh-induced masseter rigidity?*
c. What associated *perioperative changes* would increase your concern with respect to the MH susceptibility of a patient who had an episode of *masseter rigidity* that did not progress to MH?
d. Should one cancel an elective procedure if the patient develops *trismus* after *SCh?* Why or why not?
e. Is the *SCh-induced increase in jaw tension* prevented by treatment with: (1) a paralyzing dose of *NDR?* (2) a defasciculating dose of NDR?
f. Contrast the responses of normal and *MH-susceptible muscle* to 3% halothane.
g. Contrast the responses of normal and *MH-susceptible muscle* to caffeine.
h. Why isn't the caffeine-halothane contracture test *(CHCT)* 100% specific for *MH susceptibility?* How do the North American and European tests differ?
i. How is the muscle specimen for the CHCT obtained?
j. If a patient with a positive CHCT test does not develop MH on subsequent exposure to potentially triggering agents, does this mean that there was a *false-positive CHCT result?*
k. Summarize the normal role of *calcium in muscle contraction* and the modulating role of the sarcoplasmic reticulum.
l. Is there evidence that *inhalational agents* alter *calcium* release?
m. Should the *MH-susceptible patient* avoid *coffee?*
n. Should the *MH-susceptible patient* avoid *aminophylline?*
o. Can the *MH-susceptible patient* lead a *normal life?*
p. Is the *abnormality of calcium control in MH* limited to skeletal muscle?
q. What is the *differential diagnosis of a CK level above 1,000 IU?*
r. What is the potential significance of the *ryanodine receptor* and/or the locus for glucose phosphate isomerase?
s. Can increased *sympathetic activity* elicit an *MH episode?*
t. Must an anesthetic machine with vaporizers be replaced by a *"new clean machine"* for use in an *MH-susceptible patient?*
u. What is *MHAUS?*
v. What are the negative consequences of falsely *labeling a patient* (and his or her family) as *MH susceptible?*

Answers ◆

a. *Succinylcholine* commonly causes *increased jaw tension*. The *masseter* is designed for tonic contractions and thus may be more likely than most other muscles to demonstrate increased tone. The increased tension generally is not detected.[60] However, reduced mean mouth opening and significantly increased jaw stiffness ("*spasm*") are not uncommon, especially in children receiving halothane and SCh.[54,62] Administration of *SCh during halothane anesthesia* in children is associated with up to a 1% incidence of spasm. Other factors may contribute. A recent study in cats showed that jaw (and to a lesser extent tibialis muscle) contraction may be augmented by elevated *catecholamines*[49]: the relative strength of SCh-induced jaw contracture increased 600% in cats that received epinephrine, 1 µg · kg^{-1}.[49]

b. Apparent *masseter rigidity may be due to* light anesthesia with inadequate relaxation, temporomandibular joint dysfunction, a marked nonpathologic response of the jaw muscles to SCh,[54,55] MH, denervation, or a myopathy such as myotonia or polymyositis.[18,67–71] It is more likely to indicate MH or myotonia if other muscles are rigid, and it is more likely to represent MH if systemic signs such as hypercarbia are present. Postoperatively, MH may be distinguished from other disorders by biopsy and electromyogram testing. Five of the approximately 64 patients in one series who presented with intraoperative masseter rigidity were found to have myotonia congenita but were not MH susceptible, according to in vitro assessment of biopsy specimens.[69]

c. The *likelihood that masseter spasm is indicative of MH* or that it will be associated with a positive contracture test is increased if there is evidence of *muscle damage* or *systemic changes*. The following points should be considered:

   1. Generalized rigidity, ventricular arrhythmias, cyanosis, and postoperative myoglobinuria were commonly observed in patients who tested positive for MH.[72]
   2. In two series, 76–95% of patients with generalized rigidity had a positive result on the contracture test.[72,125]
   3. In a retrospective review of approximately 110 cases of masseter spasm that did not progress to MH,[69] the likelihood of a positive caffeine, halothane, or caffeine plus halothane contracture test was 29% if the patient had masseter spasm alone, 57% if the patient had masseter spasm plus signs of metabolic changes (increased temperature or heart rate, arrhythmias), and 76% if there was masseter spasm with a CK level >1,500 IU and myoglobinuria.[69]
   4. In a survey of patients referred for testing after masseter rigidity, a *perioperative CK* was >20,000 IU in six of 30 who tested positive and in none of 22 who tested negative.[75]
   5. Testing for *myoglobinuria* alone is not specific. Myoglobinuria is not uncommon after SCh and halothane.[126,127] In referred patients, four of 14 contracture-positive patients and three of 14 contracture-negative patients had myoglobinuria.[68,75]

6. There is a relatively high incidence of an underlying myopathy in patients with masseter spasm who test negative for MH.[68,75]

Thus, despite the associations, none of the clinical symptoms can be regarded as a specific sign of MH. "The in vitro contracture tests remain essential for confirming or rejecting the diagnosis of MH in less pronounced or abortive cases."[72] Additionally, it should be noted that a positive contracture test has a specificity of only 85% (question h).

d. Opinions have differed as to whether the increased *risk of MH following trismus* should lead one to *cancel nonemergency surgery*. Gronert and others have recommended *judicious monitoring* of end-tidal CO_2, blood gases, blood pressure, ECG, temperature, urine color, and muscle tone. Should any changes occur suggesting an abnormal metabolic response, the procedure should be halted if at all possible and treatment for MH instituted. Otherwise the procedure may be continued.[128] Others have even suggested that the inhalational agent may be continued in the context of "jaw stiffness"[57] and spasm[63] (a controversial step) so long as vigilant monitoring is maintained. Littleford and colleagues reported that continuing the triggering agents in 57 cases of isolated masseter spasm resulted in no increase in long-term morbidity,[63,129] although several patients had myoglobinuria, acidosis, and/or increased CK levels, which may indeed have indicated a severe systemic response.[130]

In contrast, others have recommended a more cautious approach.[18,64,68,73–76,130,131] They contend that, for an elective procedure, the additional problems that might be engendered by continuing the anesthetic are not justified, and they recommend that elective surgery be postponed and a biopsy obtained. Their concern is that "once end-tidal CO_2 begins to rise dramatically and the diagnosis of MH is made, the delay in mixing and in delivering dantrolene in sufficient quantities will produce injury and death."[130] Simply observing the patient for 10–20 minutes is not sufficient, since MH typically becomes apparent 20–40 minutes after spasm and may recrudesce hours later.[65,73,74]

e. Whereas the *SCh-induced increase in jaw tension* is prevented by pretreatment with a *paralyzing dose of NDR*, it is not prevented by a *defasciculating dose* of relaxant even if fasciculations are successfully prevented.[51] Insofar as such a defasciculating dose is believed to work presynaptically, this suggests that a presynaptic mechanism (e.g., SCh-induced repetitive nerve firing) is not solely responsible for SCh-induced spasm.

f. In the in vitro setting of the caffeine-halothane contracture test, *normal skeletal muscle* may respond to *3% halothane* with a small contracture (usually less than 0.5–0.6 gm). Although there are interlaboratory differences, most authorities believe that *MH-susceptible muscle will produce an isometric contracture >0.8 gm* during exposure to 3% halothane. Clearly, this induction of contracture by inhalational agents in a specific in vitro setting is different from their relaxant properties in vivo.

g. In *normal muscle*, 1–2 mM of *caffeine* increases cytoplasmic Ca^{2+} and typically increases *twitch tension* without *contracture*; contractures are not noted until doses above 4 mM are administered. In MH-susceptible muscle, 0.3–1.5 mM of caffeine elicits a 1-gm isometric contracture (i.e., the "contracture vs. caffeine" dose-response curve is shifted to the left).[78,82,132] A muscle may be classified as *MH susceptible* if there is *a contracture of >0.3 gm in response to 2 mM of caffeine*.

h. Interpretation of the *CHCT* is hampered by a 15% incidence of *false-positive results*. In 1987, the *North American Malignant Hyperthermia Group* of MH diagnostic centers proposed *standardized testing techniques* and guidelines. Assessment of low-risk subjects to determine the incidence of false positives noted that 9.2% exceeded a 0.7-gm contracture threshold for *3% halothane* (n = 414) and 15.2% exceeded a 0.2-gm contracture threshold for *2 mM of caffeine*. The authors concluded that specificity may be improved by looking at responses obtained during both exposures and by increasing the threshold for caffeine from ≥0.2 gm to ≥0.3 gm.[83]

The *European MH Society* criteria differ slightly. During European testing, a positive response to caffeine is recorded when a sustained increase in basal tension (contracture) of 0.2 gm or more occurs with a caffeine concentration of 2 mM · L^{-1} as well as a contracture in response to 2% halothane in the gas phase. When the strips respond only to either caffeine or halothane, the European result is tabulated as equivocal. The methodologies also differ: European group members expose muscle to incremental doses of halothane rather than a single dose of 3% halothane.

It should be noted that responses are not necessarily uniform for all the muscle strips isolated from a single biopsy specimen.[75] Furthermore, there is large *interlaboratory variability*, and supposed false positives may occur as a result of different procedures. Additionally, there is a phenotype that develops contractures in response to a combination of caffeine and halothane but not to either agent alone. Some argue that this may constitute MH susceptibility,[69,71,133] but it is associated with a large number of false positives.[77]

Then again, *what is a false positive?* In many patients who developed masseter spasm, the triggering agent itself was removed or the anesthetic was discontinued; hence an MH episode may have been aborted. Furthermore, a low-risk subject still may have a finite risk of being MH susceptible such that a positive response of the biopsy specimen may not necessarily be a false-positive response. A positive CHCT may also indicate another disorder: seven of 18 patients with myopathic disorders and three of seven with neuropathic disorders had positive halothane contracture tests.[81]

i. *Muscle strips* are obtained by biopsy of proximal leg muscle (quadriceps femoris or vastus lateralis).[36] Muscle from this region responds similarly to the adductor pollicis over a wide range of stimulating frequencies.[134] The strips are mounted in tissue baths and stimulated at a relatively slow rate. Then the potentially offending agent is added.

   The biopsy may be performed under regional anesthesia (spinal, epidural, or femoral nerve block) or under general anesthesia with non-triggering agents. It is done at the hospital that will be performing the testing. Local infiltration of the muscle should be avoided. In a recent survey, 22% of patients complained of residual discomfort at the biopsy site.[85] In general, biopsies are not done in children less than 6 years old because of insufficient muscle.

j. Even if a patient does not develop MH during a given exposure, he or she may nevertheless develop it during a subsequent exposure. The *risk of MH in a patient with a positive biopsy* is hard to ascertain: how willing should we be to test such results (i.e., to administer known triggering agents to a patient with a positive CHCT)? These problems have led one team of investigators to conclude, "We will probably never know if a positive muscle biopsy predicts the potential for an MH crisis"[129] (until we have a genetic test).

k. Normally, the muscle action potential causes the sarcoplasmic reticulum to release *calcium* and thereby increase cytoplasmic levels from the relaxed level of less than 10^{-7} M to between 10^{-7} and 10^{-5} M. This opposes troponin inhibition of myosin and allows *actin-myosin*–mediated contraction. *Relaxation* occurs after calcium is pumped back into the sarcoplasmic reticulum and is extruded from the cell; these actions cause Ca^{2+} levels to decrease below the mechanical threshold.

l. *Halothane, enflurane,* and *isoflurane* increase the *release of Ca^{2+}* from the *sarcoplasmic reticulum*.[7,27] It has recently been shown in vitro that halothane, enflurane, and isoflurane increase the velocity of Ca^{2+} leakage from isolated rabbit sarcoplasmic reticulum and increase ATPase activity.[26]

m. In the absence of halothane, ≥0.7 mM of *caffeine* was necessary to elicit a *contracture in MH-susceptible muscle* from four subjects.[135] This dosage is more than 20 times the exposure achieved after ingestion of 8 cups of *coffee* in a 7-hour period (0.02–0.025 mM) and more than 10 times the exposure achieved after oral ingestion of 7 mg · kg^{-1} (0.06 mM) of caffeine.[135] In the presence of 1% halothane, a contracture was observed in muscle exposed to 0.1 mM of caffeine.[135] Several days of oral caffeine ingestion likewise made pigs more susceptible to MH in response to halothane and SCh.[136] However, the risk associated with coffee is largely theoretical.

n. In the absence of halothane, ≥1.5 mM of *theophylline* was necessary to elicit a *contracture in muscle strips* from four MH-susceptible subjects.[135] This is 10 times the maximum therapeutic level. In the presence of 1% halothane, a small contracture was produced by theophylline, 0.25 mM (2 × the therapeutic level). Thus, it has been suggested that the administration of theophylline or aminophylline in the presence of halothane may *increase the likelihood of an MH response* in the MH-susceptible patient.[135] Again, the risk may be largely theoretical.

o. The patient who is MH susceptible can lead an *essentially normal life* but should avoid triggering anesthetic agents and possibly haloperidol (and related drugs), severe exercise in hot conditions, and exposure to halogenated hydrocarbons (such as bromochlorodifluoromethane in fire extinguishers).[137] Such individuals may have muscle pains, fatigue, and fever (which respond to dantrolene). They should wear a Medic Alert bracelet and notify their physicians of their condition, as should untested relatives of a patient with MH.

p. *Calcium abnormalities* may exist in and affect cardiac muscle, smooth muscle, nerves, platelets,[138] lymphocytes, monocytes,[139] and pancreatic islet cells (leading to an increased glucose-induced insulin response).[140] However, it is unclear as to whether the same abnormalities that exist in skeletal muscle also exist in other muscles, blood cells, or organs. For example, the myocardial abnormalities noted during acute MH episodes may simply be a consequence of acute autonomic and metabolic disturbances.[141]

q. A *CK level >1,000 IU* may be found with MH,[87-89,91,92,108] central core disease,[92] muscular dystrophy,[92,116] myositis,[142] hyperkalemic periodic paralysis,[92] and such life-threatening situations as acute myocardial infarction, seizures, delirium tremens, severe trauma, and fulminant thyroid storm. Elevated levels may also be noted after electrical countershock, electroconvulsive therapy, cerebral trauma, aerobic exercise (77 IU before exercise to approximately 900 IU and as high as 3,473 IU after exercise),[143] and in marathon runners (35 IU before the race, 730 IU after the marathon but with a positive MB fraction in 50%).[144] CK levels may also be slightly higher during pregnancy.[145] They are increased moderately after surgery and after SCh-induced fasciculations (Table 19-1). Hence, an elevated CK does not predict MH susceptibility with high specificity or even high sensitivity.[87-89,91,92] However, it may help identify susceptible individuals in some families with a history of MH[88,89,108]: high resting CK levels—approximately 200 IU vs. 41 IU in controls—generally were found in patients with the most severe halothane contracture and morphological abnormality.[89] "The likelihood of MH susceptibility in patients with persistently elevated serum levels of CK is great enough to warrant a thorough neurologic examination together with muscle biopsy for in vitro testing for MH susceptibility."[91]

r. The *ryanodine receptor* is a portion of the *sarcoplasmic reticulum* calcium release channel.[149,150] It is so named because it *binds to the plant alkaloid ryanodine* with high specificity. In MH-susceptible swine, this

TABLE 19-1
CK Levels

	Pre	Post
Minor gynecologic or dental surgery[146]	96	275
Thoracic/abdominal surgery[147]	13	117
Full-blown MH episode	normal or increased	often >20,000
Succinylcholine for minor surgery:[148]		
If intense fasciculations	19	99
If no fasciculations	24	24

receptor is more prone to ryanodine inhibition of contractile activity. The receptor has been sequenced in man, and is reportedly a major site of action for halothane and caffeine.[151] It has been proposed that mutations of the *genes on chromosome 19* that code this receptor may result in predisposition to MH. However, studies in more than 50 MH-positive families turned up only one family with a possible defect on chromosome 19. Recent evidence suggests linkage to a *different locus*.[106] Other patterns of inheritance[107,110] may reflect a *multitude of disorders with a tendency to induce excessive myoplasmic Ca^{2+} and contractures* in response to inhalational anesthetics and SCh. Abnormalities of glucose phosphate isomerase, phosphorylases, and lipases have been proposed.[23,28–31] Eventually, molecular genetics may permit the specific diagnosis of MH.[105]

s. *Sympathetic activity* contributes to the signs and symptoms of an MH crisis[19] and may even contribute to masseter spasm.[49] It has been implicated in stress-induced hyperthermia in pigs. But there is still no direct evidence to suggest that the sympathetic nervous system initiates MH in humans.

t. It has been reported that a *"new machine"* is not necessarily required for the MH-susceptible patient. There is evidence that removal or sealing of vaporizers, replacement of the fresh gas outlet hose, and use of a disposable circle after a flush of 10 L/min for 5–15 minutes are sufficient.[152–154]

u. The Malignant Hyperthermia Association of the United States (*MHAUS*) is an organization with a 24-hour number (209–634–4917) for emergency calls as well as public information.

v. The importance of appropriate labeling of patients as MH-susceptible was emphasized in a recent review.[155] Indiscriminate labeling soon leads to significant numbers of patients who will have to be managed as MH susceptible, requiring deviation from the current practice of frequent potent inhalational anesthetic administration. This may compromise management of difficult airways (including epiglottitis), full stomachs, asthma, or tetralogy of Fallot, and restrict eligibility for insurance.[155]

References ◆

1. Denborough MA, Lovell RRH: Anaesthetic deaths in a family. Lancet 2:45, 1960
2. Allen PD, Ryan JF, Jones DE, et al: Sarcoplasmic reticulum calcium uptake in cryostate sections of skeletal muscle from malignant hyperthermia patients and controls (correspondence). Muscle Nerve 9:474, 1986
3. Denborough MA: The pathopharmacology of malignant hyperpyrexia. Pharmacol Ther 9:357–365, 1980
4. Kim DH, Sreter FA, Ohnishi ST, Ryan JF, Roberts J, Allen PD, Meszaros LG, Antoniu B, Ikemoto N: Kinetic studies of Ca^{2+}: release from sarcoplasmic reticulum of normal and malignant hyperthermia susceptible pig muscles. Biochim Biophys Acta 775:320–327, 1984
5. Lopez JR, Alamo L, Caputo C, Wikinski J, Ledezma D: Intracellular ionized calcium concentration in muscles from humans with malignant hyperthermia. Muscle Nerve 8:355–358, 1985
6. Nelson TE, Flewellen EH: Rationale for dantrolene vs. procainamide for treatment of malignant hyperthermia. Anesthesiology 50:118–122, 1979
7. Nelson TE: Abnormality in Ca^{2+} release from skeletal sarcoplasmic reticulum in pigs susceptible to malignant hyperthermia. J Clin Invest 72:862–873, 1983
8. Stadhouders AM, Viering WAL, Verburg MP, et al: *In vivo* induced malignant hyperthermia in pigs: III. Localization of calcium in skeletal muscle mitochondria by means of electromicroscopy and microprobe analysis. Acta Anaesthesiol Scand 28:14, 1984
9. Gronert GA, Theye RA: Halothane-induced porcine malignant hyperthermia: metabolic and hemodynamic changes. Anesthesiology 44:36, 1976
10. Gronert GA, Mott J, Lee J: Aetiology of malignant hyperthermia. Br J Anaesth 60:253, 1988
11. Gronert GA: Malignant hyperthermia. Anesthesiology 53:395, 1980
12. Lucke JN, Hall GM, Lister D: Porcine malignant hyperthermia: I. Metabolic and physiological changes. Br J Anaesth 48:297–304, 1976
13. Verburg MP, Oerlemans FTJJ, van Bennekom CA, Gielen MJM, deBruyn CHMM, Crul JF: *In vivo* induced malignant hyperthermia in pigs: I. Physiological and biochemical changes and the influence of dantrolene sodium. Acta Anaesthesiol Scand 28:1–8, 1984
14. Halsall PJ, Cain PA, Ellis FR: Retrospective analysis of anaesthetics received by patients before susceptibility to malignant hyperpyrexia was recognized. Br J Anaesth 51:949, 1979
15. Strazis KP, Fox AW: Malignant hyperthermia: a review of published cases. Anesth Analg 77:297–304, 1993
16. Donlon JV, Newfield P, Streter FA, et al: Implications of masseter spasm after succinylcholine. Anesthesiology 49:298–301, 1978
17. Ellis FR, Harriman DGF, Keaney NP, Kyei-Mensah K, Tyrrel JH: Halothane-induced muscle contracture as a cause of hyperpyrexia. Br J Anaesth 43:721–722, 1971
18. Fletcher FE, Rosenberg H: *In vitro* interaction between halothane and succinylcholine in human skeletal muscle: implications for malignant hyperthermia and masseter muscle rigidity. Anesthesiology 63:190–194, 1985
19. Gronert GA, Theye RA: Pathophysiology of hyperkalemia induced by succinylcholine. Anesthesiology 43:89–99, 1975
20. Ording H: Incidence of malignant hyperthermia in Denmark. Anesth Analg 64:700–704, 1985
21. Boheler J, Hamrick JC Jr, McKnight RL, et al: Isoflurane and malignant hyperthermia (letter). Anesth Analg 61:712–713, 1982
22. Pan TH, Wollak AR, DeMarco JA: Malignant hyperthermia associated with enflurane anesthesia. Anesth Analg 54:47–49, 1975
23. Cheah KS, Cheah AM, Waring JC: Phospholipase A2 activity, calmodulin, Ca^{2+} and meat quality in young and adult halothane-sensitive and halothane-insensitive British Landrace pigs. Meat Sci 17:37, 1986
24. Gronert GA, Milde JH, Taylor SR: Porcine muscle responses to carbacol, alpha and beta adrenoreceptor agonist, halothane or hyperthermia. J Physiol 307:319, 1980
25. Ohnishi ST, Taylor S, Gronert GA: Calcium-induced Ca^{2+} release from sarcoplasmic reticulum of pigs susceptible to malignant hyperthermia: the effects of halothane and dantrolene. FEBS Lett 161:103, 1983

26. Blanck TJJ, Peterson CV, Baroody B, Tegazzin V, Lou J: Halothane, enflurane, and isoflurane stimulate calcium leakage from rabbit sarcoplasmic reticulum. Anesthesiology 76:813–821, 1992
27. Nelson TE, Sweo T: Ca^{2+} uptake and Ca^{2+} release by skeletal muscle sarcoplasmic reticulum: differing sensitivity to inhalational anesthetics. Anesthesiology 69:571–577, 1988
28. Cheah KS, Cheah AM: Skeletal muscle mitochondrial phospholipase A2 and the interaction of mitochondria and sarcoplasmic reticulum in porcine malignant hyperthermia. Biochim Biophys Acta 638:40, 1981
29. Fletcher JE, Rosenberg H, Michaux K, et al: Triglyceride lipase, not phospholipase A2, activity is elevated in skeletal muscle from malignant hyperthermia susceptibles. Anesthesiology 69:A413, 1988
30. McCarthy TV, Healy JMS, Heffron JJA, Lehane M, Deufel T, Lehmann-Horn F, Farrall M, Johnson K: Localization of the malignant hyperthermia susceptibility locus to human chromosome 19q12–13.2. Nature 343:562–564, 1990
31. Willner JH, Woods DS, Cerri C, et al: Increased myophosphorylase A in malignant hyperthermia. N Engl J Med 303:138–140, 1980
32. Britt BA: Dantrolene. Can Anaesth Soc J 31:61–75, 1984
33. Harrison GG: Dantrolene--dynamics and kinetics. Br J Anaesth 60:279, 1988
34. Morgan KG, Bryant SH: The mechanism of action of dantrolene sodium. J Pharmacol Exp Ther 201:138–147, 1977
35. Wingard DW, Bobko S: Failure of lidocaine to trigger porcine malignant hyperthermia. Anesth Analg 58:99–103, 1979
36. Berkowitz A, Rosenberg H: Femoral block with mepivacaine for muscle biopsy in malignant hyperthermia patients. Anesthesiology 62:651–652, 1985
37. Harrison GG, Morrell DF: Response of MHS swine to IV infusion of lignocaine and bupivacaine. Br J Anaesth 52:385, 1980
38. Ording H, Nielsen VG: Atracurium and its antagonism by neostigmine (plus glycopyrrolate) in patients susceptible to malignant hyperthermia. Br J Anaesth 58:1001, 1986
39. Gronert GA, Thompson RL, Onofrio BM: Human malignant hyperthermia: awake episodes and correction by dantrolene. Anesth Analg 59:377–378, 1980
40. Gronert GA, Milde JH: Variations in onset of porcine malignant hyperthermia. Anesth Analg 60:499–503, 1981
41. Landers DF, Hon CA, Platts A, Becker GL: Effects of pretreatment with droperidol, haloperidol or trifluoperazine on skeletal muscle contracture *in vitro*. Anesthesiology 71:A815, 1989
42. Fletcher JE, Rosenberg H: *In vitro* studies of droperidol for use in human malignant hyperthermia. Anesthesiology 63:A302, 1985
43. Andersson K: Effects of chlorpromazine, imipramine and quinidine on the mechanical activity of single skeletal muscle fibers of the frogs. Acta Physiol Scand 85:532, 1982
44. Gronert GA, Ahern CP, Milde JH, et al: Effect of CO_2, calcium, digoxin, and potassium on cardiac and skeletal muscle metabolism in malignant hyperthermia susceptible swine. Anesthesiology 64:24–28, 1986
45. Britt BA, Webb GE, LeDuc C: Malignant hyperthermia induced by curare. Can Anaesth Soc J 21:371, 1974
46. Williams CH, Roberts JT, Hoech GP, et al: The fulminant hyperthermia-stress syndrome: total neuromuscular blockade with dimethyl curare prevents the development of the syndrome in susceptible pigs. J Thermal Biol 3:104, 1978
47. Lister D, Hall GM, Lucke JN: Porcine malignant hyperthermia: III. Adrenergic blockade. Br J Anaesth 48:831–837, 1976
48. Leary NP, Ellis FR: Masseteric muscle spasm as a normal response to suxamethonium. Br J Anaesth 64:488–492, 1990
49. Pryn SJ, Van Der Spek AFL: Comparative pharmacology of succinylcholine on jaw, eye and tibialis muscle. Anesthesia 73:A859, 1990
50. Plumley MH, Bevan JC, Saddler JM, Donati F, Bevan DR: Dose-related effects of succinylcholine on the adductor pollicis and masseter muscles in children. Can J Anaesth 37:15–20, 1990
51. Smith CE, Saddler JM, Bevan JC, Donati F, Bevan DR: Pre-treatment with non-depolarizing neuromuscular blocking agents and suxamethonium-induced increases in resting jaw tension in children. Br J Anaesth 64:577–581, 1990

52. Saddler JM, Bevan JC, Plumley MH, Polomeno RC, Donati F, Bevan DR: Jaw muscle tension after succinylcholine in children undergoing strabismus surgery. Can J Anaesth 37:21–25, 1990
53. Smith CE, Donati F, Bevan DR: Effects of succinylcholine at the masseter and adductor pollicis muscles in adults. Anesth Analg 69:158–162, 1989
54. Van Der Spek AFL, Fang WB, Ashton-Miller JA, et al: Increased masticatory muscle stiffness during limb flaccidity associated with succinylcholine administration. Anesthesiology 69:11, 1988
55. Van Der Spek AFL, Fang WB, Ashton-Miller JA, Stohler CS, Carlson DS, Schork MA: The effects of succinylcholine on mouth opening. Anesthesiology 67:459–465, 1987
56. Van Der Spek AFL, Reynolds PI, Fang WB, Ashton-Miller JA, Stohler CS, Schork MA: Changes in resistance to mouth opening induced by depolarizing and nondepolarizing neuromuscular relaxants. Br J Anaesth 64:21–27, 1990
57. Van Der Spek AFL, Spargo PM, Nahrwold ML: Masseter spasm and malignant hyperthermia are not the same thing (letter). Anesthesiology 64:291–292, 1986
58. Butler-Browne GS, Eriksson P-O, Laurent C, Thornell L-E: Adult human masseter muscle fibers express myosin isozymes characteristic of development. Muscle Nerve 11:610–620, 1988
59. Carlsöö S: Motor units and action potentials in masticatory muscles. Acta Morphol Neerl Scand 2:13–19, 1958
60. Brandom BW: Atracurium and succinylcholine on the masseter muscle (editorial). Can J Anaesth 37:7–11, 1990
61. Gallant EM, Gronert GA, Taylor SR: Cellular membrane potential and contractile threshold in mammalian skeletal muscle susceptible to malignant hyperthermia. Neurosci Lett 28:181–186, 1982
62. Carroll JB: Increased incidence of masseter spasm in children with strabismus anesthetized with halothane and succinylcholine. Anesthesiology 67:559–561, 1987
63. Littleford JA, Patel LR, Bose D, Cameron CB, McKillop C: Masseter muscle spasm in children: implications of continuing the triggering anesthetic. Anesth Analg 72:151–160, 1991
64. Schwartz L, Rockoff MA, Koka BV: Masseter spasm with anesthesia: incidence and implications. Anesthesiology 61:772–775, 1984
65. Allen GC, Rosenberg GC: Malignant hyperthermia susceptibility in adult patients with masseter muscle rigidity. Can J Anaesth 37:31–35, 1990
66. Christian AF, Ellis FR, Halsall PJ: Is there a relationship between masseteric muscle spasm and malignant hyperpyrexia? Br J Anaesth 62:540–544, 1989
67. Davies DD: Hypertonic syndrome associated with suxamethonium administration (correspondence). Br J Anaesth 42:656, 1970
68. Ellis FR, Halsall PJ: Suxamethonium spasm: a differential diagnostic conundrum. Br J Anaesth 56:381–384, 1984
69. Ellis FR, Halsall PJ, Christian AS: Clinical presentation of suspected malignant hyperthermia during anaesthesia in 402 probands. Anaesthesia 45:838–841, 1990
70. Flewellen EH, Nelson E: Masseter spasm induced by succinylcholine in children: contracture testing for malignant hyperthermia. Report of six cases. Can Anaesth Soc J 29:42–49, 1982
71. Flewellen EH, Nelson TE: Halothane-succinylcholine induced masseter spasm: indicative of malignant hyperthermia susceptibility? Anesth Analg 63:693–697, 1984
72. Hackl W, Mauritz W, Schemper M, Winkler M, Sporn P, Steinbereithner K: Prediction of malignant hyperthermia susceptibility: statistical evaluation of clinical signs. Br J Anaesth 64:425–429, 1990
73. Rosenberg H: Trismus is not trivial (editorial). Anesthesiology 67:453–455, 1987
74. Rosenberg H: Management of patients in whom trismus occurs following succinylcholine. Anesthesiology 68:654–655, 1988
75. Rosenberg H, Fletcher JE: Masseter spasm rigidity and malignant hyperthermia susceptibility. Anesth Analg 65:161–164, 1986
76. Rosenberg H, Reed S, Heiman T: Masseter spasm, rhabdomyolysis and malignant hyperthermia (abstract). Anesthesiology 53:S248, 1980
77. Rosenberg H, Reed S: In vitro contracture tests for susceptibility to malignant hyperthermia. Anesth Analg 62:415–420, 1983

78. Kalow W, Britt BA, Terreau ME, Haist C: Metabolic error of muscle metabolism after recovery from malignant hyperthermia. Lancet 2:895–898, 1970
79. Moulds RFW, Denborough MA: Identification of susceptibility to malignant hyperpyrexia. Br J Med 4:245–247, 1974
80. Ording H: Diagnosis of susceptibility to malignant hyperthermia in man. Br J Anaesth 60:287–302, 1988
81. Heiman-Patterson TD, Rosenberg H, Fletcher JE, Tahmoush AJ: Halothane-caffeine contracture testing in neuromuscular diseases. Muscle Nerve 11:453–457, 1988
82. Nelson TE, Denborough MA: Studies on normal human skeletal muscle in relation to the pathopharmacology of malignant hyperpyrexia. Clin Exp Pharmacol Physiol 4:315–322, 1976
83. Larach MG, Landis JR, Bunn JS, Diaz M, The North American Malignant Hyperthermia Registry: Prediction of malignant hyperthermia susceptibility in low-risk subjects. Anesthesiology 76:16–27, 1992
84. Allen GC, Rosenberg H, Fletcher JE: Safety of general anesthesia in patients previously tested negative for malignant hyperthermia susceptibility. Anesthesiology 72:619–622, 1990
85. Ording H, Hedengran AM, Skovgaard LT: Evaluation of 119 anaesthetics received after investigation for susceptibility to malignant hyperthermia. Acta Anaesthesiol Scand 35:711–716, 1991
86. Isaacs H, Badenhorst M: False-negative results with muscle caffeine halothane contracture testing for malignant hyperthermia. Anesthesiology 79:5–9, 1993
87. Amaranath L, Lavin TJ, Trusso A, Boutros AR: Evaluation of creatinine phosphokinase screening as a predictor of malignant hyperthermia. Br J Anaesth 55:531–533, 1983
88. Britt BA, Endrenyi L, Peters PL, Kwong FH-F, Kadijevic L: Screening of malignant hyperthermia susceptible families by creatine phosphokinase measurement and other clinical investigations. Can Anaesth Soc J 23:263–284, 1976
89. Ellis FR, Clarke IMC, Modgill M, Currie S, Harriman DGF: Evaluation of creatinine phosphokinase in screening patients for malignant hyperpyrexia. Br Med J 3:511–513, 1975
90. Kaplan AM, Bergeson PS, Gregg SA, Curless RG: Malignant hyperthermia associated with myopathy and normal muscle enzymes. J Pediatr 91:431–434, 1977
91. Lingaraju N, Rosenberg H: Unexplained increases in serum creatine kinase levels: its relation to MH susceptibility. Anesth Analg 72:702–705, 1991
92. Paasuke RT, Brownell AKW: Serum creatine kinase level as a screening test for susceptibility to malignant hyperthermia. JAMA 255:769–771, 1986
93. Olgin J, Argov Z, Rosenberg H, Tuchler M, Chance B: Noninvasive evaluation of malignant hyperthermia-susceptibility with phosphorus nuclear magnetic resonance spectroscopy. Anesthesiology 68:507–513, 1988
94. Payen J-F, Bosson J-L, Bourdon L, Jacquot C, Le Bas J-F, Stieglitz P, Benabid A-L: Improved noninvasive diagnostic testing for malignant hyperthermia susceptibility from a combination of metabolites determined *in vivo* with ^{31}P-magnetic resonance spectroscopy. Anesthesiology 78:848–855, 1993
95. Olgin J, Rosenberg H, Allen G, Seestedt R, Chance B: A blinded comparison of noninvasive, *in vivo* phosphorus nuclear magnetic resonance spectroscopy and the *in vitro* halothane/caffeine contracture test in the evaluation of malignant hyperthermia susceptibility. Anesth Analg 72:36–47, 1991
96. Barany M, Siegel IM, Venkatasubramanian PN, Mok E, Wilbur AC: Human leg neuromuscular diseases: P-31 MR spectroscopy. Radiology 172:503–508, 1989
97. Edwards RHT, Wilkie DR, Dawson MJ, Gordon RE, Shaw D: Clinical use of nuclear magnetic resonance in the investigation of myopathy. Lancet 1:722–731, 1982
98. Younkin DP, Berman P, Sladky J, Chee C, Bank W, Chance B: ^{31}P NMR studies in Duchenne muscular dystrophy: age-related metabolic changes. Neurology 37:165–169, 1987
99. Laschuk MJ, Lee RJ, Zochodne DW, Drieger AL, Gordon K, Thompson T: 31P NMR measured exercise-induced skeletal muscle acidosis in MHS individuals (abstract). Can J Anaesth 34:S65-S66, 1987
100. Jones PIE, Britt BA, Steward DJ, et al: Tourniquet test as a predictor of malignant hyperthermia susceptibility. Anesth Analg 60:256, 1981
101. Roberts JF, Ryan JF, Ali HH, et al: Abnormally high regional oxygen consumption in

malignant hyperthermia patients induced by a non-anesthetic stress (ten minutes ischemia to the upper extremity). Anesthesiology 57:A229, 1982
102. Britt BA, Scott EA, Kleiman A, et al: Failure of the tourniquet-twitch test as a diagnostic or screening test for malignant hyperthermia. Anesth Analg 66:1047, 1986
103. Urwyler A, Ellis FR, Halsall PJ, Hopkins PM: Muscle relaxation rates in individuals susceptible to malignant hyperthermia. Br J Anaesth 65:421–423, 1990
104. Britt BA, Kalow W: Malignant hyperthermia: a statistical review. Can Anaesth Soc J 17:293–315, 1970
105. Levitt RC: Prospects for the diagnosis of malignant hyperthermia susceptibility using molecular genetic approaches. Anesthesiology 76:1039–1048, 1992
106. Levitt RC, Nouri N, Jedlicka A, McKusick VA, Marks A, Shutack JG, Fletcher JE, Rosenberg H, Meyers DA: Evidence for genetic heterogeneity in malignant hyperthermia susceptibility. Genomics 11:543–547, 1991
107. McPherson E, Taylor CA Jr: The genetics of malignant hyperthermia: evidence for heterogeneity. Am J Med Genet 11:273–285, 1982
108. Brownell AK: Malignant hyperthermia's relationship to other diseases. Br J Anaesth 60:303–308, 1988
109. Heiman-Patterson TH, Natter H, Rosenberg H, et al: Malignant hyperthermia susceptibility in X linked muscle dystrophies. Pediatr Neurol 2:356, 1986
110. King JO, Denborough MA, Zapf PW: Inheritance of malignant hyperpyrexia. Lancet 1:365–370, 1972
111. McPherson EW, Taylor CA: The King syndrome: malignant hyperthermia, myopathy and multiple anomalies. Am J Med Genet 8:159, 1981
112. Steenson AJ, Torkelson RD: King's syndrome with malignant hyperthermia: potential outpatient risks. Am J Dis Child 141:271–273, 1987
113. Denborough MA, Dennett X, Anderson RM: Central-core disease and malignant hyperpyrexia. Br Med J 1:272–273, 1973
114. Eng GD, Epstein BS, Engel K, McKay R: Malignant hyperthermia and central core disease in a child with congenital dislocating hip. Arch Neurol 35:189–197, 1978
115. Fletcher R, Blennow G, Olsson AK, et al: Malignant hyperthermia in a myopathic child: prolonged postoperative course requiring dantrolene. Acta Anaesthesiol Scand 26:431, 1982
116. Isaacs H, Barlow M: Malignant hyperpyrexia during anaesthesia: possible correlation with subclinical myopathy. Br Med J 1:275, 1970
117. Brownell AKW, Passuke RT, Elash A, et al: Malignant hyperthermia in Duchenne muscular dystrophy. Anesthesiology 58:180–182, 1983
118. Kelfer HM, Singer WD, Reynolds RN: Malignant hyperthermia in a child with Duchenne muscular dystrophy. Pediatrics 71:118–119, 1983
119. Caroff SN, Rosenberg H, Fletcher JE, et al: Malignant hyperthermia susceptibility in neuroleptic malignant syndrome. Anesthesiology 67:20, 1987
120. Weinberg S, Twersky RS: Neuroleptic malignant syndrome. Anesth Analg 62:845–880, 1983
121. Rampton AJ, Kelly DA, Shanahan EC, et al: Occurrence of malignant hyperpyrexia in a patient with osteogenesis imperfecta. Br J Anaesth 56:1443, 1984
122. Newberg LA, Lambert EH, Gronert GA: Failure to induce malignant hyperthermia in myotonic goats. Br J Anaesth 55:57, 1983
123. Jardon OM: Physiologic stress, heat stroke, malignant hyperthermia—a perspective. Milit Med 147:8–14, 1982
124. Denborough MA, Galloway GJ, Hopkinson KC: Malignant hyperpyrexia and sudden infant death. Lancet 2:1068–1069, 1982
125. Larach MG, Rosenberg H, Larach DR, Broennle AM: Prediction of malignant hyperthermia susceptibility by clinical signs. Anesthesiology 66:547–550, 1987
126. Asari H, Inoue K, Maruta H, Hirose Y: The inhibitory effect of intravenous d-tubocurarine and oral dantrolene on halothane-succinylcholine-induced myoglobinemia in children. Anesthesiology 61:332–333, 1984
127. Ryan JF, Kagen LJ, Hyman AI: Myoglobinemia after a single dose of succinylcholine. N Engl J Med 285:824–827, 1971
128. Gronert GA: Management of patients in whom trismus occurs following succinylcholine (letter). Anesthesiology 68:653–654, 1988
129. Patel LR, Bose D, Littleford JA: Masseter muscle spasm in children (letter). Anesth Analg 73:362–363, 1991

130. Rosenberg H, Shutack JG: Masseter muscle spasm in children (letter). Anesth Analg 73:361–362, 1991
131. Schwartz L, Rockoff M, Kok BV: Masseter spasm and malignant hyperthermia (letter). Anesthesiology 64:292–293, 1986
132. Nelson TE, Flewellen EH: Malignant hyperthermia: diagnosis, treatment and investigations of a skeletal muscle lesion. Tex Rep Biol Med 38:105–120, 1979
133. Nelson TE, Flewellen EH, Gloyna DF: Spectrum of susceptibility to malignant hyperthermia--diagnostic dilemma. Anesth Analg 62:545–552, 1983
134. Edwards RHT, Young A, Hosking GP, Jones DA: Human skeletal muscle function: description of tests and normal values. Clin Sci 52:283–290, 1977
135. Flewellen EH, Nelson TE: Is theophylline, aminophylline, or caffeine (methylxanthines) contraindicated in malignant hyperthermia susceptible patients? Anesth Analg 52:115–118, 1983
136. Chapin JW, Chang GL, Wingard DW: Coffee (caffeine) and porcine malignant hyperthermia. Anesthesiology 55:A292, 1981
137. Denborough MA, Hopkinson KC: Firefighting and malignant hyperthermia. Br Med J 296:1442–1443, 1988
138. Rosenberg H, Fisher CA, Reed SB, et al: Platelet aggregation in patients susceptible to malignant hyperthermia. Anesthesiology 55:621–624, 1981
139. Klip A, Elliott ME, Frodis W, et al: Anaesthetic induced increase in ionized calcium in blood mononuclear cells from malignant hyperthermia patients. Lancet 1:463, 1987
140. Denborough MA, Warne GL, Moulds RFW, Tse P, Martin FIR: Insulin secretion in malignant hyperpyrexia. Br Med J 3:493–495, 1974
141. Kawamoto M, Yuge O, Kikuchi H, et al: No myocardial involvement in nonrigid malignant hyperthermia. Anesthesiology 64:93, 1986
142. Brownlow K, Elevitch FR: Serum creatine phosphokinase isoenzyme (CPK_2) in myositis: a report of six cases. JAMA 230:1141–1144, 1974
143. Nicholson GA, Morgan GJ, Meerkin M, Strauss ER, McLeod JG: The effect of aerobic exercise on serum creatine kinase activities. Muscle Nerve 9:820–834, 1986
144. Oliver LR, De Waal A, Retief FJ, Marx JD, Kriel JR, Human GP, Potgieter GM: Electrocardiographic and biochemical studies on marathon runners. S Afr Med J 53:783–787, 1978
145. Isherwood DM, Ridley J, Wilson J: Creatine phosphokinase (CPK) levels in pregnancy: a case report and a discussion of the value of CPK levels in the prediction of possible malignant hyperpyrexia. Br J Obstet Gynaecol 82:346–349, 1975
146. Eisenberg M, Balsley S, Katz RL: Effects of diazepam on succinylcholine-induced myalgia, potassium increase, creatinine phosphokinase elevation, and relaxation. Anesth Analg 58:314–317, 1979
147. Dixon SH, Fuchs JCA, Ebert PA: Changes in serum creatine phosphokinase activity following thoracic, cardiac, and abdominal operation. Arch Surg 103:66–68, 1971
148. Charak DS, Dhar CL: Suxamethonium-induced changes in serum creatine phosphokinase. Br J Anaesth 53:955–957, 1981
149. Lai FA, Erickson HP, Rousseau E, Liu Q-Y, Meissner G: Purification and reconstitution of the calcium release channel from skeletal muscle. Nature 331:351–391, 1988
150. Timmerman M, Ashley C: Excitation-contraction coupling: bridging the gap. J Muscle Res Cell Motil 9:367–369, 1988
151. Zorzato F, Fiji J, Otsu K, Phillips M, Green NM, La FA, Meissner G, MacLennan DH: Molecular cloning of cDNA encoding human and rabbit forms of the Ca^{2+} release channel (ryanodine receptor) of skeletal muscle sarcoplasmic reticulum. J Biol Chem 265:2244–2256, 1990
152. Beebe JJ, Sessler DI: Preparation of anesthesia machines for patients susceptible to malignant hyperthermia. Anesthesiology 69:395, 1988
153. Ritchie PA, Cheshire MA, Pearce NH: Decontamination of halothane from anaesthetic machines achieved by continuous flushing with oxygen. Br J Anaesth 60:859, 1988
154. McGraw TT, Keon TP: Malignant hyperthermia and the clean machine. Can J Anaesth 36:530–532, 1989
155. Larach MG: Should we use muscle biopsy to diagnose malignant hyperthermia susceptibility? (editorial). Anesthesiology 79:1–4, 1993

20

DAVID G. SILVERMAN | HENRY ROSENBERG

Malignant Hyperthermia: Signs, Symptoms, and Treatment

◆ SIGNS AND SYMPTOMS

The first signs of *malignant hyperthermia* (MH) commonly are manifestations of the *hypercarbia* that results from the *hypermetabolic state:* an increase in end-tidal carbon dioxide ($EtCO_2$) and in the partial pressure of carbon dioxide in venous and arterial blood ($PvCO_2$ and $PaCO_2$); increased heat in the CO_2 absorber, and exhaustion of soda lime; tachypnea (unless ventilation is controlled), tachycardia, and dysrhythmias. We also commonly see hyperthermia, muscle rigidity, and cyanosis.[1-7] Fever alone is not diagnostic, as it may result from multiple causes. *Laboratory findings* include acidosis and possibly hypoxemia, hyperkalemia, hypercalcemia followed by hypocalcemia, abnormal clotting studies (disseminated intravascular coagulation), increased creatine kinase (CK) levels (>20,000 IU), myoglobinemia, and myoglobinuria. Signs and symptoms often occur precipitously but may not become evident until several hours after the start of surgery.[8]

◆ TREATMENT

Dantrolene, a hydantoin derivative used to treat spasticity, is the drug of choice for prophylaxis and treatment.[9-14] It *impedes Ca^{2+}-dependent muscle contraction* and thereby alters the strength-duration curve[12] and shortens the time of contraction,[15] probably by limiting sarcoplasmic reticulum release of Ca^{2+} or interfering with voltage-dependent charge movement in the T-system.[16-18] It recently has been confirmed that dantrolene decreases myoplasmic Ca^{2+} in vivo, especially in MH-susceptible patients[18] (Table 20-1). It does not affect the neuromuscular junction (NMJ) per se.[17]

Dantrolene, 1 mg · kg^{-1}, *decreases mechanomyographic twitch height* to 60% of normal and decreases grip strength[19]; 2.2–2.5 mg · kg^{-1}, which produces a plasma level of approximately 4 µg · mL^{-1}, decreases twitch height to 25% of normal. Tetanic fade is affected to a lesser degree,[15] and there is

TABLE 20-1
Effects of Dantrolene on Ca^{2+} Concentration (μM)

	Ca^{2+} Concentration (μM)	
Dantrolene Dose ($mg \cdot kg^{-1}$)	Patients with Normal Muscle	Patients Susceptible to Malignant Hyperthermia
0	0.112	0.485
0.5	0.096	0.325
1.5	0.077	0.233
2.5	0.068	0.092

Source: Data derived from Lopez JR, Gerardi A, Lopez MJ, Allen PD: Effects of dantrolene on myoplasmic free [Ca^{2+}] measured *in vivo* in patients susceptible to malignant hyperthermia. Anesthesiology 76:711–719, 1992.

relative respiratory sparing.[17] Although in routine doses dantrolene has not been found to cause dangerous muscle weakness in normal individuals, it should be used cautiously in patients with neuromuscular disorders.[20] As expected, dantrolene may increase the effects of neuromuscular blocking agents[21]; however, in normal patients, it does not affect the ability to reverse them. In usual clinical doses, dantrolene has little effect on myocardial contractility.[10]

Dantrolene is effective against MH because it reduces Ca^{2+}-induced hyperactivity, relieves spasticity, and may reduce MH-induced arrhythmias. It causes complete relaxation of caffeine-, halothane-, and succinylcholine (SCh)-induced contractures in MH-susceptible muscle,[22] and it reduces SCh-induced chemical changes and myalgias.[23] Even in normal individuals, dantrolene may reduce halothane and SCh-induced myoglobinemia.[24]

A typical *oral pretreatment regimen* consists of 1–1.5 mg $\cdot$ kg^{-1} orally q.i.d. (5 mg $\cdot$ kg^{-1} $\cdot$ day^{-1}). Higher doses may be indicated but are associated with a greater incidence of gastrointestinal disturbances and muscle weakness (i.e., stumbling and stuttering).[16,19] A 5-year-old girl with an underlying muscular disorder developed signs of upper airway obstruction during oral prophylaxis.[20,25] *Intravenous (IV) pretreatment* is more controllable. It typically entails 1–2.4 mg $\cdot$ kg^{-1} given IV over 30–120 minutes[19]; however, this protocol may cause weakness, nausea, and vomiting.

Because patients with myopathies may be prone to developing significant muscle weakness with dantrolene and because MH-susceptible patients have been safely anesthetized (with nontriggering agents) without dantrolene,[26-28] *pretreatment generally is not indicated* so long as triggering agents are avoided and emergency treatment is available. Vigilance is essential regardless of the anesthetic regimen. Fortunately, apparently no one has died when such vigilance is maintained, triggering agents are avoided, and dantrolene is available.

Each *vial of dantrolene* contains 20 mg of drug and 3 gm of *mannitol* to provide isotonicity. Dantrolene should be administered via the central venous pressure line when possible, as it is very *alkaline* (the pH of 9.5 promotes dissolving). Ideally, *the drug should be diluted in water* (60 mL per dantrolene vial). Large bottles of D5W can be used. Saline should not be used, as the solute may oppose dissolution. Warming the vial may accelerate dissolution. Azumolene is a preparation that does not require such mixing; however, it causes more hepatic toxicity than traditional dantrolene preparations and currently is not approved for use.

During a crisis, typical procedures include the following:

1. Remove all sources of a possible *triggering agent.* Stop the anesthesia and discontinue surgery as soon as possible. Change the tubing and/or machine.
2. Call for *help.*
3. *Hyperventilate* the patient with 100% oxygen to decrease $PaCO_2$ and increase oxygenation.
4. Administer *dantrolene,* 2.5 mg · kg^{-1} IV, repeated as needed or followed by a rapid infusion of an additional 7.5 mg · kg^{-1}. Most cases will respond to 3–5 mg · kg^{-1}. Alternatively, one may infuse 1 mg · kg^{-1} · min^{-1} until relief of adverse signs is detected and then repeat half the initial dose at 4-hour intervals until all signs and symptoms have resolved. If the episode does not resolve within several minutes, then an additional 10 mg · kg^{-1} (and possibly much higher doses) should be used, or a rapid infusion may be titrated to effect. According to the North American Malignant Hyperthermia Registry, the mean initial dose in 73 reports of dantrolene usage in likely and almost certain cases of MH was 2.3 mg · kg^{-1} (with a range of 0.2–10.0 mg · kg^{-1}; the mean total dose in these patients was 5.6 mg · kg^{-1} (0.9–33.9 mg · kg^{-1}).[29] If MH is suspected, dantrolene should not be withheld out of fear of exacerbating other causes of fever and tachycardia; it has been shown to be "safe" in the context of sepsis.[30] Dantrolene may also be used during a cesarean section; the fetal:maternal partition ratio is approximately 0.4.[31]
5. *If severe hyperthermia is present,* cool the patient by packing in ice, infusing cooled saline, and possibly lavaging the stomach, rectum, and peritoneum. Otherwise, avoid excess cooling, as this leads to shivering and peripheral ischemia, which may decrease heat loss.
6. *If acidosis is severe and unresolving,* consider administering sodium bicarbonate. Otherwise, it may be best to avoid the Na^+ and bicarbonate load (which is also provided by the dantrolene solution).
7. Maintain *urine output* with fluids (but not lactated Ringer's solution, as it contains K^+ and Ca^{2+}) and diuretics. An output of ≥0.2 mL · kg^{-1} · hr^{-1} should prevent myoglobin cast formation.
8. Administer *procainamide* (≤1 gm/70 kg/30 min) if arrhythmias persist

after dantrolene.[13] In addition to being an antiarrhythmic, procaine inhibits abnormal drug-induced contractures in MH-susceptible muscle in vitro (but not as effectively as dantrolene).[32] Procainamide may be infused until the arrhythmias have resolved, unless the QT interval is prolonged by 50% or more. Such prolongation indicates significant cardiac depression, which may be treated with isoproterenol. The safety of other antiarrhythmics has not been proven; lidocaine and other amide local anesthetics have been used safely. *Avoid calcium channel blockers,* as they provide little confirmed benefit, may exacerbate the effects of hyperkalemia, and may promote marked cardiovascular depression in the context of dantrolene therapy.[33–37]

9. *Maintain cardiac output,* which may be compromised in the context of acidosis, hyperkalemia, hemoconcentration, arrhythmias, and their treatment.[2,38]
10. Treat *hyperkalemia* (with insulin, 0.1–0.2 units · kg^{-1}, and dextrose, 0.5–1.0 mg · kg^{-1}), *hypoglycemia* (which may result from the hypermetabolic state), *hypovolemia, coagulopathy,* and related abnormalities. If hypokalemia develops, treat it slowly because of potentially decreased renal function and the possibility that a marked increase in K^+ may retrigger an MH episode.
11. *Monitor for at least 24–48 hours.* An MH crisis can recrudesce after apparently successful resolution of the initial episode. Recrudescence is especially likely if all parameters have not fully returned to normal (e.g., heart rate). In the North American MH Registry report, approximately 25% of patients had an MH recrudescence despite a mean initial dantrolene dose of 2.3 mg · kg^{-1}.[29] *Dantrolene should be continued* for several doses.[6,9,19,39] The dosing interval should be titrated to symptoms, taking into account that the $t_{1/2}$ of dantrolene given IV is 12 hours and that therapeutic plasma levels (>2.5 µg · mL^{-1}) typically persist for 4–6 hours after 2.5 mg · kg^{-1} IV.[16,40] This may be achieved with repeated oral administration; a single dose of 2 mg · kg^{-1} achieved a level of 2.08 ± 0.07 µg · mL^{-1}.[23]

Discussion Questions ◆

a. Is *increased temperature* the first sign of an *MH crisis?*
b. What factors contribute to *tachycardia and arrhythmias* during an MH crisis?
c. Why might a patient become *cyanotic* during an MH crisis?
d. Why, in theory, might each of the following hamper *identification of an MH crisis:* (1) controlled ventilation by hand, (2) pancuronium, (3) ketamine.

e. Is a *venous* or an *arterial blood gas value* more likely to identify MH? Why?
f. How can one rapidly *distinguish myoglobin from hemoglobin* in the urine?
g. What is the differential diagnosis of *increased end-tidal* CO_2?
h. Can an MH episode occur without intense *muscle contractions?*
i. Following a motorbike accident, a teenage boy undergoing general anesthesia with spontaneous ventilation via a Bain circuit develops *hypercarbia, arrhythmias, acidosis, elevated CK levels, and myoglobinuria.* Is this MH? Why or why not?
j. Is *postoperative fever* a strong indicator of MH susceptibility?
k. Compare the responses of the *mechanomyogram and the electromyogram to dantrolene* in normal subjects.
l. Would you expect *dantrolene* to reduce *myoplasmic* Ca^{2+} levels?
m. Is it reasonable to anesthetize an MH-susceptible patient who has not received *dantrolene prophylaxis?*
n. Summarize the potential *side effects of dantrolene therapy.*
o. Can dantrolene be used safely in an *MH-susceptible parturient?*
p. What is the *neuroleptic malignant syndrome?* How is it treated?
q. Is the patient with *neuroleptic malignant syndrome* more susceptible to SCh-induced *hyperkalemia?*

Answers ◆

a. The *first signs* of an MH crisis often include muscle rigidity, hypercarbia, and tachycardia. These signs commonly occur before an increase in temperature is noted. However, no single sign is 100% sensitive and 100% specific.[41]
b. *Tachycardia and dysrhythmias* may result from hypermetabolism, hyperthermia, acidosis, hypercarbia, hyperkalemia, hyper- and hypocalcemia, hypoxemia, and increased sympathetic activity.
c. *Cyanosis* may result from (1) the hypermetabolic state, which causes increased oxygen extraction (even if arterial oxygenation is near normal), (2) catecholamine-induced vasoconstriction, and (3) in severe cases, as a result of arterial hypoxemia due to cardiorespiratory collapse.
d. In response to the effects of *increased* $PaCO_2$ (e.g., increased respiratory drive, tachycardia), an anesthesia care giver providing *ventilation by hand* may hyperventilate the patient. This may delay laboratory detection of the increased CO_2 production. *Pancuronium* and *ketamine* cause tachycardia, which may mask MH-induced tachycardia.
e. A *venous sample* is more reflective of increased carbon dioxide production than is an *arterial sample* because the increased CO_2 content of venous blood has not been reduced by the lungs. The earliest detectable changes during an MH episode are increasing lactate and CO_2 in venous

blood (or end-tidal exhaled gas). Arterial blood reflects an increase in CO_2 more slowly, especially in the presence of hyperventilation; however, arterial blood gas samples also provide valuable information about oxygen and pH.

f. After centrifugation, the supernatant is pink if there is *hemoglobinuria* and clear if there is *myoglobinuria*.

g. The differential diagnosis of *increased EtCO_2* includes hypoventilation, a nonfunctioning machine valve or exhausted CO_2 absorber, hyperthyroidism or fever, and excess CO_2 production due to MH.

h. It is possible for an MH episode to occur without intense muscle *contractures* if the amount of *myoplasmic calcium* is sufficient to increase metabolic activity but not to elicit detectable contractures.

i. Although *hypercarbia* and *acidosis* may be manifestations of MH, they may also be a consequence of hypoventilation. Similarly, although *elevated CK levels* and *myoglobinuria* may be manifestations of MH, they may also be a consequence of muscle trauma. All of these findings may be likely in an anesthetized patient who is breathing spontaneously with a Bain circuit after a motorbike accident.[1]

j. An otherwise unexplained *postoperative fever* may be associated with MH susceptibility,[42] but is not necessarily a reliable indicator.[1,43] In one report, biopsy specimens from 5 of 28 patients who underwent testing because of apparently isolated postoperative fever developed contractures during exposure to 3% halothane.[42] In another series of 32 probands who presented for muscle biopsy because of postoperative fever, only one had a positive contracture test; he specifically had been told previously that he was "allergic to halothane."[1] The authors of the latter series noted that their concern would be increased if the patient reported prolonged (2–3 days) muscle stiffness and red/brown urine in the immediate postoperative period.[43]

k. The *mechanomyogram* is sensitive to the direct muscle relaxant properties of *dantrolene*.[17,44] In contrast, the *electromyogram* essentially remains normal, as dantrolene does not impede nerve conduction or transmission across the NMJ.

l. It recently has been confirmed *in vivo* that dantrolene decreases myoplasmic Ca^{2+}, especially in MH-susceptible patients. By limiting sarcoplasmic release of Ca^{2+}, it impedes Ca^{2+}-dependent muscle contraction (Table 20-1).[18]

m. In the past, most anesthesiologists elected to "play it safe" and therefore *pretreated the MH-susceptible patient with dantrolene*. Many now believe that such pretreatment is not necessary so long as a nontriggering technique is employed, end-expired CO_2 is monitored, and dantrolene is readily available. The decision not to treat has been prompted in large part by the weakness and gastrointestinal upset that may accompany prophylactic regimens.

n. *Dantrolene* may cause *muscle weakness* and possible respiratory obstruction, especially in the patient with a clinical myopathy. It may also cause thrombophlebitis, gastrointestinal upset, and *increased serum K^+*. According to the North American MH Registry, phlebitis occurred in 9%, gastrointestinal upset in 6%, muscle weakness in 24%, and respiratory failure in 6% of 85 patients who received IV dantrolene to treat a likely MH episode.[29] Prolonged use may cause *cholestasis*. In the context of a *calcium channel blocker* such as verapamil, it may cause marked hypotension.

o. Dantrolene *crosses the placenta*.[31,45–47] Its half-life in the neonate is approximately 20 hours.[31] Nevertheless, it still may be employed relatively safely in the parturient at term,[31,49] and typically it does not affect newborn Apgar scores.[31] Of note, there is evidence that dantrolene may enhance bupivacaine toxicity.[50]

p. The *neuroleptic malignant syndrome* (NMS) is a drug-induced syndrome with signs and symptoms similar to those of MH. It is due to *central dopamine inhibition* (in striatum and frontal limbic systems). Such inhibition is induced by the use of butyrophenones (especially haloperidol), phenothiazines, monoamine oxidase inhibitors, and possibly lithium in NMS-susceptible individuals. Because it is caused by drugs that diminish central dopamine activity, it may also be precipitated by acute discontinuation of levodopa.

NMS is characterized by: rigidity, akinesis, and other extrapyramidal disturbances; agitation; high fevers; rhabdomyolysis; elevated CK levels; acidosis; tachycardia and hypertension; delirium, stupor, and coma; and a 10% mortality.[50–52] Muscle strips from patients with an episode of NMS were more likely to develop halothane-induced contractures in one study[53] but this was not verified in another investigation.[54] Although the signs and symptoms may be similar to those of acute MH, the onset of and recovery from NMS are much slower (usually following a course of several days). It typically begins with dysarthria, with progressive dysfunction over the next 24–72 hours.

The *treatment of NMS* includes discontinuing drugs, treating symptoms and signs, and maintaining urine output. Muscle rigidity may be alleviated with NDRs. However, *dantrolene*[55] may be the drug of choice, because (1) it is most effective if the rigidity is due to contractures (e.g., MH-like), (2) it can reduce muscle tone without paralysis, and (3) it will reduce the fever. The administration of *bromocriptine,* a dopamine receptor agonist, should be considered if the patient still exhibits signs of joint stiffness or CNS changes.[55]

q. SCh may induce a *hyperkalemic response* in the NMS patient with active rhabdomyolysis.[56] However, in patients undergoing electroconvulsive therapy after recovery from NMS, the syndrome or its consequences were not precipitated when SCh was administered.[57]

References

1. Ellis FR, Halsall PJ, Christian AS: Clinical presentation of suspected malignant hyperthermia during anaesthesia in 402 probands. Anaesthesia 45:838–841, 1990
2. Gronert GA, Theye RA: Halothane-induced porcine malignant hyperthermia: metabolic and hemodynamic changes. Anesthesiology 44:36, 1976
3. Gronert GA: Malignant hyperthermia. Anesthesiology 53:395, 1980
4. Gronert GA, Milde JH: Variations in onset of porcine malignant hyperthermia. Anesth Analg 60:499–503, 1981
5. Neubauer KR, Kaufman RD: Another use for mass spectrometry: detection and monitoring of malignant hyperthermia. Anesth Analg 64:837–839, 1985
6. Rutberg H, Hakanson E: Malignant hyperthermia: clinical course and metabolic changes in two patients. Acta Anaesthesiol Scand 30:211–214, 1986
7. Verburg MP, Oerlemans FTJJ, van Bennekom CA, Gielen MJM, deBruyn CHMM, Crul JF: In vivo induced malignant hyperthermia in pigs: I. Physiological and biochemical changes and the influence of dantrolene sodium. Acta Anaesthesiol Scand 28:1–8, 1984
8. Murphy AL, Conlay L, Ryan JF, et al: Malignant hyperthermia during a prolonged anesthetic for reattachment of a limb. Anesthesiology 60:149, 1984
9. Allen GC, Cattran CB, Peterson RG, et al: Plasma levels of dantrolene following oral administration in malignant hyperthermia-susceptible patients. Anesthesiology 69:900–904, 1988
10. Britt BA: Dantrolene. Can Anaesth Soc J 31:61–75, 1984
11. Kolb ME, Horne ML, Martz R: Dantrolene in human malignant hyperthermia. Anesthesiology 56:254–262, 1982
12. Morgan KG, Bryant SH: The mechanism of action of dantrolene sodium. J Pharmacol Exp Ther 201:138–147, 1977
13. Nelson TE, Flewellen EH: Rationale for dantrolene vs. procainamide for treatment of malignant hyperthermia. Anesthesiology 50:118–122, 1979
14. Aldrete JA: Advances in the diagnosis and treatment of malignant hyperthermia. Acta Anaesthesiol Scand 25:477–483, 1981
15. Krarup C: The effect of dantrolene on the enhancement and diminution of tension evoked by staircase and by tetanus in rat muscle. J Physiol 311:389–400, 1981
16. Harrison GG: Dantrolene—dynamics and kinetics. Br J Anaesth 60:279, 1988
17. Nott NW, Bowman WC: Actions of dantrolene sodium on contractions of the tibialis anterior and soleus muscles of cats under chloralose anaesthesia. Clin Exp Pharmacol Physiol 1:113–122, 1974
18. Lopez JR, Gerardi A, Lopez MJ, Allen PD: Effects of dantrolene on myoplasmic free [Ca^{2+}] measured in vivo in patients susceptible to malignant hyperthermia. Anesthesiology 76:711–719, 1992
19. Flewellen EH, Nelson TE, Jones WP, Arens JF, Wagner DL: Dantrolene dose-response in awake man: implications for management of malignant hyperthermia. Anesthesiology 59:275–280, 1983
20. Watson CB, Reierson N, Norfleet EA: Clinically significant muscle weakness induced by oral dantrolene sodium prophylaxis for malignant hyperthermia. Anesthesiology 65:312–314, 1986
21. Driessen JJ, Wuis EW, Gieden JM: Prolonged vecuronium neuromuscular blockade in a patient receiving oral dantrolene. Anesthesiology 62:523–524, 1985
22. Austin KL, Denborough MA: Drug treatment of malignant hyperpyrexia. Anaesth Intensive Care 5:207–213, 1977
23. Laurence AS, McKean JF: Dantrolene and suxamethonium: myalgia, biochemical changes and serum dantrolene levels following oral dantrolene pre-treatment in laparoscopy patients. Eur J Anaesthesiol 7:493–500, 1990
24. Asari H, Inoue K, Maruta H, Hirose Y: The inhibitory effect of intravenous d-tubocurarine and oral dantrolene on halothane-succinylcholine-induced myoglobinemia in children. Anesthesiology 61:332–333, 1984
25. Watson CB, Norfleet EA: Dantrolene prophylaxis and neuromuscular disorders. Anesthesiology 66:702–703, 1987
26. Derkay CS, Grundfast KM: Management of otolaryngic patients susceptible to malignant hyperthermia without dantrolene. Otolaryngol Head Neck Surg 105:680–686, 1991

27. Hackl W, Mauritz W, Winkler M, Sporn P, Steinbereithner K: Anaesthesia in malignant hyperthermia-susceptible patients without dantrolene prophylaxis: a report of 30 cases. Acta Anaesthesiol Scand 34:534–537, 1990
28. Ording H, Hedengran AM, Skovgaard LT: Evaluation of 119 anaesthetics received after investigation for susceptibility to malignant hyperthermia. Acta Anaesthesiol Scand 35:711–716, 1991
29. Larach MG, Simon LJ, Allen GC: Safety and efficacy of dantrolene sodium for the treatment of malignant hyperthermia events. Anesthesiology 79:A1079, 1993
30. Beebe DS, Belani KG, Tuohy SE, Sweeney MF, Gillingham K, Komanduri V, Palahniuk RJ: Is dantrolene safe to administer in sepsis? The effect of dantrolene after endotoxin administration in dogs and rats. Anesth Analg 73:289–294, 1991
31. Shime J, Gare D, Andrews J, Britt B: Dantrolene in pregnancy: lack of adverse effects on the fetus and newborn infant. Am J Obstet Gynecol 159:831, 1988
32. Moulds RFW, Denborough MA: Procaine in malignant hyperpyrexia. Br Med J 4:526–528, 1972
33. Carter JC, Gergis SD, Carter A, et al: The caffeine-halothane challenge test and calcium blockers. Anesthesiology 59:A226, 1983
34. Durbin CG, Fisher NA, Lynch C III: Cardiovascular effects in dogs of intravenous dantrolene alone and in the presence of verapamil. Anesthesiology 59:A227, 1983
35. Gallant EM, Foldes FF, Rempel WE, et al: Verapamil is not a therapeutic adjunct to dantrolene in porcine malignant hyperthermia. Anesth Analg 64:601–606, 1985
36. Gronert GA, Ahern CP, Milde JH, et al: Effect of CO_2, calcium, digoxin, and potassium on cardiac and skeletal muscle metabolism in malignant hyperthermia susceptible swine. Anesthesiology 64:24, 1986
37. Rubin AS, Zablocki AD: Hyperkalemia, verapamil and dantrolene. Anesthesiology 66:246, 1987
38. Hall GM, Lucke JN, Orchard C, Lovell R, Lister D: Porcine malignant hyperthermia: VIII. Leg metabolism. Br J Anaesth 54:941–947, 1982
39. Fletcher R, Blennow G, Olsson AK, et al: Malignant hyperthermia in a myopathic child: prolonged postoperative course requiring dantrolene. Acta Anaesthesiol Scand 26:431, 1982
40. Lerman J, McLeod ME, Strong HA: Pharmacokinetics of intravenous dantrolene in children. Anesthesiology 70:625, 1989
41. Hackl W, Mauritz W, Schemper M, Winkler M, Sporn P, Steinbereithner K: Prediction of malignant hyperthermia susceptibility: statistical evaluation of clinical signs. Br J Anaesth 64:425–429, 1990
42. Allen GC, Larach MG: Does postoperative fever predict susceptibility to malignant hyperthermia (MH)? Anesthesiology 79:A1078, 1993
43. Halsall PJ, Ellis FR: Does postoperative pyrexia indicate malignant hyperthermia susceptibility? Br J Anaesth 68:209–210, 1992
44. Lee C, Katz RL: Neuromuscular pharmacology: a clinical update and commentary. Br J Anaesth 52:173–188, 1980
45. Glassenberg R, Cohen H: Intravenous dantrolene in a pregnant malignant hyperthermia susceptible (MHS) patient. Anesthesiology 51:A404, 1984
46. Morrison DH: Placental transfer of dantrolene. Anesthesiology 59:265, 1983
47. Weingarten AE, Korsh JI, Neuman GC, et al: Postpartum uterine atony after intravenous dantrolene. Anesth Analg 66:269–270, 1987
48. Douglas MJ, McMorland GH: The anaesthetic management of the malignant hyperthermia susceptible parturient. Can Anaesth Soc J 33:371–378, 1986
49. Rosenblatt R, Tallman RD, Weaver J, Wang Y: Dantrolene potentiates the toxicity of bupivacaine. Anesthesiology 61:A209, 1984
50. Caroff SN: The neuroleptic malignant syndrome. J Clin Psychiatry 41:679, 1980
51. Guze BH, Baxter LR: Neuroleptic malignant syndrome. N Engl J Med 313:163–166, 1985
52. Weinberg S, Twersky RS: Neuroleptic malignant syndrome. Anesth Analg 62:845–880, 1983
53. Caroff SN, Rosenberg H, Fletcher JE, et al: Malignant hyperthermia susceptibility in neuroleptic malignant syndrome. Anesthesiology 67:20, 1987
54. Adnet PJ, Krivosic-Horber RM, Adamantidis MM, Haudecoeur G, Adnet-Bonte CA,

Saulnier F, Dupuis BA: The association between neuroleptic malignant syndrome and malignant hyperthermia. Acta Anaesthesiol Scand 33:676–680, 1989
55. Granato JR, Stern BJ, Ringel A, et al: Neuroleptic malignant syndrome: successful treatment with dantrolene and bromocriptine. Ann Neurol 14:89, 1983
56. George AL Jr, Wood CA Jr: Succinylcholine-induced hyperkalemia complicating the neuroleptic malignant syndrome (letter). Ann Intern Med 106:172, 1987
57. Addonizio G, Susman VL: ECT as a treatment alternative for patients with symptoms of neuroleptic malignant syndrome. J Clin Psychiatry 48:102, 1987

21

DAVID G. SILVERMAN

Myasthenia Gravis and the Myasthenic Syndrome

◆ MYASTHENIA GRAVIS

Myasthenia gravis (MG) causes a *fluctuating weakness* that may be limited to the eyes but also may be more widespread and involve the bulbar and ventilatory muscles (often the cranial nerves of the oropharynx). It is characterized by *decreased acetylcholine (ACh) receptors*,[1-5] possibly owing to autoimmune lysis by circulating antibodies.[2,3,6,7] ACh receptor destruction may occur presynaptically as well as postsynaptically. The antibody-induced block or destruction is sufficient to reduce miniature end-plate potentials to a degree that is sufficient to cause *rate-related failure of neuromuscular transmission*.[2,8,9]

Myasthenia gravis is characterized by *decreased twitch response and fade* during rapid stimulation (e.g., at ≥3 Hz),[10] *particularly after exercise*.[11] The mechanogram may be more sensitive than the electromyogram, suggesting a possible concomitant effect on contractility.[10] Although presynaptic activity is not necessarily normal,[11] the amount of ACh release does not appear to be decreased.[12]

Myasthenia gravis may be aggravated by pulmonary infections, sedation, anesthesia (especially with general anesthetics with relaxant properties), and surgery. It typically is associated with *thymomas*, rheumatoid arthritis, lupus, hypothyroidism, pernicious anemia, myocarditis, and polymyositis. The thymus gland is involved in the majority of cases, and thymectomy may be helpful.[13] However, the benefits may not be evident immediately postoperatively.[13] Myasthenia gravis often is associated with *cardiovascular dysfunction*, with focal myocarditis and dysrhythmias.[14]

The patient with MG typically receives *pyridostigmine (Mestinon)*,[15] usually given in a dose of 60 mg orally every 6 hours. Its effect reaches a peak at about 2 hours and lasts about 4 hours, and it accumulates with repeated doses. The intravenous (IV) equivalent is 1/30th to 1/60th of the total daily oral dose in divided doses. The equivalent doses of neostigmine are approximately 0.5 mg IV or 0.7–1.0 mg IM. Be aware that cholinergic crisis is possible. Patients may also be taking steroids and azathioprine for immunosuppression. *Steroids* may facilitate spontaneous release of ACh as well as decrease the amplitude of miniature end-plate potentials; *azathioprine* may alter the effects of nondepolarizing agents (Chap. 9).

It may be safest to perform a *regional anesthetic technique* in the patient with MG. However, high doses of *ester-type local anesthetics* may exacerbate MG, perhaps because they are metabolized by cholinesterases. In addition to avoiding neuromuscular blocking agents, a successful regional technique avoids inhalational agents, which may have increased neuromuscular effects in the patient with MG.[16]

As expected, the patient with MG is *extremely sensitive to nondepolarizing agents* (NDRs).[17-30] This sensitivity is most evident in the presence of volatile anesthetics, antiarrhythmics, antibiotics, and other agents that may affect neuromuscular function (Chap. 9).[16,31,32] Patients in whom MG is well-controlled or in apparent remission exhibit a wide range of sensitivities,[33,34] including relatively normal responses. NDR sensitivity can be quantified with the *curare test*. After the forearm is isolated with a tourniquet, a very small dose of NDR (e.g., 1% of the ED_{95}) is given IV. In the classic test, the tourniquet is released at 4–5 minutes, and trains of stimuli are applied 1, 11, and 21 minutes after the release; MG is characterized by pronounced persistent fade and decreased grip strength.[18] One can titrate relaxant according to this test or start with 1–10% of the generally recommended dose and increase the dosage as tolerated. The diagnosis of MG can also be aided by the *Tensilon test:* the patient with MG shows clear improvement after IV administration of 2–10 mg of edrophonium (Tensilon). It might be best to avoid this test during pregnancy, as it theoretically may promote stimulation of uterine cholinergic receptors and precipitate premature labor.

Doses of NDR for the patient with MG typically begin as low as 0.03 mg · kg^{-1} for *d*-tubocurarine and 0.005 mg · kg^{-1} for pancuronium. As little as 2 mg of tubocurarine may produce a clinical block.[30] Atracurium[19-25] and vecuronium[17,26,27] have been used successfully. The former may be preferable: 25% of the normal atracurium dose has been used for intraoperative paralysis, with only slight prolongation of the RI_{25-75} recovery index (from 12 minutes to 17 minutes).[25] It has been recommended that vecuronium be titrated by administering 0.005 mg · kg^{-1} increments[26]; there is a wide range of prolongation of vecuronium-induced block (up to 700%).[17]

The effects of depolarizing agents also are affected by MG, but to a lesser degree than the effects of NDRs.[30] *Succinylcholine* (SCh) may be given as a bolus[28] or infusion[29] in the patient with MG. There often is decreased sensitivity to SCh[30,35-37] or decamethonium,[36,38] with the sensivity varying among the muscles of a given patient. In patients with MG in whom anticholinesterase therapy was withheld on the morning of surgery, SCh, 1 mg · kg^{-1}, provided an adequate depolarizing block that was slightly delayed, to 81 seconds (range, 54–138 seconds), compared to 56 seconds (range, 34–82 seconds) in controls.[37] Resistance is most evident after relatively low doses (e.g., 0.5 mg · kg^{-1}).[37] The *dose-response curve is shifted to the right,* and the ED$_{50}$, ED$_{90}$, and ED$_{95}$ for SCh are 2–2.6 times higher than in normals (when a cumulative dose and infusion technique are used[35]). Such findings have led to the recommendation that at least 1.5–2.0 mg · kg^{-1} be administered to produce rapid onset of paralysis.[35] The increased requirements may be most pronounced in apparently uninvolved muscles. There is also an increased tendency toward SCh-induced phase 2 block.[28–30,35–39] There does not appear to be an increased tendency toward hyperkalemia or malignant hyperthermia. In contrast to the decreased sensitivity to SCh that characterizes MG, an increased and prolonged response to SCh may occur if there is a *residual effect of the anticholinesterase therapy* used to treat the disorder[40] or if pseudocholinesterase levels are reduced to less than 20% of normal as a result of plasma exchange.[41–44] When all of these factors are taken into account, "the use of succinylcholine in patients with myasthenia gravis has generally been without incident."[35]

◆ MYASTHENIC SYNDROME

The myasthenic syndrome (commonly referred to as the *Eaton-Lambert myasthenic syndrome, ELMS*) is another immune-mediated disorder of the NMJ.[7,8,45] In contrast to MG, ELMS is characterized by a *prejunctional defect* of the presynaptic Ca^{2+} channels.[7,45–48] The associated decrease in ACh release *(decreased number of quanta)* causes failure of neuromuscular transmission,[12] similar to the effects of elevated Mg^{2+}, botulism, and perhaps neomycin.[46] The size of each ACh quantum, the postsynaptic ACh receptor number, ACh receptor sensitivity, and the miniature end-plate potential evoked by each quantum essentially are normal.[45,46]

In contrast to MG, *ELMS improves with rapid stimulation and exercise.*[8] It affects proximal muscles (e.g., pelvic girdle muscles) first, and it is associated with *pronounced sensitivity to SCh.* Admittedly, the increase in strength on exertion is transient and may be followed by fatigue. Both disorders are characterized by *increased sensitivity to NDRs.* ELMS is not helped by anticholinesterases to the same extent as MG is[8,46]; it is more likely to be helped by drugs that increase ACh release (guanidine and 4-aminopyridine).[49–51] The syndrome typically is associated with oat cell (and other small cell) carcinoma, the classic *Eaton-Lambert syndrome,*[46] and may be associated with other disorders such as amyotrophic lateral sclerosis.[52]

◆ VON RECKLINGHAUSEN'S DISEASE

Patients with *von Recklinghausen's disease* (neurofibromatosis) may exhibit mixed features of the above-mentioned disorders. They have an increased sensitivity to nondepolarizing agents that *resembles* MG more than ELMS.[53] They may be resistant to SCh[53] or overly sensitive.[54,55]

Discussion Questions ◆

a. The patient with *myasthenia gravis* may have decreased ability to generate neostigmine-induced postactivation repetition. What does this suggest about *motor neuron function?*
b. What factors might dissuade you from *extubating the trachea* of a patient with *MG* at the conclusion of a *thymectomy?*
c. Why might one wish to exercise extra caution with *beta blockers* in the patient with *MG?*
d. How does recent *plasmapheresis* affect the subsequent anesthetic management of the patient with MG?
e. Is it safe to use an *ester-type local anesthetic* for spinal anesthesia in the patient with MG? Why or why not?
f. Outline a *management plan* for anesthetizing the patient with *MG for a thymectomy*, taking into account that thymectomy may alleviate some of the symptoms of MG.
g. Compare the responses to *relaxants* in patients with *MG and myasthenic syndrome.*
h. Describe the *electromyogram* in the patient with *MG.*
i. How do *electromyogram* responses differ in the *myasthenic syndrome* and MG?

Answers ◆

a. In addition to the postsynaptic component, MG may also have a presynaptic component; the decreased ability to generate neostigmine-induced *postactivity repetition* (described in Chap. 15) suggests nerve dysfunction.[56] Because the nerve itself can transmit nerve impulse trains of 200 Hz, the presynaptic component of MG probably is limited to the presynaptic terminal (perhaps presynaptic cholinoceptors).[56]
b. In addition to patient strength and ability to protect the airway, factors to consider *prior to tracheal extubation* include the *type of incision* (sternal vs. transcervical),[57] any underlying pulmonary disease, abnormal airway anatomy, possible nerve damage secondary to surgery, high metabolic needs (oxygen requirements), altered fluid and electrolyte status, cardiovascular dysfunction, and obesity. Discriminant analysis identified four *preoperative factors* in patients undergoing thymectomy via a *sternal incision*. In order of decreasing importance, these factors were (1) duration of MG longer than 6 years, (2) the presence of respiratory disease, (3) a pyridostigmine requirement greater than 750 mg/day, and (4) a vital capacity less than 2.9 L.[58] In contrast, after the

transcervical approach only eight of 23 patients with the above-mentioned preoperative criteria for postoperative ventilatory support required mechanical ventilation.[57]

c. *Beta blockers* and related antiarrhythmic agents can augment neuromuscular block and may thereby worsen MG (Chap. 9).[32] Beta blockers can also potentiate the cholinergic effects of anticholinesterase therapy and may exacerbate conduction abnormalities.

d. *Plasmapheresis* may alleviate symptoms in the patient with poorly controlled MG.[59] It is important to check *electrolyte levels* afterward and to be aware that, although they are replaced, *clotting factors* may be altered. Plasmapheresis can markedly decrease *plasma cholinesterase levels* and thereby cause prolongation of SCh-induced (and perhaps mivacurium-induced) block.[49-52] In addition, plasmapheresis may decrease the plasma levels of certain *medications*.

e. High doses of *ester-type local anesthetics* may exacerbate MG, perhaps because these anesthetics are metabolized by cholinesterases. However, the low doses used for spinal anesthesia are safe.

f. The following are reasonable steps to take in the patient with MG who is *undergoing thymectomy:*

   1. *Discontinue anticholinesterases* the night prior to surgery if tolerable to the patient (i.e., unless discontinuation would lead to profound weakness with dyspnea and difficulty swallowing). Anticholinesterases interfere with the use of nondepolarizing and depolarizing relaxants intraoperatively and may be excessive if surgery proves to be helpful. If preoperative weakness is encountered or anticipated, then continue anticholinesterase therapy until the morning of surgery.
   2. Provide *steroids* (if the patient has been receiving them).
   3. Use relaxant judiciously. Succinylcholine, 1.5–2.0 mg · kg^{-1}, may be used to facilitate tracheal intubation, but infusion may lead to phase 2 block. If NDRs are indicated, titrate the dose to neuromuscular response with the aid of a nerve stimulator. Try to avoid long-lasting agents.
   4. *Extubate* the trachea once adequate strength (with ability to protect the airway and sustain adequate ventilation) is confirmed. Err on the side of conservatism.
   5. *Restart anticholinesterase* at one-half or less of the preoperative dosage. Monitor ventilation. Supplement anticholinesterase therapy as indicated with edrophonium until effective titration has been accomplished. Remember that reversal is not totally benign (Chap. 15): prolonged depolarizing block has been documented after reversal of vecuronium with 3 mg of neostigmine.[60]
   6. Consider *plasmapheresis*[59] to remove immune factor if there is marked exacerbation postoperatively. The improvement often begins within a few days of initiating the exchange and continues for several days.[59]

g. The *Eaton-Lambert myasthenic syndrome* increases sensitivity to both *depolarizing and nondepolarizing muscle relaxants*. MG increases sensitivity to NDRs and causes an inconsistent response to depolarizing agents; phase 2 block commonly develops.

h. The *electromyogram in MG reveals* fade by the second stimulus when testing is at ≥3 Hz; by the fifth stimulus at 3 Hz, the response may be reduced to 10%.[11] A *progressive decrement in the amplitude* of the compound muscle action potential has also been noted with myotonia, poliomyelitis, amyotrophic lateral sclerosis, polyneuropathies, polymyositis, and McArdle's syndrome.[11]

i. *Electromyographic findings* differ between MG and the Eaton-Lambert myasthenic syndrome: (1) the response to a single stimulus is relatively normal in MG, while the amplitude of the action potential is severely decreased in ELMS; and (2) whereas exercise causes progressive fade in MG, it first causes fade but then causes strengthening that temporarily persists after stimulation (i.e., facilitation) in ELMS.

References ◆

1. Cull-Candy SG, Miledi R, Trautman A: End-plate currents and acetylcholine noise at normal and myasthenic human end-plates. J Physiol (Lond) 287:247–265, 1979
2. Drachman DB: Myasthenia gravis (Part 1). N Engl J Med 298:136–142, 186–193, 1978
3. Drachman DB, Kao I, Pestronk A, Toyka KV: Myasthenia gravis as a receptor disorder. Ann NY Acad Sci 274:226–234, 1976
4. Fambrough DM, Drachman DB, Satyamurti S: Neuromuscular junction in myasthenia gravis: decreased acetylcholine receptors. Science 182:293–295, 1973
5. Vincent A, Newsom-Davis J: Alpha bungarotoxin and anti-acetylcholine receptor antibody binding to the human acetylcholine receptor. In Ceccarelli B, Clementi F (eds): Advances in Pharmacology. New York, Raven Press, 1979, pp 269–278
6. Vincent A: Neuroimmunology of myasthenia gravis. Brain Behav Immun 2:346–351, 1988
7. Zweiman B, Arnason BG: Immunologic aspects of neurological and neuromuscular diseases. JAMA 258:2970–2973, 1987
8. Engel AG: Myasthenia gravis and myasthenic syndromes. Ann Neurol 16:519–534, 1984
9. Ito Y, Miledi R, Vincent A, Newsom-Davis J: Acetylcholine receptors and end-plate electrophysiology in myasthenia gravis. Brain 101:345–368, 1978
10. Botelho SY: Comparison of simultaneously recorded electrical and mechanical activity in myasthenia gravis patients and in partially curarized normal humans. Am J Med 19:693–696, 1955
11. Ozdemir C, Young RR: The results to be expected from electrical testing in the diagnosis of myasthenia gravis. Ann NY Acad Sci 274:203–222, 1976
12. Cull-Candy SG, Miledi R, Trautmann A, Uchitel OD: On the release of transmitter at normal, myasthenia gravis and myasthenic syndrome affected human end-plates. J Physiol (Lond) 299:621–638, 1980
13. Scadding GK, Thomas HC, Havard CWH: Myasthenia gravis: acetylcholine-receptor antibody titres after thymectomy. Br Med J 1:1512, 1977
14. Hofstad H, Ohm O, Mork SJ, et al: Heart disease in myasthenia gravis. Acta Neurol Scand 70:176, 1984
15. Flacke W: Treatment of myasthenia gravis. N Engl J Med 288:27–31, 1973
16. Eisenkraft JB, Papatestas AE, Sivak M: Neuromuscular effects of halogenated agents in patients with myasthenia gravis. Anesthesiology 61:A307, 1984

17. Buzello W, Noeldge G, Krieg N, Brobmann GF: Vecuronium for muscle relaxation in patients with myasthenia gravis. Anesthesiology 64:507–509, 1986
18. Brown JC, Charlton JE: A study of sensitivity to curare in myasthenic disorders using a regional technique. J Neurol Neurosurg Psychiatry 38:27–33, 1975
19. Ward S, Wright DJ: Neuromuscular blockade in myasthenia gravis with atracurium besylate. Anaesthesia 39:51–53, 1984
20. Baraka A: Atracurium in myasthenics undergoing thymectomy. Anesth Analg 63:1127–1130, 1984
21. Bell CF, Florence AM, Hunter JM, et al: Atracurium in the myasthenic patient. Anaesthesia 39:961–968, 1984
22. MacDonald AM, Keen RI, Pugh ND: Myasthenia gravis and atracurium. Br J Anaesth 56:651–654, 1984
23. Vacanti CA, Ali HH, Schweiss JF, et al: The response of myasthenia gravis to atracurium. Anesthesiology 62:692–694, 1985
24. Greene SJ, Shanks CA, Ronai AK, Ramseur A: Atracurium-induced neuromuscular blockade in five myasthenic patients. Anesth Analg 64:221, 1985
25. Ramsey FM, Smith GD: Clinical use of atracurium in myasthenia gravis: a case report. Can Anaesth Soc J 32:642–645, 1985
26. Eisenkraft JB, Book WJ, Papatestas AE: Sensitivity to vecuronium in myasthenia gravis: a dose-response study. Can J Anaesth 37:301–306, 1990
27. Nilsson E, Meretoja OA: Vecuronium dose-response and maintenance requirements in patients with myasthenia gravis. Anesthesiology 73:28–32, 1990
28. Azar I: The response of patients with neuromuscular disorders to muscle relaxants: a review. Anesthesiology 61:173–187, 1984
29. Ginsberg H, Varejes L: The use of a relaxant in myasthenia gravis. Anaesthesia 10:177–178, 1955
30. Foldes FF, McNall PG: Myasthenia gravis: a guide for anesthesiologists. Anesthesiology 23:837–872, 1962
31. Bennett EJ, Schmidt GB, Patel KP, Grundy EM: Muscle relaxants, myasthenia, and mustards? Anesthesiology 46:220–221, 1977
32. Weisman SJ: Masked myasthenia gravis. JAMA 141:917–920, 1949
33. Lake CL: Curare sensitivity in steroid-treated myasthenia gravis: a case report. Anesth Analg 57:132, 1978
34. Fillmore RB, Herren AL, Pirlo AF: Curare sensitivity in myasthenia gravis (letter). Anesth Analg 57:515, 1978
35. Eisenkraft JB, Book WJ, Mann SM, Papatestas AE: Resistance to succinylcholine in myasthenia gravis: a dose-response study. Anesthesiology 69:760–763, 1988
36. Johnson BR, Kim YI, Sanders DB: Neuromuscular blocking properties of suxamethonium and decamethonium in normal and myasthenic rat muscle. J Neurol Sci 59:431–440, 1983
37. Wainwright AP, Brodrick PM: Suxamethonium in myasthenia gravis. Anaesthesia 42:950–957, 1987
38. Churchill-Davidson HC, Richardson AT: Neuromuscular transmission in myasthenia gravis. J Physiol 122:252–263, 1953
39. Churchill-Davidson HC: Abnormal response to muscle relaxants (condensed). Proc R Soc Med 48:621–624, 1955
40. Abel M, Eisenkraft JB, Patel N: Response to suxamethonium in a myasthenic patient during remission. Anaesthesia 46:30, 1991
41. Dau PC, Lindstrom JM, Cassel CK, Denys EH, Shev EE, Spitler LE: Plasmapheresis and immunosuppressive drug therapy in myasthenia gravis. N Engl J Med 297:1134–1140, 1977
42. Lumley J: Prolongation of suxamethonium following plasma exchange. Br J Anaesth 52:1149–1150, 1980
43. Wood GJ, Hall GM: Plasmapheresis and plasma cholinesterase. Br J Anaesth 50:945–949, 1978
44. Patterson JL, Walsh ES, Hall GM: Progressive depletion of plasma cholinesterase during daily plasma exchange. Br Med J 2:580, 1979
45. Vincent A, Lang B, Newsom-Davis J: Autoimmunity to the voltage-gated calcium channel underlies the Lambert-Eaton myasthenic syndrome, a paraneoplastic disorder. Trends Neurosci 12:496–502, 1989

46. Elmqvist D, Lambert EH: Detailed analysis of neuromuscular transmission in a patient with the myasthenic syndrome sometimes associated with bronchogenic carcinoma. Mayo Clin Proc 43:689–713, 1968
47. Lang B, Newsom Davis J, Peers C, Prior C, Wray D: The effect of myasthenic syndrome antibody on presynaptic calcium channels in the mouse. J Physiol 390:257–270, 1987
48. Peers C, Lang B, Newson-Davis J, Wray DW: Selective action of myasthenic syndrome antibodies on calcium channels in a rodent neuroblastoma x glioma cell line. J Physiol 421:293–308, 1990
49. Agoston S, van Weerden T, Westra P, Broekert A: Effects of 4-aminopyridine in Eaton Lambert syndrome. Br J Anaesth 50:383–385, 1978
50. Oh SJ, Kim KW: Guanidine hydrochloride in the Eaton-Lambert syndrome (electrophysiologic improvement). Neurology 23:1084–1090, 1973
51. Telford RJ, Hollway TE: The myasthenic syndrome: anaesthesia in a patient treated with 3 • 4 diaminopyridine. Br J Anaesth 64:363–366, 1990
52. Mulder DW, Lambert EH, Eaton LM: Myasthenic syndrome in patients with amyotrophic lateral sclerosis. Neurology 9:627–631, 1959
53. Baraka A: Myasthenic response to muscle relaxants in von Recklinghausen's disease. Br J Anaesth 46:701–703, 1974
54. Magbagbeola JAO: Abnormal responses to muscle relaxant in a patient with von Recklinghausen's disease (multiple neurofibromatosis) (letter). Br J Anaesth 42:710, 1970
55. Manser J: Abnormal responses in von Recklinghausen's disease (letter). Br J Anaesth 42:183, 1970
56. Roe RD, Riker WF, Standaert FG: Motor nerve ending disorder in myasthenia gravis. Neurology 38:293–297, 1988
57. Eisenkraft JB, Papatestas AE, Kahn CH, et al: Predicting the need for postoperative mechanical ventilation in myasthenia gravis. Anesthesiology 65:79–82, 1986
58. Leventhal S, Orkin FK, Hirsh RA: Prediction of the need for postoperative mechanical ventilation in myasthenia gravis. Anesthesiology 53:26–30, 1980
59. Pinching AJ, Peters DK, Newsom Davis J: Remission of myasthenia gravis following plasma exchange. Lancet 2:1373–1376, 1976
60. Kim J-M, Mangold J: Sensitivity to both vecuronium and neostigmine in a sero-negative myasthenic patient. Br J Anaesth 63:497–500, 1982

22   DAVID G. SILVERMAN

Nerve Injury, Burns, and Trauma

◆ OVERVIEW OF ACETYLCHOLINE RECEPTOR PROLIFERATION

It may be best to view the neuromuscular response to injury, burns, and trauma in terms of (1) the *degree* of acetylcholine receptor (AChR) proliferation, (2) the *location* of AChR proliferation (intra- vs. extrajunctional), and (3) the *nature* of the AChRs (normal receptors vs. immature receptors).

The location, degree, and nature of change at the muscle membrane are highly dependent on the severity and duration of the insult. Typically, a decrease in ACh release (or prolonged AChR inhibition) initially results in *increased AChR density at the end-plate.*[1-11] This probably is a consequence of AChR proliferation, but it may simply be due to end-plate contraction. The increase in density is not necessarily indicative of major injury. It may be noted after several days of inactivity of a limb,[10-14] or as a consequence of decreased ACh release after chronic diphenylhydantoin therapy[1,6,15] or long-term infusion of a nondepolarizing relaxant (NDR)[1,2,4,16] or local anesthetic[17,18] (Chap. 9).

After *severe injuries* (e.g., denervation, major burn, major trauma), there not only is proliferation of normal AChRs within the end-plate but also a change in the *nature and location of new "extrajunctional" receptors (EJRs)*[19-32] as the neural trophic influences are lost[9,19,24-26] and muscle activity declines.[23,27,28] Although normal receptors contain two alpha, one beta, one delta, and one *epsilon* subunit, EJRs contain two alpha, one beta, one *gamma,* and one delta subunit.[27,30-33] EJRs have markedly increased sensitivity to ACh and dicholines,[19-21,26,34-39] with altered single-channel conductance and prolonged channel opening.[8,31,36-39] In addition, as they proliferate extrajunctionally along the muscle surface, EJRs allow *muscle depolarization without the modulating influence of the insulating rim of dual-gated Na^+ channels that surround the end-plate* (question h in Chap. 2).

The findings are not clear-cut, however. Denervation does not necessarily lead to cessation of all production of normal AChRs.[40-42] The synthesis of normal AChRs will increase if the muscle is innervated, reinnervated, or stimulated frequently.[9,23,25, 27-39,33,37,40,41,43]

◆ ACETYLCHOLINE RECEPTOR PROLIFERATION AND MUSCLE RELAXANTS

The proliferation of AChRs at the end-plate causes increased sensitivity to ACh. Proliferation of EJRs causes increased and even life-threatening sensitivity to depolarizing agents such as SCh and decreased effectiveness of NDRs.[1–10,12–14,20,26,34–36,44–82]

Of greatest potential significance to the anesthesiologist is the EJR-induced potential for *hyperkalemia and contractures after SCh administration.*[10,20,26,34,35,45–50,53–73] In denervated skeletal muscle with EJR proliferation, the increased sensitivity and prolonged response to SCh as well as the diffuse chemosensitivity of the denervated muscle membrane may lead to (1) a mass depolarization with a burst of muscle action potentials (MAPs), (2) diffusely increased membrane permeability to Na^+ and K^+, with an increase in Na^+-K^+ exchange, (3) increased oxygen consumption, and (4) contractures. The latter results from direct stimulation of the muscle membrane by SCh without modulation by dual-gated Na^+ channels between contractions (more aptly termed *contracture* in this setting). This exaggerated response to SCh typically is not preceded by increased SGOT or CPK levels[56] or microscopic evidence of membrane disruption,[83] although such evidence of rhabdomyolysis may result from SCh administration.

The exaggerated *response to SCh* is dose related, and its magnitude may be lessened but not necessarily eliminated by using a smaller dose. It may be prevented by first inducing total paralysis with a large dose of an NDR.[73] However, a small (defasciculating) dose of an NDR does not reliably provide protection against SCh-induced hyperkalemia in these settings. This may be attributable in part to hyposensitivity to NDRs as well as hypersensitivity to SCh.

Several disorders have been associated, to varying degrees, with a propensity for SCh-induced hyperkalemia and/or contractures. The effects of denervation, diffuse neuronal injury, prolonged immobility, intracranial disorders, burns, and trauma are discussed below. Muscle disorders are discussed in Chapter 23.

It has been reported that AChR proliferation may account for approximately 70% of the increase in ED_{95} of an NDR after a lower motor neuron injury.[5] Potential mechanisms include (1) the increase in absolute number and/or density of junctional receptors, which increases the margin of safety postsynaptically[5–7] before competitive block can be achieved; and, more importantly, (2) proliferation of extrajunctional receptors, which provide a "sink" that binds NDR molecules, while being markedly less susceptible to antagonism by NDRs[8,44,51,52,74] and decidedly more responsive to ACh and dicholines such as SCh.[16,19–21,26,34–39]

In addition, the insults that alter AChR density may be associated with increased plasma concentrations of alpha$_1$-acid glycoprotein (Chap. 10).

Binding to this protein decreases the free fraction of relaxant[6] and hence its availability. (This has been shown to contribute to the decreased response to NDRs during chronic phenytoin therapy[1,6,84] and following extensive trauma and burns[1,6,85] [Chap. 10].) Finally, injuries to the nerve and junction may cause decreased acetylcholinesterase activity, which allows ACh to compete more effectively with an NDR.

◆ DENERVATION

As suggested above, *lower and upper motor denervation* both may lead to EJR proliferation with extrajunctional chemosensitivity and SCh-induced hyperkalemia and/or contractures.

Lower motor neuron destruction (e.g., single extremity paralysis or brachial plexus injury) causes Wallerian degeneration and AChR proliferation within a few hours. EJR proliferation typically predisposes to SCh-induced hyperkalemia and contractures in 3–8 days; these effects peak at 14 days.[1,34,55,60] The duration of the danger period has not been well documented but typically lasts for at least several months. Following systemic *administration of SCh,* the venous blood from a denervated extremity typically has an increase in K$^+$ concentration that is approximately 4–7 mEq · L^{-1} above the normal increase of 0.5 mEq · L^{-1}.[55,60] Even the intact limb may be prone to slightly increased K$^+$ release (approximately 1.5 mEq · L^{-1}).[55]

The effect of lower motor denervation on the *response to NDRs* is less clear-cut. As noted earlier, denervation-induced EJR proliferation should lead to increased requirements for NDRs; however, other factors, such as loss of facilitatory input to the NMJ, may predominate. Thus, the response is not always predictable.

Following *upper motor neuron destruction,* as in a stroke or cord transection, the risk of SCh-induced hyperkalemia may be attributable to the subsequent effects on lower motor neurons.[86-88] The resultant *lower neuron damage* is evidenced by fibrillation potentials, fewer single fiber motor units, positive sharp waves, and decreased electromyographic (EMG) conduction.[87-89] Extrajunctional chemosensitivity (i.e., *EJR proliferation*) is evident. The risk of *SCh-induced hyperkalemia* is time dependent[90]; the onset tends to be slightly slower than after direct lower motor neuron injury. It is prominent by the time *spasticity* has appeared, and reaches a peak in *10–21 days.* Serial EMGs after a stroke showed that fibrillation and sharp waves first appeared during the second week and peaked in 3–10 weeks.[86] The high risk probably persists as long as evidence of progressive dysfunction is present; it is especially marked in the first 6 months.[46,47,60] The risk is less clear-cut after return of some function.[86] Modest increases in EJRs have been noted 3 years after a spinal cord injury.[91] In a series of patients monitored after stroke, denervation activity on the EMG decreased as spasticity and volitional activity increased, presumably due to reestablishment of trophic influences. In some patients, however, denervation activity persisted for the entire 1-year study period.[86]

After a *stroke,* the functioning muscles on the paralyzed side typically exhibit increased *dose requirements for NDRs.*[75-79,92,93] This increased need may be attributable to the AChR proliferation described earlier, as well as to axonal sprouting[93] and destruction of central inhibitory pathways (which primarily inhibit nerve-to-muscle conduction).[92] With the regional curare test (described for myasthenia gravis in Chap. 21), the relative resistance to tubocurarine was evident in as little as 3 days or as long as 5 years after a stroke had occurred.[92] This is most common when the weakness that accompanies a stroke predominates. However, when hyperreflexia and hypertonia predominate (due to interruption of central inhibitory pathways), there may be an exaggerated response to NDRs.[92]

In addition to the changes on the paralyzed side, the *opposite side* may also evince "hyposensitivity" (albeit far less) to NDRs.[14,75,77-79] Hyposensitivity on the opposite side may be due to loss of central inhibitory pathways, to bilateral changes as a result of crossing pathways, to global CNS damage (e.g., cerebral edema), and/or to decreased patient activity.

The patient with a *meningomyelocele* may have altered responses to NDRs but typically does not develop SCh-induced hyperkalemia (question f).[94]

◆ DIFFUSE NEURONAL DISEASE

The effects of diffuse neuronal disease may be less well-defined than the effects of discrete lesions.[95-98] It is important to appreciate that *"conflicting" features* may be interacting:

1. The NMJs and neighboring muscle sites associated with injured nerves are characterized by AChR (especially EJR) proliferation. This may lead to hyposensitivity to NDRs and the potential for SCh-induced hyperkalemia or contractures.
2. Affected neurons that are still viable may have decreased ACh synthesis and release, with increased fade and increased sensitivity to NDRs.[50,92,95,99]
3. The NMJs of intact nerves are normal; however, they are reduced in number, and hence there is decreased neuromuscular reserve.
4. There is the potential for collateral sprouting from surviving fibers.[93]
5. There may be disproportionate destruction of central facilitatory or inhibitory pathways.[92]

Such a conflicting picture is typical of *amyotrophic lateral sclerosis* (ALS),[95,96] a degenerative disorder of motor ganglia and pyramidal tracts (question d). This disorder is characterized by weakness and possible spasticity. There is muscle atrophy with a reduction in the number of motor units.[93] SCh may elicit contractures.[100] Clinically, however, we often encounter increased rather than decreased sensitivity to NDRs. The increased sensitivity is consistent with the observation that ALS may be characterized by fade in response to tetanic stimulation, an effect that may improve after cholinesterase administration.[99] Such myasthenic-like dysfunction may be due to decreased ACh synthesis as a result of degeneration of spinal cord ganglia.[95] The sensitivity of patients with ALS to NDRs may also be attributable to their decreased neuromuscular reserve as a result of destruction of a large number of motor units. The increased sensitivity could also result from disproportionate injury to central facilitatory pathways.

The above problems may also occur with *multiple sclerosis* (MS), a disorder characterized by focal plaques of demyelination throughout the central nervous system.[97] This leads to decreased neural activity at the associated NMJs, with the *potential for AChR proliferation*.[80] *EJR proliferation* in patients with MS often is of a relatively mild degree; it depends on the extent of disease. The altered nerve function leads to pronounced weakness and to spasm and myotonia-like contractures that may be helped by quinine or diphenylhydantoin.[98] The receptor proliferation *may lead to hyposensitivity to NDRs and exaggerated responses to SCh*.[46,80,98] There is one report of SCh-induced hyperkalemia in a patient with MS.[46] The lack of other reports suggests a relatively low susceptibility of MS patients to such a crisis.[46,50,101,102] The five patients who received SCh in a series of 11 patients with MS did not develop any SCh-related problems[102]; postoperative exacerbations were most closely associated with pyrexia rather than with a specific anesthetic agent.[102]

Patients with *polyneuropathies* may be prone to SCh-induced hyperkalemia.[58,61,62,72] In addition, polyneuropathies may have features resembling myasthenic syndrome or myasthenia gravis.[103] Thus, NDRs may cause intense, prolonged paralysis. *Guillain-Barré syndrome,* an acute polyneuritis that may occur after an otherwise benign viral illness, leads to weakness and predisposes to SCh-induced hyperkalemia.[62] SCh-induced hyperkalemia was reported in a patient 3 weeks after apparent recovery from Guillain-Barré disease.[62] *Tetanus,* a presynaptic disorder caused by *Clostridium tetani,* likewise leads to weakness and may predispose to SCh-induced hyperkalemia.[59] *Poliomyelitis,* a viral disease of the motor ganglia that causes denervation-induced muscle changes, is now rare in the Western world. Patients recovering from poliomyelitis may evidence fade and exaggerated responses to NDRs.[50,104] Several years after the acute illness, clinically unaffected upper extremities displayed a twofold increase in NDR sensitivity; recovery times were not affected.[105]

In addition, *abnormal responses to SCh* may be obtained with severe prolonged systemic infections,[56,106-108] Friedreich's ataxia,[109] prolonged periodic paralysis,[110,111] metastatic rhabdomyosarcoma (with proliferation of immature receptors),[112] and uremia.[59,72]

In some neurological and traumatic states, the pathophysiological process affecting nerve and muscle can continue for prolonged periods.[72,113,114] An exaggerated sensitivity to SCh may persist well beyond the initial insult.[46,62,63] It also should be noted that many of the disorders are *associated with autonomic dysfunction,* perhaps due to denervation of organs associated with reflex mechanisms.[115]

◆ IMMOBILITY AND DISUSE

Immobility and *disuse* may lead to muscle weakness[13,116–118] and AChR proliferation,[3,9–14,18,119–121] indicating that these changes may occur despite persistence of some neural activity.[121] Likewise, prolonged treatment with a local anesthetic[17,18] or an NDR[1,2,4,16] may lead to graded denervation-like changes. There is evidence to suggest that the metabolic changes in immobilized muscles have a retrograde effect on motor nerves, causing neurological dysfunction.[121] With respect to NDR-induced block, *"conflicting" features* once again may be interacting: (1) *muscle atrophy* decreases the patient's neuromuscular reserve, leading to increased sensitivity, and (2) the *AChR proliferation* provides a "sink" for NDRs, leading to overall hyposensitivity to NDRs.[3,11,12,14,81] The increase in EJRs is of lesser magnitude than that which occurs in denervated muscle.[121] Thus, although SCh-induced elevations in K^+ and VO_2 are increased in immobilized muscle,[10,33,54,67,122] such elevations typically are less pronounced than in denervated muscle.[64] Severe SCh-induced hyperkalemia is not likely unless there is effective immobilization (e.g., by spica cast or total bed rest) for more than 10 days.[10,64]

In contrast to immobility, *increased conditioning* may lead to a lessening of receptor density and increased sensitivity to NDRs.[123]

◆ INTRACRANIAL DISORDERS

In contrast to stroke, several intracranial disorders affect brain function but tend not to affect motor nerves. Nevertheless, SCh-induced hyperkalemia has been reported in diffuse intracranial lesions (which in many cases may have been attributable to prolonged bed rest).[68,124–129] *Closed head injury* or ruptured *cerebral aneurysm* may lead to SCh-induced hyperkalemia,[125,126] most likely as a consequence of subsequent immobility.[126,128,129] *Parkinson's disease,* which is characterized by loss of dopaminergic fibers in the basal ganglia, does not typically alter the response to neuromuscular blocking agents.[46,92,130] In one case, an increase in K^+ from 4.2 to 7.6 mEq · L^{-1} was reported (during infusion of 800 mg of SCh over 30 minutes),[131] but hyperkalemia has not been noted in other series.[46,130] *Huntington's chorea,* which is characterized by atrophy of the basal ganglia, likewise does not tend to predispose to pathological response; however, it may be associated with pseudocholinesterase deficiency[132] and sensitivity to NDRs.[133] *Creutzfeldt-Jakob disease,* an acute viral disorder that results in rapid intellectual deterioration and myoclonus, may affect lower motor neuron function[134,135] and thus may predispose to SCh-induced hyperkalemia. It may also induce autonomic dysfunction.[136]

Children with *cerebral palsy* have decreased sensitivity to NDRs[137] but a relatively low likelihood of developing SCh-induced hyperkalemia (question f).[138]

◆ BURNS

Burns cause local tissue damage as well as local and widespread neuropathic changes. Evidence of burn-induced neural injury includes fibrillation potentials, reduced nerve conduction,[139,140] and AChR proliferation.[7,82,141] Fifteen percent of burned patients exhibit reduced motor-conduction velocities in two or more nerves.[139] Especially when the burn injury involves more than 30% of body surface area, there may be AChR proliferation in unburned (as well as burned) regions, with altered response to relaxants.[1,7,142–147]

Burns are notorious for predisposing to marked *SCh-induced hyperkalemia* and related dysrhythmias.[1,63,67,148–152] Serum K^+ concentrations may increase by 6 mEq · L^{-1} after administration of SCh to the burned patients,[150] as compared to an increase of 0.5 mEq · L^{-1} in normal subjects. *Possible mechanisms* include EJR proliferation (as with neuronal destruction),[7,82,141] leaky membranes, altered Ca^{2+} flux in damaged muscle fibers, and burn-induced neuropathies. SCh-induced hyperkalemia is not restricted to patients with widespread burns, having been noted in a patient with only an 8% burn.[153] The increased K^+ release appears to arise from nonburned as well as burned areas of the body.[63] As with denervation, we are concerned not so much with the *number of receptors* as with their *immature nature* and their *extrajunctional location*. The use of a low dose of SCh may decrease the likelihood of critical hyperkalemia[154]; however, the situation remains unpredictable.[1] Pretreatment with a defasciculating dose of a *nondepolarizing agent* does not prevent the hyperkalemic response.

Burns are also associated with a markedly *increased sensitivity to the neuromuscular blocking effects of SCh* (increased depth of block, increased duration), such that 0.1 mg · kg^{-1} may induce complete twitch inhibition.[154] This effect may be attributable to local tissue changes as well as a systemic *decrease in pseudocholinesterase* (which typically lasts for several weeks after a major burn).[153,155]

The risk of *SCh-induced hyperkalemia* is time-related. On *days 1 and 2*, administration of SCh is probably safe, but one should nevertheless be cautious in the context of a major burn. On *days 3–28* the risk of a hyperkalemic response is greatest.[149,151,153,154] During *months 2–6* the risk is still high. At *1 year* the risk is less clear-cut; the likelihood of hyperkalemia is greatest if healing is not complete.

Following a major burn, there is *decreased sensitivity to NDRs,* typically in proportion to the extent of injury.[142,144,145,147,156–161] The plasma levels for a given degree of twitch depression may be 400% of normal, and durations of action are markedly reduced.[142,157,159,160] Evidence for a persistent defect was noted by the slight hyposensitivity to metocurine in a patient 1 year after complete recovery from a 45% burn.[161] Other patients have shown normal responses to atracurium and vecuronium 3 years post burn.[144,145]

The hyposensitivity to NDRs may also be attributable in part to *increased protein binding*.[1,85] As noted earlier, *alpha$_1$-acid glycoprotein* is an acute-phase reactant that binds to relaxant and decreases the amount of free relaxant. However, although plasma binding of tubocurarine in burn patients was 170% of control, this accounted for only part of the increased dose requirements.

◆ MAJOR TRAUMA

Following major soft tissue trauma, SCh again may induce *hyperkalemia*.[59,162,163] An 84% SCh-induced increase in serum K$^+$ has been reported several days after major injury, but not on day 1.[162] The peak response typically is noted at 20 days.[163] Direct *muscle injury*, cold injury with subsequent immobilization, irradiation, or irritation of muscle by a foreign substance all may result in supersensitivity to agonists.[164–166]

Discussion Questions ◆

a. Summarize the *effect of denervation* on the location, number, and type of *postsynaptic acetylcholine receptors* (AChRs).
b. Following a *stroke,* are requirements for NDRs increased on the contralateral *(unparalyzed) side* and/or at the diaphragm? Why or why not?
c. On *reversal of an NDR* in a patient with major *denervation or a burn* injury, what is the likelihood that the increased ACh level will provide a response similar to that seen with SCh (e.g., hyperkalemia, contractures)? Will the response be clinically significant?
d. Does *amyotrophic lateral sclerosis* predispose to: (1) SCh-induced hyperkalemia? (2) weakness in response to a small dose of NDR? Explain.
e. Can a nondepolarizing agent be used to treat the stiffness and spasms associated with *Clostridium*-induced *tetanus?*
f. Is a 3-year-old child with *cerebral palsy* or a *meningomyelocele* at the same risk for SCh-induced hyperkalemia as the person with a 3-month-old cord transection or amyotrophic lateral sclerosis? Why or why not?
g. Does a *ruptured cerebral aneurysm* predispose to SCh-induced hyperkalemia?
h. Why might it be dangerous to administer SCh to a patient who has been *immobilized for many days* in an ICU?
i. If a patient demonstrates *hyposensitivity to an NDR* 1 year after a *burn*

injury, does this mean that he or she would evidence SCh-induced hyperkalemia? Why or why not?

Answers ◆

a. Within a few days of a *denervating injury*, there is marked AChR proliferation (presumably in response to the acute decline in ACh release). The initial AChR proliferation probably occurs predominantly at the end-plate. However, the loss of a trophic influence from the nerve terminal allows *extrajunctional proliferation* of immature receptors (EJRs). These receptors have markedly increased sensitivity to ACh and SCh, and the underlying muscle is prone to contractures and an outpouring of K^+ since its firing is not modulated by an end-plate (see also answer h in Chap. 2).

b. On the side *contralateral* to that paralyzed by a *stroke*, the response to NDR may be decreased because of (1) *disuse atrophy* if the patient is bedridden (disuse atrophy is characterized by receptor proliferation and decreased response to NDRs); (2) some descending motor fibers may be uncrossed; (3) the possibility of global injury (e.g., cerebral edema, which will affect descending pathways from both sides of the brain); and (4) predominant loss of central inhibitory pathways. Fortunately, in the typical case, the *diaphragm is virtually unaffected*. However, because of *extremity "resistance"* to NDRs, following administration of an NDR the adductor pollicis may suggest incomplete block or recovery while the diaphragm may be paralyzed.[12] This is a reversal of the usual relationship (Chap. 3).

c. *Reversal of nondepolarizing block* in the patient with extensive *denervation* typically is not associated with hyperkalemia or contractures. Possible explanations include the following: (1) ACh does not elicit the prolonged receptor channel opening that is induced by SCh, or (2) the ACh that accumulates in intact junctions (where it must compete with remaining NDR) as a result of reversal may not gain access to the abnormal receptors that lie extrajunctionally. Nevertheless, reversal may not be totally benign. Increased contractions have been reported in a patient with progressive muscular dystrophy and in a patient with myotonia.[167]

d. *Amyotrophic lateral sclerosis* (ALS) is a degenerative disease of motor cells and, as such, is associated with a *proliferation of EJRs* as well as *increased overall sensitivity to NDRs*. At first glance, these features appear to be inconsistent. As expected, the EJR proliferation leads to *SCh-induced contractures* and possibly *hyperkalemia*. The somewhat surprising feature is that these patients are highly susceptible to NDRs, even though EJR proliferation serves as a "sink" for NDR molecules. The increased susceptibility to NDR-induced weakness may be due to (1) myasthenic dysfunction, perhaps a consequence of injury-induced reduction of ACh release; (2) the patient's lack of neuromuscular reserve, with inability to withstand block of even a small fraction of the remaining healthy NMJs; and (3) possibly a disproportionate destruction of facilitatory pathways as a result of spinal cord damage. As little as 1.5 mg of *d*-tubocurarine (less than 5% of the ED_{95}) has caused difficulty swallowing in the patient with ALS.[95,96]

e. The stiffness and spasms associated with *Clostridium-induced tetanus* can be effectively treated with a *nondepolarizing agent* (and mechanical ventilation).[168] Both *C. botulinum* and *C. tetani* block ACh release[169]; however, *C. tetani* primarily affects central synapses and cause spasticity and convulsions. Peripherally, the functional denervation may lead to AChR proliferation of a nature and magnitude sufficient to provoke *SCh-induced hyperkalemia*.

f. A child with *cerebral palsy*[138] is far *less likely to develop SCh-induced hyperkalemia* than a patient with a 3-month-old denervation injury or ALS. Perhaps this is because exposure to SCh in the patient with cerebral palsy is likely to occur several years after injury, i.e., beyond the time of peak effect. Additionally, cerebral palsy causes less acute lower motor neuron effects than does a denervating injury. Nevertheless, children with cerebral palsy manifested a resistance to nondepolarizing block with vecuronium (which was only partly attributable to their phenytoin therapy[137]).

The above is also true for children with *meningomyelocele*, a disorder with lower as well as upper motor neuron destruction.[94] Again, *time appears to be a critical factor*. Additionally, fetal denervation may limit muscle development and thus the susceptibility to SCh-induced K^+ release.[94]

g. Recent evidence suggests that an acutely *ruptured cerebral aneurysm does not predispose to SCh-induced hyperkalemia*. The mean increase in serum potassium was 0.4 mmol · L^{-1} in 34 patients.[129] It appears that previous reports of SCh-induced hyperkalemia were attributable to the patients being bedridden for weeks after the acute hemorrhage.

h. Several factors may interact to increase the likelihood of *SCh-induced hyperkalemia* in a patient who has been *immobilized in an ICU*: major trauma, sepsis, prolonged immobilization (disuse atrophy), drug interaction with other medications, and prolonged drug-induced paralysis may lead to AChR proliferation and an exaggerated response to SCh. (The high incidence of neuropathies and myopathies is discussed in Chap. 11.)

i. *Hyposensitivity to NDRs* has been reported *1 year after a major burn injury*,[161] but appears to be of far lesser degree than at 1–6 months after injury. The hyposensitivity to NDRs suggests that one or more of the following have persisted: (1) AChR proliferation at the end-plate, (2) ACh proliferation extrajunctionally, and/or (3) increased $alpha_1$-acid glycoprotein concentrations (and hence increased NDR protein binding). Hyposensitivity to an NDR does not necessarily indicate that the nature, magnitude, and location of AChR proliferation are such that they would result in a pathological response to SCh. However, SCh-induced hyperkalemia may be likely if there is persistent EJR proliferation. Hence, one cannot say with certainty that SCh would be safe.[1]

References ◆

1. Martyn JAJ, White DA, Gronert GA, Jaffe RS, Ward JM: Up-and-down regulation of skeletal muscle acetylcholine receptors: effects on neuromuscular blockers. Anesthesiology 76:822–843, 1992
2. Chang CC, Chuang ST, Huang MC: Effects of chronic treatment with various neuromuscular blocking agents on the number and distribution of acetylcholine receptors in the rat diaphragm. J Physiol (Lond) 250:161–173, 1975
3. Gronert GA, Matteo RS, Perkins S: Canine gastrocnemius disuse atrophy: resistance to paralysis by dimethyl tubocurarine. J Appl Physiol 57:1502–1506, 1984
4. Hogue CW, Ward JM, Itani MS, Martyn JAJ: Tolerance and up-regulation of acetylcholine receptors follows chronic infusion of d-tubocurarine. J Appl Physiol 72:1326–1331, 1992
5. Hogue CW, Itani MS, Martyn JAJ: Resistance of d-tubocurarine in lower motor neuron injury is related to increased acetylcholine receptors at the neuromuscular junction. Anesthesiology 73:703–709, 1990
6. Kim CS, Arnold FJ, Itani MS, Martyn JAJ: Decreased sensitivity to metocurine during long-term phenytoin therapy may be attributable to protein binding and acetylcholine receptor changes. Anesthesiology 77:500–506, 1992
7. Kim C, Martyn JA, Fuke N: Burn injury to trunk of rat causes denervation-like responses in gastrocnemius muscle. J Appl Physiol 65:1745–1751, 1988
8. Lorkovic H: Acetylcholine-induced currents in denervated mouse soleus muscle: effects of antagonists. Neuropharmacology 29:573–577, 1990
9. Fambrough DM: Control of acetylcholine receptors in skeletal muscle. Physiol Rev 59:165–227, 1979
10. Fung DL, White DA, Jones BR, Gronert GA: The onset of disuse-related potassium efflux to succinylcholine. Anesthesiology 75:650–653, 1991
11. Gronert GA: Disuse atrophy with resistance to pancuronium. Anesthesiology 55:547–549, 1981
12. Waud BE, Waud DR: Tubocurarine sensitivity of the diaphragm after limb immobilization. Anesth Analg 65:493–495, 1986
13. Solandt DA, Partridge RC, Hunter J: The effect of skeletal muscle fixation on skeletal muscle. J Neurophysiol 6:17–22, 1943
14. Waud BE, Amaki Y, Waud DR: Disuse and d-tubocurarine sensitivity in isolated muscles. Anesth Analg 64:1178–1182, 1985
15. Martyn JAJ, Kim CS: Decreased sensitivity to metocurine during chronic phenytoin may be due to protein binding and receptor changes. Anesthesiology 75:A640, 1991
16. Berg DK, Hall ZW: Increased extrajunctional acetylcholine sensitivity produced by chronic post-synaptic neuromuscular blockade. J Physiol 244:659–676, 1975
17. Libelius R, Sonesson B, Stamenovic BA, et al: Denervation-like changes in skeletal muscle after treatment with a local anesthetic (Marcaine). J Anat 106:297–309, 1970
18. Sokoll MD, Sonesson B, Thesleff S: Denervation changes produced in an innervated skeletal muscle by long continued treatment with a local anesthetic. Eur J Pharmacol 4:179–187, 1968
19. Miledi R: The acetylcholine sensitivity of frog muscle fibres after complete or partial denervation. J Physiol (Lond) 151:1–23, 1960
20. Axellson J, Thesleff S: A study of supersensitivity in denervated mammalian skeletal muscle. J Physiol (Lond) 147:178, 1959

21. Katz B, Miledi R: The development of acetylcholine sensitivity in nerve free segments of skeletal muscle. J Physiol (Lond) 170:389–396, 1964
22. Schuetze SM, Role LW: Developmental regulation of nicotinic acetylcholine receptors. Annu Rev Neurosci 10:403–457, 1987
23. Brenner HR, Rudin W: On the effect of muscle activity on the end-plate membrane in denervated mouse muscle. J Physiol 410:501, 1989
24. Levitt-Gilmour TA, Salpeter MM: Gradient of extrajunctional acetylcholine receptors early after denervation of mammalian muscle. J Neurosci 6:1606, 1986
25. Dreyer F: Acetylcholine receptor. Br J Anaesth 54:115–130, 1982
26. Thesleff S: Effects of motor innervation on the chemical sensitivity of skeletal muscle. Physiol Rev 40:734–752, 1960
27. Goldman D, Brenner HR, Heinemann S: Acetylcholine receptor alpha-, beta-, gamma-, and delta-subunit mRNA levels are regulated by muscle activity. Neuron 1:329, 1988
28. Laufer R, Changeux JP: Activity-dependent regulation of gene expression in muscle and neuronal cells. Mol Neurobiol 3:1, 1989
29. Salpeter MM, Cooper DL, Levitt-Gilmour T: Degradation rates of acetylcholine receptors can be modified in the postjunctional plasma membrane of the vertebrate neuromuscular junction. J Cell Biol 103:1399, 1986
30. Gu Y, Hall ZW: Characterization of acetylcholine receptor subunits in developing and denervated mammalian muscle. J Biol Chem 263:12878–12885, 1988
31. McCarthy MP, Earnest JP, Young EF, Choe S, Stroud RM: The molecular neurobiology of the acetylcholine receptor. Annu Rev Neurosci 9:383–413, 1986
32. Schuetze SM: Embryonic and adult acetylcholine receptors: molecular basis of developmental changes in ion channel properties. Trends Neurosci 9:386–388, 1986
33. Goudsouzian NG, Standaert FG: The infant and myoneural junction. Anesth Analg 65:1208–1217, 1986
34. Gronert GA, Lambert EH, Theye RA: The response of denervated skeletal muscle to succinylcholine. Anesthesiology 39:13–22, 1973
35. MacLagan J, Vrobva G: A study of the increased sensitivity of denervated and reinnervated muscle to depolarizing drugs. J Physiol (Lond) 182:131–143, 1966
36. Lorkovic H: Sensitivity of rodent skeletal muscles to dicholines: dependence on innervation and age. Neuropharmacology 28:373–377, 1989
37. Fischbach GD, Schuetze SM: A postnatal decrease in acetylcholine channel open time at rat endplates. J Physiol (Lond) 303:125–137, 1980
38. Gu Y, Franco A Jr, Gardner PD, Lansman JB, Forsayeth JR, Hall ZW: Properties of embryonic and adult muscle acetylcholine receptors transiently expressed in COS cells. Neuron 5:147–157, 1990
39. Reiser G, Miledi R: Changes in the properties of synaptic channels opened by acetylcholine in denervated frog muscle. Brain Res 479:83, 1989
40. Goldman D, Carlson BM, Staple J: Induction of adult-type nicotinic acetylcholine receptor gene expression in noninnervated regenerating muscle. Neuron 7:649, 1991
41. Shyng SL, Salpeter MM: Effect of reinnervation on the degradation rate of junctional acetylcholine receptors synthesized in denervated skeletal muscles. J Neurosci 10:3905, 1990
42. Shyng SL, Salpeter MM: Degradation rate of acetylcholine receptors inserted into denervated vertebrate neuromuscular junctions. J Cell Biol 108:647, 1989
43. Rotzler S, Brenner HR: Metabolic stabilization of acetylcholine receptors in vertebrate neuromuscular junction by muscle activity. J Cell Biol 111:655, 1990
44. Beranck R, Vyskocil F: The action of tubocurarine and atropine on normal and denervated rat skeletal muscle. J Physiol (Lond) 188:53–66, 1967
45. Azar I: The response of patients with neuromuscular disorders to muscle relaxants: a review. Anesthesiology 61:173–187, 1984
46. Cooperman LH: Succinylcholine-induced hyperkalemia in neuromuscular disease. JAMA 213:1867–1871, 1970
47. Cooperman LH, Strobel GE Jr, Kennell EM: Massive hyperkalemia after administration of succinylcholine. Anesthesiology 32:161–164, 1970
48. Snow JC, Kripke BJ, Sessions GP, et al: Cardiovascular collapse following succinylcholine in a paraplegic patient. Paraplegia 11:119, 1973

49. Jenkinson DH, Nichols JG: Contractures and permeability changes produced by acetylcholine in depolarized denervated muscle. J Physiol (Lond) 159:111–127, 1961
50. Azar I: Complications of neuromuscular blockers: interaction with concurrent diseases. Anesthesiol Clin North Am 11:409–429, 1993
51. Morris CE, Wong BS, Jackson MB, et al: Single-channel currents activated by curare in cultured embryonic rat muscle. J Neurosci 3:2525, 1983
52. Trautmann A: Curare can open and block ionic channels associated with cholinergic receptors. Nature 298:272, 1982
53. Fiacchiano F, Bricchi M, Lasio G: Monitoring curarisation in tetraparesis. Anaesthesia 45:128–131, 1990
54. Stone WA, Beach TP, Hamelberg W: Succinylcholine-induced hyperkalemia in dogs with transected sciatic nerve and spinal cord. Anesthesiology 32:515–520, 1970
55. John DA, Tobey RE, Homer LD, Rice CL: Onset of succinylcholine-induced hyperkalemia following denervation. Anesthesiology 45:294–299, 1976
56. Kohlschutter B, Baur H, Roth F: Suxamethonium-induced hyperkalemia in patients with severe intra-abdominal infections. Br J Anaesth 48:557–561, 1976
57. Stone WA, Beach TP, Hamelberg W: Succinylcholine—danger in the spinal-cord-injured patient. Anesthesiology 32:168, 1970
58. Smith RB: Hyperkalaemia following succinylcholine administration in neurological disorders: a review. Can Anaesth Soc J 18:199–201, 1971
59. Roth F, Wuthrich H: The clinical importance of hyperkalemia following suxamethonium administration. Br J Anaesth 41:311–316, 1969
60. Tobey RE, Jacobsen PM, Kahle CT, et al: The serum potassium response to muscle relaxants in neural injury. Anesthesiology 37:332, 1972
61. Fergusson RJ, Wright DJ, Willey RF, et al: Suxamethonium is dangerous in polyneuropathy. Br Med J 282:298–299, 1981
62. Feldman JM: Cardiac arrest after succinylcholine administration in a pregnant patient recovered from Guillain-Barré syndrome. Anesthesiology 72:942–944, 1990
63. Birch AA Jr., Mitchell GD, Playford GA, Lang CA: Changes in serum potassium response to succinylcholine following trauma. JAMA 210:490–493, 1969
64. Gronert GA, Theye RA: Effect of succinylcholine on skeletal muscle with immobilization atrophy. Anesthesiology 40:268–271, 1974
65. Jones R, Vrbova G: Two factors responsible for the development of denervation hypersensitivity. J Physiol (Lond) 236:517–538, 1974
66. Brooke MM, Donovon WH, Stolov WC: Paraplegia: succinylcholine-induced hyperkalemia and cardiac arrest. Arch Phys Med Rehabil 59:306, 1978
67. Gronert GA, Theye RA: Pathophysiology of hyperkalemia induced by succinylcholine. Anesthesiology 43:89–99, 1975
68. Smith RB, Grenvik A: Cardiac arrest following succinylcholine in patients with central nervous system injuries. Anesthesiology 33:558–560, 1970
69. Tobey RE: Paraplegia, succinylcholine and cardiac arrest. Anesthesiology 32:359, 1970
70. Walker DE, Barry JM, Hodges CV: Succinylcholine-induced ventricular fibrillation in the paralyzed urology patient. J Urol 113:111, 1975
71. Beach TP, Stone WA, Hamelberg W: Circulatory collapse following succinylcholine: report of a patient with diffuse lower motor neuron disease. Anesth Analg 50:431–437, 1971
72. Walton JD, Farman JV: Suxamethonium hyperkalaemia in uraemic neuropathy. Anaesthesia 28:666–668, 1973
73. Baraka A: Antagonism of succinylcholine-induced contracture of denervated muscles by d-tubocurarine. Anesth Analg 60:605, 1981
74. Colquhoun D, Sheridan RE: The effect of tubocurarine competition on the kinetics of agonist action on the nicotinic receptor. Br J Pharmacol 75:77–86, 1982
75. Shayevitz JR, Matteo RS: Decreased sensitivity to metocurine in patients with upper motoneuron disease. Anesth Analg 64:767–772, 1985
76. Laycock JR, Smith CE, Donati F, et al: Sensitivity of the adductor pollicis and the diaphragmatic muscles to atracurium in a hemiplegic patient. Anesthesiology 67:851, 1987
77. Graham DH: Monitoring neuromuscular block may be unreliable in patients with upper motor-neuron lesions. Anesthesiology 52:74, 1980

78. Iwasaki H, Namika A, Omote K, et al: Response differences of paretic and healthy extremities to pancuronium and neostigmine in hemiplegic patients. Anesth Analg 64:864–866, 1985
79. Moorthy SS, Hilgenberg JC: Resistance to nondepolarizing muscle relaxants in paretic upper extremities of patients with residual hemiplegia. Anesth Analg 59:624–627, 1980
80. Brett RS, Schmidt JH, Gage JS, Schartel SA, Poppers PJ: Measurement of acetylcholine receptor concentration in skeletal muscle from a patient with multiple sclerosis and resistance to atracurium. Anesthesiology 66:837–839, 1987
81. Fung D, Perkins S, Gronert G, Matteo R: Disuse resistance to metocurine. Anesthesiology 71:A786, 1989
82. Lagasse RS, Schmidt JH, Dilger JP, Gage JS, Schartel SA, Brett RS: Acetylcholine receptor concentration and resistance to atracurium in patients with thermal injury. Anesth Analg 70:S222, 1990
83. Hegab E-S, Schiff HI, Smith DJ, Turndorf N: An electron microscopic study of normal and chronically denervated rat skeletal muscle following succinylcholine challenge. Anesth Analg 53:650–656, 1974
84. Abramson FP, Lutz MP: The effects of phenytoin dosage on the induction of α_1-acid glycoprotein and antipyrine clearance in the dog. Eur J Drug Metab Pharmacokinet 11:135–143, 1986
85. Kremer JM, Wilting J, Janssen LH: Drug binding to human α_1-acid glycoprotein in health and disease. Pharmacol Rev 40:1–47, 1988
86. Benecke R, Berthold A, Conrad B: Denervation activity in the EMG of patients with upper motor neuron lesions: time course, local distribution and pathogenetic aspects. J Neurol 230:143–151, 1983
87. Krueger KC, Waylonis GW: Hemiplegia: lower motor neuron electromyographic findings. Arch Phys Med Rehabil 54:360–364, 1973
88. McComas AJ, Sica REP, Upton ARM, Aruilera N: Functional changes in motoneurones of hemiparetic patients. J Neurol Neurosurg Psychiatry 36:183–193, 1973
89. Takebe K, Narayan G, Kukulka C, Basmajian JV: Slowing of nerve conduction velocity in hemiplegia: possible factors. Arch Phys Med Rehabil 56:285–289, 1975
90. Yoshioka K, Miyata Y: Changes in distribution of the extrajunctional acetylcholine sensitivity along muscle fibers during development and following cordotomy in the rat. Neuroscience 9:437–443, 1983
91. Eldridge L, Liebhold M, Steinbach JH: Alterations in cat skeletal neuromuscular junctions following prolonged inactivity. J Physiol (Lond) 313:529–545, 1981
92. Brown JC, Charlton JE: Study of sensitivity to curare in certain neurological disorders using a regional technique. J Neurol Neurosurg Psychiatry 38:34–45, 1975
93. Wohlfart G: Collateral regeneration from residual motor nerve fibers in amyotrophic lateral sclerosis. Neurology 7:124, 1957
94. Dierdorf SF, McNiece WL, Rao CC, Wolfe TM, Means LJ: Failure of succinylcholine to alter plasma potassium in children with myelomeningocoele. Anesthesiology 64:272–273, 1986
95. Mulder DW, Lambert EH, Eaton LM: Myasthenic syndrome in patients with amyotrophic lateral sclerosis. Neurology 9:627–631, 1959
96. Rosenbaum KJ, Neigh JL, Stobell GE: Sensitivity to non-depolarizing muscle relaxants in amyotrophic lateral sclerosis: report of two cases. Anesthesiology 35:638–641, 1971
97. Powell HC, Lampert PW: Pathology of multiple sclerosis. Neurol Clin 1:631, 1983
98. Weintraub MI, Megaled MS, Smith BH: Myotonic-like syndrome in multiple sclerosis. NY State J Med 70:677–679, 1970
99. Lambert EH, Mulder DW: Electromyographic studies in amyotrophic lateral sclerosis. Proc Mayo Clin 32:441, 1957
100. Orndahl G, Sternberg K: Myotonic human musculature: stimulation with depolarizing agents. Mechanical registration of the succinylcholine, succinylmonocholine, and decamethonium. Acta Med Scand 172:389, 1962
101. Frost PM: Anaesthesia and multiple sclerosis. Anaesthesia 26:104, 1971
102. Seimbowicz E: Multiple sclerosis and surgery. Anaesthesia 31:1211, 1976
103. Baginsky RG: A case of peripheral polyneuropathy displaying myasthenic EMG patterns. Electroencephalogr Clin Neurophysiol 25:397, 1968

104. Hodes R: Electromyographic study of defects of neuromuscular transmission in human poliomyelitis. Arch Neurol Psychiatry 60:457, 1948
105. Gyermek L: Increased potency of nondepolarizing relaxants after poliomyelitis. J Clin Pharmacol 30:170–173, 1990
106. Khan TZ, Khan RM: Changes in serum potassium following succinylcholine in patients with infections. Anesth Analg 62:327–331, 1983
107. Roelofs RI, Cerra F, Beilka N, et al: Prolonged respiratory insufficiency due to acute motor neuropathy: a new syndrome? Neurology 33(suppl 2):240, 1983
108. Witt NJ, Zochodne DW, Bolton CF, Grand'Maison F, Wells G, Young B, Sibbald WJ: Peripheral nerve function in sepsis and multiple organ failure. Chest 99:176–184, 1991
109. Kume M, Sin T, Oyama T: Anesthetic experience with a patient with Friedreich's ataxia: a case report. Jpn J Anesthesiol 25:877–880, 1976
110. Flewellen EH, Bodensteiner JB: Anesthetic experience in a patient with hyperkalemic periodic paralysis. Anesth Rev 7:44, 1980
111. Siler JN, Discavage WJ: Anesthetic management of hypokalemic periodic paralysis. Anesthesiology 43:489, 1975
112. Krikken-Hogenberk LG, deJong JR, Bovill JG: Succinylcholine-induced hyperkalemia in a patient with metastatic rhabdomyosarcoma. Anesthesiology 70:553–555, 1989
113. Dalakas MC, Elder G, Hallett M, Ravits J, Baker M, Papadopoulos N, Albrecht P, Sever J: A long term follow-up study of patients with post-poliomyelitis neuromuscular symptoms. N Engl J Med 314:959–963, 1986
114. Schott GD: Induction of involuntary movements by peripheral trauma: an analogy with causalgia. Lancet 2:712–716, 1986
115. Krone A, Reuther P, Fuhrmeister U: Autonomic dysfunction in polyneuropathies: a report of 106 cases. J Neurol 230:111, 1983
116. Duchateau J, Hainaut K: Electrical and mechanical changes in immobilized human muscle. J Appl Physiol 62:2168, 1987
117. Gogia P, Schneider VS, LeBlanc AD, et al: Bed rest effect on extremity muscle torque in healthy men. Arch Phys Med Rehabil 69:1030, 1988
118. Muller EA: Influence of training and of inactivity on muscle strength. Arch Phys Med Rehabil 51:449, 1970
119. Fiamengo SA, Savarese JJ: Use of muscle relaxants in intensive care units. Crit Care Med 19:1457–1459, 1991
120. Fischbach GD, Robbins N: Effect of chronic disuse of rat soleus neuromuscular junctions on postsynaptic membrane. J Neurophysiol 34:562–569, 1971
121. Booth FW: Effect of limb immobilization on skeletal muscle. J Appl Physiol 52:1113, 1982
122. Hemming AE, Charlton S, Kelly P: Hyperkalemia, cardiac arrest, suxamethonium, and intensive care (letter). Anaesthesia 45:990, 1990
123. Gronert GA, White DA, Shafer SL, Matteo RS: Exercise produces sensitivity to metocurine. Anesthesiology 70:973–977, 1989
124. Cowgill DB, Mostello LA, Shapiro HM: Encephalitis and a hyperkalemic response to succinylcholine. Anesthesiology 40:409–411, 1974
125. Stevenson PH, Birch AA: Succinylcholine induced hyperkalemia in a patient with a closed head injury. Anesthesiology 51:89–90, 1979
126. Frankville DD, Drummond JC: Hyperkalemia after succinylcholine administration in a patient with closed head injury without paresis. Anesthesiology 67:264, 1987
127. Thomas ET: Circulatory collapse following succinylcholine: report of a case. Anesth Analg 48:333, 1969
128. Iwatsuki N, Kuroda N, Amaha K, et al: Succinylcholine-induced hyperkalemia in patients with ruptured cerebral aneurysms. Anesthesiology 53:64–67, 1980
129. Manninen PH, Mahendran B, Gelb AW, Merchant RN: Succinylcholine does not increase serum potassium levels in patients with actively ruptured cerebral aneurysms. Anesth Analg 70:172–175, 1990
130. Muzzi DA, Black S, Cucchiara RF: The lack of effect of succinylcholine on serum potassium in patients with Parkinson's disease (letter). Anesthesiology 71:322, 1989
131. Gravlee GP: Succinylcholine-induced hyperkalemia in a patient with Parkinson's disease. Anesth Analg 59:444–446, 1980

132. Propert DN: Pseudocholinesterase activity and phenotypes in mentally ill patients. Br J Psychiatry 134:477, 1979
133. Lamont AMS: Brief report: anaesthesia and Huntington's chorea. Anaesth Intensive Care 7:189, 1979
134. MacMurdo SD, Jakymec AJ, Bleyaert AL: Precautions in the anesthetic management of a patient with Creutzfeldt-Jakob disease. Anesthesiology 60:590, 1984
135. Sadeh M, Goldhammer Y, Chagnac Y: Creutzfeldt-Jakob disease associated with peripheral neuropathy. Isr J Med 26:220, 1990
136. Khurana RK, Garcia JH: Autonomic dysfunction in subacute spongiform encephalopathy. Arch Neurol 38:114–117, 1981
137. Moorthy SS, Krishna G, Dierdorf SF: Resistance to vecuronium in patients with cerebral palsy. Anesth Analg 73:275–277, 1991
138. Dierdorf SF, McNiece WL, Rao CC, Wolfe TM, Krishna G, Means LJ, Haselby KA: Effect of succinylcholine on plasma potassium in children with cerebral palsy. Anesthesiology 62:88–90, 1985
139. Henderson B, Koepke GH, Feller I: Peripheral polyneuropathy among patients with burns. Arch Phys Med Rehabil 52:149–151, 1971
140. Mitts A, Schreifer T, Martyn JAJ: Electromyographic studies of patients with thermal injury. Anesthesiology 65:A294, 1986
141. Kim C, Fuke N, Jeevendra Martin JA: Burn injury to rat increases nicotinic acetylcholine receptors in the diaphragm. Anesthesiology 68:401–406, 1988
142. Dwersteg JF, Pavlin EG, Heimbach DM: Patients with burns are resistant to atracurium. Anesthesiology 65:517, 1986
143. Marathe PH, Haschke RH, Slattery JT, Zucker JR, Pavlin EG: Acetylcholine receptor density and acetylcholinesterase activity in skeletal muscle of rats following thermal injury. Anesthesiology 70:654–659, 1989
144. Mills AK, Martyn JAJ: Neuromuscular blockade with vecuronium in paediatric patients with burn injury. Br J Clin Pharmacol 28:155–159, 1989
145. Mills AK, Martyn JAJ: Evaluation of atracurium neuromuscular blockade in paediatric patients with burn injury. Br J Anaesth 60:450–455, 1988
146. Martyn JAJ, Tomera JF: Acetylcholine receptor density and acetylcholinesterase enzyme activity in skeletal muscle of rats following thermal injury (correspondence). Anesthesiology 71:625–627, 1989
147. Tomera JF, Martyn JAJ, Hoaglin DC: Neuromuscular dysfunction in burns and its relationship to burn size, hypermetabolism and immunosuppression. J Trauma 28:1499–1504, 1988
148. Belin RP, Karleen CI: Cardiac arrest in the burned patient following succinylcholine administration. Anesthesiology 27:516–518, 1966
149. Lowenstein E: Succinylcholine administration in the burned patient. Anesthesiology 27:494–496, 1966
150. Schaner PJ, Brown RL, Kirksey TD, et al: Succinylcholine-induced hyperkalemia in burned patients. Anesth Analg 48:764–770, 1969
151. Tolmie JD, Joyce TH, Mitchell GD: Succinylcholine danger in the burned patient. Anesthesiology 28:467–470, 1967
152. Finer BL, Nylen BO: Cardiac arrest in the treatment of burns, and report on hypnosis as a substitute for anesthesia. Plast Reconstr Surg 27:49, 1961
153. Viby-Mogensen J, Hanel HK, Hansen E, Sorensen B, Graae J: Serum cholinesterase activity in burned patients: II. Anaesthesia, suxamethonium and hyperkalaemia. Acta Anaesthesiol Scand 19:169–179, 1975
154. Brown TCK, Bell B: Electromyographic responses to small doses of suxamethonium in children after burns. Br J Anaesth 59:1017–1021, 1987
155. Viby-Mogensen J, Hanel HK, Hansen E, Sorensen B, Graae J: Serum cholinesterase activity in burned patients: I. Biochemical findings. Acta Anaesthesiol Scand 19:159–168, 1975
156. Martyn JA, Liu LM, Szyfelbein SK, Ambalavanar ES, Goudsouzian NG: The neuromuscular effects of pancuronium in burned children. Anesthesiology 59:561–564, 1983
157. Mills A, Martyn JAJ: Evaluation of vecuronium neuromuscular blockade in pediatric patients with thermal injury (abstract). Anesth Analg 66:S119, 1987

158. Martyn JAJ, Goldhill DR, Goudsouzian NG: Clinical pharmacology of muscle relaxants in patients with burns. J Clin Pharmacol 26:680–685, 1986
159. Martyn JAJ, Szyfelbein SK, Ali HH, et al: Increased d-tubocurarine requirement following major thermal injury. Anesthesiology 52:352–355, 1980
160. Marathe PH, Dwersteg JF, Pavlin EG, et al: Effect of thermal injury on the pharmacokinetics and pharmacodynamics of atracurium in humans. Anesthesiology 70:752, 1989
161. Martyn JAJ, Matteo RS, Szyfellelbein SK, et al: Unprecedented resistance to neuromuscular blocking effects of metocurine with persistence after complete recovery in a burned patient. Anesth Analg 61:614, 1982
162. Mazze RI, Escue HM, Houston JB: Hyperkalemia and cardiovascular collapse following administration of succinylcholine to the traumatized patient. Anesthesiology 31:540–544, 1979
163. Kopriva C, Ratliff J, Fletcher JR, Van Tassel P, Stout R: Serum potassium changes after succinylcholine in patients with acute massive muscle trauma. Anesthesiology 34:246, 1971
164. Cairoli VJ, Ivankovich AD, Vucicevic D, Patel K: Succinylcholine-induced hyperkalemia in the rat following radiation injury to muscle. Anesth Analg 61:83–86, 1982
165. George AL Jr, Wood CA Jr: Succinylcholine-induced hyperkalemia complicating the neuroleptic malignant syndrome (letter). Ann Intern Med 106:172, 1987
166. Laycock JRD, Loughman E: Suxamethonium-induced hyperkalaemia following cold injury. Anaesthesia 41:739–741, 1986
167. Buzello W, Krieg N, Schlickewei A: Hazards of neostigmine in patients with neuromuscular disorders. Br J Anaesth 54:529–534, 1982
168. Orko R, Rosenberg PH, Himberg JJ: Intravenous infusion of midazolam, propofol and vecuronium in a patient with severe tetanus. Acta Anaesthesiol Scand 32:590–592, 1988
169. Simpson LL: Molecular pharmacology of botulinum toxin and tetanus toxin. Annu Rev Pharmacol Toxicol 26:427–453, 1986

23

DAVID G. SILVERMAN / HENRY ROSENBERG

Other Muscle Disorders

In addition to malignant hyperthermia, a variety of clinical and subclinical myopathies may be associated with markedly abnormal responses to relaxants.[1,2]

◆ MUSCULAR DYSTROPHY

Duchenne's muscular dystrophy is an X-linked recessive disorder that is characterized by proximal muscle weakness and pseudohypertrophy in early childhood and typically progresses to ventilatory failure and death by the end of the second decade. The *diffuse muscle injury* is associated with an *elevated creatine kinase level* and a tendency toward massive *release of potassium*. Degeneration of the respiratory muscles leads to respiratory insufficiency and a decreased ability to cough, with a restrictive pattern on *pulmonary function* tests. The *heart* may exhibit conduction abnormalities, a prominent R wave in the right precordium (due to right outflow tract obstruction as a result of an obstructive cardiomyopathy), and myocardial muscle and valvular changes. Muscular dystrophy may also affect the *smooth muscle* of the gastrointestinal tract, causing gastric dilation and decreased gastrointestinal motility.

Clearly, the *patient is prone to weakness* as a consequence of loss of muscle reserve. Otherwise, *nondepolarizing relaxants* (NDRs) elicit an essentially normal response,[3,4] possibly of prolonged duration.[5] A tonic response to reversal with neostigmine has been reported.[6]

The administration of *succinylcholine* (SCh) in the context of clinical as well as subclinical muscular dystrophy has been associated with *contractures, hyperkalemia* (with cardiac arrest), and other evidence of *rhabdomyolysis*.[4,7–15] The incidence (approximately 6 per year) of SCh-induced cardiac arrest in patients with undiagnosed Duchenne Dystrophy has led to a recent FDA decision to consider SCh contraindicated in children and young adults unless there is a definite indication for its use (Chap. 18). There are isolated case reports of responses that resembled (and may have been) *malignant hyperthermia* in association with this disorder.[7,14,16–19] One may also see *ventilatory insufficiency* as a result of *delayed muscle weakness* 5–36 hours after anesthesia with SCh.[7] Halothane and other *inhalational agents* exacerbate SCh-induced destruction and may sometimes lead to muscle destruction and hyperkalemic cardiac arrest, even in the absence of SCh.[14,20,21]

◆ MYOTONIA

The myotonias are a group of disorders of the muscle membrane that cause a sustained muscle contraction after muscle stimulation. The electromyogram (EMG) is characterized by *postactivity muscle contractures,* with rapid bursts of potential ("myotonic aftercharges," "dive-bomber" sounds on the loudspeaker) in response to tapping or moving an EMG needle. Contractures may be brought on by activity, direct stimulation, exogenous depolarizing agents,[22,23] and possibly cold (especially in paramyotonia). Eventually, *muscle atrophy* and associated weakness predominate. The two major types are myotonia dystrophica and myotonia congenita.

Myotonia dystrophica (Steinert's or Hoffmann's disease) presents as a *systemic disorder* in the mid-teens. A gene abnormality on chromosome 19, expansion of repeated adenosine-guanine-cytosine trinucleotide sequences, causes an enzymatic defect that alters muscle function.[24] Clinical severity is related to the number of repeated sequences. Abnormalities include cataracts, testicular atrophy, a low IQ, cholelithiasis, and a "hatchet face" appearance due to muscle wasting; *high creatine kinase levels;* diffuse *endocrine abnormalities* (decreased thyroid and adrenal function, diabetes); altered gut motility[25]; and myocardial dysfunction (especially *cardiac conduction abnormalities* of the His-Purkinje system, with ventricular irritability, heart block, and Stokes-Adams attacks).[26,27] Patients with myotonia dystrophica frequently develop postoperative pulmonary *complications* (since they lack ventilatory muscle reserve), may have reduced responsiveness to hypoxia, and may develop excessive sedative-induced respiratory depression.[28–31] *Aspiration* is more likely as a result of prolonged depression and weakness of pharyngeal and laryngeal muscles and of the esophageal sphincter.[25,30,32,33] Thus, this disorder may pose multiple problems for the anesthesiologist.[31,34–36]

Myotonia congenita (Thomsen's disease) is nondystrophic, and is less systemic in nature and less life-threatening than myotonia dystrophica. It apparently is due to a gene abnormality on chromosome 7, which causes an ion channel defect. The disorder appears in early childhood and is characterized by *generalized weakness despite apparent hypertrophy.* It may manifest as difficulty swallowing because of oropharyngeal dysfunction.

Succinylcholine should be avoided in patients with *myotonia.*[31,35–43] It may induce contractures, in the context of which it may be virtually impossible to provide adequate ventilation even after SCh is discontinued. The SCh-induced release of K^+ may also alter muscle function: a large increase typically increases the occurrence of spontaneous myotonic discharges.[31]

Myotonia may be associated with *malignant hyperthermia;* however, the relationship is uncertain.[44] Both myotonia dystrophica and myotonia congenita typically are associated with *masseter spasm* after SCh.[34,45,46] The cause of the masseter spasm may be distinguished by EMG or biopsy.

Nondepolarizing relaxants generally may be used safely[41]; a normal response is suggested by the regional curare test.[5] However, excessive muscle weakness and especially prolonged duration may be noted.[47] Careful titration is essential. Reversal has been "safe"; however, prolonged block has been reported after attempted reversal of nondepolarizing block with neostigmine.[6,31] In addition, because myotonic muscle has increased sensitivity to acetylcholine (ACh),[23] an excess of reversal theoretically may disturb myotonic musculature. The use of a short-acting NDR, without the need for subsequent reversal, may prove useful. Prior to the recent introduction of mivacurium, an intermediate-acting agent such as atracurium was recommended.[48–50] One should seek to minimize respiratory depression and shivering.

◆ MYOSITIS

Polymyositis and dermatomyositis are characterized by skeletal muscle weakness, which may be accompanied by dysphagia, arthritis, decreased cervical and mandibular mobility, Raynaud's disorder, pulmonary interstitial fibrosis, myocarditis, and ST-segment abnormalities.[51–54] Pulmonary disease is a major cause of morbidity and mortality. The EMG is characterized by muscle fiber *fibrillation, sharp wave activity,* and *decreased muscle action potentials.*[53] Histological examination shows perivascular inflammatory infiltrates and muscle fiber degeneration. These disorders theoretically may lead to *hyperkalemia* in response to SCh. Patients with myositis have decreased muscular reserve and tend to be sensitive to NDRs; they may exhibit a myasthenia-like syndrome with prolonged weakness.[55]

◆ FAMILIAL PERIODIC PARALYSIS

Familial periodic paralysis is a symptom complex of nondystrophic, ion channel disorders that are characterized by *episodes of muscle paralysis* lasting hours to days. Paralysis often is induced during periods of rest after exercise and often is associated with an abnormal response to K^+.[56,57]

There are actually three varieties of *familial periodic paralysis:* hyperkalemic, hypokalemic, and normokalemic. If patients with *hyperkalemic periodic paralysis* develop hyperkalemia, they may develop prolonged paralysis. This may be induced by potassium administration, cold exposure, glucocorticoids, and stress. Patients with the *hypokalemic variety* are extremely sensitive to low K^+ levels; weakness may occur before the serum K^+

level has dropped below normal. This may be precipitated by stress, hypothermia, carbohydrate loading, high salt intake, diuretic therapy, and alkalosis.

These disorders pose the potential for an *SCh-induced myotonic response* and also for SCh-induced hyperkalemia,[56,58] in proportion to the extent of disease-induced muscle wasting. It is important to determine whether the contractures and paralysis are the result of SCh administration or are simply an exacerbation of the disease itself. The disorders are also associated with cardiac dysrhythmias.

Discussion Questions ◆

a. Is the patient with *muscular dystrophy* at increased risk for pulmonary *aspiration* of gastric contents?
b. What is the most likely cause of a *cardiac arrest* following a thiopental-SCh induction in the patient with *muscular dystrophy*? How should it be treated?
c. In the absence of SCh, might halothane trigger *hyperkalemia* in the patient with *Duchenne's muscular dystrophy*?
d. How does muscle from a patient with *Duchenne's muscular dystrophy* respond to the *caffeine-halothane contracture test*?
e. Why might the administration of a *respiratory depressant* be contraindicated in a patient with *myotonia dystrophica*?
f. Do patients with *myotonia* have increased susceptibility to *aspiration pneumonitis*?
g. Why might one elect to use a *regional anesthetic* in the patient with *myotonia dystrophica*?
h. How might one treat a *contracture* that results from intraoperative muscle manipulation in the patient with *myotonia*?
i. What special problems does *pregnancy* pose to the patient with *myotonia*?
j. Why might one elect to avoid SCh in the patient with *familial periodic paralysis*?
k. Distinguish between *fibrillations* and *fasciculations* on the *EMG*.
l. Compare the effects of *denervation* and *myopathy* on the number and size of *motor unit action potentials*.
m. Define *contracture*.

Answers ◆

a. The patient with *muscular dystrophy* may have *pharyngeal weakness* as well as gastric dilation and decreased gastrointestinal motility. The patient thus is at increased risk for pulmonary *aspiration* of gastric contents. Such features and the associated risk are more common in more advanced cases (i.e., after 8–10 years of age).

b. In the patient with a subclinical or clinical *myopathy* such as muscular dystrophy, *SCh may precipitate* extensive *rhabdomyolysis* and severe hyperkalemia (as is often the case for malignant hyperthermia as well). This may result in cardiac arrest. Bradycardic cardiac arrest after SCh administration in a young male should be presumed to be secondary to hyperkalemia in a child with Duchenne's muscular dystrophy. The myopathy may be subclinical; the child may be asymptomatic until age 5. Emergency therapy should include dextrose, 0.5–1.0 gm · kg^{-1}; regular insulin, 0.1–0.2 units · kg^{-1}; calcium chloride, 0.5–1.0 mg · kg^{-1}, and dantrolene if malignant hyperthermia is suspected (Chap. 20).

c. *Anesthetic disasters* related to *Duchenne's muscular dystrophy* can occur in the absence of SCh.[14] *Inhalational anesthesia* has been implicated in malignant hyperthermia, cardiac arrest, unexplained arrhythmias, and fevers. In addition to potentiating SCh-induced hyperkalemia and creatine kinase release, halothane may produce these changes to a lesser degree when administered as the sole agent.

d. The *caffeine-halothane contracture test* may induce contractures in muscle strips from patients with muscular dystrophy and other myopathic disorders.[59,60] The muscles are abnormal and may respond to precipitating agents such as SCh with systemic contractures, masseter spasm, and/or rhabdomyolysis. Alternatively, masseter spasm and rhabdomyolysis can occur in a patient with muscular dystrophy despite a negative caffeine-halothane contracture test.[59]

e. In addition to abnormal muscle function, the patient with *myotonia dystrophica* may have a *central component* that decreases the response to carbon dioxide (sleep apnea pattern, hypersomnolence). The myotonic patient is particularly sensitive to thiopental and related sedatives as a result of central and/or peripheral dysfunction.[28,31] Hence, sedatives and other respiratory depressant drugs should be used with caution.

f. Tracheal *aspiration* of gastric or pharyngeal contents is more likely in patients with *myotonia* because they often have thoracic and pharyngeal muscle weakness. This leads to a high incidence of postoperative pulmonary complications.[31]

g. A *regional anesthetic* may be indicated for the patient with *myotonia*[61] because it should obviate administration of SCh or of an anticholinesterase (to reverse nondepolarizing block). It also may avoid the need for large doses of respiratory depressants such as thiopental. In addition, a regional technique may be less disturbing to already disturbed cardiac and endocrine function, and less likely to be associated with aspiration.

h. Administration of an NDR cannot be relied on to *prevent or treat a myotonic response*,[37,41,62] for the primary defect lies beyond the neuromuscular junction. However, isolated cases have been cited in which 15 and 30 mg of tubocurarine counteracted a myotonic response to SCh.[39] Even dantrolene cannot necessarily prevent a contracture.[63] One should avoid local irritation and rely on direct infiltration with local anesthetic or quinine, or intravenous infusion of quinidine.[22,62] Symptomatic treatment with agents such as phenytoin, quinidine, and procainamide must be undertaken cautiously in light of the patient's propensity for depressed atrioventricular conduction.[40]

i. *Myotonia-associated weakness* may be exacerbated during *pregnancy*[64] and may aggravate the effects of the decrease in functional residual capacity that accompanies pregnancy. Despite the added risk of intercostal weakness, regional anesthesia still may be performed effectively.[61] After delivery, the neuromuscular function of both the neonate and the mother should be assessed.

j. Especially with the hyperkalemic form of *familial periodic paralysis*, the response to *SCh* is variable and may include myotonic contractures and even hyperkalemia.[56,58]

k. *Fibrillation potentials* probably represent the action potentials of *single muscle fibers;* they are observed regularly beginning 2–3 weeks after denervation and persist up to many years. They may also be seen with myositis or muscular dystrophy. *Fasciculations* involve entire motor units; they are seen with *anterior horn cell diseases* such as amyotrophic lateral sclerosis, progressive spinal muscular dystrophy, and progressive neuropathic (peroneal) muscular atrophy (Charcot-Marie-Tooth disease) *as well as in healthy people*. Repetitive fasciculations characterize *myokymia,* which may be seen in normal subjects but also in patients with tetany, uremia, and thyrotoxicosis.[65]

l. *Diseases of the lower motor neuron* are characterized by motor unit action potentials that are reduced in number (i.e., *motor units are lost*); they may also be associated with delayed conduction (increased latency). *Diseases of muscle* are characterized by motor unit action potentials that are reduced in size, since *some muscle fibers of a given motor unit are lost,* but the units themselves are still present.

m. A *contracture* is a prolonged muscle shortening of increased tension that arises from an initial depolarization but is not subsequently associated with repeated muscle action potentials. This abnormal state of muscle tension may be precipitated by an agonist (such as ACh or SCh) or mechanical stimulation, or it may occur spontaneously. Contractures have been observed in a number of disorders, including denervation injuries, multiple sclerosis, amyotrophic lateral sclerosis, muscular dystrophy, and myotonia.[66]

In contrast to a contracture, a *summated tetanic contraction* results from summation of individual contractions, each of which is preceded by initiation of a muscle action potential at the end-plate.

References ◆

1. Azar I: The response of patients with neuromuscular disorders to muscle relaxants: a review. Anesthesiology 61:173–187, 1984
2. Gamburg C, Rosenberg H: Neuromuscular diseases, myopathies, and anesthesia. Curr Rev Clin Anesth 8:170–175, 1988
3. Cobham IG, Davis HS: Anesthesia for muscular dystrophy patients. Anesth Analg 43:22–29, 1964
4. Richards WC: Anaesthesia and serum creatinine phosphokinase levels in patients with Duchenne's pseudohypertrophic muscular dystrophy. Anaesth Intensive Care 1:150–153, 1972
5. Brown JC, Charlton JE: Study of sensitivity to curare in certain neurological disorders using a regional technique. J Neurol Neurosurg Psychiatry 38:34–45, 1975
6. Buzello W, Krieg N, Schlickewei A: Hazards of neostigmine in patients with neuromuscular disorders. Br J Anaesth 54:529–534, 1982
7. Smith CL, Bush GH: Anaesthesia and progressive muscular dystrophy. Br J Anaesth 57:1113–1118, 1985
8. Delphin E, Jackson D, Rothstein P: Use of succinylcholine during elective pediatric anesthesia should be reevaluated. Anesth Analg 66:1190–1192, 1987
9. Genever EE: Suxamethonium-induced cardiac arrest in unsuspected pseudohypertrophic muscular dystrophy. Br J Anaesth 43:984–986, 1971
10. Henderson WAV: Succinylcholine induced cardiac arrest in unsuspected Duchenne muscular dystrophy. Can Anaesth Soc J 31:444–446, 1984
11. Lenter SPK, Thomas PR, Withington PS, et al: Suxamethonium associated hypertonicity and cardiac arrest in suspected pseudohypertrophic muscular dystrophy. Br J Anaesth 54:1331–1332, 1982
12. Linter SPK, Thomas PR, Withington PS, et al: Suxamethonium associated hypertonicity and cardiac arrest in unsuspected pseudohypertrophic muscular dystrophy. Br J Anaesth 54:1331–1332, 1982
13. Miller ED, Sanders DB, Rowlingson JC, et al: Anesthesia-induced rhabdomyolysis in a patient with Duchenne's muscular dystrophy. Anesthesiology 48:146, 1978
14. Sethna NF, Rockoff MA: Cardiac arrest following inhalation induction of anaesthesia in a child with Duchenne's muscular dystrophy. Can Anaesth Soc J 33:799–802, 1986
15. Lewandowski KB: Strabismus as a possible sign of subclinical muscular dystrophy predisposing to rhabdomyolysis and myoglobinuria: a study of an affected family. Can Anaesth Soc J 29:372, 1982
16. Brownell AKW, Passuke RT, Elash A, et al: Malignant hyperthermia in Duchenne muscular dystrophy. Anesthesiology 58:180–182, 1983
17. Kelfer HM, Singer WD, Reynolds RN: Malignant hyperthermia in a child with Duchenne muscular dystrophy. Pediatrics 71:118–119, 1983
18. Rosenberg H, Heiman-Patterson T: Duchenne's muscular dystrophy and malignant hyperthermia: another warning. Anesthesiology 59:362, 1983
19. Wang JM, Stanley TM: Duchenne muscular dystrophy and malignant hyperthermia—two case reports. Can Anaesth Soc J 33:492–497, 1986
20. Pearson CM, Beck WS, Bladh WH: Idiopathic paroxysmal myoglobinuria. Arch Intern Med 99:376, 1957
21. Rubiano R, Chang J-L, Carroll J, Sonbolian N, Larson CE: Acute rhabdomyolysis following halothane anesthesia without succinylcholine. Anesthesiology 67:856–857, 1987
22. Landau WM: Essential mechanism in myotonia: an electromyographic study. Neurology 2:369–388, 1952
23. Orndahl G: Myotonic human musculature: stimulation with depolarizing agents. I. Mechanical registration of the effects of acetylcholine and choline. Acta Med Scand 172:739–751, 1962
24. Pizzuti A, Friedman DL, Caskey CT: The myotonic dystrophy gene Arch Neurol 50:1173–1179, 1993
25. Harvey JC, Sherbourne DH, Siegel CI: Smooth muscle involvement in myotonic dystrophy. Am J Med 39:81–91, 1965
26. Forsberg H, Olofson B-O, Eriksson A, et al: Cardiac involvement in congenital myotonic dystrophy. Br Heart J 63:119, 1990

27. Perloff JK, Stevenson WG, Roberts NK, et al: Cardiac involvement in myotonic muscular dystrophy (Steinert's disease): a prospective study of 25 patients. Am J Cardiol 54:1074, 1984
28. Dundee JW: Thiopentone in dystrophica myotonica. Anesth Analg 31:257–259, 1952
29. Jammes Y, Pouget J, Grimaud C, et al: Pulmonary function and electromyographic study of respiratory muscles in myotonic dystrophy. Muscle Nerve 8:586, 1985
30. Pruzanski W, Profis A: Pulmonary disease in myotonic dystrophy. Am Rev Respir Dis 91:874–879, 1965
31. Aldridge LM: Anaesthetic problems in myotonic dystrophy. Br J Anaesth 57:1119–1130, 1985
32. Hannon VM, Cunningham AJ, Hutchinson M, et al: Aspiration pneumonia and coma—an unusual presentation of dystrophica myotonia. Can Anaesth Soc J 33:803, 1986
33. Pierce JW, Creamer B, MacDermott V: Pharynx and oesophagus in dystrophia myotonica. Gut 6:392–395, 1965
34. Dalal FY, Bennett EJ, Raj PP, Lee DG: Dystrophia myotonica: a multisystem disease. Can Anaesth Soc J 19:436–444, 1972
35. Talmage EA, McKechnic FB: Anesthetic management of patients with myotonia dystrophica. Anesthesiology 20:717–719, 1959
36. Ravin M, Newmark Z, Saviello G: Myotonia dystrophica, an anesthetic hazard: two case reports. Anesth Analg 54:216, 1975
37. Baraka A, Haddad C, Afifi A, et al: Control of succinylcholine-induced myotonia by d-tubocurarine. Anesthesiology 33:669–670, 1970
38. Cody JR: Muscle rigidity following administration of succinylcholine. Anesthesiology 29:159–162, 1968
39. Durant NN, Katz RL: Suxamethonium. Br J Anaesth 54:195–208, 1982
40. Kaufman L: Anaesthesia in dystrophica myotonia. Proc R Soc Med 53:183–185, 1960
41. Mitchell MM, Ali HH, Savarese JJ: Myotonia and neuromuscular blocking agents. Anesthesiology 49:44–48, 1978
42. Paterson IS: Generalized myotonia following suxamethonium. Br J Anaesth 34:340–342, 1962
43. Thiel RE: The myotonic response to suxamethonium. Br J Anaesth 39:815–821, 1967
44. Newberg LA, Lambert EH, Gronert GA: Failure to induce malignant hyperthermia in myotonic goats. Br J Anaesth 55:57, 1983
45. Britt BA, Kalow W: Malignant hyperthermia: a statistical review. Can Anaesth Soc J 17:293–315, 1970
46. Morley JB, Lambert TF, Katulas BA: A case of hyperpyrexia with myotonia congenita. In: Excerpta Medica International Congress Series, vol 295. Princeton, NJ, Excerpta Medica, p 543
47. Diefenbach C, Lynch J, Abel M, Buzello W: Vecuronium for muscle relaxation in patients with dystrophia myotonica. Anesth Analg 76:872–874, 1993
48. Boheimer N, Harris JW, Ward S: Neuromuscular blockade in dystrophica myotonica. Anaesthesia 40:872–874, 1985
49. Nightingale P, Healey TEJ, McGuiness K: Dystrophic myotonica and atracurium. Br J Anaesth 57:1131–1135, 1985
50. Stirt JA, Stone DJ, Weinberg G, et al: Atracurium in a child with myotonic dystrophy. Anesth Analg 64:369–370, 1985
51. Caro I: Dermatomyositis as a systemic disease. Med Clin North Am 73:1181, 1989
52. Dickey BF, Myers AR: Pulmonary disease in polymyositis/dermatomyositis. Semin Arthritis Rheum 14:60, 1984
53. Hochberg MC, Feldman D, Stevens MB: Adult onset polymyositis/dermatomyositis: an analysis of clinical and laboratory features and survival in 76 patients with a review of the literature. Semin Arthritis Rheum 15:168, 1986
54. Tazelaar HD, Viggiano RW, Pickersgill J, et al: Interstitial lung disease in polymyositis and dermatomyositis. Am Rev Respir Dis 141:727, 1990
55. Flusche G, Unger-Sargon J, Lambert DH: Prolonged neuromuscular paralysis with vecuronium in a patient with polymyositis. Anesth Analg 66:188–190, 1987
56. Flewellen EH, Bodensteiner JB: Anesthetic experience in a patient with hyperkalemic periodic paralysis. Anesth Rev 7:44, 1980

57. Siler JN, Discavage WJ: Anesthetic management of hypokalemic periodic paralysis. Anesthesiology 43:489, 1975
58. Gronert GA, Theye RA: Pathophysiology of hyperkalemia induced by succinylcholine. Anesthesiology 43:89–99, 1975
59. Heiman-Patterson TD, Rosenberg H, Fletcher JE, Tahmoush AJ: Halothane-caffeine contracture testing in neuromuscular diseases. Muscle Nerve 11:453–457, 1988
60. Takagi A, Sunohara N, Ishihara T, Nonaka I, Sugita H: Malignant hyperthermia and related neuromuscular diseases: caffeine contracture of the skinned muscle fibers. Muscle Nerve 6:510–514, 1983
61. Cope DK, Miller JN: Local and spinal anesthesia for cesarean section in a patient with myotonic dystrophy. Anesth Analg 65:687–690, 1986
62. Geshwind N, Simpson JA: Procaine amide in the treatment of myotonia. Brain 78:81–91, 1955
63. Phillips DC, Ellis FR, Exley KA, et al: Dantrolene sodium and dystrophia myotonica. Anaesthesia 39:568–573, 1984
64. Paterson RA, Tousignant M, Skene DS: Caesarean section for twins in a patient with myotonic dystrophy. Can Anaesth Soc J 32:418–421, 1985
65. Eaton LM, Lambert EH: Electromyography and electric stimulation of nerves in diseases of motor unit: observations on myasthenic syndrome associated with malignant tumors. JAMA 163:1117–1124, 1957
66. Azar I: Complications of neuromuscular blockers: interaction with concurrent diseases. Anesthesiol Clin North Am 11:409–429, 1993

Index

Page numbers followed by *t* and *f* indicate tables and figures, respectively.

Abdominal relaxation, adequacy of, 65, 72
Abductor digiti quinti (minimi) muscles
 innervation of, 25
 monitoring
  during onset of block, 33
  perioperative, 64–65
 sensitivity to neuromuscular relaxants, 28, 33, 53
Accelerography, 55
Acetylcholine, 1–2, 2*f*, 4
 mobilization, and fade, in response to NDRs, 38*f*, 38–39
 and neuromuscular blocking agents, structural similarities, 11, 12*f*
 and nondepolarizing block, 11, 13
 quantum content, of vesicles, 1, 7
 receptors. *See also* Cholinoceptors
  decreased, in myasthenia gravis, 324
  proliferation, 332–348
  subunits, 2, 3*f*
 release
  from presynaptic terminal, 1, 5–6
  use-dependent rundown of, 4, 17
 structure of, 11, 12*f*
Acetylcholinesterase, 2, 3*f*, 3, 13
ACh. *See* Acetylcholine
Acid base/lytes, effects
 on nondepolarizing block, 128*t*–131*t*
 on pseudocholinesterase and succinylcholine, 265*t*
Acidosis
 differential diagnosis of, 319
 effect on nondepolarizing block, 123*t*
 intracellular, in diagnosis of malignant hyperthermia susceptibility, 300
 metabolic, effect on nondepolarizing block, 130*t*–131*t*
Acrylates, formation from atracurium, 149–150
Actin, 4, 6
Action potential(s). *See also* Muscle action potential(s)
 compound, 58
 nerve, 1
Adductor pollicis force translation monitor, 53–55
Adductor pollicis muscle
 innervation, 26
 monitoring
  perioperative, 64–65
  during recovery from block, 33
 posttetanic count, 31, 58
 sensitivity to neuromuscular relaxants, 25–26, 28, 29*f*, 31, 53, 58
 and monitoring depth of block, 58
 single twitch stimulation, monitoring, during intubation, 44
 twitch height, and receptor occupancy, 16
Aging. *See* Elderly; Old age
Airway muscles, sensitivity to neuromuscular relaxants, 26, 28
Airway protection, adequacy of, 65, 73
Airway resistance, during neuromuscular block, 32
Albumin, serum, effect on nondepolarizing block, 123*t*–124*t*
Alcuronium
 cardiovascular effects of, 143, 144*t*, 174
 dosages and durations of, 172*t*, 174
 elimination of, 174
 pharmacology of, 174
 pretreatment prior to succinylcholine, 282*t*
Alfentanil, pretreatment prior to succinylcholine, 282*t*
Alkalosis, effect on nondepolarizing block, 123*t*
Allergic reaction, 146
Alloferin. *See* Alcuronium
All-or-none phenomenon, 1–3, 6, 16
Alpha$_1$-acid glycoprotein, effect on nondepolarizing block, 113, 123*t*–124*t*, 333–334, 339
Alpha subunits, 2, 3*f*, 332
Aminoglycosides
 effect on nondepolarizing block, 105*t*
 neuromuscular effects, opposed by calcium, 112
Aminophylline
 neuromuscular effects of, 160
 and risk of malignant hyperthermia, 305–306
Aminopyridine, effect on nondepolarizing block, 6, 104*t*
Amyotrophic lateral sclerosis, neuromuscular effects of, 335–336, 340–341
Analgesia, with neuromuscular block, in ICU, 70
Analgesics, intravenous, effect on pseudocholinesterase and succinylcholine, 261*t*
Anaphylaxis
 with relaxants, 146–147, 157
 with thiopental plus relaxant, 157
Anatomy, of neuromuscular transmission, 1–10, 2*f*–3*f*
Anectine. *See* Succinylcholine
Anesthesia
 deaths related to, 70
 nitrous-narcotic-NDR, 72
Antagonists, fractional occupancy by, 16
Antiarrhythmics, effect on nondepolarizing block, 106*t*
Antibiotics
 effects
  on nondepolarizing block, 104*t*–105*t*, 112
  on pseudocholinesterase and succinylcholine, 259*t*
 neuromuscular effects, opposed by calcium, 112
Anticholinesterase(s). *See also specific anticholinesterase*
 in asthma, 228
 effects
  on bronchomotor tone and airway secretions, 228
  gastrointestinal, 228
  on nondepolarizing block, 105*t*, 112
  on phase 1 block, 243
  on pseudocholinesterase and succinylcholine, 258*t*
 long-term exposure to, effects on neuromuscular block, 230
 overdose and toxicity, 221–222, 229
  neuromuscular effects, 222
 reversal of mivacurium, 202–203
 reversal of phase 2 block, 243, 246
 reversal of relaxants, 217–230
Anticonvulsants, effect on nondepolarizing block, 105*t*–106*t*, 112

Index

Antiemetics, effect on nondepolarizing block, 106t
Antihistamines, effects with NDRs, 156
Antimuscarinic(s). *See also* Atropine; Glycopyrrolate
  in prevention of succinylcholine-induced bradycardia, 277
  reversal of relaxants, 219, 228–229
Antineoplastics, effects
  on nondepolarizing block, 106t
  on succinylcholine and pseudocholinesterase, 258t
Antirheumatic drugs, effect on nondepolarizing block, 106t
Anxiolytics, effect on nondepolarizing block, 110t
Apnea, with succinylcholine, and pseudocholinesterase activity, 267
Arduan. *See* Pipecuronium bromide
Arrhythmia(s)
  differential diagnosis of, 319
  in malignant hyperthermia, 318
Arterial pressure, atracurium effect on, 145, 145t
Aspiration of gastric contents
  with muscular dystrophy, 352
  with myotonia, 353
Aspirin
  mitigation of histamine's effects, 146
  pretreatment prior to succinylcholine, 282t
  vasodilatory action of tubocurarine blocked by, 157
Asthma
  atracurium and, 187
  and reversal of relaxants, 228
  steroid administration and, 160
Atracurium
  and asthma, 187
  cardiovascular effects of, 144, 144t, 186–187
  in children, 185
    dose-response relationship for, 132–133, 133t
  clearance, 96
  clinical duration (Dur$_{25}$), 98, 100
  dosages and durations of, 172t, 184
  effect on mean arterial pressure/heart rate, 145, 145t
  in elderly, 184, 191
  histamine release with, 145, 145t, 186–187
  hypotension with, prevention of, 187
  increased dose, side effects of, 82
  infusion rate for, 95, 185, 203, 203t
  long-term use in ICU, 152
  metabolism, 184
  metabolites, 149–150, 152, 185. *See also*
    Laudanosine
  in obstetrics, 147–148
  pharmacology of, 184–187, 187t, 191
  and pheochromocytoma, 187
  plus thiopental, potential toxicity, 157
  presynaptic block with, 13
  pretreatment prior to succinylcholine, 282t
  for rapid-sequence intubation, 158
  recovery from, 98, 100
    train-of-four monitoring during, 192
  recovery index for, 98
  in renal failure, 226–227
  structure of, 11, 12f, 185
  weakness or paralysis after, with long-term use in ICU, 152
Atrophy, disuse, effects
  on nondepolarizing block, 124t
  on succinylcholine and pseudocholinesterase, 263t
Atropine
  for anticholinesterase toxicity, 222
  with edrophonium, administration of, 228
  effects on barrier pressure of esophageal sphincter, 228
  neostigmine with, 219–220
  pharmacology of, 219
  reversal of relaxants with, 228–229

dose for, 219
Autonomic dysfunction, 337
Azathioprine, in myasthenia gravis, 324–325

Bambuterol, effect on succinylcholine and pseudocholinesterase, 259t
Barbiturates
  and malignant hyperthermia, 298
  pretreatment prior to succinylcholine, 282t
Barrier pressure, of esophageal sphincter, and reversal of relaxants, 228
Becker's muscular dystrophy, and malignant hyperthermia susceptibility, 300
Benzodiazepine(s)
  for anticholinesterase toxicity, 222
  effect on nondepolarizing block, 110t
Benzylisoquinolonium, structure of, 11. *See also specific agent*
Beta agonists
  effect on nondepolarizing block, 107t
  neuromuscular effects of, 160
Beta blockers
  effects
    on nondepolarizing block, 106t
    on pseudocholinesterase and succinylcholine, 260t, 284
    on serum potassium, 284
  in myasthenia gravis, 328
Beta subunits, 2, 3f, 332
Biophase, 78
  neuromuscular blocking agents in, effects of potency, 88–89
Bradycardia, with succinylcholine, 277
Bradyphylaxis
  with depolarizing relaxants, 243, 245
  with succinylcholine infusion, 96
Buffered diffusion, 79
  effects of potency, 88–89
Burn(s)
  effects
    on nondepolarizing block, 124t
    on pseudocholinesterase and succinylcholine, 264t
  neuromuscular response to, 338–339, 341–342
Butyryl cholinesterase. *See* Pseudocholinesterase

Ca. *See* Calcium
Caffeine-halothane contracture test, 353
  for malignant hyperthermia, 299–300, 303–305
Calcium
  abnormalities, in malignant hyperthermia, 306
  decreased, effect on nondepolarizing block, 128t
  effect
    on neuromuscular effects of antibiotics, 112
    on nondepolarizing block, 128t–129t
  increased
    effect on nondepolarizing block, 128t–129t
    effect on succinylcholine and pseudocholinesterase, 267t
  in muscle contraction, 4, 305
  myoplasmic, dantrolene effects on, 315t, 315, 319
  in presynaptic nerve terminal, 1, 2f, 4–6
  pretreatment prior to succinylcholine, 282t
  release, and inhalational agents, 305
Calcium–calmodulin binding, 6
Calcium channel(s)
  fast (P), 1, 5
  slow (L), 1, 5
  voltage dependent, 5
Calcium channel blockers
  effects
    on nondepolarizing block, 107t
    on pseudocholinesterase and succinylcholine, 259t
  mechanism of action, 5

Carbamazepine, effect on nondepolarizing block, 112–113
Carbon dioxide, end-tidal, 65
  curare cleft on tracing of, 74
  in diagnosis of malignant hyperthermia, 314, 318–319
  increased, differential diagnosis of, 319
Cardiac arrest, hyperkalemia-precipitated, 299
Cardiopulmonary bypass, effect on nondepolarizing block, 124t
Cardiovascular drugs
  effect on nondepolarizing block, 106t–107t
  effect on pseudocholinesterase and succinylcholine, 259t–260t
Cardiovascular effects
  of nondepolarizing relaxants, 143–144, 144t, 174, 186–187
  of succinylcholine, 276–278
  of d-tubocurarine, 143, 144t, 156
Central core disease, and malignant hyperthermia susceptibility, 300
Central nervous system, nondepolarizing relaxant effects on, 149
Cerebral aneurysm, neuromuscular effects of, 337, 341
Cerebral blood flow
  and nondepolarizing relaxant use, 149
  with succinylcholine, 278
Cerebral palsy
  effect on nondepolarizing block, 124t
  neuromuscular effects of, 338, 341
Cesarean section
  nondepolarizing block for, 147–148
  dose selection and priming with, 87–88
  rapid-sequence induction for, relaxant selection for, 158–159
Channel block, 14–15, 17, 239
Children. See also Infant(s); Neonate(s)
  antimuscarinics for, 229
  atracurium in, 185
  dose-response relationship for, 132–133, 133t
  depolarizing block in, 245
  doxacurium in, 177
  mivacurium in, 204
  nondepolarizing block in, 127t
  dose-response relationships for, 132–133
  pseudocholinesterase in, 264t
  rapid-sequence intubation in, 88
  rocuronium in, 207
  succinylcholine in, 242, 245, 264t, 283
  adverse effects of, 277
  vecuronium in, 81, 189
Chlorpromazine
  effect on nondepolarizing block, 110t
  effect on pseudocholinesterase and succinylcholine, 261t
  pretreatment prior to succinylcholine, 283t
Cholinesterase
  assay, in organophosphate poisoning, 230
  exogenous, administration of, 243–244
  inhibition, with nondepolarizing relaxant use, 149
  reversible carbamylation, 230
Cholinesterase inhibitors, 14, 149
Cholinoceptors
  occupancy, by neuromuscular blocking agents, 11, 13, 17
  presynaptic, in acetylcholine mobilization, 4
Chronic disease state, effect on succinylcholine and pseudocholinesterase, 263t
Cimetidine, 156–157
Clearance
  of nondepolarizing relaxants, 96, 100–101
  in renal failure, 133

Clindamycin, effect on nondepolarizing block, 105t
Clinical duration, 98, 100
Closed-channel block, 14
Closed head injury, neuromuscular effects of, 337
Clostridium botulinum, effect
  on nondepolarizing block, 111t
  on pseudocholinesterase and succinylcholine, 262t
Clostridium tetani
  effect
    on nondepolarizing block, 111t
    on succinylcholine and pseudocholinesterase, 262t
  neuromuscular effects of, 336, 341
Compound action potential, 58
Contracture(s), 354
  definition of, 354
  succinylcholine-induced
    disorders associated with, 333–339
    in muscular dystrophy, 349
  versus summated tetanic contraction, 354
Cortical motor evoked potentials, effect of neuromuscular block on, 32
Coughing, prediction, assessment of posttetanic count for, 58
Creatine kinase
  increased
    differential diagnosis of, 306, 319
    neuromuscular effects of, 150, 160
  levels, in muscular dystrophy, 349
  measurement of, in diagnosis of malignant hyperthermia, 300
  release, succinylcholine-induced, 283
  reduction of, 282t, 283, 286
Creutzfeldt-Jakob disease, neuromuscular effects of, 337–338
Critical illness, effects
  on nondepolarizing block, 124t
  on pseudocholinesterase and succinylcholine, 262t
Curare cleft, on end-tidal CO_2 tracing, 74

Dantrolene
  effects
    on myoplasmic calcium, 315t, 315, 319
    on nondepolarizing block, 107t
  EMG with, 59, 319
  and malignant hyperthermia, 298–299
  MMG with, 59, 319
  placental transfer of, 320
  pretreatment prior to succinylcholine, 282t
  prophylactic therapy with, 319
  side effects of, 314–315, 320
  therapy, for malignant hyperthermia, 314–317, 319–320
Decamethonium, 13, 242–243
  histamine release with, 145
  mechanism of action, 7, 239–240, 242
  negative features of, 243
  neuromuscular effects of, 13
  renal excretion of, 242
  structure of, 13
Defasciculation, prior to rapid-sequence induction, risks with, 286. See also Nondepolarizing relaxant(s), defasciculating dose
Delta subunits, 2, 3f, 332
Denervation
  effect on succinylcholine and pseudocholinesterase, 264t
  neuromuscular response to, 333–335, 340
Depolarization, 1–4
  end-plate, with depolarizing relaxants, 14, 239, 245
Depolarizing block, 13–14
  phase 1, 239, 243–246

Index

persistent, 243
phase 2, 14, 239, 243–246
    fade, 44–45
    reversal, 243
stimulation patterns with, 37, 38f
and tetanic stimulation, 245
Depolarizing relaxant(s), 1–4, 239–254. *See also* Decamethonium; Succinylcholine
    bradyphylaxis with, 243, 245
    in children, 245
    effects, in myasthenia gravis, 325–326
    end-plate depolarization with, 14, 239, 245
    flaccid paralysis with, 14
    masseter spasm with, 241
    mechanism of action, 11, 239–240
    muscle action potential with, 239, 245
    muscle tension with, 14
    neuromuscular effects of, 239–254
    onset, muscle differences in, 28
    presynaptic effects of, 14, 240, 247
    recovery from, muscle differences in, 28
    sensitivity to, 28
        of eye muscles, 32
        muscle differences in, 28
    structure of, 11, 12f
    tachyphylaxis with, 243–245
Dermatomyositis, 351
Desensitization, 14–15, 239
Diaphragm
    fatigue, 7
    muscle fiber types of
        in full-term newborn and children, 7
        in premature infant, 7
    sensitivity to neuromuscular relaxants, 27–28, 29f, 31
Diazepam, effect on succinylcholine and pseudocholinesterase, 260t
Dibucaine number, 256–258, 267
Diffuse neuronal disease, neuromuscular response to, 333, 335–337
Dimethyltubocurarine. *See also* Metocurine
    histamine release with, 173
    pharmacology of, 173
    structure of, 12f
Diphenhydramine, effects on histamine release with NDRs, 156
Diphenylhydantoin, 14. *See also* Phenytoin
Disuse atrophy
    effect on nondepolarizing block, 124t
    effect on pseudocholinesterase and succinylcholine, 264t
    in ICU patients, 150–151
    neuromuscular response to, 337
Docking proteins, 1, 6
Double-burst stimulation, 41f–42f, 42–43, 46
    effect of stimulating current intensity on, 24, 30–31
    in evaluation of depth of block, 52
    first burst of impulses in, duration of, 46
    mechanical fade in, 46
Doxacurium
    cardiovascular effects, 144, 144t
    in children, 177
    clearance, 176
        in renal failure, 133
    dosages and durations of, 172t, 176
    in elderly, 176
    histamine release with, 145
    pharmacology of, 176–178
    in renal disease, 176
    in renal failure, 226–227
    structure of, 11, 12f
    time to maximum block for, 79

Doxapram, effect on nondepolarizing block, 107t
Droperidol
    effect on nondepolarizing block, 106t
    and malignant hyperthermia, 298
Dual block, 239
Duchenne's muscular dystrophy, 349, 353
    and malignant hyperthermia susceptibility, 300
Dur_{10}, monitoring, 97–98
Dur_{25}, 98, 100
Dur_{95}, 98, 100

Eaton-Lambert syndrome, 326, 329
Echothiophate eye drops, effect on succinylcholine and pseudocholinesterase, 258t
Eclampsia
    pseudocholinesterase in, 264t
    succinylcholine in, 264t
ED_{95}
    definition of, 85
    units of, 85
Edrophonium
    atropine with, administration of, 228
    contraindications to, 224
    dosage (dose requirement), 219–220
    effect on pseudocholinesterase and succinylcholine, 259t
    glycopyrrolate with, 229
    indications for, 224
    mechanism of action, 217
    onset, 220
    pharmacology of, 218t
    reversal of relaxants with, 220–221, 224, 228
EJRs. *See* Extrajunctional receptors
Elderly
    atracurium in, 184, 191
    doxacurium in, 176
    pancuronium in, 174
    pipecuronium in, 175
    rocuronium in, 207
    vecuronium in, 190
Electrode(s)
    for electromyography, 53, 55t, 56f, 60
        active recording, placement of, 60
        grounding, placement of, 60
        reference recording, placement of, 60
    needle, 30
    for neurostimulation, 23, 30
        placement, 25
    surface, limitations of, 30
Electromyography, 53, 54f, 55t, 55, 56f, 57
    electrode placement for, 60
    fibrillation versus fasciculation on, 354
    intraoperative, limitations of, 69, 72–74
    intraoperative monitoring with, 58
    latency, of artifact versus muscle action potential, 58
    in myasthenia gravis, 329
    in myasthenic syndrome, 329
    in myotonia, 350
    response to direct muscle stimulation, versus nerve-to-muscle transmission, 58
    sensitivity to tetanic fade, 59
Elimination, of nondepolarizing relaxant, 96
Elimination constant, 96
Elimination half-life, 95–96
    of nondepolarizing relaxants, 171
EMG. *See* Electromyography
End-plate, of neuromuscular junction, 2–3, 3f
    depolarization
        with depolarizing relaxants, 14, 239, 245
        persistent, 17
    in neonate, 18
    sensitivity of, to nondepolarizing block, 16

End-plate potential, 2, 6
  miniature, 2, 6
  summated, 2, 6
Enflurane
  effect on depolarizing block, 244
  neuromuscular effects of, 69
Epinephrine, effect on nondepolarizing block, 107t
Epsilon subunits, 2, 3f, 18, 332
Esmeron. See Rocuronium
Esmolol, effect on succinylcholine and pseudocholinesterase, 259t
Esophageal sphincter, opening pressure, and reversal of relaxants, 228
Evan's myopathy, and malignant hyperthermia susceptibility, 300
Evoked response
  fade of, 4
  monitoring, 51–63
    active recording electrode placement for, 60
    compound action potential in, 58
    electromyography for, 53, 54f, 55t, 55, 56f, 57
    gel bridge in, 60
    mechanomyography for, 53–57
    posttetanic count in, 51–52, 52t, 58
    reference recording electrode placement for, 60
    tactile means, 51–52, 52t, 58
    transducer overload in, 59
    visual means, 51–52, 52t, 58
Extracellular fluid volume, 85, 132
Extrajunctional receptors
  proliferation, 17
  response to nerve injury, burns, and trauma, 332–348
Eye, extrinsic muscles of, sensitivity to nondepolarizing relaxants, 32

Facial nerve
  intracranial stimulation of, 32
  stimulation of, 26
Fade, 4, 13, 37, 38f, 38–39. See also Train-of-four
  in assessment of recovery, 98–99
  identification of, 51, 58
  mechanical, in double-burst stimulation, 46
  mechanisms of, 13, 17
  with nondepolarizing block, 44
  in phase 2 block, 44–45
  tetanic, 59
    degree of block and, 44–45
    end-plate current decline in, 44–45
Familial periodic paralysis, 351–352, 354
  hyperkalemic, 351–352, 354
    and malignant hyperthermia susceptibility, 300
  hypokalemic, 351–352
  normokalemic, 351–352
Fasciculation(s), 14
  on EMG, 354
  succinylcholine-induced, 240, 281
    reduction of, 282, 283t, 286
Fatigue, muscular resistance to, 7
Fazadinium, cardiovascular effects, 143
Fentanyl
  effect on depolarizing block, 244
  induction, cardiovascular effects of vecuronium in, 191
  pretreatment prior to succinylcholine, 282t
Fetus
  plasma levels of relaxant attained in, 157–158
  uptake of nondepolarizing relaxant(s), 147–148, 148t, 157–158
Fever, postoperative, 319
Fibrillation, on EMG, 354
Flaxedil. See Gallamine
Fluoride number, 257

Fractional occupancy, by antagonists, 16
Friedreich's ataxia, abnormal responses to succinylcholine in, 336

Gallamine, 88, 156
  cardiovascular effects, 143, 144t
  clinical duration (Dur_{25}), 98
  contraindications to, 173
  dosages and durations of, 172t
  onset, 88
  pharmacology of, 173
  presynaptic block with, 13
  pretreatment prior to succinylcholine, 282t
  in renal failure, 133, 226–227
  structure of, 173
  vagolytic effects of, 156
Gamma subunit, 17, 332
Ganglionic blockers, effect on nondepolarizing block, 107t
Gastrointestinal system, succinylcholine effect on, 280–281
Gel bridge, 60
Genitourinary function, succinylcholine effect on, 280–281
Geography, effect on nondepolarizing block, 124t
Glucocorticoids, effect on pseudocholinesterase and succinylcholine, 260t
Glycopyrrolate
  dose, during reversal, 219
  with edrophonium, 229
  neostigmine with, 219–220
  pharmacology of, 219
  reversal of relaxants with, 229
Guillain-Barré syndrome, neuromuscular effects of, 336

Halothane, and malignant hyperthermia, 297–299
Hand grip, assessment, intraoperative, 66–68
Head lift
  assessment, intraoperative, 66–68
  as indicator of readiness for tracheal extubation, 66
Heart rate, atracurium effect on, 145, 145t
Heat stroke, and malignant hyperthermia susceptibility, 300
Hemidiaphragm preparation, rat, 15
Hexafluorenium, effect on pseudocholinesterase and succinylcholine, 262t
Hexamethonium, 11, 17
  presynaptic block with, 13, 17
Histamine H_1-receptor antagonists, 146, 156
Histamine H_2-receptor antagonists, 146, 156–157
  effect on nondepolarizing block, 107t–108t
  effect on succinylcholine and pseudocholinesterase, 262t
Histamine H_3-receptor antagonists, 156–157
Histamine N-methyltransferase, 145
  inhibition, 156
Histamine release
  with atracurium, 145, 145t, 186–187
  with decamethonium, 145
  with dimethyltubocurarine, 173
  with doxacurium, 145
  with mevocurium, 145
  with mivacurium, 145–146, 146t, 204
  with nondepolarizing relaxants, 144–147, 145t–146t, 156
  with succinylcholine, 145, 277
  with d-tubocurarine, 145, 157
Hoffmann's disease, 350
Hofmann elimination, 149–150, 185
Huntington's chorea, neuromuscular effects of, 337
Hypercarbia
  differential diagnosis of, 319

Index

effect on nondepolarizing block, 124*t*
Hyperkalemia. *See also* Familial periodic paralysis, hyperkalemic
 cardiac arrest precipitated by, 299
 in malignant hyperthermia, management of, 317
 succinylcholine-induced, 277–278, 283, 284, 333
  in muscular dystrophy, 349
  with nerve injury, burns, and trauma, 333–339
  and neuroleptic malignant syndrome, 320
Hyperparathyroidism, effect on nondepolarizing block, 124*t*
Hyperthermia, malignant. *See* Malignant hyperthermia
Hyperthyroidism, effect on succinylcholine and pseudocholinesterase, 263*t*
Hypoalbuminemia, effect on nondepolarizing block, 123*t*
Hypocarbia, effect on nondepolarizing block, 124*t*
Hypoperfusion, effect on nondepolarizing block, 124*t*
Hypoproteinemia, effect on pseudocholinesterase and succinylcholine, 263*t*
Hypotension
 with alcuronium, 174
 with atracurium, prevention of, 187
 with tubocurarine, 157
Hypothenar eminence
 monitoring EMG responses at, during onset of block, 33
 muscles
  electromyography of, 58
  sensitivity to nondepolarizing relaxant, 58–59
Hypothermia, effect on nondepolarizing block, 124*t*, 131–132

Immobility, muscle, neuromuscular response to, 337
Immunosuppressives, effect on nondepolarizing block, 108*t*
Impedance, in neurostimulation, 23
Infant(s). *See also* Neonate(s)
 depolarizing block in, 245
 nondepolarizing block in
  dosages, 132–133
  dose-response relationships for, 132–133
Infection(s). *See also* Sepsis
 prolonged systemic, abnormal responses to succinylcholine in, 336
Infusion
 continuous, recovery time after, 96–97
 of nondepolarizing relaxant, dosages, 95–96
 plasma to NMJ concentration gradient during, 100
Infusion rate, of nondepolarizing relaxants, 81
Inhalational anesthetics
 calcium release and, 305
 effect
  on depolarizing block, 244
  on nondepolarizing block, 14–15, 44, 109*t*–110*t*
  on pseudocholinesterase and succinylcholine, 260*t*
  residual, during recovery from neuromuscular block, 69–70
Injection site, for neuromuscular block, 15
Injury, effect
 on nondepolarizing block, 124*t*–125*t*
 on succinylcholine and pseudocholinesterase, 264*t*
Innervation ratio, 5
Inorganic phosphate/ATP ratio, 300
Inorganic phosphate/phosphocreatine ratio, 300
Inspiratory capacity, tetanic stimulation as indicator of, 44
Intensive care unit, patients, problems contributing to neuromuscular dysfunction and myopathy, 159–160
Intercostal muscle(s), muscle fiber types of, 7
Intermediate-acting nondepolarizing relaxant(s), 172*t*, 184–199
Interosseous muscles, innervation of, 25
Intracranial disorders, neuromuscular response to, 337–338
Intracranial pressure
 increased, rapid tracheal intubation with, 285
  vecuronium for, 191–192
 succinylcholine effect on, 278–279, 284
Intragastric pressure, succinylcholine effect on, 280, 286
Intraocular pressure
 with depolarizing block, 32
 succinylcholine and, 6, 279–280, 285
Intraoperative monitoring, of relaxation, 64–68, 67*t*
 limitations of, 68–70
Intravenous administration, of nondepolarizing relaxants, 78–94
Intubation. *See also* Tracheal intubation
 rapid-sequence, 88
 with rocuronium, 205–206, 210

Jaw muscle. *See also* Masseter muscle
 rigidity, with succinylcholine, in malignant hyperthermia, 241, 298–299
 tension, with succinylcholine, 240, 301–302

Ketamine
 effect
  on nondepolarizing block, 109*t*
  on succinylcholine and pseudocholinesterase, 260*t*
 and malignant hyperthermia, 298
King Denborough syndrome, and malignant hyperthermia susceptibility, 300
Kyphoscoliosis, and malignant hyperthermia susceptibility, 300

Lactate, muscle levels of, 300
Laryngeal muscle(s), sensitivity to neuromuscular relaxants, 27–28, 31
 and monitoring depth of block, 58
Laudanosine, 186, 187*t*
 effects, 185–186
  on cardiovascular system, 187
  on central nervous system, 149, 186
 fetal:maternal ratio for, 148
 formation, 149–150, 185–186
Leg lift, assessment, intraoperative, 67–68
Lidocaine, pretreatment prior to succinylcholine, 282*t*
Lidocaine seizure threshold, effects of nondepolarizing relaxant on, 149
Lincomycin, effect on nondepolarizing block, 105*t*
Lithium, effect
 on nondepolarizing block, 109*t*
 on succinylcholine and pseudocholinesterase, 261*t*
Liver failure
 effect
  on nondepolarizing block, 125*t*
  on pseudocholinesterase and succinylcholine, 263*t*
 mivacurium in, 202
 nondepolarizing block in, 150
 rocuronium in, 206
Local anesthetics
 effect
  on nondepolarizing block, 15, 109*t*
  on pseudocholinesterase and succinylcholine, 260*t*
 in myasthenia gravis, 328

364 Index

Lower motor nerve injury, with extrajunctional chemosensitivity and SCh-induced hyperkalemia and/or contractures, 334

Magnesium
  effect on nondepolarizing block, 129t
  increased
    effect on nondepolarizing block, 129t
    effect on succinylcholine and pseudocholinesterase, 266t
  presynaptic effects of, 17
Magnesium sulfate, pretreatment prior to succinylcholine, 282t
Maintenance, with nondepolarizing relaxant, 67t, 95–99, 172t
Malignant hyperthermia
  crisis
    identification of, factors affecting, 318–319
    management of, 316–317
  cyanosis in, 318
  differential diagnosis of, 319
  dysrhythmias in, 318
  effect on pseudocholinesterase and succinylcholine, 263t
  in muscular dystrophy, 349
  with myotonia, 351
  and neuroleptic malignant syndrome, compared, 320
  pathophysiology of, 297
  prevalence of, 300
  risk factors for, 300, 302–303
  signs of, 314, 318
  succinylcholine and jaw muscle rigidity in, 298–299, 302–303
  susceptibility, 297–298
    and anesthetic administration, 307
    appropriate diagnosis of, importance of, 307
    effect on patient's life, 306
    sympathetic activity and, 307
  symptoms of, 314, 318
  tachycardia in, 318
  tests for, 299–300, 303
  treatment of, 314–317, 319–320
  triggering agents, 297–298
  without muscle contractions, 319
Malignant Hyperthermia Association of the United States, 307
Malnutrition, effect on nondepolarizing block, 125t
Mannitol, effect on nondepolarizing block, 109t
MAP. See Muscle action potential(s)
Margin of safety, with nondepolarizing block, 11, 16
Masseter muscle
  local injection of pancuronium into, 15
  muscle twitch tension, with succinylcholine onset, 240
  rigidity, succinylcholine-induced, 302
  sensitivity to neuromuscular relaxant, 27
  spasm
    with depolarizing relaxant, 241
    with halothane and succinylcholine, 302
    and malignant hyperthermia, 302–303
  succinylcholine effect on, 301–302
    in malignant hyperthermia, 298–299
    in myotonia, 351
Mast cell, histamine release from, 157
Maximal current, neurostimulation, 23–24, 26f
Maximum expiratory pressure, 66
  sensitivity to neuromuscular block, 69
Maximum inspiratory pressure
  relationship to clinical signs, with neuromuscular block, 66, 67t
  sensitivity to neuromuscular block, 66, 69

Mechanical fade, in double-burst stimulation, 46
Mechanical ventilation
  neuromuscular relaxation for, 150–155. See also Nondepolarizing relaxant(s), long-term use
  monitoring, 70–72
  and steroid administration, 160
  weaning from, guidelines for, 66
Mechanomyography, 53–57
  intraoperative, limitations of, 69, 72–74
Meningomyelocele, neuromuscular effects of, 335, 341
Mestinon. See Pyridostigmine
Metabolic acidosis, effect on nondepolarizing block, 130t–131t
Metabolic alkalosis, effect on nondepolarizing block, 131t
Metoclopramide, effect
  on nondepolarizing block, 106t
  on succinylcholine and pseudocholinesterase, 261t
Metocurine. See also Dimethyltubocurarine
  cardiovascular effects, 144, 144t
  clearance, in renal failure, 133
  clinical duration (Dur$_{25}$) of, 98
  dosages and durations of, 172t
  long-term use in ICU, 152
  structure of, 11
Metronidazole, effect on nondepolarizing block, 105t
Metubine. See Metocurine
Mevocurium, histamine release with, 145
MHAUS, 307
Miniature end-plate potential, 2, 6
Mivacron. See Mivacurium
Mivacurium
  cardiovascular effects, 144t
  in children, 204
  clearance, 96, 200–202
  clinical duration (Dur$_{25}$) of, 98
  continuous infusion, 203
  dosages and durations of, 100, 172t, 200–201
  histamine release with, 145–146, 146t, 204
  increased dose, side effects of, 82
  in infants, 205
  infusion, 208
  infusion rate for, 95, 203, 203t
  intersubject variability with, 201
  in liver failure, 202
  metabolism, 100–101, 200–202
  nerve stimulator use with, 209
  onset, 209
  pharmacology of, 200–204, 201f, 203t, 208–210
  in rapid-sequence induction for Cesarean section, 158–159
  recovery from, 202–204, 208–209
  recovery index, 98, 201, 203
  reversal, 200, 202–203, 208–209
  structure of, 11, 12f
MMG. See Mechanomyography
Monitoring. See also Evoked response, monitoring
  depth of block, in ICU, 153–154
  with nondepolarizing relaxant, 67t, 97–99, 172t
Monoamine oxidase inhibitors, effect on pseudocholinesterase and succinylcholine, 260t
Morphine, effect on nondepolarizing block, 110t
Motor action potentials, effects of denervation versus myopathy on, 354
Motor nerve
  Na$^+$/K$^+$ pump, 4–5
  sodium/potassium pump in, 5
Motor unit, overview of, 1
Multi-organ failure, nondepolarizing block in, 150
Multiple sclerosis
  acetylcholine receptor proliferation in, 336

Index

sensitivity to relaxants in, 336
Muscarinic effects, 219
  in adults versus children, 229
Muscle(s)
  contraction, 1. *See also* Tetanic contraction
    and rate of neurostimulation, 4
  contraction times, 7
  denervated, receptors in, 17–18
  differential response to relaxants, by muscle type, 7, 26–28, 32–33
  disuse, neuromuscular response to, 337
  imbalances, and malignant hyperthermia susceptibility, 300
  immobility, neuromuscular response to, 337
  movement, control of, 5
  nonstriated, effects nondepolarizing relaxants on, 147
  perioperative changes, with succinylcholine, 281–283
Muscle action potential(s), 2–4
  with depolarizing relaxants, 239, 245
  generation of, 17, 37
    all-or-none, 1–3, 6, 16
Muscle fiber(s)
  necrosis, with long-term use of NDRs, 150
  tonic, 6–7
  twitch, 6–7
  type I (slow-twitch, red), 7
  type II, 7
  types of, 6–7
Muscle relaxants, neuromuscular response to, 332–334
Muscle tension, and depolarizing block, 14
Muscular dystrophy, 349–350, 352–353
  pathophysiology of, 349
Myalgias, succinylcholine-induced, reduction of, 282t, 283, 286
Myasthenia gravis, 324–326
  clinical features of, 324
  effect on succinylcholine and pseudocholinesterase, 263t
  electromyography in, 329
  motor neuron dysfunction in, 327
  nondepolarizing relaxant administration in, 325–326
  pyridostigmine therapy for, 324
  succinylcholine administration in, 325–326
  thymectomy in, 327–328
  tracheal extubation in, 327–328
Myasthenic syndrome, 326, 329
  electromyography in, 329
Myoglobin release, succinylcholine-induced, 283
  reduction of, 282t, 283, 286
Myoglobinuria, differential diagnosis of, 319
Myopathy
  in ICU patients, with long-term nondepolarizing relaxant use, 70–71, 150–155, 159–160
  and malignant hyperthermia susceptibility, 300
  postparalysis, 150
  steroid-induced, 160
Myosin, 4
Myositis, 351
Myotonia, 350–351, 353–354
  aspiration of gastric contents in, 353
  and malignant hyperthermia susceptibility, 300
  regional anesthesia in, 353
Myotonia congenita, 350–351
Myotonia dystrophica, 350–351, 353

Na. *See* Sodium
Narcotics, effect on nondepolarizing block, 109t–110t
NDRs. *See* Nondepolarizing relaxant(s)
Needle electrodes, 30
Neonate(s)
  end-plate receptor types in, 18

nondepolarizing block in, 85–86, 127t
  premature, nondepolarizing block in, 127t
Neostigmine
  with atropine, 219–220
  dosage, and previous physostigmine administration, 230
  dosage (dose requirement), 219
  effect
    on neuromuscular effects of antibiotics, 112
    on succinylcholine and pseudocholinesterase, 264t
  with glycopyrrolate, 219–220
  mechanism of action, 217
  pharmacology of, 218t, 219–220
  in renal failure, 227
  reversal of mivacurium, 202–203, 208–209
  reversal of relaxants with, 219–220, 230
Nerve branch, 1
Nerve bundle, 1
Nerve fiber, 1
  threshold for firing, 1
Nerve gas, toxicity, 222, 229–230
Nerve stimulator(s)
  features of, 23, 24t
  use
    in ICU, 71
    with mivacurium, 209
Nerve stimulator impulse, 23
  pulse duration, 6
Nerve terminal, 1
  presynaptic, 1, 2f
Neurofibromatosis, 326–327
Neuroleptic malignant syndrome
  clinical features of, 320
  and hyperkalemic response to succinylcholine, 320
  and malignant hyperthermia, compared, 320
  pathogenesis of, 320
  treatment of, 320
Neurological medications, effect on pseudocholinesterase and succinylcholine, 260t–261t
Neuromuscular block
  in denervated muscle, 17–18
  depth of
    clinical ED_{100} and, 86
    evaluation of, 52
  injection sites, 15
  laboratory models, 15
  mechanisms of, 11–22
  in neonate, 18
  recovery from, monitoring, 65
  residual, 70, 74
  reversal, readiness for, assessment of, 65
  underestimation of, 39
Neuromuscular blocking agents. *See also* Depolarizing relaxant(s); Nondepolarizing relaxant(s); *specific agent*
  and acetylcholine, molecular similarity, 11, 12f
  in biophase, effects of potency, 83–89
  buffered diffusion, effects of potency, 88–89
  onset, effects of potency, 88–89
  structure of, 11, 12f
  tissue:blood partition coefficient, 86
Neuromuscular junction, 1
  end-plate, postsynaptic receptor channels of, 2–3, 3f
Neuromuscular monitoring, and receptor occupancy, 40t, 41
Neuromuscular relaxation, monitoring
  in intensive care unit, 70–72
  intraoperative, 64–68, 67t
  limitations of, 68–70
  for mechanical ventilation, 70–72

Neuromuscular transmission
  anatomy of, 1–10, 2f–3f
  physiology of, 1–10, 2f–3f
Neuronal disease, diffuse, neuromuscular response to, 333, 335–337
Neuropathy, effect on pseudocholinesterase and succinylcholine, 263t
Neurostimulation. *See also* Single twitch stimulation; Tetanic stimulation
  electrode placement, 25
  features of, 23–36, 24t
  frequency
    and apparent depth of block, 43–44
    and apparent rate of block onset, 44
  impedance in, 23
  maximal current, 23–24, 26f
  patterns
    with depolarizing block, 37, 38f
    with nondepolarizing block, 37–47, 38f, 40t, 41f–42f
  prerelaxant baseline, 37
  skin temperature in, 25
  stimulus intensity
    constant current, 23–24, 27f
    effect on twitch height, 23–24, 30
    maximal current for, 23–24
    supramaximal current, 24
  stimulus strength for, 23, 24f
  supramaximal current, 24–25, 27f
  ulnar nerve stimulation, 25–26
Nicotinic effects, 219
Nitrous-narcotic-NDR anesthesia, 72
Nitrous oxide, effect
  on nondepolarizing block, 109t
  on pseudocholinesterase and succinylcholine, 260t
NMJ. *See* Neuromuscular junction
Nondepolarizing block, 11–13
  acid-base/lytes and, 128t–131t
  acidosis and, 123t
  albumin level and, 123t–124t
  alcohol effect on, 15
  alkalosis and, 123t
  alpha$_1$-acid glycoprotein effect on, 123t–124t
  antibiotic effect on, 15
  barbiturate effect on, 15
  burns and, 124t
  calcium channel blocker effect on, 15
  calcium effect on, 128t–129t
  cardiopulmonary bypass effect on, 124t
  cerebral palsy and, 124t
  for cesarean section, 87–88
  in critical illness, 124t
  disuse atrophy and, 124t
  dose-response relationships, in infant, child, and adult, 132–133
  end-plate sensitivity to, 16
  features of, 11, 13
  flaccid paralysis of, 11
  geographical effects on, 124t
  with hypercarbia, 124t
  hyperparathyroidism and, 124t
  hypoalbuminemia and, 123t
  with hypocarbia, 124t
  hypoperfusion and, 124t
  hypothermia and, 124t, 131–132
  injuries affecting, 124t–125t
  liver failure and, 125t
  magnesium effect on, 125t, 129t
  malnutrition and, 125t
  margin of safety with, 11, 16
  metabolic acidosis and, 130t–131t
  metabolic alkalosis and, 131t
  motor nerve injury and, 124t–125t
  naloxone effect on, 15
  naltrexone effect on, 15
  neuropathy and, 124t
  obesity and, 125t
  in old age, 126t–127t
  onset, monitoring of orbicularis oculi during, 32–33
  PaCO$_2$ effect on, 129t–130t
  patient status and conditions and, 123–142, 124t–131t
  in pediatrics, 127t
  phenothiazine effect on, 15
  phosphate effect on, 129t
  postpartum, 126t
  potassium effect on, 129t
  prednisolone effect on, 15
  in pregnancy, 125t–126t
  in premature neonate, 127t
  recovery from, time to effective, 217–218
  in renal failure, 127t–128t, 133, 150
  reversal, evaluation for, 52
  in sepsis, 128t
  serum proteins and, 123t–124t
  stimulation patterns with, 37–47, 38f, 40t, 41f–42f
  succinylcholine effects on
    with existing block, 246–247
    with subsequent block, 246–247
Nondepolarizing relaxant(s)
  administration of
    in myasthenia gravis, 325–326
    timing principle of, 83
  aminosteroidal, 11
  in biophase, 78
  bolus dose, 81
  buffered diffusion and, 79
  cardiovascular effects, 143–144, 144t
  central nervous system effects, 149
  clearance of, 96, 100–101
    renal, 101, 133
  clinical duration (Dur$_{25}$), 171, 172t
  combination therapy, 82
    recovery time after, 97
  curariform, 11
  defasciculating dose
    effect on succinylcholine requirement and duration, 246
    and succinylcholine effect on intraocular pressure, 279, 285
    and succinylcholine-induced fasciculations, 281–283
    and succinylcholine-induced increase in jaw tension, 303
  dosage, 81–82, 172t
    increased, 81–82, 86–87
    with long-term use in ICU patients, 151
    in myasthenia gravis, 325
    in neonate, 85–86
    for pediatric patients, 132–133
    in rapid-sequence induction for Cesarean section, 158–159
  dosages and durations of, 172t
  drug selection, 81–82
  effect on succinylcholine and pseudocholinesterase, 261t
  effects, on nonstriated muscle, 147
  elimination half-life of, 171
  fetal:maternal ratios, 147, 157–158
  fetal uptake of, 148, 148t, 157–158
  high-dose, 81
  histamine release with, 144–147, 145t–146t
  incremental dose, for maintenance, 96
  infusion, dosage, 95–96

Index

infusion rate, 81
intermediate-acting, 172t, 184–199
  administration during recovery from long-acting NDR, 97, 101
  dosages and durations of, 172t, 184
  ED_{95}, with cumulative dosing, 210
intravenous administration, 78–94
of long duration, 171–183, 172t
long-lasting, recovery from, 98
long-term effects of, 143–170, 144t–146t, 148t
long-term use
  disuse atrophy and myopathy with, 70
  guidelines/recommendations for, 154–155
  metabolite accumulation with, 70
  monitoring, 70–71, 74
  titration of relaxant in, 74
magnitude of effect, 79, 80f, 81
maintenance and recovery with, monitoring of, 67t, 97–99, 172t
maintenance with, 67t, 95–99, 172t
and malignant hyperthermia, 298
mechanism of action, 11
metabolites
  potentially harmful, 149–150
  and prolonged paralysis in ICU patients, 159
in myotonia, 351
for neonate, 85–86
in obstetrics, 147–148, 148t
  dose-to-delivery interval, 147–148
onset, 78–94, 80f
  with bolus dose, 81
  and dosage increase, 86–87
  with high dose, 81
  lag, 79–80
  muscle differences in, 28
placental transfer of, 147
potentiation of each other, 82
preganglionic nicotinic receptor block with, 143–144
presynaptic binding, 13
presynaptic effects of, 13, 17
priming dose, 82–83, 87
  in rapid-sequence induction for Cesarean section, 158–159
prior, effect on current nondepolarizing relaxants, 110t
for rapid-sequence intubation, 88
receptor occupancy, 11, 13, 17, 78–81, 80f
  clinical signs and, 73–74
  and twitch height depression, 86
recovery from, muscle differences in, 28
recovery kinetics with, 96–97, 97f
renal elimination of, 210
response to, in muscular dystrophy, 349–350
reversal, 217–238
  adequacy of, 226, 228
  with anticholinesterases, 217–230. *See also specific anticholinesterase*
  with antimuscarinic agents, 219, 228–229
  with apparent 100% recovery, 225
  in asthma, 228
  with edrophonium, 220–221, 224, 228, 230
  factors affecting, 217–218, 225
  gastrointestinal effects of, 228
  guidelines for, 224–225
  with neostigmine, 219–220, 230
  neuromuscular function after, 224
  with pancuronium, 224
  precautions with, 225–226
  priming dose of reversal agent for, 227
  with pyridostigmine, 220
  requirement for, versus electing not to administer, 225–226

selection of agent for, and depth of block, 224
sensitivity to, 25–28
  of eye muscles, 32
  muscle differences in, 26–28, 32
  in myasthenia gravis, 325, 329
  in myasthenic syndrome, 329
short-acting, 200–204, 201f, 203t, 208–210
  dosages and durations of, 172t
  ED_{95}, with cumulative dosing, 210
structure of, 11, 12f
sympathomimetic effects, 143–144
systemic effects, 143–170, 144t–146t, 148t
umbilical vein–umbilical artery gradient for, 148, 158
vagolytic effects of, 143–144, 156
variation in response to, 81–83, 87
volume of distribution, 85
Norcuron. *See* Vecuronium
Nuromax. *See* Doxacurium

Obesity
  effect on pseudocholinesterase and succinylcholine, 264t
  nondepolarizing block and, 125t
  vecuronium and, 190
Obstetrics
  nondepolarizing block in, 125t–126t, 147–148, 148t, 157–158
  pseudocholinesterase in, 264t
  succinylcholine in, 264t
Old age. *See also* Elderly
  nondepolarizing block and, 126t–127t
  pseudocholinesterase activity in, 265t
Ondansetron, effect on nondepolarizing block, 106t
Open-channel (use-dependent) block, 14
Oral contraceptives, effect on pseudocholinesterase and succinylcholine, 264t
Orbicularis oculi muscle
  monitoring
    during onset of block, 32–33
    perioperative, 65
  sensitivity to neuromuscular relaxants, 28, 29f
ORG 9426. *See* Rocuronium
Organophosphate insecticides
  effect on succinylcholine and pseudocholinesterase, 258t
  toxicity, 221–222, 229
    cholinesterase assay in, 230
Oropharynx, sensitivity to neuromuscular relaxants, 27
Osteogenesis imperfecta, and malignant hyperthermia susceptibility, 300
Oxime(s), indications for, 229

$PaCO_2$, effect on nondepolarizing block, 129t–130t
Pancuronium, 11, 17
  cardiovascular effects, 143, 144t, 144
  cholinesterase inhibition with, 149
  clinical duration (Dur_{25}), 98
  3-desacetyl derivative, 159. *See also* Pancuronium, metabolites
  dosages and durations of, 172t, 174
  effect on succinylcholine and pseudocholinesterase, 265t
  in elderly, 174
  elimination of, 174
  infusion rate for, 95
  metabolites, 174
    and prolonged paralysis in ICU patients, 159
  in obstetrics, 147–148
  onset, 88
  pharmacology of, 173–174, 177
  plus thiopental, potential toxicity, 157

Pancuronium *(cont.)*
  presynaptic block with, 13, 17
  pretreatment prior to succinylcholine, 282t
  recovery from, train-of-four monitoring during, 192
  in renal failure, 133, 226–227
  reversal, 224
    with antimuscarinic agent, 219
  structure of, 11, 12f, 173
  sympathomimetic effects of, 173
  vagolytic effects of, 156, 173
  weakness or paralysis after, with long-term use in ICU, 151–152
Paralysis. *See also* Familial periodic paralysis
  flaccid
    with depolarizing relaxant, 14
    with nondepolarizing relaxant, 11
  long-term, in ICU patients, 150–155
  prolonged periodic, abnormal responses to succinylcholine in, 336
Parkinson's disease, neuromuscular effects of, 337
Patient, status and condition of, effect on nondepolarizing block, 123–142, 124t–131t
Pavulon. *See* Pancuronium
Peak expiratory flow rate, correlation with neuromuscular function, 68–69
Peak tetanic tension, 59
Pectus excavatum, and malignant hyperthermia susceptibility, 300
Penicillins, effect on nondepolarizing block, 105t
Perioperative medications, effect on pseudocholinesterase and succinylcholine, 261t–262t
Peroneal nerve, stimulation of, 26
Pharmacokinetics/pharmacodynamics of nondepolarizing relaxant
  aminopyridine effect on, 6, 104t
  antiarrhythmic effect on, 106t
  antibiotic effect on, 104t–105t, 112
  anticholinesterase effect on, 105t, 112
  anticonvulsant effect on, 105t–106t, 112
  antiemetic effect on, 106t
  antineoplastic effect on, 106t
  antirheumatic drug effect on, 106t
  anxiolytic effect on, 110t
  benzodiazepine effect on, 110t
  beta$_2$ agonist effect on, 107t
  beta blocker effect on, 106t
  calcium channel blocker effect on, 107t
  cardiovascular drug effect on, 106t–107t
  chlorpromazine effect on, 110t
  clindamycin effect on, 105t
  Clostridium botulinum effect on, 111t
  Clostridium tetani effect on, 111t
  dantrolene effect on, 107t
  doxapram effect on, 107t
  droperidol effect on, 106t
  epinephrine effect on, 107t
  ganglionic blocker effect on, 107t
  H$_2$ antagonist effect on, 107t–108t
  immunosuppressive effect on, 108t
  inhalational anesthetic effect on, 44, 109t–110t
  ketamine effect on, 109t
  lincomycin effect on, 105t
  lithium effect on, 109t
  local anesthetic effect on, 15, 109t
  mannitol effect on, 109t
  metoclopramide effect on, 106t
  metronidazole effect on, 105t
  monitoring, 67t, 97–99, 172t
  morphine effect on, 110t
  multiple compartment hypothesis, 13
  narcotic effect on, 109t–110t
  nitrous oxide effect on, 109t
  ondansetron effect on, 106t
  penicillin effect on, 105t
  physostigmine effect on, 110t
  polymyxin effect on, 105t
  prior nondepolarizing relaxant effect on, 110t
  propofol effect on, 108t–109t
  sedative effect on, 110t
  snake alpha-bungarotoxin effect on, 112t
  steroid effect on, 15, 110t–111t
  succinylcholine effect on, 111t
  tetracycline effect on, 105t
  tetrodotoxin effect on, 112t
  theophylline effect on, 111t
  thiopental effect on, 108t
  time to maximum block, 78
  toxin effect on, 111t–112t
  vancomycin effect on, 105t
  vasodilator effect on, 106t
Pharyngeal muscles
  sensitivity to neuromuscular relaxants, 31–32
  weakness, during recovery from neuromuscular block, 69
Phase 1 block. *See* Depolarizing block
Phase 2 block. *See* Depolarizing block
Phenothiazines, and malignant hyperthermia, 298
Phenytoin
  effect
    on nondepolarizing block, 112–113
    on succinylcholine and pseudocholinesterase, 260t
  pretreatment prior to succinylcholine, 282t
Pheochromocytoma, atracurium and, 187
Phosphate, decreased, effect on nondepolarizing block, 129t
Phosphocreatine, muscle levels of, 300
Phosphodiesterase inhibitors, effect on succinylcholine and pseudocholinesterase, 263t
Phosphodiester/phosphocreatine ratio, 300
Phospholine. *See* Echothiophate eye drops
Physiology of neuromuscular transmission, 1–10, 2f–3f
Physostigmine
  effect
    on nondepolarizing block, 110t
    on pseudocholinesterase and succinylcholine, 258t
  previous administration, neostigmine dosage and, 230
Pipecuronium
  cardiovascular effects, 144, 144t
  dosages and durations of, 172t
  in elderly, 175
  lyophilized, 175
  metabolite, 175
  pharmacology of, 175
  in renal failure, 175, 226–227
  reversibility, with anticholinesterase, 175
  structure of, 11, 12f
Plasma cholinesterase. *See* Pseudocholinesterase
Plasmapheresis, in myasthenia gravis, 328
Plasma protein binding, effect on pharmacokinetics and pharmacodynamics, 113
Poliomyelitis, neuromuscular effects of, 336
Polymyositis, 351
Polymyxins, effect on nondepolarizing block, 105t
Polyneuropathy, neuromuscular effects of, 336
Posterior tibial nerve, stimulation of, 26
Postjunctional membrane, 2, 3f
Postsynaptic receptor channels, 2–3, 3f
Postsynaptic receptors, occupancy, in nondepolarizing block, 11, 13, 17
Posttetanic count, 39
  assessment, advantages of, 58

Index

cough, evoked response monitoring, 58
  evaluation of, 51–52, 52t
  in laryngeal adductor, 31, 58
Posttetanic facilitation, 13
  with nondepolarizing block, 38f, 39, 45
  in unblocked neuromuscular junction, 59–60
Potassium
  decreased, effect on succinylcholine and pseudocholinesterase, 265t
  effect on nondepolarizing block, 129t
  levels, in muscular dystrophy, 349
  in motor nerve, 2, 5–6
  serum, beta blockers and, 284. See also Hyperkalemia
Pralidoxime, for anticholinesterase overdose/toxicity, 222, 229
Pregnancy
  myotonia-associated weakness in, 354
  nondepolarizing block in, 125t–126t
  pseudocholinesterase in, 264t
  succinylcholine in, 264t
Presynaptic membrane, 1, 2f
  calcium, 4–5
  calcium binding, 1, 2f
  sodium, 1, 2f
Presynaptic nerve terminal, 1, 2f, 4–5
  fast calcium channel, 1, 4–5
  slow calcium channel, 1, 4–5
Priming dose, of nondepolarizing relaxant, 82–83, 87
Propanidid, effect on succinylcholine and pseudocholinesterase, 260t
Propofol, effect on nondepolarizing block, 108t–109t
Protein, serum, effect on nondepolarizing block, 123t–124t
Protein kinase II, calcium/calmodulin-dependent, 6
Pseudocholinesterase
  abnormal forms of, 256
  acid base/lytes and, 265t
  activity, 256–257
    medications affecting, 258t–262t
    in old age, 264t
  antibiotic effect on, 258t
  anticholinesterase effect on, 258t
  antineoplastic effect on, 258t
  assay, 256
  atypical allele, 243, 246
    and mivacurium metabolism, 202
  atypical alleles, 256–258
  bambuterol effect on, 259t
  burns and, 263t
  cardiovascular drugs and, 259t
  in children, 264t
  chronic disease state and, 263t
  critical illness and, 262t
  deficiency, effect on duration of succinylcholine, 267
  denervation and, 263t
  dibucaine number, 256–258
  disuse atrophy and, 263t
  in eclampsia, 264t
  fluoride number, 257
  genetics, 256–257, 257t
  glucocorticoid effect on, 260t
  hyperthyroidism and, 263t
  hypoproteinemia and, 263t
  inhalational anesthetics and, 260t
  inhibition
    by neostigmine, 231
    with pancuronium, 149
    by pyridostigmine, 231
  injury and, 263t

  intravenous analgesics and, 260t
  liver failure and, 263t
  malignant hyperthermia and, 263t
  metabolism of succinylcholine, 255–275
  mivacurium metabolism, 200–202
  myasthenia gravis and, 263t
  in neonate, 264t
  neurological medications and, 260t
  nondepolarizing relaxants and, 261t
  obesity and, 264t
  in obstetrics, 264t
  oral contraceptives and, 264t
  patient status and, 262t–266t
  perioperative medications and, 261t–262t
  phosphodiesterase inhibitors and, 262t
  post partum, 264t
  in pregnancy, 264t
  production in liver, 256
  psychiatric disorders and, 265t
  renal transplant and, 265t
  sepsis and, 265t
  toxin effect on, 262t
Psychiatric disorder(s), effect on pseudocholinesterase and succinylcholine, 265t
Psychotropic medications, effect on pseudocholinesterase and succinylcholine, 260t–261t
Ptosis, and malignant hyperthermia susceptibility, 300
Pyridostigmine
  advantages of, 220
  dosage (dose requirement), 219
  effect on pseudocholinesterase and succinylcholine, 258t
  mechanism of action, 217
  for myasthenia gravis, 324
  pharmacology of, 218t
  pretreatment, and nerve gas exposure, 230
  in renal failure, 226–227
  reversal of relaxants, 220–221

Quaternary amines, 11
Quelicin. See Succinylcholine
Quinidine, effect on pseudocholinesterase and succinylcholine, 260t

Rapid-sequence induction
  defasciculation prior to, risks with, 286
  with nondepolarizing relaxant, 88
  vecuronium versus rocuronium for, 209–210
Rat, hemidiaphragm preparation, 15
Receptor
  junctional, 2, 3f
  occupancy
    and neuromuscular monitoring, 40t, 40–41
    by nondepolarizing relaxants, 11, 13, 17, 73–74, 78–81, 80f, 86
    by succinylcholine, 17
Recovery index, 98
Recovery kinetics, with nondepolarizing relaxant, 96–97, 97f
Rectus abdominis muscle, sensitivity to neuromuscular relaxants, 27–28
Recurarization, in renal failure, 226–227
Recurrent laryngeal nerve, stimulation of, 26
Redistribution, of nondepolarizing relaxants, 100
Refractory period
  motor nerve, 4, 6
  neuromuscular, 4, 6
Regional anesthesia, in myotonia, 353
Regurgitation, risk, with succinylcholine, 280, 286
Renal failure
  atracurium in, 226–227
  clearance in, 133

Renal failure *(cont.)*
  doxacurium clearance in, 133
  gallamine in, 133, 226–227
  mivacurium in, 202
  neostigmine in, 227
  nondepolarizing block in, 127*t*–128*t*, 133, 150
  pancuronium in, 133, 226–227
  pipecuronium in, 175, 226–227
  and prolonged paralysis in ICU patients, 159
  pyridostigmine in, 226–227
  recurarization in, 226–227
  and relaxant-induced myopathy, 153–154
  reversal of relaxants in, 226–227
  rocuronium in, 206–207
  succinylcholine and, 282, 284
  vecuronium in, 190–191
Renal transplant, effect on succinylcholine and pseudocholinesterase, 265*t*
Repolarization, 2–4
Respiratory depression, postoperative, prolonged, 227, 227*t*
Respiratory muscles, sensitivity to neuromuscular relaxants, 26, 31
Resting potential, 1, 5
Rhabdomyolysis, 353
  succinylcholine-induced, 281–282
  in muscular dystrophy, 349
  in myopathy, 353
Rhabdomyosarcoma, metastatic, abnormal responses to succinylcholine in, 336
RI_{25-75}, 98
Rocuronium, 159, 205–210
  cardiovascular effects, 143–144, 144*t*
  cardiovascular profile of, 207
  in children, 207
  clearance, 206–207
  dosages and durations of, 172*t*, 206
  duration of action, 100
  in elderly, 207
  in hepatic failure, 206
  high-dose, 209–210
  infusion rate for, 207
  intubating conditions with, 205–206, 210
  lag time with, 205
  metabolite of, 206
  muscle sensitivity to, differences in, 28
  onset, 88, 205–206, 209
  pharmacology of, 205–210
  potency of, 205
  for rapid-sequence intubation, 159
  redistribution, 100, 206
  in renal failure, 206–207
  structure of, 11, 12*f*
  time to maximum block for, 79
Ryanodine receptor, 306–307

Salicylates, pretreatment prior to succinylcholine, 282*t*
Sarcoplasmic reticulum, calcium release from, 4
SCh. *See* Succinylcholine
Sedation, with neuromuscular block, in ICU, 70–71
Sedatives, effect on nondepolarizing block, 110*t*
Sepsis
  effect on pseudocholinesterase and succinylcholine, 266*t*
  nondepolarizing block in, 128*t*, 150
Single twitch, 4, 7
Single twitch stimulation, 37, 38*f*, 44
  twitch height, 45
Skin resistance, and neurostimulation, 23, 25*f*
Skin temperature, in neurostimulation, 25
Skin tests, for sensitivity to relaxants, 157

Snake alpha-bungarotoxin, effect on nondepolarizing block, 112*t*
Sodium, in presynaptic nerve terminal, 1, 2*f*, 4–5
Sodium channel(s)
  dual-gated, 3, 14, 17, 239, 245
  voltage-sensitive, 3
Sodium/potassium pump, in motor nerve, 5
Squint, and malignant hyperthermia susceptibility, 300
Status of patient, effect on nondepolarizing block, 123–142, 124*t*–131*t*
Steady-state concentration, 95
Steinert's disease, 350
Steroid(s)
  administration of, in ICU patients, 152–154, 160
  effect on nondepolarizing block, 15, 110*t*–111*t*
  high-dose, effects on neuromuscular function, 160
  in myasthenia gravis, 324–325
Stimulus strength, for neurostimulation, 23, 24*f*
Strabismus, and malignant hyperthermia susceptibility, 300
Stretching, preoperative, as pretreatment prior to succinylcholine, 282*t*
Stroke
  neuromuscular effects of, 335, 340
  neuromuscular response to, 340
Succinylcholine, 13, 240–242
  abnormal response to
    in muscular dystrophy, 349–350, 353
    in myotonia, 350–351, 353
    with nerve injury, burns, and trauma, 333–339
    in periodic paralysis, 352, 354
  acid base/lytes and, 266*t*
  administration, in myasthenia gravis, 325–326
  antibiotic effect on, 258*t*
  anticholinesterase effect on, 258*t*
  antineoplastic effect on, 258*t*
  apnea with, and pseudocholinesterase activity, 267
  bambuterol effect on, 259*t*
  bradycardia with, 277
  burns and, 263*t*
  cardiovascular drugs and, 259*t*
  cardiovascular effects of, 276–278
  in children, 242, 245, 264*t*, 282
    adverse effects of, 277
  chronic disease state and, 263*t*
  clearance, 255
  continuous infusion of, 242
  creatine kinase release with, reduction of, 282*t*, 286
  critical illness and, 262*t*
  denervation and, 263*t*
  disuse atrophy and, 263*t*
  dose-response curve with, 241
  duration, and pseudocholinesterase levels, 256
  in eclampsia, 264*t*
  effects
    after edrophonium, versus after pyridostigmine or neostigmine, 231
    on existing nondepolarizing block, 111*t*, 246–247
    on intracranial pressure, 278–279, 284
    on subsequent nondepolarizing block, 111*t*, 247
    in von Recklinghausen's disease, 326–327
  elimination, 255
  elimination kinetics, 241
  end-plate depolarization with, 245
  fasciculations with, reduction of, 282*t*, 283, 286
  gastrointestinal effects, 280–281
  genitourinary effects, 280–281
  glucocorticoid effect on, 260*t*
  histamine release with, 145, 277

Index

hyperkalemia with, and neuroleptic malignant syndrome, 320
hyperthyroidism and, 263t
hypoproteinemia and, 263t
infusion, 208
  complications of, 96
  dosage, 96
infusion rate for, 96, 203, 203t
infusion requirements, 242
inhalational anesthetics and, 244, 260t
injury and, 263t
intramuscular administration, 15, 241
  bradycardia with, 277
intraocular pressure and, 6, 279–280, 285
intravenous analgesics and, 261t
intubating conditions, 241
jaw muscle rigidity with, in malignant hyperthermia, 298–299
in liver failure, 263t
and malignant hyperthermia, 297–299
malignant hyperthermia and, 263t
mechanism of action, 17, 239–240
medications affecting, 258t–262t
metabolism, 241, 255–275
myalgias with, reduction of, 282t, 283, 286
myasthenia gravis and, 264t
myoglobin release with, 283
  reduction of, 282t, 283, 286
in neonate, 264t
neurological medications and, 260t–261t
neuromuscular effects of, 240–242, 246
nondepolarizing relaxants and, 261t
obesity and, 264t
in obstetrics, 264t
onset, 14, 81, 240–241
oral contraceptives and, 264t
patient status and, 262t–266t
perioperative medications and, 261t–262t
perioperative muscle changes with, 281–283
persistent block with, 243–244
phosphodiesterase inhibitors and, 262t
placental transfer of, 280–281
plasma levels, and reversal of block, 246
plus thiopental, potential toxicity, 157
postpartum use of, 265t
in pregnancy, 265t
presynaptic effects of, 240, 247
pretreatment prior to, 277–280, 282t, 285
psychiatric disorders and, 265t
receptor occupancy, 17
recovery from, 242
redistribution, 255
in renal failure, 282, 284
renal transplant and, 265t
requirements, in adults versus children, 245
respiratory effects, 280–281
response to, in muscular dystrophy, 349–350
self-taming dose, as pretreatment, 282t
sensitivity to
  in different muscles, 241–242
  in myasthenic syndrome, 326
sepsis and, 265t
structure of, 12f, 13
with thiopental, precipitate of, potential toxicity, 277
toxin effect on, 263t
undesirable effects of, 276–296
and volatile anesthetics, 244
Sudden infant death syndrome, 300
Supramaximal current, for neurostimulation, 24–25, 27f
Surface area-adjusted dosage, 85–86, 132
Surface electrodes, limitations of, 30

Suxamethonium. *See* Succinylcholine
Synaptophysin, 1, 6
Syncurine. *See* Decamethonium
Systemic effects, of nondepolarizing relaxant, 143–170, 144t–146t, 148t

Tachyphylaxis, with depolarizing relaxants, 243–245
Tensilon test, 325
Tetanic contraction (response), 4, 7–8, 37–39
  summated, 4, 6–8, 37, 245
  versus contracture, 354
Tetanic stimulation, 37–39, 38f
  depolarizing block and, 245
  EMG versus MMG responses during, 59
  fade during, 37–39, 38f, 59
  as indicator of inspiratory capacity, 44
  response to, 4, 7–8
  and train-of-four, comparison of, 44–45
Tetanus
  recovery during, 59
  for tracheal extubation, 68
Tetracycline(s)
  effect on nondepolarizing block, 105t
  neuromuscular effects, opposed by calcium, 112
Tetrodotoxin, effect on nondepolarizing block, 112t
Theophylline
  effect on nondepolarizing block, 111t
  and risk of malignant hyperthermia, 305–306
Thiopental
  effect
    on nondepolarizing block, 108t
    on pseudocholinesterase and succinylcholine, 261t
  plus relaxant
    anaphylaxis with, 157
    precipitate of, potential toxicity, 157, 191
  plus succinylcholine, precipitate of, potential toxicity, 277
Thomsen's disease, 350
Thumb tension, resting preload, 54
  effects of, by mode of stimulation, 60
Thymectomy, in myasthenia gravis, 327–328
Tidal volume, 65
  intraoperative, correlation with neuromuscular block, 68–69
Time to maximum block, 78
Timing principle, for nondepolarizing relaxant administration, 83
Tissue:blood partition coefficient, for neuromuscular blocking agents, 86
Toxins, effect
  on nondepolarizing block, 111t–112t
  on pseudocholinesterase and succinylcholine, 263t
Tracheal extubation
  in ICU, 71–72
  in myasthenia gravis, 327–328
  readiness for, indicators of, 66
  tetanus for, 68
Tracheal intubation
  rapid, with increased intracranial pressure, 285
  vecuronium for, 191–192
  relaxation for, monitoring, 64–65, 67t
  single twitch stimulation monitoring during, 44
Tracrium. *See* Atracurium
Train-of-four stimulation, 38f, 40t, 40–42, 45–46
  effect of stimulating current intensity on, 24, 30–31
  in evaluation of depth of block, 52
  fade, 40, 51
  mechanographic response to, 46
  versus tetanic stimulation, 45–46
  T_4/T_1 ratio, 30–31, 40–41, 45–46, 58

Train-of-four stimulation (cont.)
  during course of neuromuscular block, 46
  cutoff value, adequacy of, 69, 72–74
  at given T_1 depression, during onset versus recovery, 99–100
  recovery, after recovery of T_1, 101, 224
  during recovery, 192, 224
  for tracheal extubation, 68, 98–99
Transducer overload, 59
Trauma, neuromuscular response to, 339
Trimethaphan, effect on pseudocholinesterase and succinylcholine, 265t
Trismus, 299, 303
Troponin, 4
d-Tubocurarine (Tubocurarine), 11, 17
  cardiovascular effects, 143, 144t, 156
  clearance, 96
  clinical duration (Dur_{25}), 98
  dosages and durations of, 171–172, 172t
  histamine release with, 145, 157
  hypotension with, 157
  and malignant hyperthermia, 298
  mechanism of action, 7
  in obstetrics, 147–148
  onset, 88
  peripheral vasodilation with, 156
  pharmacology of, 171–172
  presynaptic block with, 13, 17
  presynaptic effects of, 17
  pretreatment prior to succinylcholine, 283t
  recovery from, train-of-four monitoring during, 192
  recovery index for, 98
  reversal, with antimuscarinic agent, 219
  structure of, 11, 12f
Twitch response. See also Single twitch
  lack of, 51
  posttetanic count and, 51–52, 52t

Ulnar nerve stimulation, 25–26, 31
  in perioperative monitoring, 64
Umbilical vein–umbilical artery gradient, for relaxant, 148, 158
Upper motor nerve injury
  effect on nondepolarizing block, 124t–125t
  with extrajunctional chemosensitivity and SCh-induced hyperkalemia and/or contractures, 334
Uremia, abnormal responses to succinylcholine in, 336

Vancomycin, effect on nondepolarizing block, 105t
Vasodilators, effect on nondepolarizing block, 106t
Vecuronium
  cardiovascular effects of, 144, 144t, 188
    in high-dose fentanyl induction, 191
  in children, 189
  clearance, 96
  clinical duration (Dur_{25}), 98
  3-desacetyl derivative, 159. See also Vecuronium metabolites
  dosages and durations of, 172t

duration of action, 100
  in elderly, 190
  elimination, 101
  high-dose, 82
    in children, 81
    for rapid-sequence intubation, 158
  infusion rate for, 95, 188–189, 203, 203t
    in pediatric patients, 189
  infusions, prolonged effect after, 188
  metabolite, 189–191
    and prolonged paralysis in ICU patients, 159
  muscle sensitivity to, differences in, 28, 29f
  in neonates and infants, 189
  and obesity, 190
  onset, 88
  pharmacology of, 188–192
  presynaptic block with, 13
  pretreatment prior to succinylcholine, 283t
  for rapid intubation, in patient with increased intracranial pressure, 191–192
  recovery from, 98
    train-of-four monitoring during, 192
  recovery index for, 98
  redistribution, 100–101, 188
  in renal failure, 190–191
  structure of, 11, 12f, 188
  weakness or paralysis after, with long-term use in ICU, 151–152
Ventilatory abnormalities, in muscular dystrophy, 349–350
Ventilatory capacity, recovery of, indicators of, 65–69, 73
Ventilatory depression, anesthesia-related, 69–70, 73
Ventilatory function
  and neuromuscular function, relationship of, 69
  during nondepolarizing block, 31–32
Visual disturbances, after nondepolarizing block, 32
Vital capacity
  intraoperative, significance of, 69
  during neuromuscular block, 26–27, 32
  sensitivity to neuromuscular block, 65–66
Vitamin E, pretreatment prior to succinylcholine, 282t
Vocal cord(s)
  movement, prediction, assessment of posttetanic count for, 58
  relaxation, 31
    for laser surgery, 65
Volatile anesthetics
  effect on pseudocholinesterase and succinylcholine, 260t
  and malignant hyperthermia, 297
Volume of distribution, 85
von Recklinghausen's disease, 326–327

Weakness
  after atracurium, with long-term use in ICU, 152
  with dantrolene therapy, 314–315, 320
  in myasthenia gravis, 324
  myotonia-associated, in pregnancy, 354
  residual, after reversal of relaxant, 226